Obesity
Theory and Therapy

Second Edition

Obesity

Theory and Therapy

Second Edition

Editors

Albert J. Stunkard, M.D.

Professor
Department of Psychiatry
University of Pennsylvania
Philadelphia, Pennsylvania

Thomas A. Wadden, Ph.D.

Professor
Department of Psychology
Syracuse University
Syracuse, New York

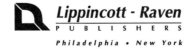

Lippincott - Raven
P U B L I S H E R S
Philadelphia • New York

Printed in the United States of America

9 8 7 6 5 4 3

Library of Congress Cataloging-in-Publication Data

Obesity: theory and therapy / editors, Albert J. Stunkard,
  Thomas A. Wadden.—2nd ed.
    p. cm.
  Includes bibliographical references and index.
  ISBN 0-88167-884-8
  1. Obesity. I. Stunkard, Albert J., 1922–   . II. Wadden, Thomas A.
  [DNLM: 1. Obesity. WD 210 O113]
RC628.O32 1992
616.3'98—dc20
DNLM/DLC
for Library of Congress   92-21813

Care has been taken to confirm the accuracy of the information presented and to describe generally accepted practices. However, the authors, editors, and publisher are not responsible for errors or omissions or for any consequences from application of the information in this book and make no warranty, express or implied, with respect to the contents of the publication.

The authors, editors, and publisher have exerted every effort to ensure that drug selection and dosage set forth in this text are in accordance with current recommendations and practice at the time of publication. However, in view of ongoing research, changes in government regulations, and the constant flow of information relating to drug therapy and drug reactions, the reader is urged to check the package insert for each drug for any change in indications and dosage and for added warnings and precautions. This is particularly important when the recommended agent is a new or infrequently employed drug.

Some drugs and medical devices presented in this publication have Food and Drug Administration (FDA) clearance for limited use in restricted research settings. It is the responsibility of the health care provider to ascertain the FDA status of each drug or device planned for use in their clinical practice.

For Margaret and Jan

With deepest love and affection

Contents

Contributing Authors

John E. Blundell, Ph.D. *BioPsychology Group, Department of Psychology, University of Leeds, Leeds LS2 9JT, United Kingdom*

Peter J. Brown, Ph.D. *Department of Anthropology, Emory University, Atlanta, Georgia 30322*

Kelly D. Brownell, Ph.D. *Department of Psychology, Yale University, New Haven, Connecticut 06520*

Arnold W. Cohen, M.D. *Department of Obstetrics and Gynecology, Division of Maternal-Fetal Medicine, University of Pennsylvania Medical Center, Philadelphia, Pennsylvania 19104*

Cornelius Doherty, M.D. *Department of Surgery, University of Iowa College of Medicine, 200 Hawkins Drive, Iowa City, Iowa 52246*

Johanna T. Dwyer, D.Sc., R.D. *Tufts University Medical School, and Frances Stern Nutrition Center, New England Medical Center Hospitals, Box 783, 750 Washington Street, Boston, Massachusetts 02111*

Leonard H. Epstein, Ph.D. *Department of Psychiatry, University of Pittsburgh School of Medicine, 3811 O'Hara Street, Pittsburgh, Pennsylvania 15213*

Carlos M. Grilo, Ph.D. *Department of Psychology, Yale University, New Haven, Connecticut 06520*

Luis Hernandez, M.D. *Department of Psychology, Princeton University, Princeton, New Jersey 08540; Current Address: Department of Physiology, University of Los Andes, Avenue Don Tulio, 5101-A Merida, Venezuela*

Bartley G. Hoebel, Ph.D. *Department of Psychology, Princeton University, Princeton, New Jersey 08540*

Richard E. Keesey, Ph.D. *Departments of Psychology and Nutritional Sciences, University of Wisconsin, 1202 West Johnson Street, Madison, Wisconsin 53706*

Reinhold G. Laessle, Ph.D. *Center of Psychobiological and Psychosomatic Research, Department of Psychoendocrinology, University of Trier, Building D, P.O. Box 3825, D5500 Trier, Federal Republic of Germany*

Clare L. Lawton, Ph.D. *BioPsychology Group, Department of Psychology, University of Leeds, Leeds LS2 9JT, United Kingdom*

Edward A. Lew, A.M., F.S.A. *Department of Medicine, Columbia University College of Physicians and Surgeons, St. Luke's-Roosevelt Hospital Center, New York, New York 10025; Current Address: 1750 Jamaica Way, Unit 213, Punta Gorda, Florida 33950*

Diana Lu, M.S., R.D. *Frances Stern Nutrition Center, New England Medical Center Hospitals, Box 783, 750 Washington Street, Boston, Massachusetts 02111*

Edward E. Mason, M.D., Ph.D., F.A.C.S. *Department of Surgery, University of Iowa College of Medicine, 200 Hawkins Drive, Iowa City, Iowa 52246*

Joanne M. Meyer, Ph.D. *Department of Human Genetics, Medical College of Virginia, Virginia Commonwealth University, Box 3, MCV Station, Richmond, Virginia 23298*

Arthur M. Nezu, Ph.D. *Department of Mental Health Sciences, Hahnemann University, Broad and Vine Streets, Philadelphia, Pennsylvania 19102-1192*

Michael G. Perri, Ph.D. *Department of Clinical and Health Psychology, University of Florida, P.O. Box 100165, Gainesville, Florida 32610-0165*

Karl M. Pirke, M.D., Ph.D. *Center of Psychobiological and Psychosomatic Research, Department of Psychoendocrinology, University of Trier, Building D, P.O. Box 3825, D5500 Trier, Federal Republic of Germany*

Eric Ravussin, Ph.D. *National Institute of Diabetes and Digestive and Kidney Diseases, National Institutes of Health, 4212 North 16th Street, Room 541A, Phoenix, Arizona 85016*

Anthony Sclafani, Ph.D. *Department of Psychology, Brooklyn College of the City University of New York, Brooklyn, New York 11210*

Trevor Silverstone, D.M., F.R.C.P., F.R.C.Psych. *Department of Psychological Medicine, Medical College of St. Bartholomew's Hospital, University of London, West Smithfield, London EC1 7BE, United Kingdom*

Lars Sjöström, M.D., Ph.D. *Department of Medicine, Sahlgren's Hospital, University of Göteborg, S-413 45 Göteborg, Sweden*

Joy D. Steinfeld, M.D. *Department of Obstetrics and Gynecology, Division of Maternal-Fetal Medicine, University of Pennsylvania Medical Center, Philadelphia, Pennsylvania 19104; Current Address: Department of Obstetrics and Gynecology, Division of Maternal-Fetal Medicine, Cooper Hospital, University Medical Center, 3 Cooper Plaza, Suite 211, Camden, New Jersey 08103*

Albert J. Stunkard, M.D. *Department of Psychiatry, University of Pennsylvania, 3600 Market Street, Philadelphia, Pennsylvania 19104-2648*

Boyd A. Swinburn, M.B., Ch.B., F.R.A.C.P. *Department of Community Health, University of Auckland, New Zealand*

C. Barr Taylor, M.D. *Department of Psychiatry, Stanford University School of Medicine, Stanford, California 94305-5490*

Theodore B. VanItallie, M.D. *Department of Medicine, Columbia University College of Physicians and Surgeons, St. Luke's-Roosevelt Hospital Center, New York, New York 10025; Current Address: P.O. Box 1560, Boca Grande, Florida 33921*

Thomas A. Wadden, Ph.D. *Department of Psychology, Syracuse University, 430 Huntington Hall, Syracuse, New York 13244*

Preface to the First Edition

Why another book on obesity? The answer is straightforward: to provide an authoritative account of what we know about obesity today.

This volume follows in the tradition of the superb general accounts of obesity by Mayer and by Bray. As when these earlier works were published, new information about obesity is scattered over such a wide body of literature that it is largely inaccessible, except to the specialist. The time seemed ripe to collect in one place an account of the current status of the treatment of obesity and our understanding of the disorders that underlie it.

Obesity is written for clinicians. This objective does not preclude others using it to good purpose. But it has been designed specifically for that large and growing number of persons who are trying to apply the latest fruits of knowledge to the care of obese people. Throwing off the heritage of years of indifference and even despair about the treatment of obesity, more and more clinicians are approaching their obese patients with new hope. This hope is born of two ongoing developments of the recent past: the increasing number of increasingly effective treatments and our growing understanding of the nature of the disorder.

The organization of *Obesity* reflects the sources of this hope—basic science and treatment. The first nine chapters on basic mechanisms are selective rather than comprehensive. Their topics were chosen for two reasons: the research they describe is new and exciting and it is clinically relevant. Five of these chapters describe recent advances in classical disciplines—genetics, cellular anatomy, neurophysiology, conditioning, and pharmacology. Two chapters deal with new ideas about set points and dietary obesity, and two with psychological issues. The fifteen chapters on treatment include five on psychological and social measures, three on diet, and two on surgery. Five other chapters describe the use of medication and of exercise, the treatment of children and pregnant women, and an algorithm for the evaluation of obese patients.

We have been fortunate in the stature of the contributors to this volume. Not only are they authorities in the fields they describe—in most instances they are *the* authority. I am most grateful to them.

Albert J. Stunkard

Preface

The preface to the first edition began with the question, "Why another book on obesity?" Such a question is far less likely to be raised today. A number of recent professional conferences have highlighted the conflict inherent in the obvious ill effects of obesity (with the need to control it) and the limited success of our treatments. We have seen the demedicalization of obesity with the rise of commercial weight loss programs, and then their decline, leaving both professionals and lay persons uncertain as to where to turn. The proliferation of diets, both sensible and bizarre, continues apace, but is now buffeted by the growing anti-diet movement. The preoccupation of the great majority of young women with their weight has become so common as to constitute a "normative discontent" while the smaller number of women further out on the distribution curve, who binge and vomit, shows no evidence of decline.

The clinician who seeks to help obese persons is thus faced with a bewildering panoply of often conflicting injunctions. In any number of situations it is not clear what is to be done. This edition of *Obesity*, like the first edition, is written primarily for the clinician. The need for a new edition appears greater than ever.

To meet this need we have followed the outline of the earlier edition, seeking to address the latest findings on the theory and therapy of obesity. The result is a volume that should give the clinician the background to face the many challenges presented by this disorder. The first ten chapters on theory present a selection of some of the most important developments in our understanding of the nature of human obesity. This development still does not permit a treatment directed toward the etiology of obesity, but it does provide the clinician with an understanding of the factors that contribute to the patient's weight problems. The eleven chapters on treatment provide an up-to-date review of the major modalities of treatment, illustrating the progress that has been made in recent years and noting, realistically, the limitations of current treatment.

A particular pleasure for both of us in the editing of this volume has been the opportunity to collaborate on this, as on many previous endeavors. We thank the contributors for their superb chapters that maintain this volume at the high level of its predecessor.

Albert J. Stunkard
Thomas A. Wadden

Obesity
Theory and Therapy

Second Edition

Obesity: Theory and Therapy, Second Edition,
edited by A. J. Stunkard and T. A. Wadden.
Raven Press, Ltd., New York © 1993.

1

Introduction and Overview

Albert J. Stunkard

Department of Psychiatry, University of Pennsylvania,
Philadelphia, Pennsylvania 19104-2648

Eleven years ago the first edition of this volume celebrated the scope and diversity of the new research that was transforming our understanding of obesity. At that time it was still possible to contain within one volume a large part of these research findings. Such is no longer the case. The flood of new research —as much in the past decade as in the previous 50 years—has placed a premium on the careful selection of topics. The authors of the ten chapters on research have been asked to reflect in some depth upon particularly exciting new findings. Some authors had contributed chapters to the first edition; their new chapters illustrate the remarkable progress that has been made since then. Others describe new areas of research or old areas that have expanded dramatically. Together these ten chapters present an interweaving of fact and theory that yields an ever more coherent picture of obesity. It is a source of deep satisfaction to see investigators in very different fields, working with very different tools, develop such remarkably complementary systems. The scope and diversity of these systems is bringing us ever closer to the day when basic research on obesity can make a difference in the care of patients.

THEORY

Impact of Body Weight, Body Composition, and Adipose Tissue Distribution on Morbidity and Mortality

It seems fitting to begin this volume on obesity with a description of the ill effects of this disorder. Obesity is of concern primarily because of these ill effects, because it is a serious medical condition. Yet ill-informed voices have been heard recently from many quarters denying that obesity causes death and disability and even ascribing its ill effects to the results of treatment. It is thus salutary to be reminded of why we are concerned with this disorder, and this reminder could not come from a better informed and more careful source than Lars Sjöström of the Department of Medicine of Sahlgren's Hospital in Gothenberg, Sweden.

Sjöström begins with a thorough review of the studies that have examined the relation between obesity, as indexed by the body mass index (weight in kilograms/height in meters^2) and morbidity and mortality. He points out that some of the early studies that failed to find such an association had serious limitations—small sample sizes, short duration, and failure to control for smoking or intermediate risk factors. The more recent studies of larger populations, studied for longer periods of time with appropriate controls, have all found dramatic increases in morbidity and mortality. The question of the ill effects of obesity has been clearly answered.

Sjöström goes on to point out that the body mass index itself has limitations in its confounding of fatness and shortness, each of which confer risk to different degrees. He proceeds to describe the early studies of the association of regional fat distribution with morbidity and mortality. It was the Gothenburg group that first showed the greater predictive power of the waist/hip ratio over the body mass index in coronary heart disease in both men and women. Now the Gothenburg group has already moved far beyond such gross measures of body fat distribution to increasingly sophisticated computerized tomographic (CT) studies, which reveal the distribution of fat throughout the body. The use of multiple CT scans has enabled Sjöström to make highly accurate estimates of the volume of three key compartments—lean body mass, subcutaneous adipose tissue, and visceral adipose tissue. He points out that only visceral adipose tissue is associated with the multiple metabolic disorders, including diabetes, hypercholesterolemia, hypertriglyceridemia, and hypertension. He proposes a simple clinical measure that provides much of the information yielded by multiple CT scans. It is the sagittal trunk diameter at the level of the iliac crest of persons lying on their back. It is easily measured as the distance from the examination table to a carpenter's level placed over the abdomen. Apparently visceral fat is the primary contributor to this diameter, and subcutaneous fat has little impact. The simplicity and potential importance of this new measure suggests that it may soon become a standard clinical measure of obesity, and it seems likely that we will soon be learning more about its significance from future epidemiologic studies, like those that have proved so fruitful in Gothenburg in the past.

Basic Neural Mechanisms of Feeding and Weight Regulation

Hoebel and Hernandez's chapter on "Basic Neural Mechanisms of Feeding and Weight Regulation" shows in a particularly dramatic way how much we have learned during the past decade. For the clinician, whose progress has been slower, it is both overwhelming and stimulating. It is overwhelming because of the vast new complexities that have been added to the already complex neural systems known 10 years ago. New transmitters have been discovered and new functions for old ones. It is also stimulating, because patterns are emerging, and we are learning to understand the mechanisms that underlie the complex behaviors leading to obesity.

The old puzzle as to what initiates bouts of overeating seems to be yielding to a disarmingly simple explanation—a decrease in energy utilization. This decrease appears to be independent of the fuel that is being utilized. New complexities also emerge, along with questions that had been recognized only dimly 10 years ago. For example, it has become apparent that not only energy but also macronutrients are regulated and that highly specialized systems subserve the control of nutrient intake. These systems utilize newly recognized neuropeptides with specific functions. Galanin, for example, stimulates intake of fats, while neuropeptide Y (as well as norepinephrine) stimulates intake of carbohydrates.

The new understanding of macronutrient selection does not stop here. It has become clear in rats, and may well be true in humans, that the newly recognized power of circadian rhythms extends also to macronutrient intake. Upon awakening, in the early dark period, rats show a strong preference for carbohydrates, with the rapid energy that they provide. The awesome circuitry underlying this preference is already understood. Thus the paraventricular nucleus stimulates corticotrophic-releasing factor, which, in turn, releases adrenocorticotrophic hormone and, through it, corticosterone. Corticosterone not only stimulates carbohydrate metabolism directly but it also feeds back to the PVN to potentiate the binding of both norepinephrine and neuropeptide Y to receptors that mediate carbohydrate intake.

Hoebel and Hernandez outline a number of other integrative circuits that underlie some of the classical findings of behavioral psychology. As he puts it, "Pavlov conditioned salivary secretion; we have conditioned neurotransmitter secretion." Pavlovian conditioning can be viewed as the learning of the relations among environmental events. The authors show how this view has been expanded to include the learning of both the nutritional value and the toxic qualities of foods. The nucleus accumbens is a critical area for such learning, with an increase in dopamine release during feeding and a decrease in dopamine release during nausea, so what is learned in these situations is the control of dopamine release in the nucleus accumbens, facilitating both locomotion and reinforcement. Thus the classical conditioning of dopamine (and other neurotransmitters) alters the animal's instrumental responses for food. This conditioning of neurotransmitter release may provide the long-sought link between Pavlovian (respondent) conditioning and Skinnerian (operant) conditioning. Dopamine in the nucleus accumbens could be the link. Complex as they may appear, neural systems and neurotransmitters will ultimately have a simplifying function, as they resolve old puzzles and lay the basis for an even more thorough understanding of eating and obesity.

Psychological Aspects of Appetite

The chapter on "Pharmacological Aspects of Appetite" by Blundell and Lawton illustrates how several chapters that describe apparently unrelated aspects of obesity are in reality closely related. The authors reflect the evolutionary perspective presented later by Brown in noting that during the course of human evolution scarcity rather than abundance has been the usual problem. The result, as they point out, is that "the operation of the (energy) regulation system is not symmetrical; there is a strong defense against undernutrition and only weak response to the effects of overnutrition." Blundell and Lawton comment on the resulting overconsumption of "the abundant supply of palatable, high energy dense food," a problem that is dissected later by Sclafani in his chapter on "Dietary Obesity." The pharmacological aspects of appetite likewise have close connections with the "Neural Mechanisms of Feeding and Weight Regulation" (Hoebel and Hernandez).

A leitmotif of this chapter is that "appetite is not a unitary phenomenon" but instead consists of such components as hunger, macronutrient selection, and hedonics. "Hunger," we are reminded, is "a nagging irritating feeling that prompts thought of food and reminds us that the body needs energy"; as such, it is a "biologically useful sensation." Despite our familiarity with hunger, we know little about its neurochemical substrate and even our usual association of hunger with food intake is belied in certain circumstances—for example, by drugs that do not exert equal action on hunger and food intake.

In some ways we know more about the newly discovered control of macronutrient selection than about our old friend hunger. Blundell and Lawton place particular emphasis on the events taking place within the paraventricular nucleus (which is also singled out for special attention by Hoebel and Hernandez). They note the influence in the paraventricular nucleus of neuropeptide Y and α-2 adrenergic agonists in stimulating carbohydrate intake and the effects of serotonin agonists in suppressing carbohydrate intake. These findings lend support to Wurtman's hypothesis that plasma ratios of the serotonin-precursor tryptophan to other large neutral amino acids determine brain serotonin activity. According to this theory, the ingestion of carbohydrates, which enhances this ratio and thereby the levels of brain serotonin, acts as a feedback to inhibit further carbohydrate intake.

The ingestion not only of carbohydrate, but also of fat, may be separately controlled, although not as precisely. Blundell and Lawton, as do Hoebel and Hernandez, point to the role of galanin in simulating fat intake. The independent control of fat intake is further supported by the anorexic action of an agent that is believed to act primarily on fat digestion—the activation peptide of pancreatic procolipase. The possibility of intervening pharmacologically in the control of fat intake is particularly attractive since, as Ravussin and Swinburn point out in their chapter on "Energy Metabolism," the intake of fat is poorly controlled and fat intake is not necessarily proportional to fat oxidation. The resulting excess of fat intake over fat expenditure, uncontrolled by feedback mechanisms, is a strong candidate possibility for the weight gain that leads to obesity. Here is a circumstance in which pharmacological assistance to a weak regulatory mechanism could pay large dividends.

A third component of appetite is the hedonic or pleasure value of foods and eating. Sweet taste has long been recognized as a stimulus to eating and as a reward. It now appears that opioid peptides act to increase food intake by enhancing preferences for sweet foods. Support for this view is provided by the reduction of food intake produced by opioid receptor antagonists such as naloxone and naltrexone. These agents apparently reduce food intake by decreasing the perceived pleasantness of a sweet solution without having any effect upon hunger. By contrast, serotonin agonists reduce hunger (and food intake) with no effect on the pleasantness of sweet tastes. Such pharmacologic dissection provides an elegant example of the dissociation of appetite into such components as hunger, macronutrient selection, and hedonics.

Blundell and Lawton point out a major problem in developing drugs for the control of eating and obesity. It is the difficulty in determining whether the *actions* of an agent are due to some nonspecific blockade of eating or whether they actually affect the processes that match food intake to nutritional requirements. The authors believe that it is "useful to regard potential appetite-suppressant drugs not as blockers of eating but as agents that amplify and exploit the mechanisms of the natural anorexigenic agent—food." Our rapidly evolving understanding of this mechanism gives hope that, after the dearth of the past two decades, we may look forward to a number of new pharmacologic agents for the control of eating and obesity.

and body weight. These studies have led him to conclude that energy balance is regulated in organisms (including human) for both normal and elevated body weight. He adds support to the view that in obesity energy metabolism and body weight are controlled at an elevated level. This level is controlled by a set point that not only determines the regulated level of body weight but also actively defends that level in the face of pressures to raise or lower it. It has been argued that it is impossible to assess a body weight set point in humans, as it is for animals. In answer to this argument, Keesey proposes that the body weight set point of a person is that weight at which resting energy expenditure is consonant with the value predicted by Kleiber's equation relating energy expenditure to body weight—kcal/day = 65.5 ± 1.4 body weight$_{kg}^{.75}$.

Keesey proposes two tests of this definition of a body weight set point. The first is the finding that, under normal circumstances, body weight raised to the $\frac{3}{4}$ power predicts energy expenditure. The second is the presence of compensatory adjustments of energy expenditure when weight is gained or lost.

Keesey has subjected two types of organisms—dietary obese and lateral hypothalamic lean rodents to these tests. When food intake is decreased or increased, both overweight and underweight rodents show a compensatory change in the constant in the Kleiber equation—to 43.3 in the case of weight reduction and to 77.5 in the case of weight gain. Keesey maintains that the generality of the findings linking body weight to energy expenditure makes it possible to move beyond animal experiments to clinical applications of set-point theory. Precisely such reasoning has gone into Ravussin and Swinburn's prediction of weight changes as a function of energy expenditure. There appears to be an increasing consensus on how energy metabolism and body weight are related.

Physiological Regulation of Body Energy

In his chapter, Keesey reviews his 20 years of study of the regulation of energy balance

Energy Metabolism

The subject of energy metabolism follows quite logically from Keesey's discussion of the physiological regulation of body energy, moving from a more general description of regulation to a more precise elucidation of its components and how they contribute to the development of obesity in humans. Ten years ago it was possible for a volume on obesity not to consider the issue of energy metabolism. This is no longer the case. The rapid increase in our understanding of energy metabolism has transformed our view of obesity, and the scholarly review by Ravussin and Swinburn illustrates the importance of its role. These authors demonstrate the failings of the traditional energy balance equation (change in energy stored = energy intake − energy expenditure) and show that there is no theoretical need for so-called luksuskonsumption." Instead, they show that the appropriate equation is *rate* of change in energy stores = *rate* of change in energy intake − *rate* of change in energy expenditure. This equation helps to show why periods of positive energy balance result in only small increases in body weight and how the increase in body weight reestablishes the equilibrium between energy expenditure and body weight. In this perspective weight gain can be viewed not only as a consequence of an initial positive energy balance but also as the mechanism whereby energy balance is restored. The precision of this mechanism is illustrated by the fact that energy balance may be maintained during a 10-year period, during which 10 million kilocalories of (intermittent and variable) energy intake are matched with 10 million kilocalories of (continuous and variable) energy expenditure.

An important development in our understanding of energy balance is the recognition that there are separate balances for the three major macronutrients, carbohydrate, protein, and fat. The intake of carbohydrate and protein is very tightly controlled so that no significant excess intake over expenditure occurs and stores of these nutrients remain in balance. By contrast, the intake of fat is not well controlled and fat intake is not necessarily proportional to fat oxidation. Energy balance is thus virtually equivalent to fat balance. A chronic imbalance of fat intake in relation to fat oxidation can occur and is the most likely cause of the weight gain that leads to obesity.

The implications of these findings for the treatment of obesity are clear and favorable. They indicate that there should be no compensation, or increase in appetite for fat, when dietary fat is reduced. This theoretical rationale is supported by a growing number of empirical studies. They show that weight loss can occur with reduction of fat intake only and that this weight loss is associated with little pressure to regain the weight, as so often occurs in weight loss resulting from a reduction in total calories.

Ravussin and Swinburn propose an imaginative concept of the risk factors for weight gain. It is known that obese persons have a relatively high metabolic rate, a low respiratory quotient (the ratio of carbohydrate to fat oxidation), and insulin insensitivity. According to Ravussin and Swinburn, risk factors for weight gain consist of the exact opposite. They cite studies showing that a low metabolic rate, a high respiratory quotient, and increased insulin sensitivity all independently predict weight gain. Furthermore, this weight gain appears to serve a teleologic function; it is associated with "normalization" of the three functions.

Dietary Obesity

In his chapter on dietary obesity in the first edition of this book, Sclafani described the kind of dietary intake that gives rise to obesity. Ten years of research has made it possible to move beyond such descriptions to an understanding of the mechanisms leading to dietary obesity. In this effort Sclafani provides an important link to the chapter by Ravussin and Swinburn, implicating fat intake in the pathogenesis of obesity and showing how fat comes to be such an important part of the diets of developed countries. A common explanation for the high fat contents of current diets is that they are "palatable." Sclafani shows, however, that the traditional definition of palatability is circular. For example, diets that promote overeating were described as palatable, while overeating, in turn, was "explained" by the palatability of the diet.

Sclafani moves beyond this tautology to show that palatability (as measured by food choice and food consumption) is actually the result of two different processes. One is the innate preference for tastes such as sweetness and oiliness; the other is learned preferences that derive from postingestional consequences. The preferences for the fats in our diet result from both innate and conditioned preferences. Sclafani's sophisticated analysis shows that we are by no means locked into automatic and unconditioned preferences for fat; we are not doomed to struggle helplessly against our biological heritage. Instead, understanding the mechanism of conditioned food preferences should free us to develop more palatable low-fat foods and more effective behavioral programs.

Genetics and Human Obesity

The chapter on "Genetics and Human Obesity" makes it clear how very far our knowledge of this subject has progressed in the decade since the first edition of this book, which dealt largely with how genetic factors *might* influence human obesity. The present chapter by Meyer and Stunkard describes how genetic factors *do* influence human obesity. A series of family studies has firmly established the *familial* nature of human obesity. However, family members share environments as well as genes, and family studies by themselves cannot distinguish between the contributions of these two kinds of influence. Adoption and twin studies can disentangle these contributions, and studies of adoptees and of twins have made considerable progress in assessing these contributions.

Since adoptees do not share a "family environment" with their biologic parents, any similarity between parents and offspring is due solely to the genes that they share. By contrast, the similarity between adoptees and their adoptive parents reflects only the environment that they share. Two "full" adop-

tion studies, (studies that include information about both biologic parents as well as about adoptive parents) have been carried out. Each reveals a significant contribution of the biologic parents. By contrast, there is only a weak contribution of the adoptive mother, and it is present only while the adoptees are living with her. In adult life, no trace of the childhood rearing environment remains. The environment in which the adoptees live as adults does, however, have a significant impact upon their body weight.

Twin studies, which compare the similarity of identical twins with that of fraternal twins, provide a different type of information about the roles of genes and environment. A growing number of twin studies have confirmed the strong influence of genetic factors in human obesity. They could not, however, assess the contribution of the rearing environment since it was shared by the twin pairs. A special kind of twin study, of identical twins who had been reared apart, not only confirmed the importance of genetic factors but also the lack of influence of the childhood rearing environment. Furthermore, the importance of the current environment is illustrated by the fact that the correlation between pairs of identical twins is considerably less than 1.0.

Studies of genetic factors in human obesity are focusing on the nature of the contribution of genes and environment. These studies have already found evidence for interactions between genetic and environmental influences. They suggest that the most parsimonious model views obesity as the result of unfavorable environmental influences acting upon genetically predisposed individuals. Studies of the interaction of genetic and environmental factors will be immeasurably aided by the identification of major genes predisposing to obesity. Complex segregation analyses have already found evidence of major genes for obesity, and linkage studies attempting to locate such genes are already under way. At the present time, however, we know enough to help patients to a better understanding of their obesity. The information about the influence of genetic factors, for example, can help to relieve the shame and guilt that so many obese people feel about their weight, while the importance of environmental factors provides them with the hope that they may be able to control their weight.

Restrained Eating

The concept of restrained eating described by Pirke and Laessle may well be the most important recent psychological contribution to our understanding of eating and obesity. This concept of restrained eating was introduced in the 1970s by Herman and Polivy, who suggested that dietary restraint, or the tendency for persons to eat less than they would like to in order to control their weight, may account for many of the differences in behavior between obese and nonobese persons. The idea of restraint has featured prominently in research on anorexia nervosa and bulimia nervosa in recent years and far less in obesity. Much of this latter research has been carried out by Pirke and his group in Germany. One important contribution was the assessment of dietary restraint in persons in the natural environment. These studies revealed a paradox—although restrained eaters eat less than unrestrained eaters, their body mass index and body weight are higher. This finding could, of course, be the result of underreporting of food intake by restrained eaters. Accordingly, Pirke and Laessle measured the energy expenditure of their subjects by the powerful new doubly labeled water method. Despite their greater body mass index and greater weight, restrained eaters expended less energy than did unrestrained eaters. Since these subjects were studied while they were in energy balance, their energy intake must also have been lower.

In thorough studies of the biological associations of restrained eating, Pirke and Laessle found a shortened luteal phase of the menstrual cycle in restrained eaters. By reducing the period of elevated plasma progesterone and elevated body temperature, this shortened luteal phase may contribute to a less-ened energy need among restrained eaters. The authors note that restrained eating and dieting may be necessary conditions for the development of binge eating, but they are clearly not sufficient causes. In research for a greater predictive power of the concept of restraint, they support the idea of dividing restraint into "rigid" and "flexible" components, as proposed by Westenhoefer. In their view, "rigid," as opposed to "flexible," restraint has greater predictive power than undifferentiated restraint.

Psychosocial Consequences of Obesity and Dieting

The chapter on "Psychosocial Consequences of Obesity and Dieting" by Wadden and Stunkard describes the transformation in our views of the relationship between psychopathology and obesity. Older views had ascribed human obesity largely to psychopathological determinants. This view has changed 180 degrees in direction, and now the psychopathology of obese individuals is viewed not as a cause but as a consequence of obesity—specifically a consequence of the prejudice and discrimination to which obese individuals are subjected in our society. The authors document this prejudice and discrimination and note the remarkable resiliency of obese individuals, as illustrated by the fact that their level of general psychopathology appears no greater than that of any group seeking medical treatment. Psychopathology specific to obesity, however, does occur and is manifested in two ways—severe disparagement of the body image and binge eating without compensation. Disparagement of the body image represents an extreme of the "normative discontent" experienced by most women in our society and it is the source of great suffering. "Binge-eating disorder" is a newly established diagnosis recognizing behaviors that had been insufficiently recognized in the past. Persons with this disorder manifest a number of differences from other obese persons, and they will require different treatment from that provided by commercial weight-loss programs. The high prevalence of binge-eating disorder, between 25 and 50% of persons entering treatment for obesity means that the development of new therapies for these persons must be a high priority.

Cultural Perspectives on the Etiology and Treatment of Obesity

Peter Brown's chapter on "Cultural Perspectives on the Etiology and Treatment of Obesity" examines the relationship between culture and obesity from an anthropological perspective. The chapter is a particularly valuable complement to that on genetics, with its traditional dichotomy of genetic and environmental influences. Instead of the undifferentiated concept of "environment," Brown proposes the more differentiated concept of culture, "the learned patterns of behavior and beliefs of a social group." Such a redefinition is of great value in understanding the wide variety of potential gene–environment interactions and correlations.

Brown's first goal is to examine the biocultural evolution of the genetic and behavioral origins of obesity, which he traces back to the hunter-gatherer period. During this period, which constituted 99% of human history, food shortages were ubiquitous. Even today, 29% of primitive societies undergo food shortages severe enough to result in deaths by starvation. Under these circumstances, natural selection has favored persons who could effectively store calories in times of surplus. Women, in particular, have been favored, not only for their ability to withstand the stress of food shortages for themselves, but also for their fetuses and nursing children. The greater fat stores of women than men may well have arisen through such natural selection.

Brown's second goal is to identify cultural beliefs and behaviors that may predispose individuals to obesity. Understanding these beliefs and behaviors is of critical importance in the prevention and treatment of obesity in different social and ethnic groups. Brown documents the persistence of behaviors and

attitudes appropriate to a hunter-gatherer society in developing countries today. A dramatic illustration is the "fattening huts" for upper-class pubescent girls in traditional West African society. Regarding attitudes, he notes that 81% of the primitive societies rate "plumpness" or being "filled out" as an attribute of female beauty.

The thin ideal of female beauty in developed societies today is a very recent occurrence, and it goes hand in hand with the stigmatization of obesity and the development of anorexia nervosa and bulimia. Clearly, understanding these different cultural values will improve the communication of healthcare providers with persons of both minority and majority status. Such understanding has frequently been missing in approaches to ethnic minorities in which obesity is valued. In a sense it has been missing also in the too ready acceptance of the cultural beliefs of members of dominant Western societies, for it is beliefs about the desirability of thinness that predispose individuals, particularly women of upper social class, to the excessive concern about their weight and to the development of anorexia nervosa and bulimia.

THERAPY

The 15 clinical chapters provide a wealth of information about the treatment of obesity. Since this information is of a type more familiar to the reader with clinical interests than is that in the chapters on basic mechanisms, only the high points will be discussed.

"The Treatment of Obesity: An Overview" by Thomas Wadden begins the section on therapy with a scholarly account of the treatment options available for all but the tiny minority of severely obese persons for whom surgical treatment is indicated. Wadden's chapter provides a useful conceptual model of current treatments for obesity that integrates a classification based on body weight with features of a stepped-care approach and a third level that addresses individual treatment preferences. Wadden notes the importance of preparing patients for therapy and discusses in some detail the elements and results of a conventional behavioral approach. His account of the results obtained with very-low-calorie diets, an area in which he is a leader, describes the poor maintenance of weight losses while proposing modifications of these diets that may produce better long-term results. This chapter concludes with a number of important suggestions for future directions in the treatment of obesity.

Van Itallie and Lew's chapter on "Estimation of the Effect of Obesity on Health and Longevity" helps to translate the extensive findings of Sjöström's chapter into clinical guidelines that can be used by physicians to assess the health risks of individual patients.

The chapter on "Popular Diets for Weight Loss" by Dwyer was a particularly well-received contribution in the first edition of this book. The extensively revised chapter in this edition by Dwyer and Lu reviews the physiological and psychological means by which diets work and provides a critical analysis of ten popular weight-loss programs and nine popular diet books. The weaknesses and the (sometimes gross) inadequacies of programs and books are noted, and the clinician is provided with a reliable guide as to which programs and books can be confidently recommended to patients.

The chapter on "The Metabolic and Psychological Importance of Exercise in Weight Control" by Grilo, Brownell, and Stunkard provides an exhaustive review of the relationship between physical activity and obesity. The strong inverse relationship between physical activity and body weight is described, as is the association of physical activity with weight loss, and its even stronger relationship to the maintenance of weight loss. Recent research has moved beyond such correlational studies to experimental demonstrations of the effectiveness of physical activity in the maintenance of weight loss. This favorable demonstration makes it a matter of concern that adherence to exercise programs is so limited, and the chapter's recommendations for improving adherence are all the more valuable.

The use of appetite-suppressant medication has become progressively less common in the United States during recent years. It is, therefore, good to be reminded of "The Place of Appetite Suppressants in the Treatment of Obesity" by Silverstone, who provides a welcome discussion of this important treatment modality. In crisp, clear language he points out the value of pharmacotherapy and the characteristics of the most popular agents. He discusses an idea that is rapidly gaining acceptance—that pharmacotherapy of obesity should be carried out on a long-term basis. This could be one answer to the problem of maintenance of weight loss.

Leaders in the effort to improve maintenance of weight loss, Perri and Nezu, provide a state-of-the-art chapter on "Preventing Relapse following Treatment for Obesity." They describe the series of studies that have pioneered new approaches to the maintenance of weight loss. They point out the importance of continuing professional contact, training in relapse prevention, social support, and exercise. The most consistent finding in their studies was that structured programs of therapist contact following treatment successfully helped patients to maintain their weight losses.

Three chapters deal with the treatment of special groups—children, the morbidly obese, and pregnant women. In "New Developments in Childhood Obesity," Epstein considers the large and growing problem of childhood obesity. In his scholarly review, he discusses obesity as a developmental disorder and notes recent discoveries, such as the "adiposity rebound" in early childhood that predicts the development of obesity, and the role of genetic and nonfamilial environmental factors in the genesis of obesity. Although programs for the treatment of obesity are in their infancy, the results appear promising, particularly in the maintenance of weight loss, as revealed by Epstein's own dramatic results of a 10-year follow-up.

The chapter on "Surgery" by Mason and Doherty describes what has become the treatment of choice for severe obesity, that characterized by a body weight at least 100% over the recommended level. Although the prevalence of this disorder is very low—0.5% of the obese population—it afflicts well over one million adults in the United States and thus many physicians will have contact with patients suffering from this degree of obesity. This account by the pioneer in the development of surgical approaches to obesity will provide practitioners with a thoughtful and balanced account of this form of treatment.

The chapter on "Obstetrical Problems in the Obese Patient" by Steinfeld and Cohen provides a wealth of information about the complications of obesity, among the most common problems in obstetrics. There now seems to be agreement about the ideal amount of weight to be gained by an obese woman during pregnancy—15–25 lb rather than the 25–35 lb for a women of normal weight. There are, however, few guidelines for those who care for pregnant obese women and their many health complications. Steinfeld and Cohen provide a masterful summary of these problems, which often include serious mechanical ones arising from the mother and her often large infant, as well as the marked increase in hypertension and impaired glucose tolerance. The authors provide valuable suggestions for coping with these complications and for those encountered during delivery.

In the chapter on "Public Health Approaches to Weight Loss" Taylor and Stunkard describe the efforts to reach large numbers of persons with the hope that even small changes in individuals will produce significant results in populations. A variety of approaches are described—large-scale community interventions, worksite and school programs, and the many commercial weight-loss programs. The results of these efforts

have been modest and have directed attention to policy measures such as improving the quality of food in school lunch programs, labeling of processed food, subsidization of the production of healthy foods, and taxation of the production of unhealthy foods.

The final chapter on "Talking with Patients" by Stunkard distills the information from the various chapters dealing with theory and therapy in an effort to provide the basis for a meaningful dialogue with patients. It notes the virtues of confirming many patients in their decision not to seek treatment and helps them to understand their obesity in a way that increases their self-esteem. The goal of this chapter (as indeed is a goal of the entire book) is to help restore talking with patients to its traditional role, uniting doctor and patient in their sacred enterprise.

Looking back over what we have learned about obesity during the past decade, one cannot help but be impressed by the giant strides we have made. Large new areas of research have opened up and old areas have become increasingly productive. One might well have hoped that all this new information would have yielded the fundamental understanding necessary to bring the problem of obesity finally under control. Unfortunately, this has not been the case; the discoveries in the laboratory have yet to be translated into clinical practice. Even without a major breakthrough, however, there has been progress in treatment. Results over the short term are considerably improved, even as long-term results still elude us. So we press on into a future that looks ever brighter. The record of achievement in the pages that follow can make us proud of our increased ability to still the pain of obesity and encouraged by the promise that that ability is rapidly increasing.

Theory

Obesity: Theory and Therapy, Second Edition,
edited by A. J. Stunkard and T. A. Wadden.
Raven Press, Ltd., New York © 1993.

2

Impacts of Body Weight, Body Composition, and Adipose Tissue Distribution on Morbidity and Mortality

Lars Sjöström

Department of Medicine, Sahlgren's Hospital, University of Göteborg,
S-413 45 Göteborg, Sweden

A number of indirect techniques based on total body potassium, total body water, or body density have been used in the past to estimate body fat or adipose tissue. More direct techniques to measure adipose tissue, muscle, skeleton, skin, and visceral organs are now available. Methods for determination of fat cell weight are based on microscopic examination or osmium fixation. A valid average fat cell weight of the body can be estimated from measurements in four regions. The total fat cell number of the body is obtained by dividing body fat by the average fat cell weight.

Increase in body fat from 1 month to 1 year of age is due only to an increasing fat cell weight from 0.15 to 0.50 μg, while the expansion of body fat from 1 to 22 years of age is due to an increase in fat cell number. In adult subjects, obesity up to 30 kg body fat is usually associated with increased fat cell weight (hypertrophic obesity), while increased fat cell number and fat cell weight (hyperplastic and combined obesities) are observed in more pronounced cases of obesity. In adulthood, short-term weight changes (<2 years) are associated with changes in fat cell weight, while long-term changes are due to changes in monolocular fat cell number. Increased fat cell weight is associated with a number of metabolic disturbances, while a high fat cell number is related to early onset of obesity and poor maintenance of a reduced body weight.

The prevalences of several risk factors and diseases are dramatically increased in obesity. A number of new studies have appeared over the last decade and a review of available information reveals that all large prospective studies (n > 20,000) and several smaller investigations have found that severe obesity (body mass index, BMI $\geq$ 35 kg/m^2) is associated with an approximately twofold increase in total mortality and a severalfold increase in mortality due to diabetes, cerebro- and cardiovascular disease, and certain forms of cancer.

Indices of abdominal obesity are associated with metabolic aberrations, cardiovascular morbidity and mortality, and total mortality in several cross-sectional and longitudinal studies. Sex differences with respect to incident disease and metabolic aberrations are at least partly mediated via differences in abdominal obesity.

Body mass index represents an undefined mixture of risk index and body fat index. Since weight is positively and height negatively related to mortality, the combination of these two variables should be avoided in risk calculations. The waist/hip ratio is poorly related to the visceral adipose tissue volume as determined with multiscan computed tomography (CT) technique. By using weight, height, sagittal trunk diameter (crista level) of recumbent subjects, and CT-calibrated sex-specific equations, the components of a three-compartment model can be estimated with errors less than 20%. The compartments are lean body mass and visceral and subcutaneous adipose tissue. In contrast to BMI and the waist/hip ratio, these estimates can distinguish compartments associated with metabolic aberrations from compartments that are not.

The role of obesity as a risk factor for mortality and cardiovascular morbidity has been intensively discussed over the last 30 years. As early as the beginning of this century, insurance statistics indicated that obesity was associated with increased mortality (1), and later, two large actuarial studies (2,3) confirmed the original finding. Most population studies published during the 1960s and 1970s were not able to demonstrate relationships between overweight morbidity and mortality. However, over the last 10 to 15 years, a number of large and/or long-term studies have been able to confirm the actuarial studies. In parallel, it has been observed that certain subtypes of the obesity syndrome (hypertrophic obesity, abdominal obesity) are associated with a particularly high risk. Today, there is general agreement that obesity constitutes a major risk factor in western countries.

Since much of the controversy that has existed in the past may be related to imperfect methodology, this chapter will first deal with definitions and methods of importance for obesity–risk relationships. Some attention will then be directed to the apparent transition from the concept of adipose tissue cellularity to adipose tissue distribution. Finally, morbidity and mortality will be discussed in relation to overweight and adipose tissue distribution.

DEFINITIONS AND METHODS

Obesity is an increased amount of body fat (BF) or adipose tissue (AT), while *overweight* is an increased body weight (BW) in relation to height. Various statistical cut-off definitions have been used for obesity as well as overweight. Definitions based on mortality are available only for overweight since advanced body composition techniques have so far not been used in larger population studies. In large samples ($n > 10^5$) the relationship between mortality and body mass index (BMI, kg/m^2) is J- or U-shaped, and above average mortality rates appear at approximately $BMI \geq 28$ kg/m^2 (2–4). Marked overweight is always associated with obesity while moderate overweight is occasionally due to other conditions.

Indirect Body Composition Techniques

The majority of human body composition measurements have used indirect techniques based on different assumptions about the chemical or physical properties of fat-free mass (FFM) or lean body mass (LBM). Usually two-compartment models have been used according to:

$$BW = BF + FFM \qquad (1)$$

$$BW = AT + LBM \qquad (2)$$

In Eq. 1 BW is compartmentalized into FFM and BF. FFM is thus the nonlipid part of the body including extracellular water (ECW) and stromal vascular cells of AT as well as cell membranes, cytoplasm, and organelles of the adipocytes. In Eq. 2 BW consists of AT and LBM. LBM contains all tissues of the body except AT. In these models FFM or LBM are estimated by determining total body potassium (TBK) (5–7) or total body water (TBW) (8), using different assumptions about the potassium (5,9–13) or water (8,14,15) content of FFM or LBM. Alternatively, body density is determined by underwater weighing (16) or by means of plethysmographic techniques (17). By assuming a density of 1.1 for FFM and a density of 0.9 for BF, the percentage of BF can be calculated according to Siri's equation (18). Modified density assumptions have also been used

(19). By determining both TBK and TBW, a four-compartment model has also been used (20):

$$BW = BF + FFECS + BCM + ECW \quad (3)$$

This model assumes that the respiring (intracellular) body cell mass (BCM) contains 120 mmol K/kg. Thus BCM = TBK/120. Furthermore, it is assumed that the water content of BCM is 75%. Thus, the extracellular water (ECW) is equal to TBW − 0.75 BCM. Finally, fat-free extracellular solids (FFECS) are assumed to be 12% of ideal weight in relation to height. More recently, indirect methods based on impedance and infrared interactance have been developed to measure BF and FFM (for review, see ref. 21).

After the Chernobyl disaster in April 1986 the apparent ^{40}K content of subjects from many parts of Europe was markedly increased due to ^{134}Cs contamination. Since multiple cascades occur in the decay of ^{134}Cs but not of ^{40}K, we constructed an algorithm based on coincidence measurements, making it possible to subtract counts originating from ^{134}Cs (7).

The relationships between different body compartments according to Eqs. 1–3 are illustrated in Fig. 1. Independently of the model used (Eqs. 1–3), BF or AT are indirectly calculated by difference against BW. Furthermore, the indirect techniques are dependent on population-specific assumptions since density of FFM or LBM as well as their TBK or TBW content may vary with sex, race, age, and degree of obesity. Even if population-specific assumptions are used, the determinations of FFM and BF (or LBM and AT) are accurate only on average but not necessarily in each individual case. For instance, the water content of FFM changes with over- and dehydration and the density as well as the potassium content of FFM increases with increasing physical fitness and decreases with age (11). Several endocrine and gastrointestinal disturbances may also influence TBK and TBW content of FFM and LBM. Originally, Forbes suggested 68.1 mmol K$^+$/kg

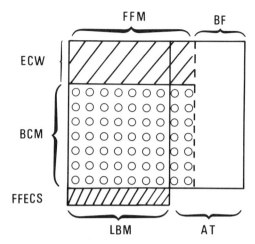

FIG. 1. Relationships between various body compartments. *FFM,* fat-free mass; *BF,* body fat; *LBM,* lean body mass; *AT,* adipose tissue; *ECW,* extracellular water; *BCM,* body cell mass; *FFECS,* fat-free extracellular solids.

FFM (5). Womersly (11) as well as the present author and colleagues (12,13) found values on the order of 64 mmol/kg for men and 62 mmol/kg for women to be more appropriate.

Indirect techniques discussed above have been used to construct equations predicting BF or FFM from weight-for-height indices (12,13,22–28), circumferences (29), skinfolds (26,30–32), and radiological (33–35) as well as ultrasound (35–37) measurements. These derived techniques are also population specific, and the sources of errors are related both to the anthropometric measuring procedures per se and to the reference methods. Finally, since the reference methods are usually based on two-compartment models, the calibrated anthropometric techniques are restricted to the same models.

Semidirect Body Composition Techniques

Direct dissections (38) or chemical analyses (9,39–43) of human cadavers are for obvious reasons limited by a number of practical and ethical considerations and, unlike the situation in studies of animals, direct examinations are not feasible in clinical studies. However, a number of techniques have recently appeared that determine body compartments or body constituents of the living human body in a more direct way. Thus body fat can be measured by equilibration with fat-soluble gases, the bone mineral content, lean tissue, and BF with dual photon absorptiometry and the nitrogen, calcium, and carbon content can be measured with neutron activation (for review, see ref. 21).

Computed tomography (CT) has been used to determine the AT area of single scans (44–53). With this procedure, relationships between the visceral AT area and various metabolic aberrations have been demonstrated. However, area determinations do not represent a true body composition technique since the body has three dimensions. For instance, it is not possible to express regional AT areas in percent of the total AT volume and, in a stricter sense, it is therefore not possible to study changes in fat patterning from area changes in a single or in a limited number of scans.

We have developed a multiscan CT technique that makes it possible to calculate total and any regional AT volume from 22 scans and the distances between the scans (12,13,21,28,54–56). Recently, this technique has been further refined so that the volume of some 20 different compartments can be determined from 28 scans and the distance between them (57–59 and Fig. 2). Using these techniques, we have performed detailed studies on the effects of growth hormone (60,61), cortisol (62), testosterone (63), weight reduction (64), and alcoholism (65) on body composition and/or adipose tissue distribution. Ethnic comparisons are being made and the CT techniques have also been used to "calibrate" anthropometric equations.

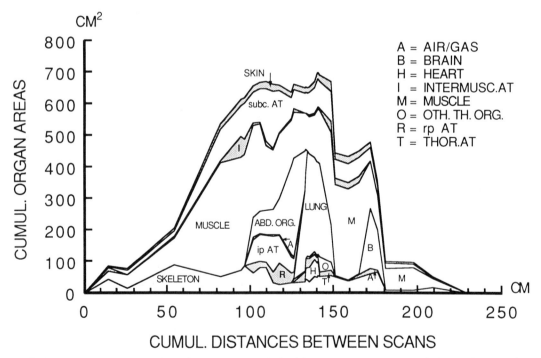

FIG. 2. Multicompartmentation of the human body. In this computer-constructed picture the cumulative organ areas in each scan are plotted versus the cumulative distance between the scans. Since cm² × cm is equal to a volume, the areas of the figure represent organ volumes. Red and yellow bone marrow are included in skeleton. The border between retroperitoneal (*rp*) adipose tissue (*AT*) (*R*) and intraperitoneal AT (*ip AT*) is approximate. Intermuscular AT (*I*) is AT tissue between muscle bundles inside the main fascia of the muscle. Copyright: Sjöström and Kvist.

CT-Calibrated Anthropometric Equations for Estimation of Lean Body Mass and Subcutaneous and Visceral Adipose Tissue

It has been claimed that the BMI [(weight, kg)/(height, m)^2] is an optimal index of the body constitution since it is minimally biased by height (23–25). We have examined several groups of subjects with the TBK technique and have found that, depending on sex, age, and degree of obesity, positive as well as negative relationships may occur between AT_{TBK} and height (28). Although these relationships have usually been fairly weak, it seems reasonable that the estimate or index of AT should demonstrate the same correlation with height as actually measured AT versus height. By using iterative correlation procedures (Fig. 3), we have found that the optimal correlation between AT_{CT} and weight/height^x (W/H^x) is obtained for x-values in the range 0.8–

1.2 (12,13). These indices demonstrate the same correlation with height as AT with height in a number of materials (28). As compared to equations based on BMI, equations based on W/H give significantly smaller absolute residuals versus actually measured AT (Fig. 4). This has also been observed in other lean and obese samples (28). In this context it should also be stressed that equations based on weight-for-height indices should estimate AT or BF in kilograms and not in percent. If percent AT or BF is estimated, the optimal exponent of height may vary severalfold from one group of subjects to another (28).

It seems reasonable that W/H should predict the degree of obesity in an optimal way since this ratio is approximately equal to volume/height (body density $\approx$ 1). Volume/height is in turn equal to the average cross-sectional area of the body. Since AT can vary several times more than any other tissue of

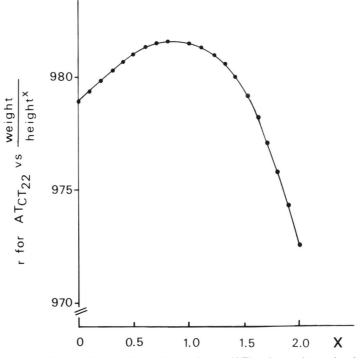

FIG. 3. Iterative correlations between the adipose tissue (*AT*) volume determined with computed tomography (CT) and various weight for height indices in 24 men. The correlation between AT determined from 22 CT scans and weight/height^x is given on the y-axis and the exponent, x, with which height is raised is given on the x-axis. The optimal correlation was obtained for W/H$^{0.9}$. Data from Kvist et al., ref. 55. Copyright: Sjöström and Kvist.

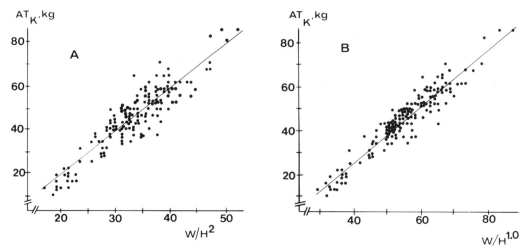

FIG. 4. The relationships between adipose tissue (*AT*) calculated from total body potassium (AT_K) and weight/height^2 (W/H^2) (**A**) or W/H (**B**) in 154 women. **A:** $R^2 \times 100 = 84.1\%$, absolute residuals 4.7 ± 3.5 kg AT. **B:** $R^2 \times 100 = 90.6\%$, absolute residuals 3.6 ± 2.7 kg AT. The residuals were significantly smaller ($p < 0.001$, paired *t* test) in the right panel. Copyright: Sjöström.

the body, the average cross-sectional area of the body could be expected to be related to the degree of obesity. Along similar lines, the dimensions of BMI would be equal to a distance, but this distance is not equal to any defined average diameter of the body since weight ($\approx$ volume) has been divided with height^2.

Table 1 sums up our published (55) "optimal" CT-calibrated equations for prediction of the total AT volume in men and women.

When comparing estimates based on weight/height with actual CT-measured total AT volumes, the errors are on the order of 10%, both in primary and cross-validation studies of both sexes. Similar errors were obtained by using weight and height as two independent predictors of total AT (12). With currently available data it was not possible to increase the explained variance further by adding other anthropometric measurements to the equation (55).

TABLE 1. *Anthropometric CT-calibrated equations and calculations to estimate LBM and the weight of subcutaneous and visceral AT*

	Primary study group		Cross validation group
	R^2 (%)	Error (%)	Error %
Males			
Total AT, liters $= 1.36 \cdot W/H - 42.0$	93	9	11
Visceral AT, liters $= 0.731 \cdot D - 11.5$	81	18	12
Females			
Total AT, liters $= 1.61 \cdot W/H - 38.3$	96	7	9
Visceral AT, liters $= 0.370 \cdot D - 4.85$	80	21	18
Males and females			
AT, kg $=$ AT, liters $\cdot 0.923$			
LBM, kg $=$ BW, kg $-$ total AT, kg			
Subcut. AT, kg $=$ total AT, kg $-$ visceral AT, kg			

Adapted from Kvist et al., ref. 55, with permission.

AT, adipose tissue; BW, body weight; CT, computed tomography; D, sagittal diameter in cm; LBM, lean body mass; W/H, weight/height in kg/m.

Lean body mass can be estimated as the difference between BW and total AT expressed in kilograms (Table 1). The conversion from lifters of AT is achieved by multiplying with the mean density (0.923) of human AT (12,13).

We have tested several hundred potential predictors of the visceral AT volume (55). Briefly, the sagittal diameter of recumbent subjects measured at the level of the iliac crest (= L_{4-5} level) seems to be the optimal predictor of the visceral AT volume. The sagittal diameter is easily obtained by measuring the distance from the examination table to a horizontal spirit level placed over the abdomen of a recumbent subject at the level of the iliac crest. The measurement is performed after a normal expiration. In the supine position intraabdominal AT is "pumping" up the abdomen in the sagittal direction, while subcutaneous AT is compressing the abdomen. This is probably the reason why the sagittal diameter is able to discriminate between visceral and subcutaneous AT at similar waist circumferences. As shown in Table 1, the errors for estimation of the visceral AT are on the order of 20% both in primary and cross-validation studies of men and women (55). The subcutaneous AT is obtained as the difference between total and visceral AT (Table 1).

Our equations have been justifiably criticized due to the small number of observations on which they are based. In men, our original equation was based on 17 subjects. In a recent follow-up, data from 37 men were collected (58). The equation based on 37 men ($y = 0.743 \cdot D - 11.8$) was almost identical to the original equation (Table 1). Similar findings were obtained in women. The equation predicting visceral AT volume in women was also adequate in six women with Cushing's syndrome, both before and after treatment (58,62). This information indicates that our original equations may be fairly robust, although more data would enhance their generalizability.

By using weight, height, and sagittal diameter, it is thus possible to estimate the components of a three-compartment model consisting of lean body mass and the weights of subcutaneous and visceral AT (Table 1). As illustrated later in this chapter, this procedure is an improvement over the use of BMI and the waist/hip ratio. BMI can not separate FFM from BF or LBM from AT. The ratio of waist to hip circumference is poorly related to the visceral AT volume (55). Both numerator and denominator of this ratio are influenced by several tissues (bone, muscle, visceral organs, and visceral and subcutaneous AT) in a way that is not fully understood.

Weight-for-Height Indices and Risk

Weight for height indices with different exponents of height may rank subjects in an entirely different manner (Table 2). Furthermore, weight is positively related to mortality (albeit with a J shape), while a negative association has been observed between height and mortality (3,4 and Fig. 5). Because of these facts (Table 2, Fig. 5), one may suspect that weight-for-height indices predicting morbidity and mortality optimally may be different from indices estimating AT or BF in an optimal way. By using an iterative regression procedure during which the exponent of height in W/H^x is gradually changed, we have in fact demonstrated that $W/H^{2.2}$ predicted myocardial infarction optimally in two different population studies of men (n = 784 and n = 10,004) (28). In one female population study (n = 1,462) $W/H^{4.8}$ predicted myocardial infarction optimally ($p = 0.004$). W/H^2 ($p = 0.02$) and W/H ($p = 0.05$) were still significant predictors while weight (=W/H^0) was not (28).

Different weight-for-height indices may thus be optimal risk predictors in different populations while AT is optimally predicted by indices being close to $W/H^{1.0}$. BMI has served both as a risk index and as an AT (or BF) index in a way that has previously not been defined. BMI thus offers an undefined mixture of risk prediction (cf. previous sentence) and AT estimation (cf. Fig. 3). This

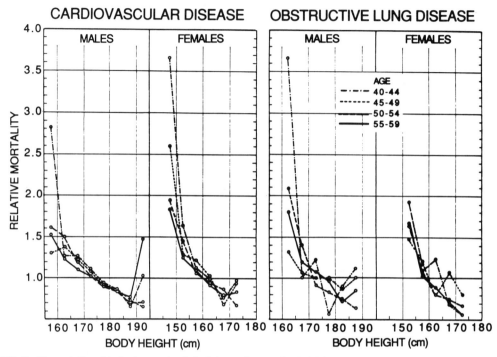

FIG. 5. The relationship between body height and mortality in high-weight (**left**) and low-weight (**right**) diseases. (From Waaler, ref. 4, with permission.)

does not seem to be critical for the detection of obesity–risk relationships in large studies but may well contribute to inconsistent results in smaller short-term studies (see below and Fig. 6). Among obese subjects, BMI reflects the negative effects of both fatness and shortness. The risks of fatness and shortness are most likely not mediated via identical mechanisms since height is negatively related to morbidity and mortality in "high-weight" as well as "low-weight" diseases (Fig. 5). Since height is negatively and weight positively related to risk, it seems more appropriate to regress incident morbidity and mor-

tality against weight and height as two independent variables rather than against BMI. Alternatively, height and weight can be used to estimate LBM and total AT with CT-calibrated equations (Table 1).

Methods for Fat Cell Weight and Number

The mean fat cell volume can be determined microscopically in frozen-cut sections of AT (66) or in collagenase liberated fat cells (67). The cell volume is converted to cell weight by multiplying it by the density of hu-

TABLE 2. *Different weight-for-height (W/H^x) indices may rank subjects differently*

Subject	BW (kg)	Height (m)	Weight-for-height index	Ranking order of subjects
A	80	1.60	W/H^1	A B C
B	85	1.65	W/H^2	B A C
C	95	1.70	W/H^3	B C A
			W/H^4	C B A

Reproduced from Sjöström, ref. 160, with permission.
BW, body weight.

man triglycerides (66). Fat cell weight of a sample can also be calculated from the triglyceride content of a sample and the number of fat cells in that sample determined by automatic counting of osmium-fixed fat cells (66,68). Osmium-fixed fat cells can also be directly sized with automatic techniques (66,69). By determining the mean fat cell weight in AT samples from gluteal, femoral, epigastric, and hypogastric regions, a valid estimate of the average fat cell weight (FCW) of the body is obtained (70,71), based in part on the fact that the FCW from different regions including intraabdominal ones are correlated (70,72). By dividing BF with the average FCW of the body, the total fat cell number (FCN) is obtained (73,74).

ADIPOSE TISSUE CELLULARITY

In adult subjects examined cross-sectionally, the monolocular FCN increases continuously and linearly over the whole body fat range while the average FCW increases up to approximately 30 kg BF (73,74). This means that moderate obesity is usually "hypertrophic," while severe obesity is "hyperplastic" or combined.

In longitudinal studies of male and female babies examined at 1, 3, 6, 9, 12, and 18 months of age, we found that the increase in BF from 0.7 kg at 1 month of age to 2.5 kg at 12 months of age was due only to an increase in FCW from 0.15 to 0.50 μg while FCN was stable at $0.6 \cdot 10^{10}$ cells (75).

A further increase in BF to 3 kg at 18 months of age was entirely due to an increase in FCN. Cross-sectional data in eight- (76) and 22- (77) year-old subjects indicate that further accumulation of fat is due to an increased monolocular FCN while the average FCW does not increase from 1 to 22 years of age. Due to methodological difficulties, some early studies arrived at other conclusions (for review, see ref. 70).

While early nutritional manipulations may have ultimate effects on FCN in some species (78–81), this does not seem to be the case in humans. Thus neither severe undernutrition during the first 11 to 18 weeks of life (82) nor extreme gestational overnutrition due to poorly controlled maternal diabetes (83) have any impact on adult adipose tissue cellularity.

In adult subjects, short-term (<1–2 years) moderate overfeeding (84) or caloric restriction (73,85–87) have an impact only on FCW while FCN seems to be unchanged. During more dramatic short-term weight reductions, obtained by gastrointestinal weight reduction surgery, both monolocular FCN and FCW are reduced (72). Similar results have also been obtained in dieting schoolgirls (76). Long-term (6 to 10 years) increase and decrease in body fat seem to be accompanied only by changes in monolocular FCN while the average FCW is unchanged (88,89). Due to these findings we have hypothesized that changes in the caloric balance initially cause a changed FCW. If the duration of the caloric imbalance is long and changes in FCW are thus marked, the altered FCW triggers changes in the monolocular FCN (88, 89). Whether a reduction in total monolocular FCN corresponds to a true disappearance of fat cells or a transformation to undetected postadipocytes is not clear. Although a discussion of pre- and postadipocytes is outside the scope of this chapter, reviews on early (70,71) and recent (90) studies have appeared.

An increased FCN seems to be statistically related to an early onset of obesity (74,91–93) but a considerable fraction of patients with late onset may have a hyperplastic obesity (85,92).

During treatment a large and rapid weight reduction can occur with hyperplastic obesity but also a short period of weight maintenance before relapse (94). Hypertrophic obesity, on the other hand, is characterized by a smaller and slower weight reduction but a longer period of weight maintenance (94). Irrespective of initial BF, the weight reduction tends to cease when the fat cell weight has reached the normal range (85). This implies that the weight reduction comes to an end at a higher body fat and body weight in hyperplastic obesity.

In vitro relationships between fat cell weight and metabolism (for review, see refs. 70, 71, 95–97) are also outside the scope of this review, while some relationships between FCW and metabolic aberrations in vivo should be mentioned briefly. Early studies indicated that hypertrophic obesity was associated with metabolic complications such as hyperinsulinemia (73,98,99), hypertriglyceridemia (100,101), and onset of diabetes mellitus in adulthood (99–101). Later, we demonstrated that associations between insulin, glucose, triglycerides, and blood pressure on the one hand and FCW on the other were typical for cells in abdominal rather than gluteal or femoral regions (102). This demonstration is in line with more recent ideas about relationships between abdominal obesity and the metabolic syndrome to be discussed below.

The same study (102) also illustrated that the waist circumference or the waist/hip circumference ratio were in fact stronger predictors of metabolic aberrations than FCW or FCN. Considering the simplicity with which adipose tissue distribution can be estimated by circumference ratios, it is not surprising that this type of measurement has dominated the epidemiological literature over the last few years. Although an overlap exists between hypertrophic and abdominal obesity (102), this overlap is not complete. In the future, it may therefore be rewarding to combine precise adipose tissue distribution techniques (12,13,54–59) with regional metabolic studies (e.g., microdialysis), regional blood flow measurements (e.g., laser doppler or xenon techniques), and determinations of regional (77,103) as well as total (73,74,98) adipose tissue cellularity.

RELATIONSHIPS BETWEEN OVERWEIGHT AND RISK

Insurance Studies

As mentioned in the introduction, a relationship between overweight and mortality has been consistently demonstrated in insurance studies (1–3). One often quoted limitation of these studies is that persons who buy life insurance are not representative of the general population (104,105). This is certainly true, and the lack of representativeness makes it hazardous to estimate the obesity-related mortality in the general population from actuarial data. However, the lack of representativeness does not affect the internal validity of insurance studies, i.e., among the 4 to 5 million policy holders of the two later studies (2,3), it was clear that obese persons had a greater mortality than individuals of average body weight.

Negative Population Studies

In spite of the strong associations shown by insurance studies, some 40% of all employee, community, and random population studies have failed to demonstrate a relationship between body weight and mortality. Other reviewers have arrived at similar percentages (106,107). Population studies are more representative of the general population than insurance studies and therefore resolution of this conflict is sorely needed. One possibility is that the negative population studies indeed reflect a smaller impact of overweight on mortality than has been concluded from insurance studies. The other possibility is an insufficient internal validity of negative population studies. Five types of reduced internal validity will be examined here.

In Fig. 6 the sizes of 51 cohorts (40 studies) have been plotted against the follow-up periods since entry into the studies. Plus signs indicate studies that found relationships between overweight and mortality while negative signs represent studies that did not. Negative studies are clearly clustered among small and/or short-term studies. All studies with more than 20,000 participants and 20 of 21 cohorts larger than 7,000 show a positive relationship between overweight and mortality. The critical follow-up period in larger studies seems to be about 5 years, although 5

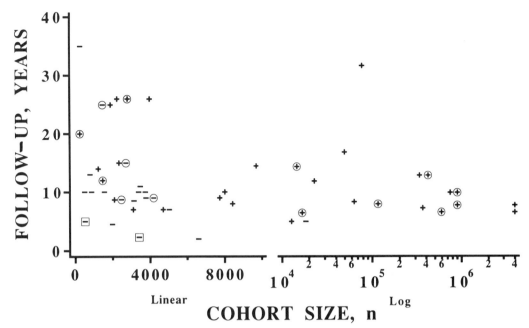

FIG. 6. Cohort size and follow-up period in relation to 40 employee, community, or random population studies finding (+) or not finding (−) a positive relationship between obesity and mortality. Encircled signs represent female cohorts and squares around signs indicate that men and women were analyzed together. For layout reasons seven cohorts have been plotted in positions deviating as little as possible from the true values. Signs for cohort sizes increasing from 0 to 5,000 in the follow-up interval 1 to 10 years correspond to references: 108 (men plus women combined), 109–112, 113 (men and women), 114, 115, 148 (men plus women combined, preliminary SOS mortality data), 117–119 (men and women), 120 (urban and rural). Signs for cohort sizes increasing from 0 to 5,000 in the follow-up interval 11 to 20 years correspond to references: 121 (women), 122–124 (women), 125 (black men and women), 126. Signs for cohort sizes increasing from 0 to 5,000 in the follow-up interval 21 to 35 years correspond to references: 127, 128 (women and men), 129 (men and women), 130. Signs for cohort sizes increasing from 5,000 to 10,000 correspond to references: 131–135. Signs for cohort sizes increasing from 10,000 to 100,000 correspond to references: 135 (women), 136, 137 (women), 138–140, 141, 143. Signs for cohort sizes increasing from 100,000 to 4,000,000 correspond to references: 142 (women), 144, 147, 144 (women), 3 (women), 4 (men and women), 2 (women and men), 3. References without comments refer to studies in men. Copyright: Sjöström.

years of follow-up was not enough to reach significance in the Whitehall study of 18,000 men (138). With decreasing cohort size, negative studies become more and more common and longer follow-up periods are required in order to achieve reproducible relationships between overweight and mortality. The need for prolonged observation periods in smaller studies is illustrated by the Framingham (2,252 men, 2,818 women; ref. 129) and Manitoba (3,983 men, ref. 130) studies, in which 26 years of follow-up were required until a positive relationship between overweight and mortality was obtained. If a study is too small, even the most prolonged observation period may not help. This is illustrated by Keys' 279 men from Minnesota, who were followed for 35 years without finding a relationship between overweight and mortality (127).

Another reason for a reduced validity of negative population studies is failure to control for smoking. Since cigarette smoking is a strong risk factor for mortality and also is more common among the lean, failure to control for smoking will produce an artifactually high mortality in lean subjects. When the mortality of obese and lean subjects is compared, the obesity-related mortality will thus be underestimated. This finding was clearly illustrated by the American Cancer Society Study in which a J-shaped relationship between mortality and BMI was observed among smokers, while a linear positive association at a lower level was seen among nonsmokers (144). In several other studies (133,134,142,145), control for smoking by multivariate analysis has led to a strengthening of the weight–mortality association. Thus studies in which overweight–mortality associations are not observed must be interpreted with caution if smoking has not been taken into account.

Failure to eliminate early mortality from the analysis is a third reason for an attenuated weight–mortality association. Clinical or subclinical illness present before entry into a study could be the reason for a reduced body weight rather than a consequence of it. This point is illustrated by data from the Build Study in Table 3 (3). The mortality ratio of subjects with initial underweight decreased over an observation period of 20 years, while the ratio of subjects with initial overweight increased with time. Failure to adjust for early mortality will thus underestimate obesity-related mortality in all comparisons with lean subjects.

A fourth reason for an insufficient internal validity of negative population studies has been inappropriate control for intermediate risk factors. Several earlier studies (111,115,120,126) found a crude relationship between overweight and mortality but concluded that obesity had no impact on mortality since the significance disappeared when controlling for conditions such as hypertension, hyperlipidemia, and diabetes. However, these conditions are not confounders but intermediate risk factors that are—at least partly—caused by obesity and through which obesity exerts its damaging effects. Therefore, it is inappropriate to control for these conditions if the aim is to examine the overall effect of obesity on mortality.

Finally, various misclassification biases may be causes for a reduced internal validity of population studies. These biases are related both to the heterogeneity of the obesity syndrome and to surrogate measures of obesity. If only certain subgroups of obese individuals are at risk, then this subgroup's risk may well be diluted below the level of statistical detection when the risk of obesity in general is considered. Patients with a preponderance of abdominal adipose tissue constitute one important subgroup (see below). Body mass index (BMI, kg/m^2) and the waist/hip circumference ratio, which are surrogate measures of obesity and adipose tissue distribution, respectively, also have considerable limitations (see Definitions and Methods). The danger with surrogate measures of obesity is illustrated by the study of men born in 1913 in which BMI was not related to total plus nonfatal myocardial infarction (122), while BF calculated from total body potassium was a significant predictor of this combined endpoint (146).

In summary so far, there are at least five reasons to question the internal validity of studies that fail to demonstrate a relationship between obesity and mortality. With rare exceptions, negative population studies are

TABLE 3. Mortality ratios in subjects with initial underweight and overweight as a function of time

	Mortality ratios by duration of policy years			
	1–5	6–10	11–15	16–22
Men 15–69 years				
≥25% underweight	1.27	1.19	1.14	1.05
15–25% overweight	1.06	1.14	1.23	1.31
Women 15–69 years				
≥25% underweight	1.67	1.28	1.34	0.90
15–25% overweight	1.06	1.03	1.13	1.12

Adapted from The Build Study, 1979, ref. 3, with permission.

small, and most of them suffer from several of the methodological limitations discussed above. The lack of relationship between BMI and mortality may thus reflect serious problems with the internal validity of negative studies, making extrapolations to the general population meaningless.

Positive Population Studies

About 60% of all employee, community, and random population studies have found a relationship between overweight and mortality. These investigations, clustered among large and long-term studies, can be identified in Fig. 6. In this section three of the most important (4,129,144) and four of the most recently studied (139,141–143) will be discussed.

In 1979, Lew and Garfinkel (144) reported on obesity in the American Cancer Society Study, which followed approximately 340,000 men and 420,000 women for 13 years, on the average. These subjects, who were 38 to 89 years old at entry, were drawn from all segments of the population although individuals who were nonwhite, of low socioeconomic class, or institutionalized were somewhat underrepresented. One important finding in the American Cancer Society Study was that the relationship of relative weight to mortality was very similar to those observed in the Build Study and in the Build and Blood Pressure Study (2,3). Given that the association between obesity and atherosclerosis has been questioned (107), it is of special interest to note that the mortality rates for coronary and cerebrovascular diseases were increased in the overweight (Fig. 7). There was a 25-fold increase in diabetes mortality among obese young women while the cancer mortality for all sites taken together was only moderately increased in the obese. However, the mortality ratios were more markedly increased for cancers of the colon (mortality ratio 1.7) and prostate (1.3) in obese men, and for cancers in gall bladder (3.6), breast (1.5), cervix (2.4), endometrium (5.4), uterus unspecified (4.7), and ovary (1.6) in obese women.

In the Framingham study (129), obesity was related to mortality and morbidity even after controlling for diabetes, hypertension, and lipids. Judged traditionally, obesity was thus an "independent" risk factor, but in fact, the residual explained variance due to obesity has two potential explanations. One possibility is imperfect measurements and thus incomplete control for the traditional risk factors used in the Framingham study. The other and more constructive explanation is that obesity exerts damaging effects via other mechanisms than those controlled for. Postulated candidates for such mechanisms are increased cardiac work load (149), altered fibrinogen levels and fibrinolytic activity (150–152), hyperinsulinemia (110,145,153, 154) and complex metabolic and endocrine aberrations associated with visceral fat accumulation (for review, see refs. 56,58).

One study is available that is not dependent on extrapolations since a whole country was examined. "The Norwegian Experience" consisted of a compulsory x-ray examination for all citizens 15 years or older (4). Baseline examinations were performed between 1967 and 1975. The original aim was to detect tuberculosis, but weight and height were also registered. All counties in Norway were examined, but two counties (covering 17% of the Norwegian population) could not be used for technical reasons. The attendance rate was 85%. Approximately 816,000 men and 902,000 women were followed for an average of 10 years and during this time almost 177,000 deaths occurred. A quadratic relationship between BMI and total mortality was observed in both sexes. As compared with the risk at BMI 23–25, the mortality was doubled in 40–50-year-old men with a BMI = 34 kg/m^2 and in women of the same age with a BMI = 38 kg/m^2. The mortalities in coronary heart disease and diabetes were similar to those reported in the American Cancer Society Study (144, cf. Fig. 7).

Four recent studies should be mentioned (139,141–143). Hoffmans reported on a U-shaped relationship between mortality and BMI in 78,612 Dutch men going through a

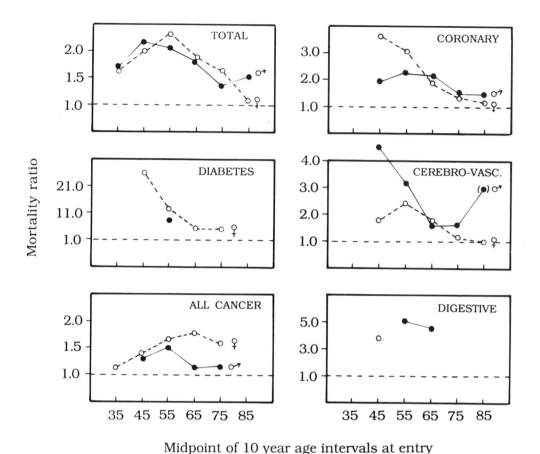

FIG. 7. Mortality ratios by cause and age for "relative weight ≥ 140"/"relative weight 90–109." Adapted from the American Cancer Society Study ref. 146 and Reproduced from Sjöström, ref. 148, with permission.

compulsory military examination at 18 years of age and then followed for 32 years (141). In this large sample, 20 years of follow-up were required before the relationship was detected. This was probably related to the low age at entry and to the fact that smoking was not controlled for. The risk ratio of obese men (BMI ≥ 26/BMI 19–19.9) was 1.95. Rissanen has observed the U-shaped relationship in another study of 22,995 males followed for 12 years (139). These men, who were 25 years and above at entry, constituted a strict random sample from all parts of Finland and from all segments of the society. Smoking and early mortality were controlled for and no inappropriate control for intermediate risk factors distorted the conclusions. The rel-

ative risk in obese men (BMI ≥ 34/BMI 22–24.9) was 1.5 (139). Manson et al. (142) have reported on 116,000 nurses from the United States who were followed for 8 years. The end point in this study was myocardial infarction plus fatal coronary heart disease combined. A linear positive relationship was observed between BMI and this endpoint. The relative risk among obese women (BMI ≥ 29/BMI < 21) was 2.5 without adjustment for smoking and 3.5 after adjustment (142). Finally, the NORA project (Nordic Risk Factor Assessment)—which is a pooling project covering 64,000 men followed for 8.4 years in The North Karelia Project, The Tromsø Heart Study, The National Screening Service in Norway, The Glostrup Study, and The Primary Prevention Study in Göteborg—found a quadratic association between BMI and total mortality and a positive linear relationship between BMI and coronary heart disease death (143). These and other studies thus indicate that the relationship between BMI and total mortality is quadratic, particularly if smoking has not been taken into account, while the association between BMI and incident cardiovascular disease and death is positive and more linear.

Among all positive studies in Fig. 6, it is certainly possible to identify some that are limited by one or several of the five shortcomings discussed above in relation to negative population studies. However, in the case of studies finding an overweight–mortality association, one can argue that this relationship was found—not due to—but in spite of shortcomings in study design. Without these shortcomings the relationship might have been even stronger. Thus validity problems of the type discussed under previous headings should normally not prevent extrapolations from positive population studies to the general population. This fact together with results from the important studies cited above (129,139,141–144) make it possible to conclude that overweight in fact has an impact on mortality in the general population. The total mortality is at least twice as high as normal in subjects with severe obesity while the mortality in specific diseases may well be 2 to 25 times higher than normal depending on disease, sex, and age.

Mortality among Extremely Obese Subjects

Studies of extremely obese subjects followed by specialized weight-control units are interesting but more difficult to evaluate with respect to generalizability. Drenick has provided data on 200 severely obese men from the United States (average weight 143.5 kg) who were admitted to a weight-control program and followed for an average period of 7.5 years (155). The age range was 23 to 70 years, with a mean of 42.7 years. In obese men aged 25 to 34, the mortality was 12 times higher than expected. With increasing age the excess mortality decreased, but at the age 65 to 74, the mortality was still twice as high as expected in this particular group of obese males.

Borelli et al. (156) have published similar observations on 264 obese (BMI ≥ 35 kg/m^2) subjects (69% women) from southern Italy who were followed for 7 years. The observed/expected mortality rate was 6.9 in women and 4.3 in men 25 to 54 years old. In 55- to 72-year-old subjects, the corresponding ratios were 3.5 and 1.6, respectively (156).

The exceedingly high relative mortality in young, severely obese subjects reported by Drenick et al. (155) and Borrelli et al. (156) seems not to be in accordance with available population data. In the American Cancer Society Study the relative mortality of obese subjects 30 to 39 years old was lower than in the age interval 40 to 59 years (Fig. 3). In the Norwegian experience 25- to 34-year-old men and women with BMI > 31 kg/m^2 had a mortality 2 times higher than subjects of average weight (4). In the Hoffmans et al. study (141) the risk ratio of obese young men (BMI ≥ 26/BMI 19–19.9) was 1.95. In a similar study, Sørensen and Sonne-Holm (147) have traced all subjects with BMI ≥ 31 kg/m^2 among 365,000 18- to 20-year-old men going through compulsory military enrollment examinations in Denmark. There were 1,320 such obese men. Over 7.3 years, 19 deaths occurred, which was 1.6 of the expected rate (147). Similarly, preliminary mortality data (148) in the intervention study Swedish Obese Subjects (116) do not support an exceedingly high mortality in young, severely obese subjects.

These comparisons indicate that the exceedingly high relative mortality among young, obese subjects observed in Drenick et al.'s (155) and Borrelli's et al.'s (156) studies may at least partly be due to selection mechanisms. On the other hand Drenick et al.'s as well as Borrelli et al.'s subjects were heavier than other young, obese groups available for comparison. The possibility can thus not be excluded that the relative mortality of young, severely obese subjects is even higher than in middle-aged severely obese subjects.

Weight Changes and Mortality

Weight gain should be associated with increased mortality since the obese state is necessarily preceded by weight increase. This simple conclusion has been elegantly quantified by Manson et al. (142) in the study of 115,886 nurses mentioned above. Subjects who had changed weight less than ±3 kg since the age of 18 served as a standard, with the relative risk of 1.0 for nonfatal myocardial infarction plus fatal coronary heart disease (combined). A weight increase of 3 to 4.9 kg resulted in a risk reduction to 0.6 and an increase of 5 to 9.9 kg in an unchanged relative risk of 1.0 (when adjusting for age and initial BMI). This is in line with Rissanen et al.'s (139) and Andres et al.'s (157) observations that the BMI associated with minimum mortality increases with age. However, weight increases of 10 to 19.9 kg and 20 to 34.9 kg from the age of 18 resulted in relative risks of 1.7 and 2.5, respectively (142). A weight increase of more than 20 kg in the preceding 4 years also resulted in a doubling of the risk (142).

Unfortunately, the number of women in Manson et al.'s (142) study with sustained weight loss was insufficient to assess the influence of weight reduction on the risk of coronary events. As a matter of fact, controlled studies with respect to this issue are lacking. Some indicative information is available, however. Marks (158) has analyzed individuals who had initially received substandard insurance due to overweight but who subsequently were issued other policies at a lower body weight. In contrast to other obese policy holders, the mortality of the weight-reduced subjects approached the standard risk (158). Similar information is also available in the Build study (3). At the Fourth International Symposium on Obesity Surgery in London in 1989, Edward Mason (159) compared the mortality in 787 vertical banded gastroplasty (VBG) patients with the mortality in Drenick et al.'s (155) conventionally treated subjects discussed above. Although it is not known if Mason's and Drenick et al.'s patients were comparable at baseline, it was interesting and encouraging to note that the annual mortality in the VBG cases (159) was one-fifth of that among Drenick's et al.'s (155) patients. The fact that the representativeness of Drenick's material can be questioned (see above) illustrates the need for prospective controlled intervention studies of obesity. Hopefully, the Swedish Obese Subjects (SOS) Study (116) and other intervention studies that may be started will elucidate questions related to risk reversibility in postobese subjects.

Morbidity and Overweight

Overweight is associated with an increased prevalence of cardiovascular risk factors (160) such as hypertension (161–163), blood lipid disturbances (162–164) and diabetes mellitus (162,163). Although controlled data on a decreasing mortality after weight reduction are lacking (see above), it is well known that obesity-related risk factors are reduced by weight reduction (165–169). From risk factor changes induced by spontaneous weight reductions in the Framingham study, it was estimated that a 10% reduction in body weight would correspond to a 20% reduction in the risk of developing coronary artery disease (165).

In contrast to prevalence and risk factor studies, considerable inconsistencies have been reported for the relationship of overweight to the incidence of cardiovascular disease (for review, see refs. 106, 107). However, as in the case of mortality studies (Fig. 6), long-term (129,130) and large (140,142) studies have usually been able to demonstrate a relationship between overweight and cardiovascular morbidity. As discussed in Definitions and Methods above, misclassifications and surrogate variables for obesity may explain why some smaller short term studies do find a relationship between overweight and

TABLE 4. *Description of the first 1,006 patients examined in the SOS project*

	Males*	Females*
No.	450	556
Age (years)	48 ± 6	48 ± 6
BMI (kg/m²)	37.6 ± 4.0	41.0 ± 4.3
Weight (kg)	119.3 ± 14.9	110.7 ± 13.6
Estimated LBM (kg)	74 ± 6	46 ± 4
Estimated total AT (kg)	45 ± 9	65 ± 11
Estimated subcut AT (kg)	37 ± 8	60 ± 10
Estimated visceral AT (kg)	8.6 ± 2.6	5.0 ± 1.2

Adapted from Sjöström et al., ref. 116, with permission.

* Age not significant; other factors $p < 0.0001$ between sexes.

AT, adipose tissue; BMI, body mass index; LBM, lean body mass.

cardiovascular morbidity while other such investigations fail to detect an association.

Overweight is also associated with increased morbidity from certain forms of cancer (170). Furthermore, serious consequences of overweight have been documented with respect to cardiac dysfunction, pulmonary problems, digestive diseases, endocrine disorders, and obstetric, orthopedic, and dermal difficulties, and with respect to social and psychological dysfunctions (171–173). In the SOS project prevalence ratios (obese/random subjects) ranged from 1.2 to 105 depending on sex, age, and risk factor, symptom, or disease under consideration (116). These comparisons were based on 450 obese men and 556 obese women (Table 4) as well as ongoing prospective population studies of men and women in Göteborg (122,124).

ADIPOSE TISSUE DISTRIBUTION AND RISK

As mentioned above, a high subgroup risk may be diluted below the level of statistical detection if the risk of obesity in general is considered. As early as 40 years ago, Jean Vague (174,175) focused on one such subgroup—upper body obesity—by comparing

the AT thickness of arms and thighs. Recently, Vague has summed up his experiences in this field (176). Some 10 years ago we (102,124) as well as Kissebah and co-workers (177) found that a preponderance of abdominal fat is associated with a number of metabolic complications. Subsequently, these original findings have been confirmed in a large number of cross-sectional (7,48,49, 53,56,58,178–184) and longitudinal (122, 124,185–191) studies. Thus it is now clear that a preponderance of abdominal AT is associated with an increased prevalence of metabolic disturbances and with an increased incidence of cardiovascular morbidity and mortality.

The mechanisms behind these associations (56,58,60–65,102,122,124,150–152,177–184,192–226,245) as well as the pathogenesis of visceral fat accumulation (179,184,192–194,217,223–228,233–244) have been elucidated to some extent, although much research remains to be done. Among several possibilities, a prevailing explanation for the relationship between risk and an increased visceral AT depot is that the resulting increase in portal free fatty acid (FFA) concentration (192–194) causes elevated hepatic gluconeogenesis (195–202) and very low-density lipoprotein (VLDL) secretion (203–204) as well as a decreased hepatic insulin clearance (178–181,205–208). The resulting hyperinsulinemia and insulin resistance, together with increased gluconeogenesis as well as an FFA-induced reduction of peripheral glucose uptake (209), will cause a reduced glucose tolerance and ultimately non-insulin-dependent diabetes. Although the clinical impact is unclear, elevated glucose levels may be related to reduced removal of low-density lipoprotein (LDL) and VLDL due to glucosylation and thus to hypercholesterolemia, hypertriglyceridemia, and low high-density lipoprotein (HDL) cholesterol levels (210). A reduced fibrinolytic activity in obesity was observed by us 20 years ago (150), and more recently, hyperinsulinemia has been shown to be positively related to the concentration of plasminogen activator inhibitor (PAI-1)

(152,211,212). High VLDL concentrations may also contribute to increased PAI-1 activity (213), a state known to be associated with myocardial infarction (214) and reinfarction in young subjects (215). Finally, hyperinsulinemia or insulin resistance may have a permissive role for the development of hypertension (see below) and high insulin levels may even promote the development of hypertension directly by increasing sodium reabsorption (216) and sympathetic tone (217). Interestingly, hypertension can be ameliorated by improving insulin sensitivity pharmacologically at a postreceptor level without changing the degree of obesity (218). Thus it seems at least hypothetically possible to link diabetes, hypertriglyceridemia, hypercholesterolemia (?), low HDL levels (?), reduced fibrinolysis, and hypertension to elevated portal FFA concentrations due to an increased visceral AT depot.

It must be pointed out, however, that carefully performed studies exist that have found weak or nonexisting relations between fat patterning and risk. This seems particularly to be the case in young subjects and with respect to hypertension (229,230). It should also be noted that the association between hypertension and hyperinsulinemia discussed above does not seem to be unconditional. Thus no relationship was found in subjects with type 2 diabetes (231), and using data on obese subjects from the SOS project (116), Smith et al. (232) found no differences in fasting insulin levels between hypertensive and nonhypertensive subjects matched for sex, age, body fat, and waist/hip ratio (see Table 2 in ref. 232). Although insulin is of direct pathogenetic importance in several situations (see above) its role may thus be limited to a more permissive (?) effect among susceptible individuals in other clinical settings. The nature of such a hypothetical susceptibility is presently unknown, although genetic backgrounds seem likely.

At least three hypotheses have been suggested to explain the differences in regional fat distribution (179,184,192–194,217,223–228,233–244). Thus, different neuroendocrine responses to stress (183,184,223–227,240), different effects of gonadal and adrenal steroids on metabolism in various AT depots (184,233–235,237–239) as well as genetic variations in tissue sensitivity (225,227,236) have been proposed. All these mechanisms may contribute to the variation in regional fat distribution. One notable sex difference seems to be that visceral adiposity is associated with a hyperandrogenic state in women (179,228) but with a hypoandrogenic state in men (184). In men, abdominal obesity as well as metabolic aberrations are improved by supplementation with androgenic steroids (63). Visceral AT is also decreased by growth hormone in subjects with pituitary insufficiency (60), while visceral AT increases after treatment of acromegaly (61). Cushing's syndrome is associated with abdominal obesity, and after treatment the visceral AT volume is drastically reduced (62). Thus, cortisol promotes visceral fat accumulation while growth hormone and testosterone (in men) have the opposite effect.

Most studies cited above have been performed with normal weight to moderately obese subjects but not exclusively with severely obese subjects. Using the CT-calibrated anthropometry described in Definitions and Methods above, we have demonstrated that adipose tissue distribution is also of great importance for metabolic aberrations in the body weight range 100 to 200 kg. For this purpose, we have used the first 1,006 subjects examined in the SOS project (Table 4) (56,58,116). The mean age was 48 in both sexes. The men were heavier than the women but had a lower BMI since they were taller. The estimated LBM was greater in men than in women, while total and subcutaneous AT were greater in women. Nevertheless, the estimated visceral AT was greater in men than in women. When examining the regression coefficients between visceral and total AT on the one hand (y) and body weight on the other (x), the visceral slope was steeper in men than in women, while the subcutaneous regression coefficient was steepest in women (not shown). In both sexes the subcutaneous slope was steeper than the visceral slope, so in relative terms the visceral AT was decreasing with increasing body weight (not shown).

Table 5 illustrates that with CT-calibrated anthropometric estimates of body composition it is possible to separate compartments related to risk factors from compartments that are not (56,58). As in most studies, both age and body weight were significantly related to systolic blood pressure. When body weight was divided into its two main compartments, we can see that the estimated total AT was related to systolic blood pressure while LBM was not. If total AT is further divided into its subcutaneous and visceral components, it appears that the estimated visceral AT was a strong predictor of systolic blood pressure while subcutaneous AT just reached significance. Age remained significant and LBM remained nonsignificant (Table 5, regression no. 3).

In both obese men and obese women the estimated visceral AT volume was significantly related to insulin, glucose, triglycerides, systolic blood pressure, and ASAT when taking age, LBM, and subcutaneous AT volume into account (56,58,245) (not shown). In obese males, cholesterol, diastolic blood pressure, dyspnea after two staircases, "coronary" electrocardiogram (ECG), intermittent claudication, and sick pensions were also related to the visceral AT volume. In obese females HDL, uric acid, ALAT, and angina pectoris were associated with the visceral AT volume. In all cases, visceral AT was a stronger predictor than subcutaneous AT (56,58,245). In several cases subcutaneous AT was not related to risk. LBM was never positively related to a risk but was negatively related to insulin in women (56,58).

Our CT-calibrated anthropometric estimates of body composition are defined in terms of compartments that are expressed in kilograms (see Definitions and Methods above). These features may have advantages over poorly defined circumference ratios, which are influenced by several body compartments in a more undefined way. This is also illustrated by Table 5. BMI gave the same information as body weight, but the waist over hip ratio was not related to systolic blood pressure in spite of the strong relationship between blood pressure and the CT-calibrated estimate of visceral AT. We have noticed that when visceral AT is the strongest predictor but subcutaneous AT still is of some importance, than the waist/hip ratio often fails to detect the importance of AT distribution, at least in this sample of very obese subjects. On the other hand, when visceral AT is the only significant body compartment predictor, then we usually obtain the same message from the waist/hip ratio as from the estimated visceral AT mass. This was the case for serum triglycerides (cf. Table 6). We may

TABLE 5. *t Ratios of indicated x variables versus systolic blood pressure (y)*[a]

	Regression no.			
	CT-calibrated			Conventional
x variable	1	2	3	4
Age	4.4	4.4	4.4	4.2
Weight	5.3			
LBM		−0.2	0.1	
Total AT		3.6		
Subcutaneous AT			2.0	
Visceral AT			3.6	
BMI				5.3
Waist/hip				0.1

Adapted from Sjöström et al., ref. 245, with permission.
[a] Multivariate regressions of 450 obese males shown in Table 4.
AT, adipose tissue; BMI, body mass index; LBM, lean body mass.

thus conclude that as compared with the waist/hip ratio, the CT-calibrated estimates of body compartments are more sensitive in detecting the metabolic importance of visceral AT.

The superiority of the estimated visceral AT mass over the waist/hip ratio is illustrated in another way in Table 6. Here the relationships between serum triglycerides and body composition were analyzed in the pooled obese sample of men and women. Neither age nor BMI was related to triglycerides (TG). However, there was a strong effect of gender (Table 6). A negative t ratio indicates lower triglycerides in women, and this effect disappeared when the estimated visceral AT was added to the equation but not when the waist/hip ratio was added. This finding indicates that the sex difference with respect to TG may at least partly be mediated via differences in visceral AT between men and women. Independently of risk factor, the importance of sex was always reduced to some extent when adding visceral AT or waist/hip (56,58). However, visceral AT had a much stronger effect in this respect. While the importance of gender completely disappeared in seven of ten cases when visceral AT was added to the equation, this occurred in only two of ten cases when waist/hip was added ($p < 0.025$, χ^2 test) (56,58). In accordance with these data, we also observed that the im-

portance of gender with respect to incident myocardial infarction disappeared when taking waist/hip into account (191). These results (56,58,191,245) thus indicate that the difference between sexes with respect to several risk factors and diseases may at least partly be mediated via the difference in visceral AT. This is easier to detect with CT-calibrated anthropometry than with conventional ratios such as waist over hip.

CONCLUSIONS

1. The morbidity and mortality of severely obese persons are dramatically increased compared to randomly selected subjects with a BMI of 20 to 25 kg/m^2.
2. Studies that have not been able to confirm this finding have been either small and/or short-term, have failed to control for smoking or early mortality, have controlled for intermediate risk factors in an inappropriate way, or have limited internal validity due to misclassification biases.
3. Traditional body composition techniques usually permit the determination of only two compartments. Body fat is obtained indirectly as the difference between body weight and fat-free mass. With a new multiscan CT method it is possible to measure directly more than 20 different organ vol-

TABLE 6. *Serum triglycerides (y) regressed versus indicated x variables in the 1,006 obese men and women shown in Table 4 (multivariate regressions and t ratios)*

| | Regression no. | | | | |
| | Conventional | | CT-calibrated | | |
x variable	1	2	3	4	5
Sex	−7.4	−3.4	−7.3	−3.2	−1.2
Age	0.2	0.2	0.1	0.0	−0.5
BMI	0.1	0.2			
Waist/hip		4.9			
Weight			−0.1		
LBM				−1.3	−1.7
Total AT				1.1	
Subcutaneous AT					−1.3
Visceral AT					5.5

Adapted from Sjöström et al., ref. 245, with permission.
AT, adipose tissue; BMI, body mass index; LBM, lean body mass.

umes with a high accuracy and reproducibility. CT-calibrated, sex-specific anthropometric equations permit estimations of lean body mass, subcutaneous adipose tissue, and visceral adipose tissue from weight, height, and sagittal trunk diameter.

4. Abdominal obesity is associated with metabolic aberrations, morbidity, and mortality in both genders. Sex differences with respect to these risks are at least partly mediated via differences in visceral adipose tissue. These associations and conditions are more easily detected with CT-calibrated anthropometric estimates of body composition than with traditional indices of overweight and adipose tissue distribution. Therefore it seems warranted to move in a direction away from BMI, waist/hip, and other ratios toward estimates (or determinations) of defined body compartments.

5. Population studies demonstrating relationships between abdominal obesity and disease have used simple indices of adipose tissue distribution. Prospective population studies with detailed baseline information on body composition including the visceral AT volume are needed in order to achieve a deeper insight in the relationships between body composition, metabolic aberrations, morbidity, and mortality.

6. A preponderance of visceral AT may be related to an even higher risk in lean than in obese individuals. Therefore detailed studies are needed on absolute and relative changes in the visceral AT volume during weight reduction. It is not sufficient to examine these questions with AT area determinations in a single or limited number of scans, since AT areas can not be expressed in percent of total AT volume. In a stricter sense, area techniques do not permit studies of (changes in) fat patterning.

7. Controlled data on postobese morbidity and mortality are entirely lacking. There-fore intervention studies of obesity are needed.

ACKNOWLEDGMENTS

Several coworkers were involved in the studies reported in this chapter. CT measurements were performed by Henry Kvist, Ulla Grangård, Lars Lönn, and Lars Jönsson at the Department of Clinical Radiology, and by Badrul Chowdhury and Per Mårin at the Department of Medicine, Sahlgrenska Hospital, Göteborg. The SOS material was collected by the staffs at 140 primary medical care centers and 10 surgical departments in Sweden (a complete list of participants provided on request) in cooperation with Lars Backman, Department of Surgery, Danderyd's Hospital, Stockholm; Bo Larsson, Marianne Sullivan, Per Hallgren, and Lauren Lissner, Department of Medicine, Lars Olbe, Department of Surgery, and Sven Lindstedt, Department of Clinical Chemistry, Sahlgrenska Hospital, Göteborg; Calle Bengtsson, Department of Primary Health Care, Göteborg; Ingmar Näslund, Department of Surgery, Örebro Hospital; Sven Dahlgren, Department of Surgery, Umeå Hospital; Egon Jonsson, Institute of Medicine, Karolinska Hospital, Stockholm; Hans Wedel, Nordic School of Public Health, Göteborg, all in Sweden, and Claude Bouchard, Physical Activity Sciences Laboratory, Laval University, Quebec, Canada. The studies are supported by grants from the Swedish Medical Research Council (B91-19M-27852-05A, B91-05239-14B, B91-19M-08338-04A), Hoffmann-La Roche, and Volvo Research Foundation.

REFERENCES

1. Association of Life Insurance Medical Directors and Actuarial Society of America. *Medico-actuarial mortality investigation.* New York: Association of Life Insurance Medical Directors and Actuarial Society of America, 1913.
2. Society of Actuaries. *Build and blood pressure study 1959.* New York: Peter F. Mallon Inc., 1959.

3. Society of Actuaries and Association of Life Insurance Medical Directors of America. *Build study 1979.* Recording and Statistical Corp., 1980.

4. Waaler HT. Height, weight and mortality: the Norwegian experience. *Acta Med Scand* 1984;Suppl 679:1–56.

5. Forbes GB, Gallup J, Hursh JB. Estimation of total body fat from potassium-40 content. *Science* 1961;133:101–2.

6. Sköldborn H, Arvidsson B, Andersson M. A new whole-body monitoring laboratory. *Acta Radiol Diagn* 1972;Suppl 233:313.

7. Kvist H, Sjöström L, Chowdhury B, et al. Body fat and adipose tissue determinations by computed tomography and by measurements of total body potassium. In: Yasumura et al., ed. *Advances in in vivo body composition studies.* New York: Plenum Press, 1990;197–218.

8. Sheng HP, Huggins RA. A review of body composition studies with emphasis on total body water and fat. *Am J Clin Nutr* 1979;32:630–47.

9. Widdowson EM. Chemical analysis of the body. In: J. Brozek, ed. *Human body composition: approaches and applications.* Oxford: Pergamon Press, 1965;31–47.

10. Boddy K, King PC, Hume R, Weyers E. The relation of total body potassium to height, weight and age in normal adults. *J Clin Pathol* 1972;25:512–7.

11. Womersley J, Durnin JVGA, Boddy K, Mahaffy M. Influence of muscular development, obesity and age on the fat free mass of adults. *J Appl Physiol* 1976;41:223–9.

12. Sjöström L, Kvist H, Cederblad Å, Tylén U. Determination of total adipose tissue and body fat in women by computed tomography, ^{40}K, and tritium. *Am J Physiol* 1986;250:E736–E745.

13. Kvist H, Chowdhury B, Sjöström L, Tylén U, Cederblad Å. Adipose tissue volume determination in males by computed tomography and ^{40}K. *Int J Obes* 1988;12:249–66.

14. Pace N, Rathbun EN. Studies on body composition. III. The body water and chemically combined nitrogen content in relation to fat content. *J Biol Chem* 1945;158:685–91.

15. Friis-Hansen B. Body water compartments in children: changes during growth and related changes in body composition. *Pediatrics* 1961;28:169–81.

16. Behnke AR, Feen BG, Welham WC. The specific gravity of healthy men: body weight/volume as an index of obesity. *JAMA* 1942;118:495–8.

17. Garrow JS, Stalley S, Diethelm R, Pittet P, Hesp R, Halliday D. A new method for measuring the body density of obese adults. *Br J Nutr* 1979;42:173–83.

18. Siri WE. Body composition from fluid spaces and density: analysis of methods. University of California Radiation Lab Rep. 3349. Donner Laboratory of Biophysics and Medical Physics, University of California, 1956.

19. Brozek J, Grande F, Andersson JT, Keys A. Densitometric analysis of body composition: revision of some quantitative assumptions. *Ann NY Acad Sci* 1963;110:113–40.

20. Bruce A, Andersson H, Arvidsson B, Isaksson B. Body composition. Prediction of normal body potassium, body water, and body fat in adults on the basis of body height, body weight and age. *Scand J Clin Lab Invest* 1980;40:461–73.

21. Sjöström L. Recent methods in the study of body composition. In: Tanner JM, ed. *Perspectives in the science of growth and development.* London: Smith-Gordon, 1989;353–66.

22. Quetelet LA. Anthropometric en mesure des différentes facultés de l'homme. Brussels: Muquardt, 1871;479.

23. Billewicz WZ, Kernsley WFF, Thomson AM. Indices of adiposity. *Br J Prev Soc Med* 1962;16:183–8.

24. Florey C Du V. The use and interpretation of ponderal index and other weight-height ratios in epidemiological studies. *J Chron Dis* 1970;23:93–103.

25. Keys AK, Fidanza F, Karvonen MJ, Kimura N, Taylor HL. Indices of relative weight and obesity. *J Chron Dis* 1972;25:329–43.

26. Womersley J, Durnin JVGA. A comparison of the skinfold method with extent of overweight and various weight-height relationships in the assessment of obesity. *Br J Nutr* 1977;38:271–84.

27. Knapik JJ, Burse RL, Vogel JA. Height, weight, per cent body fat and indices of adiposity for young men and women entering the US army. *Aviation Space Environ Med* 1983;54:223–31.

28. Sjöström L. New aspects of weight-for-height indices and adipose tissue distribution in relation to cardiovascular risk and total adipose tissue volume. In: Berry EM, Blondheim SH, Eliahou HE, Shafrir E, eds. *Recent advances in obesity research,* vol V. London: Libbey, 1987:66–76.

29. Steinkamp RC, Cohen NL, Gaffey WR, et al. Measures of body fat and related factors in normal adults. II. A simple clinical method to estimate body fat and lean body mass. *J Chron Dis* 1965;18:1279–91.

30. Matiegka J. The testing of physical efficiency. *Am J Phys Anthropol* 1922;5:223–30.

31. Durnin JVGA, Rahaman MM. The assessment of the amount of fat in the human body frame measurements of skinfold thickness. *Br J Nutr* 1967;21:681–9.

32. Durnin JVGA, Womersley J. Body fat assessed from total body density and its estimation from skinfold thicknesses: measurements on 481 men and women aged from 16 to 72 years. *Br J Nutr* 1974;32:77–97.

33. Garn SM. Roentgenogrammetric determinations of body composition. *Hum Biol* 1957;29:337–53.

34. Tanner JM. Radiographic studies of body composition in children and adults. In: Brozek J, ed. *Human body composition: approaches and applications.* Oxford: Pergamon Press, 1965;211–36.

35. Haymes EM, Lundegren HJ, Loomis JL, Buskirk ER. Validity of the ultrasonic technique as a method of measuring subcutaneous adipose tissue. *Ann Hum Biol* 1976;3:245–51.

36. Booth RAD, Goddard BA, Paton A. Measurements of fat thickness in man: a comparison of ultrasound, Harpenden calipers and electrical conductivity. *Br J Nutr* 1966;20:719–25.

37. Volz PA, Ostrove SM. Evaluation of a portable ultrasonoscope in assessing the body composition of college-age women. *Med Sci Sports Exercise* 1984;16:97–102.

38. Clarys JP, Martin AD, Drinkwater DT. Gross tissue weights in the human body by cadaver dissection. *Hum Biol* 1984;56:459–73.
39. Forbes RM, Cooper AR, Mitchell HH. The composition of the adult human body as determined by chemical analysis. *J Biol Chem* 1953;203:359–66.
40. Forbes RM, Mitchell HH, Cooper AR. Further studies on the gross composition and mineral elements of the adult human body. *J Biol Chem* 1956;223:969–75.
41. Mitchell HH, Hamilton TS, Steggerda FR, Bean HW. The chemical composition of the adult human body and its bearing on the biochemistry growth. *J Biol Chem* 1945;158:625–37.
42. Moore FD, Lister J, Boyden CM, Ball MR, Sullivan N, Dagher FJ. The skeleton as a feature of body composition. *Hum Biol* 1968;40:135–88.
43. Widdowson EM, McCance RA, Spray CM. The chemical composition of the human body. *Clin Sci* 1951;10:113–25.
44. Borkan GA, Gerzof SG, Robbins AH, Hults DE, Silbert CK, Silbert JE. Assessment of abdominal fat content by computed tomography. *Am J Clin Nutr* 1982;36:172–7.
45. Dixon AK. Abdominal fat assessed by computed tomography: sex difference in distribution. *Clin Radiol* 1983;34:189–91.
46. Enzi G, Gasparo M, Biondetti PR, Fiore D, Semisa M, Zurlo F. Subcutaneous and visceral fat distribution according to sex, age and overweight evaluated by computed tomography. *Am J Clin Nutr* 1986;44:739–46.
47. Shuman WP, Newell Morris LL, Leonetti DL, et al. Abnormal body fat distribution detected by computed tomography in diabetic men. *Invest Radiol* 1986;21:483–7.
48. Sparrow D, Borkan GA, Gerzof SG, Wisniewski C, Silbert CK. Relationship of fat distribution in glucose tolerance. Results of computed tomography in male participants of normative aging study. *Diabetes* 1986;35:411–5.
49. Fujioka S, Matsuzawa Y, Tokunaga K, Tarui S. Contribution of intra-abdominal fat accumulation to the impairment of glucose and lipid metabolism in human obesity. *Metabolism* 1987;36:54–9.
50. Seidell JC, Oosterlee A, Thijssen MAO, et al. Assessment of intraabdominal and subcutaneous abdominal fat: relation between anthropometry and computed tomography. *Am J Clin Nutr* 1987;45:7–13.
51. Baumgartner RN, Heymsfield SB, Roche AF, et al. Abdominal composition quantified by computed tomography. *Am J Clin Nutr* 1988;48:936–45.
52. Seidell JC, Oosterlee A, Deurenberg P, et al. Abdominal fat depots measured with computed tomography: effects of degree of obesity, sex and age. *Eur J Clin Nutr* 1988;42:805–15.
53. Despres JP, Nadeau A, Tremblay A, et al. Role of deep abdominal fat in the association between regional adipose tissue distribution and glucose tolerance in obese women. *Diabetes* 1989;38:304–9.
54. Kvist H, Sjöström L, Tylén U. Adipose tissue volume determinations in women by computed tomography: technical considerations. *Int J Obes* 1986;10:53–67.
55. Kvist H, Chowdhury B, Grangård U, Tylén U, Sjöström L. Total and visceral adipose tissue volumes derived from measurements with computed tomography in adult men and women: predictive equations. *Am J Clin Nutr* 1988;48:1351–61.
56. Sjöström L. Methods for measurement of the visceral adipose tissue volume and relationships between visceral fat and disease in 1000 severely obese subjects. In: Oomura Y, Tarui S, Shimazu T, Inoue S, eds. *Progress in obesity research.* London: John Libbey, 1990;323–34.
57. Chowdhury B, Kvist H, Sjöström L. Multicompartment examinations of the human body with computed tomography. *Int J Obes* 1990;14[Suppl 2] (abst).
58. Sjöström L. A computer-tomography based multi-compartment body composition technique and anthropometric predictions of lean body mass, total and subcutaneous adipose tissue. *Int J Obes* 1991;15:19–30.
59. Sjöström L, Chowdhury B, Alpsten M, Kostanty J, Kvist H, Löfgren R. A multicompartment body composition technique based on computed tomography [submitted].
60. Bengtsson B-Å, Lönn L, Edén S, et al. Effects of treatment with recombinant human growth hormone in adults with growth hormone deficiency. *J Clin Endocr Metab* 1992 (in press).
61. Brummer R-J, Lönn L, Grangård U, et al. Adipose tissue and muscle volume determination by computed tomography before and one year after adenectomy in patients with acromegaly. *Eur J Clin Invest* (in press).
62. Lönn L, Kvist H, Ernest I, Sjöström L. Changed adipose tissue distribution after treatment of Cushing's syndrome In: Ailhaud G, et al., eds. *Obesity in Europe 91.* London: John Libbey, 1992;393–396.
63. Mårin P, Holmäng S, Jönsson L, et al. The effects of testosterone treatment on body composition and metabolism in middle-aged, obese men. *Int J Obes* (in press).
64. Chowdhury B, Kvist H, Sjöström L, Andersson B, Björntorp P. Multiscan CT-determined changes in adipose tissue distribution during a small weight reduction of obese males [submitted].
65. Kvist H, Hallgren P, Jönsson L, et al. Distribution of adipose tissue and muscle mass in alcoholic men [submitted].
66. Sjöström L, Björntorp P, Vrana J. Microscopic fat cell size measurements on frozen-cut adipose tissue in comparison with automatic determinations of osmium-fixed fat cells. *J Lipid Res* 1971;12:521–30.
67. Smith U, Sjöström L, Björntorp P. Comparison between two methods to determine human adipose cell size. *J Lipid Res* 1972;13:822–4.
68. Hirsch J, Gallian E. Methods for the determination of adipose cell size in man and animals. *J Lipid Res* 1968;9:110–9.
69. Stern MP, Conrad F. An automated, direct method for measuring adipocyte cell size. *Clin Chim Acta* 1975;65:29–37.
70. Sjöström L. The contribution of fat cells to the determination of body weight. *Psychiatr Clin North Am* 1978;1:493–521.
71. Sjöström L. Fat cells and body weight. In: Stunkard

AJ, ed. *Obesity.* Philadelphia: WB Saunders, 1980;72–100.

72. Näslund I, Hallgren P, Sjöström L. Fat cell weight and number before and after gastric surgery for morbid obesity in women. *Int J Obes* 1988; 12:191–7.
73. Björntorp P, Sjöström L. Number and size of adipose tissue fat cells in relation to metabolism in human obesity. *Metabolism* 1971;20:703–13.
74. Sjöström L, Björntorp P. Body composition and adipose tissue cellularity in human obesity. *Acta Med Scand* 1974;195:201–11.
75. Häger A, Sjöström L, Arvidsson B, Björntorp P, Smith U. Body fat and adipose tissue cellularity in infants: a longitudinal study. *Metabolism* 1977;26:607–14.
76. Häger A, Sjöström L, Arvidsson B, Björntorp P, Smith U. Adipose tissue cellularity in obese school girls before and after dietary treatment. *Am J Clin Nutr* 1978;31:68–75.
77. Sjöström L, Smith U, Krotkiewski M, Björntorp P. Cellularity in different regions of adipose tissue in young men and women. *Metabolism* 1972; 21:1143–53.
78. Johnson PR, Stern JS, Greenwood MRC, et al. Effect of early nutrition on adipose cellularity and pancreatic insulin release in the Zucker rat. *J Nutr* 1973;103:738–43.
79. Knittle JL, Hirsch J. Effect of early nutrition on the development of rat epididymal fat pads: cellularity and metabolism. *J Clin Invest* 1968;47:2091–8.
80. Miller DS, Wise A. Maintenance requirement and adipocyte count of rats from large and small litters, at the same weight. *Proc Nutr Soc* 1975;34:105A.
81. Oscai LB, Spirakis CN, Wolff CA, Beck RJ. Effects of exercise and of food restriction on adipose tissue cellularity. *J Lipid Res* 1972;13:588–92.
82. Berglund G, Björntorp P, Sjöström L, Smith U. The effects of early malnutrition in men on body composition and adipose tissue cellularity at adult age. *Acta Med Scand* 1974;195:213–6.
83. Björntorp P, Enzi G, Karlsson K, Krotkiewski M, Sjöström L, Smith U. The effect of maternal diabetes on adipose tissue cellularity in man and rat. *Diabetologia* 1974;10:205–9.
84. Salans LB, Horton ES, Sims EAH. Experimental obesity in man: cellular character of the adipose tissue. *J Clin Invest* 1971;50:1005–11.
85. Björntorp P, Carlgren G, Isaksson B, Krotkiewski M, Larsson B, Sjöström L. Effect of an energy-reduced dietary regimen in relation to adipose tissue cellularity in obese women. *Am J Clin Nutr* 1975;28:445–52.
86. Bray GA. Measurement of subcutaneous fat cells from obese patients. *Ann Intern Med* 1970;73: 565–9.
87. Hirsch J, Knittle JL. Cellularity of obese and non-obese human adipose tissue. *Fed Proc* 1970;29: 1516–21.
88. Sjöström L. Can the relapsing patient be identified? In: Björntorp P, Cairella M, Howard AN, eds. *Recent advances in obesity research.* London: John Libbey & Co. Ltd, 1980;85–93.
89. Sjöström L, William-Olsson T. Prospective studies

on adipose tissue development in man. *Int J Obes* 1981;6:597–604.
90. Ailhaud G, Amri E, Barcellini-Couget S, et al. Biological signals triggering adipose cell differentiation. In: Oomura Y, Tarui S, Inoue S, Shimazu T, eds. *Progress in obesity research 1990.* London: John Libbey & Co. Ltd, 1991;201–5.
91. Brook CGD, Lloyd JK, Wolf OH. Relation between age of onset of obesity and size and number of adipose cells. *Br Med J* 1972;2:25–7.
92. Hirsch J, Batchelor B. Adipose tissue cellularity in human obesity. *Clin Endocrinol Metab* 1976; 5:299–11.
93. Salans LB, Cushman SW, Weissman RE. Studies on human adipose tissue. Adipose cell size and number in non-obese and obese patients. *J Clin Invest* 1973;52:929–41.
94. Krotkiewski M, Sjöström L, Björntorp P, et al. Adipose tissue cellularity in relation to prognosis for weight reduction. *Int J Obes* 1977;1:395–416.
95. Leibel RL, Rosenbaum M, Edens NK, Hirsch J. In vitro vs in vivo measures of lipolysis and re-esterification in human adipose tissue. In: Oomura Y, Tarui S, Inoue S, Shimazu T, eds. *Progress in obesity research 1990,* London: John Libbey & Co. Ltd, 1991;237–43.
96. Hallgren P, Raddatz E, Bergh C-H, Kucera P, Sjöström L. Oxygen consumption in collagenase-liberated rat adipocytes in relation to cell size and age. *Metabolism* 1984;33:897–900.
97. Hallgren P, Sjöström L, Hedlund H, Lundell L, Olbe L. Influence of age, fat cell weight, and obesity on the O_2 consumption of human adipose tissue. *Am J Physiol* 1989;256:E467–E474.
98. Björntorp P, Bengtsson C, Blohmé G, et al. Adipose tissue fat cell size and number in relation to metabolism in randomly selected middle-aged men and women. *Metabolism* 1971;20:927–35.
99. Björntorp P, Berchtold P, Tibblin G. Insulin secretion in relation to adipose tissue in man. *Diabetes* 1971;20:65–70.
100. Björntorp P, Gustafsson A, Persson B. Adipose tissue fat cell size and number in relation to metabolism in endogenous hypertriglyceridemia. *Acta Med Scand* 1971;190:363–7.
101. Stern MP, Olefsky J, Farquhar JW, Reaven GM. Relationship between fasting plasma lipid levels and adipose tissue morphology. *Metab Clin Exp* 1973;22:1311–7.
102. Krotkiewski M, Björntorp P, Sjöström L, Smith U. Impact of obesity on metabolism in men and women. *J Clin Invest* 1983;72:1150–62.
103. Krotkiewski M, Sjöström L, Björntorp P, Smith U. Regional adipose tissue cellularity in relation to metabolism in young and middle-aged women. *Metabolism* 1975;24:703.
104. Lew EA. Some observations on mortality studies. *J Inst Actuaries* 1977;104:221–5.
105. Bray G. *The obese patient.* Philadelphia: WB Saunders, 1976.
106. Larsson B, Björntorp P, Tibblin G. The health consequences of moderate obesity. *Int J Obes* 1981;5:97–116.
107. Barrett-Connor EL. Obesity, atherosclerosis and

coronary artery disease. *Ann Intern Med* 1985; 103:1010–9.

108. Mattila K, Haavisto M, Rajala S. Body mass index and mortality in the elderly. *Br Med J* 1986;292:867–8.

109. Cole TJ, Gilson JC, Olsen H. Bronchitis, smoking and obesity in an English and a Danish town. *Bull Physiol Pathol Respir* 1974;10:657–79.

110. Pyörälä K. Relationship of glucose tolerance and plasma insulin to the incidence of coronary heart disease: results from two population studies in Finland. *Diabetes Care* 1979;2:131–41.

111. Chapman JM, Massey FJ. The interrelationship of serum cholesterol, hypertension, body weight and risk of coronary disease. Results of the first 10 years' follow-up in the Los Angeles Heart Study. *J Chron Dis* 1964;17:933–49.

112. Paul O, Lepper MH, Phelan WH, et al. A longitudinal study of coronary heart disease. *Circulation* 1963;28:20–31.

113. Tayback M, Kumanyika S, Chee E. Body weight as a risk factor in the elderly. *Arch Intern Med* 1990;150:1065–72.

114. Heyden S, Hames CG, Bartel A, et al. Body weight and cigarette smoking as risk factors. *Arch Intern Med* 1971;128:915–9.

115. Rosenman RH, Brand RJ, Jenkins CG, Friedman M, Strauss R, Wurm M. Coronary heart disease in the Western Collaborative Group Study. Final follow-up experience of 8.5 years. *JAMA* 1975;233:872–7.

116. Sjöström L, Larsson B, Backman L, et al. Swedish Obese Subjects, SOS—recruitment to an intervention study and a selected description of the obese state. *Int J Obesity* 1992;16:465–479.

117. Westlund K, Nicolaysen R. Ten-year mortality and morbidity related to serum cholesterol. *Scand J Clin Lab Invest* 1972;30[Suppl 127]:3–24.

118. Borhain NO, Hechter HH, Breslow L. Report of a ten-year follow up of the San Francisco longshore men. *J Chron Dis* 1963;16:1251–66.

119. Tuomilehto J, Salonen JT, Marti B, et al. Body weight and risk of myocardial infarction and death in the adult population of eastern Finland. *Br Med J* 1987;295:623–7.

120. Kozarevic D, Pirc B, Racic Z, et al. The Yugoslavia Cardiovascular Disease Study. II. Factors in the incidence of coronary heart disease. *Am J Epidemiol* 1976;104:133–40.

121. Cochrane AL, Moore F, Baker LA, Haley TIL. Mortality in two random samples of women aged 55–64 followed up for 20 years. *Br Med J* 1980;2:1131–3.

122. Larsson B, Svärdsudd K, Welin L, Wilhelmsson L, Björntorp P, Tibblin G. Abdominal adipose tissue distribution, obesity and risk of cardiovascular disease and death: 13 year follow up of participants in the study of men born in 1913. *Br Med J* 1984;288:1401–4.

123. Dyer AR, Stamler J, Berkson DM, et al. Relationship of relative weight and body mass index to 14 year mortality in the Chicago Peoples Gas Company Study. *J Chron Dis* 1975;28:109–23.

124. Lapidus L, Bengtsson C, Larsson B, Pennert K, Rybo E, Sjöström L. Distribution of adipose tissue and risk of cardiovascular disease and death: a 12 year follow up of participants in the population study of women in Gothenburg, Sweden. *Br Med J* 1984;289:1261–3.

125. Wienpahl J, Ragland DR, Sidney S. Body mass index and 15-year mortality in a cohort of black men and women. *J Clin Epidemiol* 1990;43:949–60.

126. Böttiger LE, Carlsson LA. Risk factors for ischemic vascular death for men in Stockholm Prospective Study. *Atherosclerosis* 1980;36:389–408.

127. Keys A. Longevity of man: relative weight and fatness in middle age. *Ann Med* 1989;21:163–8.

128. Vandenbroucke JP, Maurity BJ, de Bruin A, et al. Weight, smoking and mortality. *JAMA* 1984; 252:2859–60.

129. Hubert HB, Feinleib M, McNamara RM, et al. Obesity as an independent risk factor for cardiovascular disease: a 26-year follow up of participants in the Framingham Heart Study. *Circulation* 1983;67:968–77.

130. Rabkin SW, Mathewson FAL, Hsu PH. Relation of body weight to development of ischemic heart disease in a cohort of young North American men after a 26 year observation period: The Manitoba Study. *Am J Cardiol* 1977;39:452–8.

131. Miller NE, Frode OH, Thelle DS, Mjös OD. High-density lipoprotein and coronary heart disease: a prospective case-control study. *Lancet* 1977; 965–7.

132. Wannamethee G, Shaper AG. Body weight and mortality in middle aged British men: impact of smoking. *Br Med J* 1989;299:1497–502.

133. Rhoads GG, Kagan A. The relation of coronary disease, stroke and mortality to weight in youth and middle age. *Lancet* 1983;1:492–5.

134. Pooling Project Research Group: relationship of blood pressure, serum cholesterol, smoking habit, relative weight and ECG abnormalities to incidence of major coronary events: final report of the pooling project. *J Chron Dis* 1978;31:201–306.

135. Comstock GW, Kandrick MA, Livesay VT. Subcutaneous fatness and mortality. *Am J Epidemiol* 1966;83:548–63.

136. Keys A. *Seven countries: a multivariate analysis of death and coronary heart disease.* Cambridge, MA: Harvard University Press, 1980.

137. Petitti DB, Wingerd J, Pellegrin F, Ramcharan S. Risk of vascular disease in women. *JAMA* 1979;242:1150–4.

138. Rose G, Hamilton PS, Keen H, et al. Myocardial ischemia, risk factors and death from coronary heart disease. *Lancet* 1977;1:105–9.

139. Rissanen A, Heliövaara M, Knekt P, Aromaa A, Reunanen A, Maatela J. Weight and mortality in Finnish men. *J Clin Epidemiol* 1989;42:781–9.

140. Paffenbarger RS, Wing AL. Chronic disease in former college students. *Am J Epidemiol* 1969; 90:527–36.

141. Hoffmans MDAF, Kromhout D, de Lezenne Coulander C. The impact of body mass index of 78,612 18-year old Dutch men on 32-year mortality from all causes. *J Clin Epidemiol* 1988;41:749–56.

142. Manson JE, Colditz GA, Stampfer MJ, et al. A prospective study of obesity and risk of coronary heart disease in women. *N Engl J Med* 1990;322:882–9.

143. Wedel H, Thelle D, Wilhelmsen L, et al. Body-mass index and mortality among men in the NORA-project. In: *Proceedings of the second international conference on preventive cardiology and the 29th annual meeting of the AHA Council on Epidemiology,* Washington DC, June 18–22, 1989, (abst).

144. Lew EA, Garfinkel L. Variations in mortality by weight among 750,000 men and women. *J Chron Dis* 1979;32:563–76.

145. Pyörälä K, Savolainen E, Lehtovirta E, et al. Glucose tolerance and coronary heart disease: Helsinki policemen study. *J Chron Dis* 1979;32:729–45.

146. Ellsinger BM, Larsson B, Welin L, Svärdsudd K, Eriksson H, Tibblin G. Is body fat mass, calculated from total body potassium determination, a stronger predictor of myocardial infarction and stroke than anthropometric indices? *Int J Obes* 1991;15[Suppl 1]18 (abst).

147. Sørensen TIA, Sonne-Holm S. Mortality in extremely overweight young men. *J Chron Dis* 1977;30:359–67.

148. Sjöström L. Mortality of severely obese subjects. *Am J Clin Nutr* 1992;55:611S–614S.

149. De Divitiis O, Fazio S, Petitto M, Maddalena G, Contaldo F, Mancini M. Obesity and cardiac function. *Circulation* 1981;64:477–82.

150. Korsan-Bengtsen K, Stenberg J, Sjöström L, Björntorp P, Sullivan L. Blood coagulation, fibrinolysis and platelet function in obese subjects at rest and after maximal exercise. *Thromb Res* 1972;1:389–406.

151. Meade TW, Chakrabarti R, Haines AP, North WR, Stirling Y. Characteristics affecting fibrinolytic activity and plasma fibrinogen concentrations. *Br Med J* 1979;1:153–6.

152. Vague P, Juhan-Vague I, Ailhaud MF, et al. Correlation between blood fibrinolytic activity, plasminogen activator inhibitor level, plasma insulin level, and relative body weight in normal and obese subjects. *Metabolism* 1986;35:250–3.

153. Ducimetiere P, Eschwege E, Papoz L, et al. Relationship of plasma insulin levels to the incidence of myocardial infarction and coronary heart disease mortality in a middle-aged population. *Diabetologia* 1980;19:205–10.

154. Weiborn TA, Wearne K. Coronary heart disease incidence and cardiovascular mortality in Busselton with reference to glucose and insulin concentrations. *Diabetes Care* 1979;2:154–60.

155. Drenick EJ, Gurunanjappa SB, Seltzer FSA, Johnson DG. Excessive mortality and causes of death in morbidly obese men. *JAMA* 1980;243:443–5.

156. Borrelli R, Isernia C, Di Biase G, Contaldo F. Mortality rate, causes and predictive factors of death in severely obese patients. *Int J Vitam Nutr Res* 1988;58:343–50.

157. Andres R, Elahi D, Tobin JD, Muller DC, Brant L. Impact of age on weight goals. *Ann Intern Med* 1985;103:1030–3.

158. Marks HH. Influence of obesity on morbidity and mortality. *Bull NY Acad Sci* 1960;36:296–312.

159. Mason E. The impact of obesity surgery on morbidity, mortality and survival. Fourth International Symposium on Obesity Surgery, London, August, 1980. *Int J Obes* 1989;13:596(abst).

160. Sjöström L. The morbidity of severely obese subjects. Speech at the NIH consensus development conference on surgical treatment of severe obesity, March 25–27, 1991. *Am J Clin Nutr* 1992;55: 508S–515S.

161. Dustan HP. Obesity and hypertension. *Ann Intern Med* 1985;103:1047–9.

162. Van Itallie TB. Health implications of overweight and obesity in the United States. *Ann Intern Med* 1985;103:983–8.

163. Stamler J. Overweight, hypertension, hypercholesterolemia and coronary heart disease. In: Mancini M, Lewis B, Contaldo F, eds. *Medical complications of obesity.* London: Academic Press, 1979;191–216.

164. Glueck CJ, Taylor HL, Jacobs D, Morrisson JA, Beaglehole R, Williams OD. Plasma high-density lipoprotein cholesterol: association with measurements of body mass. The Lipid Research Clinics Program Prevalence Study. *Circulation* 1980; 62:[Suppl IV]:IV-62–9.

165. Ashley FW JR, Kannel WB. Relation of weight change to changes in atherogenic traits: the Framingham Study. *J Chron Dis* 1974;27:103–14.

166. Kannel WB, Gordon T. Some determinants of obesity and its impact as a cardiovascular risk factor. In: Howard A, ed. *Recent advances in obesity research.* London: Newman Publishing Ltd, 1975;14–24.

167. Gleysteen JJ, Barboriak JJ. Improvement in heart disease risk factors after gastric by-pass. *Arch Surg* 1983;118:681–84.

168. Gonen B, Halverson JD, Schonfeld G. Lipoprotein levels in morbidly obese patients with massive surgically induced weight loss. *Metabolism* 1983;32:492–6.

169. Hughes TA, Twynne JT, Switzer BR, et al. Effects of caloric restriction and weight loss on glycemic control, insulin release and resistance and atherosclerotic risk in obese patients with type II diabetes mellitus. *Am J Med* 1984;77:7–17.

170. Garfinkel L. Overweight and cancer. *Ann Intern Med* 1985;103:1034–6.

171. Kral J. Morbid obesity and related health risks. *Ann Intern Med* 1985;103:1043–7.

172. Bray GA. Complications of obesity. *Ann Intern Med* 1985;103:1052–61.

173. Wadden TA, Stunkard AJ. Social and psychological consequences of obesity. *Ann Intern Med* 1985;103:1062–7.

174. Vague J. La différenciation sexuelle, facteur determineant des formes de l'obésité. *Presse Med* 1947;55:339–40.

175. Vague J. The degree of masculine differentiation of obesities: a factor determining predisposition to diabetes, arteriosclerosis, gout and uric calculous disease. *Am J Clin Nutr* 1956;4:20–34.

176. Vague J. *Obesities.* Paris: John Libbey & Co. Ltd, 1991.

177. Kissebah A, Vydelingum N, Murray R, et al. Relation of body fat distribution to metabolic complications of obesity. *J Clin Endocrinol Metab* 1982;54:254–60.

178. Peiris A, Meuller RA, Smith GA, Struve MF, Kissebah AH. Splanchnic insulin metabolism in obesity: influence of body fat distribution. *J Clin Invest* 1986;78:1648–57.

179. Peiris A, Meuller RA, Struve MF, Smith GA, Kissebah AH. Relationship of androgenic activity to splanchnic insulin metabolism and peripheral glucose utilization in premenopausal women. *J Clin Endocrinol Metab* 1987;64:162–9.

180. Evans DJ. *Body fat distribution and metabolic complications* [MD dissertation]. Cardiff: University of Cardiff, 1986.

181. Strömblad G, Björntorp P. Reduced hepatic insulin clearance in rats with dietary-induced obesity. *Metabolism* 1986;35:323–7.

182. Després JP, Trembley A, Bouchard C. Regional adipose tissue distribution and plasma lipoprotein. In: Bouchard C, Johnston F, eds. *Fat distribution during growth and later health outcomes.* New York: Alan R Liss, Inc, 1988;221–41.

183. Seidell JC, Björntorp P, Sjöström L, Sannerstedt R, Krotkiewski M, Kvist H. Regional distribution of muscle and fat mass in men—new insight into the risk of abdominal obesity using computed tomography. *Int J Obes* 1989;13:289–303.

184. Seidell JC, Björntorp P, Sjöström L, Kvist H, Sannerstedt R. Visceral fat accumulation in men is positively associated with insulin, glucose and C-peptide levels but negatively associated with testosterone levels. *Metabolism* 1990;39:897–901.

185. Stokes J, Garrison R, Kannel WB. The independent contribution of various indices of obesity to the 22-year incidence of coronary heart disease: the Framingham study. In: Vague J, ed. *Metabolic complications of human obesity.* Amsterdam: Elsevier 1985;49–57.

186. Olsson LO, Larsson B, Svärdsudd K, et al. The influence of body fat distribution on the incidence of diabetes mellitus. 13.5 year follow-up of participants in the study of men born in 1913. *Diabetes* 1985;34:1055–8.

187. Donahue RP, Abbot RD, Bloom E, Reed DM, Yano K. Central obesity and coronary heart disease in men. *Lancet* 1987;821–4.

188. Ducimetiere P, Richard J, Cambrin F. The pattern of subcutaneous fat distribution in middle-aged men and the risk of coronary heart disease: the Paris prospective study. *Int J Obes* 1986;10: 229–40.

189. Lundgren H, Bengtsson C, Blohmé G, Lapidus L, Sjöström L. Adiposity and adipose tissue distribution in relation to incidence of diabetes in women: results from a prospective population study in Gothenburg, Sweden. *Int J Obes* 1989;13:413–23.

190. Larsson B, Bengtsson C, Björntorp P, et al. Is abdominal body fat distribution a main explanation for the male/female difference in the risk of myocardial infarction? The Sixth International Congress on Obesity, Kobe, October 21–26, 1990. *Int J Obes* 1990;14[Suppl 2](abst).

191. Larsson B, Bengtsson C, Björntorp P, et al. Is abdominal body fat distribution a main explanation for the male/female difference in the risk of myocardial infarction? *Am J Epidemiol* 1992;135: 266–273.

192. Rebuffé-Scrive M, Andersson B, Olbe L, Björntorp P. Metabolism of adipose tissue in intraabdominal depots of non-obese men and women. *Metabolism* 1989;38:453–8.

193. Rebuffé-Scrive M, Andersson B, Olbe L, Björntorp P. Metabolism of adipose tissue in intraabdominal depots in obese men and women. *Metabolism* 1990;39:1021–5.

194. Bolinder J, Kager L, Östman J, Arner P. Differences at the receptor and postreceptor levels between human omental and subcutaneous adipose tissue in the action of insulin on lipolysis. *Diabetes* 1983;32:117–27.

195. Williamson JR, Kreisberg RA, Felts PW. Mechanism for the stimulation of gluconeogenesis by fatty acids in perfused rat liver. *Proc Natl Acad Sci USA* 1966;56:247–51.

196. Ruderman NB, Toeus CJ, Shafrir E. Role of free fatty acids in glucose homeostasis. *Arch Intern Med* 1969;123:299–313.

197. Blumenthal SA. Stimulation of gluconeogenesis by palmitic acid in rat hepatocytes, evidence that this effect can be dissociated from provision of reducing equivalents. *Metab Clin Exp* 1983;32:971–81.

198. Reaven G, Chang M, Ho H, Jeng CY, Hoffman BB: Lowering of plasma glucose in diabetic rats. *Am J Physiol* 1988;254:E23–E30.

199. Reaven G, Chang H, Hoffman B. Additive hypoglycemic effects of drugs that modify free-fatty acid metabolism by different mechanisms in rats with streptozocin-induced diabetes. *Diabetes* 1988;37: 28–32.

200. Ferrannini E, Barrett EJ, Bevilacqua S, DeFronzo RA. Effect of fatty acids on glucose production and utilization in man. *J Clin Invest* 1983;72:1737–44.

201. Bevilacqua S, Bonadonna R, Buzzigoli G, et al. Acute elevation of free fatty acid levels leads to hepatic insulin resistance in obese subjects. *Metabolism* 1987;36:502–8.

202. Peiris AN, Struve MF, Meuller RA, Lee MB, Kissebah AM. Glucose metabolism in obesity. Influence of body fat distribution. *J Clin Endocrinol Metab* 1988;67:760–7.

203. Carlson LA, Boberg J, Högstedt B. Some physiological and clinical implications of lipid mobilization from adipose tissue. In: Renold AE, Canlill GF Jr, eds. *Handbook of physiology. Adipose tissue. Section V.* Washington, DC: Williams & Wilkins, 1965;625–44.

204. Boström K, Borén J, Wettesten M, et al. Studies on the assembly of apo-B-100-containing lipoproteins in Hep G2 cells. *J Biol Chem* 1988;263:4434–42.

205. Faber OK, Christensen K, Kehlet H, Madsbad S, Binder C. Decreased insulin removal contributes to hyperinsulinemia in obesity. *J Clin Endocrinol Metab* 1981;56:618–21.

206. Bonora E, Zavaroni J, Coscelli C, Butturini U. Decreased hepatic insulin extraction in subjects with mild glucose intolerance. *Metabolism* 1983; 32:438–46.

207. Svedberg J, Smith U, Björntorp P, Lönnroth P. Insulin binding, degradation and action in rat hepatocytes is reduced in a dose-dependent way by free fatty acids. *Int J Obes* 1989;13[Suppl 1]:213(abst).

208. Svedberg J, Björntorp P, Smith U, Lönnroth P. Free fatty acids inhibit insulin binding, degradation and action in the isolated rat hepatocyte. *Diabetes* 1990;39:570–4.

209. Randle PJ, Garland PB, Hales CN, Newsholme EA. The glucose-fatty acid cycle. Its role in insulin sensitivity and the metabolic disturbances of diabetes mellitus. *Lancet* 1963;2:785–9.

210. Wiklund O, Witztum JL, Carew TE, Pittman RC, Elam RL, Steinberg D. Turnover and tissue sites of degradation of glucosylated low density lipoprotein in normal and immunized rabbits. *J Lipid Res* 1987;28:1098–109.

211. Juhan-Vague I, Roul C, Alessi MC, Ardissone JP, Heim M, Vague P. Increased plasminogen activator inhibitor activity in non-insulin dependent diabetic patients—relationship with plasma insulin. *Thromb Haemost* 1989;61:370–3.

212. Landin K, Tengborn L, Smith U. Elevated fibrinogen and plasminogen activator inhibitor (PAI-1) in hypertension are related to metabolic risk factors for cardiovascular disease. *J Intern Med* 1990; 227:273–8.

213. Stiko-Rahm A, Wiman B, Hamsten A, Nilsson J. Secretion of plasminogen activator inhibitor-1 from cultured human umbilical vein endothelial cells is induced by very low density lipoprotein. *Arteriosclerosis* 1990;10:1067–73.

214. Hamsten A, Wiman B, de Faire U, Blombäck M. Increased plasma levels of a rapid inhibitor of tissue plasminogen activator in young survivors of myocardial infarction. *N Engl J Med* 1985;313: 1557–63.

215. Hamsten A, de Faire U, Walldius G, et al. Plasminogen activator inhibitor in plasma: risk factor for recurrent myocardial infarction. *Lancet* 1987; 2:3–9.

216. Skøtt P, Hother-Nielsen I, Bruun NE, et al. Effects of insulin on kidney function and sodium excretion in healthy subjects. *Diabetologia* 1989; 32:694–9.

217. Landsberg L, Krieger D. Obesity, metabolism and the sympathetic nervous system. *Am J Hypertens* 1989;2:123S–132S.

218. Landin K, Tengborn L, Smith U. Treating insulin resistance in hypertension with metformin reduces both blood pressure and metabolic risk factors. *J Intern Med* 1991;229:181–7.

219. Evans DJ, Hoffman RG, Kalkhoff RK, Kissebah AH. Relationship of body fat topography to insulin sensitivity and metabolic profiles in premenopausal women. *Metabolism* 1984;33:68–75.

220. Peiris AN, Sothmann MS, Hoffmann RG, et al. Adiposity, fat distribution and cardiovascular risk. *Ann Intern Med* 1989;110:867–72.

221. Selby JV, Friedman GD, Quesenberry CP. Precursors of essential hypertension. The role of body fat distribution pattern. *Am J Epidemiol* 1989; 129:43.53.

222. Björntorp P. Abdominal obesity and development of non-insulin dependent diabetes mellitus. *Diabetes Metab Rev* 1988;4:615–22.

223. Björntorp P. Possible mechanisms relating fat distribution and metabolism. In: Bouchard C, Johnston F, eds. *Fat distribution during growth and later health outcomes.* New York: Alan R Liss, 1988;175–91.

224. Björntorp P. The associations between obesity, adipose tissue distribution and disease. *Acta Med Scand* 1988;Suppl 723:121–34.

225. Bouchard C, Bray GA, Hubbard VS. Basic and clinical aspects of regional fat distribution. *Am J Clin Nutr* 1990;52:946–50.

226. Björntorp P. "Portal" adipose tissue as a generator of risk factors for cardiovascular disease and diabetes [Editorial]. *Arteriosclerosis* 1990;10:493–6.

227. Bouchard C. Genetic factors in the regulation of adipose tissue distribution. *Acta Med Scand* 1988;Suppl 723:135–41.

228. Evans DJ, Hoffman RG, Kalkhoff RK, Kissebah AH. Relationship of androgenic activity to body fat topography, fat cell morphology and metabolic aberrations in premenopausal women. *J Clin Endocrinol Metab* 1983;57:304–10.

229. Stallones L, Meuller WH, Christensson BH. Blood pressure, fatness and fat patterning among USA adolescents from two ethnic groups. *Hypertension* 1982;4:483–6.

230. Siervogel RM, Baumgartner RN. Fat distribution and blood pressure. In Bouchard C, Johnston F, eds: *Fat distribution during growth and later health outcomes.* New York: Alan R Liss, 1988:243–61.

231. Laakso M, Sarlund H, Mykkänen L. Essential hypertension and insulin resistance in non-insulin-dependent diabetes. *Eur J Clin Invest* 1989; 19:518–26.

232. Smith U, Gudbjörnsdottir S, Landin K. Hypertension as a metabolic disorder—an overview. *J Intern Med* 1991;229[Suppl 2]:1–7.

233. Haffner SM, Katz M, Stern MP, Sunn J. Relationship of sex hormone binding globulin to overall adiposity and body fat distribution in a biethnic population. *Int J Obes* 1989;13:1–9.

234. Kirschner MA, Samojlik E, Drejka M, Szmal E, Schneider G, Ertel N. Androgen-estrogen metabolism in women with upper body versus lower body obesity. *J Clin Endocrinol Metab* 1990;70:473–9.

235. Leibel RL, Edens NK, Fried SK. Physiologic basis for the control of body fat distribution in men. *Annu Rev Nutr* 1989;9:417–43.

236. Poehlman G, Trembley A, Després JP, et al. Genotype-controlled changes in body composition and fat morphology following overfeeding in twins. *Am J Clin Nutr* 1986;43:723–31.

237. Presta E, Leibel RL, Hirsch J. Regional changes in adrenoceptor status during hypocaloric intake do not predict changes in adipocyte size or body shape. *Metabolism* 1990;39:307–15.

238. Rebuffé-Scrive M, Enk L, Crona N, et al. Fat cell metabolism in different regions in women. Effects of menstrual cycle, pregnancy and lactation. *J Clin Invest* 1985;75:1973–6.

239. Rebuffé-Scrive M, Lundholm K, Björntorp P. Glucocorticoid binding of human adipose tissue. *Eur J Clin Invest* 1985;15:267–72.

240. Seidell JC, Björntorp P, Sjöström L, Krotkiewski M, Sannerstedt R. Abdominal obesity and metabolism in men—possible role of behavioural characteristics. In: Björntorp P, Rössner S, eds. *Obesity in Europe.* London: John Libbey, 1989:91–9.

241. Shimokata H, Tobin JD, Muller DC, Elahi D, Coon PJ, Andres R. Studies in the distribution of body fat. I. Effects of age, sex and obesity. *J Gerontol* 1989;44:M66–73.

242. Shimokata H, Andres R, Coon PJ, Elahi D, Muller DC, Tobin JD. Studies in the distribution of body fat. II. Longitudinal effects of change in weight. *Int J Obes* 1989;13:455–64.

243. Shimokata H, Muller DC, Andres R. Studies in the distribution of body fat. III. Effects of cigarette smoking. *JAMA* 1990;243:1828–31.

244. Wahrenberg H, Lönnkvist F, Arner P. Mechanisms underlying regional differences in lipolysis in human adipose tissue. *J Clin Invest* 1989; 84:458–67.

245. Sjöström L, Backman L, Bengtsson C, et al. Swedish Obese Subjects, SOS—an intervention study of obesity. Relationships between cardiovascular risk factors, lean body mass, subcutaneous and visceral adipose tissue in 2451 severely obese subjects [*submitted*].

Obesity: Theory and Therapy, Second Edition,
edited by A. J. Stunkard and T. A. Wadden.
Raven Press, Ltd., New York © 1993.

3

Basic Neural Mechanisms of Feeding and Weight Regulation

Bartley G. Hoebel and Luis Hernandez

Department of Psychology, Princeton University, Princeton, New Jersey 08540

Much new information has come to light in the decade since this opening chapter was written for the first edition of *Obesity.* Technical advances in neuroscience have led to the discovery of new neurotransmitters and receptors that play crucial roles in feeding and weight regulation, which in turn opens new routes to therapy.

What we knew 10 years ago of basic principles and basic neural mechanisms is still true, but our view has expanded to include more brain and body functions, and especially a greater understanding of brain–body integration. There have been exciting discoveries in the eighties and early nineties, including (a) integrative functions of regulatory peptides such as neuropeptide Y (NPY) and cholecystokinin (CCK), which modulate feeding onset and offgo; (b) functions of dopamine and serotonin in forebrain mechanisms for feeding reinforcement; (c) new evidence bearing on sensory control of feeding and the integration of taste, gastrointestinal, hepatic, and blood-borne signals; and (d) a fresh look at the role of prenatal experience and learning in neural control of food choices and body weight maintenance.

Animals tend to maintain a very constant body weight. To understand hunger and satiety in human beings, we assume that the primitive goal of feeding behavior is to maintain the constancy of the nutrient concentration of the *milieu interieur.* The basic homeostatic mechanism must integrate internal and external energy-related stimuli and then control metabolic processes and feeding behavior. We assume that this complex homeostatic function can be broken down into simpler units of autonomic and behavioral function for the sake of understanding. With this understanding will come an accurate synthesis of feeding control systems and effective design of therapeutic measures.

Some homeostatic functions have both an automatic component, which goes on even during sleep, and a more variable behavioral component that requires arousal. For example, respiration is largely automatic, but we can also hold our breath. Temperature regulation relies heavily on both autonomic responses such as piloerection and secretion of epinephrine, and behavioral responses such as building fires or migrating to a warmer climate. Fluid balance also provides elegant examples of physiological psychology. Osmoreceptors in the hypothalamus control both fluid reabsorption and drinking behavior; blood volume receptors in the kidney control vascular functions and appetite for water and salt. Energy regulation follows a similar pattern, involving both internal and behavioral actions that the brain integrates using neural and hormonal signals.

In recent research there has been an emphasis on learned responses that anticipate homeostatic imbalances and thereby prevent the imbalance from occurring. This will be reflected in the present chapter when we discuss learned choices of dietary fat vs. carbohydrate, learned taste preferences, and learned neurotransmitter release. Plasticity of the brain even extends back to neonatal and interuterine events, which can program neuroendocrine systems for adulthood. For example, transient food deprivation in a pregnant mother can cause adult obesity in her offspring.

Energy regulation can demand very complex behavior. Some carnivores must enter into social interaction, cooperation, and pitched battle for food. On the other hand, herbivores in the ocean or in a pasture have relatively easy access to food. Collier (8) points out that the patients seen by most doctors have the behavioral repertoire of a clever, carnivorous tiger and the continual access to food of a lucky, herbivorous cow. However, this is probably not the reason why they are obese. Herbivorous animals that are restricted to food only once a day can learn to eat one big meal, and carnivores given continual access will eat many small meals. After they learn the feeding regimen, both groups maintain constant, normal body weights. Human beings also tend to maintain a stable weight for long periods.

Why do some people become obese? Overweight patients may have such palatable food that they display dietary obesity (56; see also Sclafani, *this volume*). Some may be genetically prone to obesity or to a diet that is conducive to obesity. Some individuals with normal diets and average genetic endowment may have acquired a disturbance in basic mechanisms of weight control, an abnormality in either the internal or the behavioral aspects of regulation (Fig. 1). The purpose of our analysis is to identify the different physiological mechanisms that can become exaggerated so as to appear as pathological changes in feeding and body weight. This will lay the foundation for selective, effective therapy (2,5,10–12,14,15,17–19,22–25,28–31, 35,36,38–41,55–58,60–62,66,67).

ESSENTIALS OF FEEDING CONTROL IN PRIMITIVE ANIMALS

The basic postulates of feeding research are well illustrated in the fly. This relatively simple feeding machine moves at random until it encounters food, and then extends its proboscis to eat. The tendency to extend or withdraw depends on variations in taste threshold, which in turn depend on gut fullness. Thus feeding is simply and elegantly controlled by external receptors for taste and internal receptors for gut distention. A central neural mechanism is required to integrate the

FEEDING SYSTEM

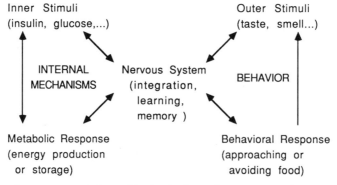

FIG. 1. Overview of energy regulation with the brain as integrator, anticipator, and controller of internal metabolic reflexes and external, behavioral responses. (Adapted from Hernandez and Hoebel, ref. 21, with permission.)

sensory signals and couple them to motor reflexes. The same process is being studied in the sea snail, *Aplysia.* If the stomach is empty, the head turns to approach the taste of seaweed, but if the stomach is full of food, then the head withdraws from the same taste (25).

The basic points to note are as follows. First the food-deprived animal becomes aroused. It starts moving. If it tastes food, it eats. Some food concentrations are more effective than others. For example, weak sugar solutions induce less eating than slightly stronger ones. If the solution is too concentrated, it counteracts the tendency to eat; this is particularly true with salty tastes, which induce eating in low concentrations and withdrawal at higher concentrations. The simple animal will eat a tasty food until its sensory receptors adapt and stop firing. When the receptors eventually disadapt, another meal may start. When the gut fills up, feeding is inhibited and the meal comes to an end even when taste neurons are firing. Thus meal frequency and the size of a meal are separately controlled, but centrally integrated.

If the neural connection from the gut to the central mechanism is cut, a fly loses its primary "satiety system," and will eat such a big meal that it may burst. In *Aplysia,* satiety is more than just stopping a meal. The animal actively turns away from food. Garden slugs have a brain complicated enough to display learned aversion. If slightly poisoned after eating, they will tend to avoid that food the next time. Computational neuroscience has recently created a computer model of the slug's neural network. Like a slug, the computer can learn what not to eat, and the model is revealing how the real network does it (16).

The fly's feeding behavior is like a thermostat: the animal initiates a pattern of feeding behavior made up of a series of reflexes whenever its energy level is low. Again like a thermostat, the on–off set point can be shifted so that the decision to start or stop feeding is regulated at a different overall level of intake. Like a home thermostat that can be adjusted to a new set point as a function of changes in humidity, shifts in daylight hours, or mental fatigue in its internal spring, so also the fly's overall level of intake can shift as a function of the quantity and quality of neural input from taste or gastric receptors.

How to reduce intake for a simple animal should be clear from the preceding discussion. One could try to (a) lower the level of locomotion, (b) hide the food, (c) diminish the taste qualities that cause approach, (d) increase the taste qualities that cause withdrawal, (e) anesthetize the taste receptors, (f) distend the stomach to alter taste responsiveness, or (g) mildly poison the beast after it eats certain foods. It is also theoretically possible to give centrally acting drugs or perform brain surgery to produce any of these effects.

Controlling the animal's access to food or the taste of food is the most direct; putting indigestible filler in the stomach is also relatively specific. Damaging a few external or internal sensory receptors might work, but is risky and often irreversible. No one has learned how to train flies to eat less, so there might be no other alternative except to keep them captive in a laboratory to control the taste or amount of food they get. If we could diagnose which feeding factor was disarranged in each individual fly, then there would be some hope for individualized therapy.

Many sensory and motor factors are involved in feeding, even in a fly. Obesity could be due to abnormalities in any one of them, or to an abnormality in the central integrative mechanism. The choice of therapy becomes a matter of deciding which factors to manipulate in each individual case. Since the mechanism that integrates feeding factors has not been elucidated in the fly, we turn to mammals.

The great advance in complicated beasts has been their ability to break out of their reflex chains. They have freed themselves on both the sensory and the motor side. Pavlov's dogs could break the sensory loop by responding with feeding reflexes to an initially neutral bell. Thorndike's cats or Skinner's rats could break the motor loop by responding with arbitrarily chosen motor patterns such as pressing a lever to get food. This sensory and motor freedom has been the breakthrough that allows vertebrates to obtain food under highly diverse conditions (51).

NEURAL MECHANISMS OF WEIGHT REGULATION

Brain research on obesity began with the study of obese people who had identifiable brain damage in the region of the pituitary. Cases continue to appear in the literature. One woman with a medial hypothalamic tumor consumed 10,000 kcal/day even after correction of most metabolic and hormonal difficulties. A related syndrome has been produced experimentally in laboratory animals, primarily the rat. At the focus of research on the physiology and psychology of energy regulation has been the hypothalamus, a central site of the lipostatic, thermostatic, and glucostatic mechanisms presumed to control energy homeostasis and the motivation to eat. Neural mechanisms of feeding in vertebrates were originally studied by just four major techniques: (a) brain lesions, (b) neuropharmacological manipulations, (c) brain stimulation, and (d) neural recording. Now we can add four others: (e) in vivo techniques for measuring neurotransmitter release, (f) techniques for labeling the neurotransmitter receptors, (g) in vivo monitoring of local brain glucose utilization as an index of neural activity, and (h) precise anatomical tracing techniques using labeled viruses that travel up sensory neurons from the stomach to the feeding areas of the cortex. Genetic mapping is on the horizon.

Evidence of a lateral hypothalamic feeding system and a medial hypothalamic satiety system was first gathered by observing the effects of variously located hypothalamic lesions in rats. Still the basis of our thinking, this dual system is now seen from a new, broader perspective. Modern neurochemistry and neuroendocrinology are largely responsible for the changes.

LESION SYNDROMES: THE ORIGINAL MODELS OF FEEDING ABNORMALITIES

Stereotaxic Lesions of the Medial Hypothalamus or Paraventricular Nucleus

Hyperphagia, Hyperinsulinemia, and Obesity

Stereotaxic lesions of the ventromedial hypothalamic (VMH) region cause overeating, which leads to obesity. The larger the lesion, within limits, the more weight the rat gains. Doubling of normal body weight is not unusual with large, accurately placed lesions. It is important to note, however, that the amount of weight gain depends on the starting weight. Teitelbaum correctly predicted that if we made rats overeat and become obese before the lesion, then they would not overeat afterwards. From this it also followed that if we would force-feed obese VMH rats to make them superobese, they would subsequently choose to undereat until they lost weight back down to their preferred obese level. The important point is that animals with this syndrome do not necessarily overeat. They simply eat in a way that maintains an unusual amount of fat in the body. Thus one major aspect of the syndrome is an upward shift in the level of body weight regulation. At an obese level, they regulate food intake beautifully (26).

Trying to reduce the body weight of some people may be asking them to live at a weight level below their own personal level of hypothalamic regulation. If a 200-pound woman acts as if she were underweight, perhaps she is, in fact, underweight relative to some higher weight level at which she would eat normally.

Patients with a high weight level have three choices. They can work at learning to enjoy it, they can fight it by trying to eat less than they want and by exercising, or they can try to shift the weight level downwards by manipulating the regulatory system. There are theoretically several ways to shift the weight level downward. One is to manipulate environmental cues. Another is to attack the orogastrointestinal tract. A third is hormonal, and a fourth is to alter the nervous system.

Hyperinsulinemia

As pointed out earlier, the sensory control of feeding involves both internal and environmental signals; medial hypothalamic lesions can affect both. The animal may become hyperinsulinemic as well as hyperphagic. This is a "chicken and egg" problem. Which comes first, the hyperinsulinemia or the hyperphagia? If food intake of lesioned rats is matched to the intake of unlesioned control animals, the hyperinsulinemia is reduced but not abolished, suggesting that the two are somewhat independent. In spite of matched food intake the lesioned rat accumulates some excess fat. This shows that hyperinsulinemia or some correlated metabolic change can increase body weight even when the quantity of food intake is normal (60,63,66).

Instead of normalizing food intake in a VMH animal, one can hold insulin level constant. Bray's (3,4) group did this by removing the pancreas and implanting a new one in the kidney capsule where it would have no innervation. In this case hypothalamic lesions caused no hyperinsulinemia at all. Therefore hypothalamic lesions normally induce hyperinsulinemia by way of a neural link with the pancreas, not a humoral link. The rats with a transplanted pancreas were slightly hyperphagic even though not hyperinsulinemic, again suggesting some degree of independence. Friedman held insulin level constant by making rats severely diabetic with alloxan and then injecting enough exogenous insulin to maintain a normal food intake and body weight. VMH lesions in these

animals caused full-fledged hyperphagia even though there was presumably no hyperinsulinemia (60). Thus we can see that medial hypothalamic lesions can directly cause both hyperinsulinemia and hyperphagia.

Parasympathetic Dominance

Medial hypothalamic lesions disrupt a host of humoral and other autonomic nervous functions in addition to that of insulin. Lesions of the VMH lead to hyperfunction of the vagus nerve as measured by gastric motility and gastric acid secretion. Given the fact that gastric motility can increase before a meal (hunger pangs), it has been proposed that increased gastric function plays an important role in hypothalamic hyperphagia. Powley and Berthoud (50) reviewed evidence that subdiaphragmatic vagotomy blocks both the hyperphagia and obesity. Vagotomy also blocks hyperinsulinemia and hypersecretion of gastric acid. Parasympathetic innervation of the pancreas and the gastrointestinal tract appears to be important in the hypothalamic obesity syndrome. At the same time that parasympathetic activity is increased, sympathetic activity is decreased (3). Equally intriguing is the fact that lesions can change the animal's reaction to external stimuli. Some medial hypothalamic lesions cause abnormal consumption of sweetened food. The animals may also eat both in the daytime and at night instead of sleeping. No one claims that these lesions are selective for just feeding, nor that the sensory changes affect food intake exclusively.

Damage to the adjacent paraventricular nucleus (PVN) or its output clearly plays a role in the VMH obesity syndrome (39). Small precise lesions show that damage to either site can cause obesity, but hyperinsulinemia and increased parasympathetic tone are due largely to destruction of the VMH. PVN lesions, on the other hand, are more likely to damage the neuropeptide cell body groups for which the PVN is well known (e.g., corticotropic releasing factor, somatostatin, growth hormone-releasing factor, and gonadotropic releasing factor).

Functionally Produced Abnormalities and Diabetes

Hyperphagia and obesity can be produced in mice by injections of gold–thioglucose. This antiinflammatory drug can cause histopathologic changes in medial hypothalamic tissue that correlate with the degree of obesity. The effect is insulin dependent. Diabetic mice are protected from gold–thioglucose lesions by an insulin deficit. Insulin therapy restores their susceptibility. It is not clear whether gold–thioglucose causes obesity by damaging glucoreceptors, or simply by nonspecific cellular or vascular damage of the medial region. In either case, it is likely that insulin gates the uptake of glucose in this region of the hypothalamus, thereby contributing to satiety and weight control in the normal animal (20). When insulin was injected in many hypothalamic sites it was discovered that the VMH is particularly sensitive for insulin-induced satiety in normal rats (44).

The glucose antimetabolite, 2-deoxy-D-glucose (2DG), causes feeding when injected systemically. The drug blocks utilization of glucose and thereby triggers excessive feeding. Injection of small amounts of 2DG directly into either the hepatic circulation or brain ventricles causes feeding. This finding suggests that cells sensitive to local metabolism are located in both the liver and the brain. Liver glucoreceptors communicate with the brain by way of the vagus nerve (21,50).

Modern imaging techniques that monitor the uptake of radioactive 2DG in the human brain will soon allow the comparison of activated brain areas in normal and obese people before and after they eat. Another approach is to give rats 2DG and then section the brain and label it for early gene products (e.g., c-Fos) that reveal the anatomical sites that responded to the glucoprivation. In this way

Ritter's group found activation of the genome of brainstem and hypothalamic nuclei that integrate energy-related signals, notably the nucleus tractus solitarus (NTS) and PVN.

Diabetics do not have a brain lesion, but their insulin deficit may be tantamount to the same thing. The severely diabetic animal that lacks insulin will be tremendously hyperphagic, but not obese. It cannot store fuel properly because glucose transport and lipogenesis are impaired, and it cannot transport glucose into the cells that signal satiety. Both the diabetic and the lesioned rat overeat sweet carbohydrate diets and reject food adulterated with quinine. On the other hand, if moderately diabetic rats are given a high fat diet, they will not be hyperphagic. This finding suggests that the satiety mechanisms do not need insulin to utilize lipids. Friedman and Stricker have suggested that the liver responds to energy utilization, per se, regardless of whether the original fuel was glucose, lipids, amino acids, or ketone bodies (15,60).

The conclusion at the present time is that medial hypothalamic damage causes both "cellular overfueling" related to hyperinsulinemia and "behavioral overfueling" due to hyperphagia. An intact vagal–pancreatic system is necessary for the hyperinsulinemia, and good tasting food is necessary for the hyperphagia. Why does body weight eventually level off? No one knows for sure. The level of circulating insulin is proportional to body weight, so perhaps the animal gains weight until there is sufficient insulin plus energy-rich metabolites to reach the insulin sensitivity threshold and the neural sensitivity threshold of the remaining receptor cell population; then insulin output and feeding are inhibited (66). At this obese level the animal will modulate its intake and maintain its weight.

One feature that distinguishes hypothalamic obesity from some other types is the permanent shift in level of weight regulation. In contrast, hyperphagia and obesity induced by tasty "junk food" goes away if the animal is returned to a diet of Purina Chow. Obesity induced by force feeding is also a temporary condition that will revert to normal when the animal can eat normally (26). Emergency eating and obesity following chronic insulin-induced hypoglycemia also revert to normal when insulin injections stop. Hypothalamic obesity, on the other hand, is permanent, unless the damage is very slight (26,36,56).

Lesions of the Lateral Hypothalamus

Hypophagia, Sensory Neglect, and Weight Loss

Lesions of the lateral hypothalamus produce deficits in feeding and weight regulation. The particular constellation of deficits depends on the exact location of the lesion and the extent to which it depletes dopamine in the striatum and nucleus accumbens. The classical case is a rat that refuses to eat or drink for days or weeks and may starve to death. If the lesion is small, asymmetric, or not very far lateral, i.e., "midlateral," the animal gradually begins to accept wet palatable food. The next stage in recovery is reappearance of weight maintenance. The animal eats sufficient food if the food is wet and sweet. Finally the animal will accept plain water during a meal, but still rejects water alone. True thirst in response to dehydration is often permanently impaired. The rat drinks to wet its mouth as it eats dry food, but acts as if plain water is aversive. These stages suggest that recovery recapitulates development of infant feeding. Milk is accepted first, water last. The role of taste in motivating the animal is paramount. Taste is so exaggerated in the lateral lesioned rat, that it is a matter of life and death. Sweet milk instead of plain chow can save its life (61).

Taste nerves have been traced from the tongue to the hypothalamus. Both anatomical and electrophysiological evidence indicate that, like most sensory systems, taste is processed in the thalamus and cortex and also projects to the hypothalamus by a short route in rats and a long route in humans. In addition, the trigeminal nerve, which serves much of the face, is indirectly connected with the hypothalamus. Hypothalamic lesions alter sensitivity in and around the mouth.

In many respects the lateral hypothalamic lesion syndrome is the mirror image of the medial lesion syndrome. The rat with a lateral lesion (LH rat) shows sensory neglect of touch, odor, and taste, whereas the rat with a medial lesion (MH rat) shows sensory enhancement. The LH rat maintains its weight at low levels; the MH rat is chronically obese (36).

The rat with a lateral hypothalamic lesion, then, appears to be subnormally responsive to both external and internal cues that promote feeding. Stricker and Zigmond suggest that these rats are not adequately activated by the stressful aspects of their emaciated condition. There may be nothing wrong with their sensory or motor apparatus that a good pinch, foot shock, or shot of amphetamine would not cure (60). Under normal circumstances, the rat is aroused to action by the physiological signs of deprivation; the lesioned rats are relatively unresponsive. This deficit shifts the level of body weight maintenance downward. The size, location, and symmetry of the lesion determine whether the rat maintains a level described as slim, skinny, emaciated, or near death. As we will discuss later, a dopamine deficit in the nigrostriatal tract may be at the root of the arousal problem, and a deficit in the mesolimbic dopamine projection to the nucleus accumbens could account for the animal's inability to find positive reinforcement in food (23,28). Studies cited below show that the lateral hypothalamus also has cell bodies involved in feeding regulation.

NEUROPHARMACOLOGICAL STUDIES OF OBESITY

Amphetamine

Modern neuropsychopharmacology focused first on brain monoamines and their roles in Parkinson's disease and schizophrenia. Norepinephrine, dopamine, and serotonin are now thought to play neuromodula-

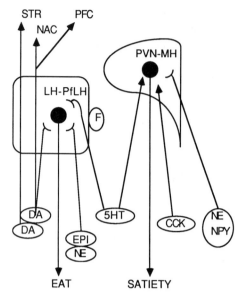

FIG. 2. Summary of selected neuropharmacological studies of feeding showing possible catecholamine interactions. Imagine looking down into the rat brain with the forebrain at the top of the page and the hindbrain at the bottom. At the left, neural projections from monoamine cell groups are shown projecting to the lateral hypothalamus (LH) and perifornical lateral hypothalamus (PfLH). They primarily inhibit the output for eating (blunt arrows). D_2 dopamine receptors, β-adrenergic receptors, and 5HT receptors in this region have been inferred from local drug injection studies lateral. to the fornix (F). This LH–PfLH region is where amphetamine releases monoamines that suppress feeding. Oomura (48) has shown that some of the LH neurons are sensitive to glucose and may contribute to eating when insulin level is high and glucose is low. Lesions here cause the classic LH starvation syndrome, but this can include damage to the dopamine (DA) fibers of passage that ascend to the striatum (STR), nucleus accumbens (NAC), and prefrontal cortex (PFC). Electrical stimulation of the PfLH can induce feeding and a feeding–reward effect manifest as electrical self-stimulation. At the right, the paraventricular nucleus (PVN) and other medial hypothalamic (MH) regions are shown where neural outputs promote satiety and inhibition of insulin secretion. Lesions of the MH cause hyperphagia, obesity, hyperinsulinemia, low sympathetic tone and may interrupt output from the PVN. Oomura has shown MH glucoreceptive neurons that are sensitive to insulin levels. Norepinephrine (NE) and neuropeptide Y (NPY) are two of the neurotransmitters that stimulate feeding in these regions, as indicated by inhibition of satiety. Serotonin (5HT)

tory roles, acting diffusely in the region of release. Many studies have demonstrated effects of monoamine deficits on one behavior or another, such as feeding, mating, or aggression. It has been difficult to establish whether the effect is specific to the behavior under study, or instead an example of nonspecific influence on overall activity level, reactivity, attention, or memory.

We were led in this work by an interest in appetite-suppressant drugs—amphetamine, fenfluramine, and phenylpropanolamine. Amphetamine injected into the lateral hypothalamus inhibits feeding partly by a β-adrenergic action. The neurotransmitter epinephrine was more potent than norepinephrine (41). Presumably the β-adrenergic receptors inhibit part of the classical lateral hypothalamic feeding system (Fig. 2). This notion fits with the observation that lateral hypothalamic lesions reduce amphetamine anorexia.

Anatomists in Sweden reported that a bundle of noradrenergic and adrenergic fibers ascend from cell groups in the midbrain and hindbrain and innervate the forebrain including the hypothalamus. We hypothesized that the "ventral noradrenergic bundle" might inhibit feeding; therefore we destroyed it selectively by injecting the catecholamine neurotoxin 6-hydroxy-dopamine into the bundle as it coursed through the midbrain. The result was overeating and increased body weight (20,26). The evidence suggested that the obesity induced by 6-hydroxy-dopamine is caused by selective depletion of catecholamine neurons that normally inhibit feeding.

Perhaps the most striking contrast to classical hypothalamic hyperphagia was the decrease in the ability of amphetamine to suppress the appetite in norepinephrine–epinephrine-depleted rats. In addition, fenfluramine, which is a serotonergic drug, became more potent (20,26,29). It is unwise to gener-

and cholecystokinin (CCK) induce satiety in part by counteracting the NE–NPY effect. (Adapted from Hoebel and Leibowitz, ref. 24, with permission.)

alize to human beings, but the implication of this finding could be very important. We have here two types of obesity; one is associated with a loss of amphetamine anorexia, the other is not. It is therefore conceivable that anorectic drugs can be used to classify various types or causes of overeating and obesity. The input path to the β-adrenergic receptors is labeled "EPI" in Fig. 2. Leibowitz found evidence for a dopamine input, labeled "DA" and a serotonergic input, "5HT," both of which inhibited feeding in the hypothalamus. Most recently an α-1 influence on satiety has been discovered in the PVN. All four of these (β, DA, 5HT, and α-1 receptors) play some role in inhibiting feeding at some time of day, depending to some degree on what macronutrient was last eaten (30,31, 41,64).

Serotonergic Anorectics: d-Fenfluramine

Blundell reports that amphetamine and fenfluramine have different effects on meal patterns in normal rats, constituting additional evidence that these drugs act on different neural substrates (1,53; see also Blundell and Lawton, *this volume*). Amphetamine caused the animals to delay the onset of large meals that they ate rapidly, whereas fenfluramine caused them to eat smaller meals at their usual time. The increased rate of eating may simply relate to the stimulant properties of amphetamine. More interesting is the possibility that fenfluramine potentiates meal termination and amphetamine retards meal initiation. This has to be an oversimplification because these drugs affect so many functions peripherally and centrally, but the concept of multiple satiety systems is an advance over the totally fallacious view that all anorectic drugs are alike.

Even isomers of fenfluramine are different. The racemic mixture is currently sold in the United States; whereas d-fenfluramine is popular in Europe. The serotonergic anorectic potency is in the d-isomer.

Major neurochemical differences between amphetamine and fenfluramine have been documented. Amphetamine potentiates catecholamines by release, reuptake block, and monoamine oxidase block. Fenfluramine does this relatively poorly, and instead causes release and reuptake block of serotonin (53). This finding suggests that one of the functions of serotonin is to inhibit feeding. The evidence for serotonin mediating satiety was extensive but contradictory until a new drug was discovered that could inhibit the firing of serotonin cells. Low doses of this compound can cause clear hyperphagia (12,22).

Nutrition and the Brain

Fernstrom, Wurtman, and others have shown that brain serotonin levels can be altered by the diet (14,67). A carbohydrate meal that releases insulin, or a direct injection of insulin, will indirectly increase the transport of tryptophan from the blood into the brain. This, in turn, boosts the synthesis of brain serotonin from tryptophan and mimics the effect of injecting serotonin into the medial hypothalamic region. In both cases, rats chose to eat less carbohydrate (28,38,40). Collier's group found that animals eating tryptophan-laced foods ate less carbohydrate, but then compensated by eating more fat; thus their total caloric intake and body weight remained the same. The two-way interaction between diet and brain chemistry is an exciting new field for study and therapy. Carbohydrate, tryptophan, and insulin team up to alter brain serotonin levels. Even if this does not lower body weight, it may have other therapeutic effects such as treating excessive carbohydrate appetite and seasonal affective disorder (SAD) (67).

Noradrenergic Anorectics: Phenylpropanolamine

There is special interest in phenylpropanolamine (PPA) as an anorectic drug because it is sold over the counter. Structurally it is closely related to norepinephrine. We explored the possibility that PPA might have a peripheral action on feeding mechanisms. The glucostatic theory of feeding control suggests that drugs with an action like insulin, or with a direct excitatory action on glucoreceptors, should curb food intake. We gave PPA to diabetic rats and mildly diabetic monkeys and found that the drug decreased their elevated blood sugar and glucosuria. PPA may increase glucose utilization. Conceivably, drugs of this type suppress feeding, in part, by an action on a glucostatic satiety mechanism. Within the hypothalamus PPA inhibits feeding by an α-1 receptor action in the PVN (64).

It is evident that different anorectic drugs can have very different effects on neurochemistry, on energy homeostasis, and on behavior. What is good for one obese patient may be poor for the next. A few of the factors to consider in choosing between drugs are: cardiovascular side effects, diabetes, arousal versus sedation, meal size versus meal frequency, and potential for abuse.

Stress

The effect of amphetamine in lateral hypothalamically lesioned rats helps to explain the neurochemistry of this starvation syndrome. Paradoxically, amphetamine, or any stimulant, will help a starving rat eat. This is probably the stimulant property of the drug at work, not its anorectic property. It is now known that dopamine depletion in the nigrostriatal tract duplicates most of the lateral hypothalamic starvation syndrome, and dopamine agonists help restore reactivity to food. A lesion in the far lateral hypothalamus interrupts the tract and depletes striatal dopamine; thus several laboratories have concluded that a striatal dopamine deficit accounts for a large part of the classical syndrome (43,59). They also agree that many behaviors besides feeding are affected. The rats are models of Parkinson's disease. Procedures that restore dopaminergic function provide a cure. In the absence of therapy these rats will starve unless the food is tasty;

they will refuse glucose unless appropriately hypoglycemic, and they will drown in water unless it is hot enough to spur them into action. They generally display ataxia and inanition (61). Another way to get them to eat is mild, chronic tail pinch, which is another form of stress.

Tail pinch-induced eating is partly dopaminergic. In a rat with a normal dopamine system, tail pinch can cause hyperphagia. This finding suggests that an overactive dopamine system might lead not only to hyperactivity, but also to hyperphagia if food is readily available. Although dopamine has been studied primarily with regard to deficits and starvation, excess dopaminergic function in parts of the striatum or accumbens is theoretically another source of obesity (31).

Damage to the dopamine pathways passing through the lateral hypothalamus does not account for all the effects of lateral hypothalamic lesions. Kainic acid was injected in the lateral hypothalamus with the intent of destroying cell bodies without harming dopamine axons that pass through. This successfully caused aphagia, adipsia, and body weight loss without extensive dopamine depletion (60). Some of the behavioral deficits of kainic acid or other excitatory amino acid neurotoxins were very much like the effects of electrolytic lesions; for example, 2DG no longer induced feeding. This is consistent with the traditional assumption that cells in the lateral hypothalamus are necessary for monitoring and integrating energy signals to induce eating and maintain normal body weight.

Chemical Neuroanatomy of Feeding

Feeding can be altered not only by infusing the hypothalamus with drugs but also with neurotransmitters. Success with locally applied neurotransmitters further proves that the hypothalamus contains synapses, not just axons, of neurons that control feeding. This is in accord with the original, lateral hypothalamic feeding theory. It is further confirmed by neural recording studies that find lateral hypothalamic cells that are inhibited by iontophoretic injection of norepinephrine and disinhibited by norepinephrine depletion (for review, see refs. 22,24–28).

The neurotransmitter for the α synapses is probably norepinephrine. The α-1 receptors apparently induce satiety and the α-2 receptors inhibit satiety. For the β synapses the neurotransmitter could be epinephrine or norepinephrine. Thus it appears that norepinephrine in the PVN can either induce or prevent feeding depending on the overall state of the system.

Circadian Neurochemistry and the Endocrine State

Circadian rhythm is an important factor in determining an animal's overall state. Many of the norepinephrine and serotonin cells in midbrain fire spontaneously in proportion to arousal state (33). The animal is behaviorally active when these cells are neurally active. It is clear that release of monoamines plays a major role in permitting the animal to process external and internal sensory information and pay attention to it. Not only does monoamine release vary with time of day, so does monoamine receptor binding. In the PVN, norepinephrine binds maximally to α-2 receptors in the early dark period when rats wake up and become active. A circadian rhythm of circulating corticosterone is partially responsible as shown by the fact that α-2 receptor binding is proportional to corticosterone levels in the blood (38–41). The PVN releases corticotropin-releasing factor (CRF), which in turn releases pituitary adrenocorticotropic hormone (ACTH), which controls the production of corticosterone. This glucocorticoid potentiates carbohydrate metabolism, and at the same time it feeds back to the PVN to potentiate α-2 receptor binding and thereby facilitate appetite. The animal gets a relatively specific appetite for carbohydrate that is induced by the action of norepinephrine and NPY binding

to neuronal receptors in the PVN. Thus when the animal wakes for "breakfast" there is a coordinated neural–hormonal receptor cascade that leads to rapid energy availability. This brain–body–behavior circuitry, as discovered by the Leibowitz laboratory, is under the control of another hypothalamic mechanism. Predictably, it is the suprachiasmatic nucleus (SCN), which contains the cells for the master circadian clock. Less is known about rhythms of neurotransmitter release and receptor changes in the lateral hypothalamus, but it is clear that sensitivity to some monoamine and peptide neurotransmitters varies with time of day (38).

Parada et al. (49) have focused on the D_2 dopamine receptor and asked why psychotic patients who receive D_2 antagonists such as haloperidol or sulperide tend to gain weight. In a new rat model of obesity, chronic sulperide caused obesity, and the effect could be obtained even with local lateral hypothalamic injections. Again, there may be combined behavioral and hormonal effects, this time involving hypothalamic control of (a) locomotion leading to food, (b) food intake, and (c) an estrogenic system that affects body weight. Thus D_2 agonists or antagonists could be theoretically useful in suppressing or inducing food intake, respectively, in selected patients; however, clinical evidence is lacking (29). Part of the problem is that dopaminergic drugs have other effects in other parts of the brain. For example, raclopride given i.p. is a D_2 antagonist that was shown to suppress the intake of a sweet solution in a manner suggesting suppression of reward properties. Similarly, pimozide i.p. caused extinction of bar-pressing responses for food. These drug actions are executed, in part, in the nucleus accumbens (25,54,65). Dopamine seems to potentiate feeding and reward in the accumbens even though it can suppress feeding in the LH. Thus a "dirty drug" like amphetamine, which releases dopamine as well as other monoamines, will be both an addictive psychostimulant in the accumbens and an appetite suppressant in the lateral hypothalamus. Sulperide is the opposite; it probably blocks locomotion and reward in the accumbens, while potentiating them in the lateral hypothalamus. Hopefully future characterization of the dopamine receptor subtypes, their rhythms, and their neurochemical synergists such as hormones and peptides will permit therapeutic control of appetite without side effects (10).

To summarize these basic neurochemical mechanisms, we have updated a diagram that indicates how monoamine systems may interact with medial and lateral hypothalamic neurons to modulate their overall function (Fig. 3). This model does not encompass all the observations that have been reported (for more comprehensive reviews, the reader is referred to refs. 5,10,12,20,22,23,25,28,37, 41,50,52,65). In brief, the far lateral hypothalamus contains dopamine fibers of the nigrostriatal tract on their way to the sensory–motor activation and orientation systems. The dopamine neurons of the mesolimbic system

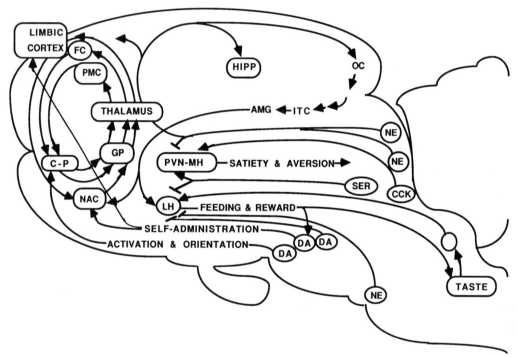

FIG. 3. Functional and neurochemical anatomy of feeding. Some of the neurotransmitters, pathways, and functions involved in feeding and its reinforcements are shown in a side view of the brain. Sharp arrows indicate excitation of the labeled function; blunt arrows are inhibition. 1. First is a system for preparedness: dorsal norepinephrine (NE) cell groups to limbic cortex, frontal cortex (FC), hippocampus (HIPP), and optic cortex (OC). 2. Visual feature detection: optic cortex to infratemporal cortex (ITC) to the amygdala (AMG). 3. Activation and orientation: substantia nigra and other dopamine (DA) inputs to caudato-putamen (C-P) for response to stress and novelty. The following additional sequence would theoretically be sufficient for feeding to occur. 4. Antisatiety: increased activity in the dorsal noradrenergic inputs to the paraventricular nucleus (PVN) and medial hypothalamus (MH) to counteract the action of serotonin (SER) and cholecystokinin (CCK) on that satiety system. 5. Decreased satiety and aversion: decreased PVN and MH output. 6. Disinhibition of feeding and its rewards: decreased activity in ascending pathways from ventral norepinephrine (NE), epinephrine (not shown), and DA cell groups, which otherwise inhibit LH feeding and reward. 7. Feeding and reward: augmented medial forebrain bundle activity including lateral hypothalamic (LH) inputs to the ventral tegmental area (DA) and other sites for enhancing food-related responses and their repetition. 8. Self-administration: excitation of DA inputs to the nucleus accumbens (NAC) to facilitate other inputs, e.g., from the AMG, and outputs to the globus pallidus (GP) for reinforcement. (Adapted from Hoebel, refs. 22 and 23, with permission.)

also pass through on their way to the nucleus accumbens and prefrontal cortex. Damage might impair self-administered reward functions. These dopamine paths are also shown at the left of the diagram in Fig. 2. A lesion here would interrupt the path and cause some degree of akinesia and aphagia. Hyperfunction might cause some type of bulimia. The LH has β-adrenergic synapses that inhibit some aspect of feeding, and may contain some of the terminations of dopamine or adrenergic neurons from ascending midbrain paths. A lesion here would destroy feeding neurons and contribute to aphagia, but selective depletion of the β-adrenergic system would disinhibit feeding and lead to obesity. The medial and paraventricular hypothalamus has α-1 and α-2 adrenergic synapses that presumably excite or inhibit satiety functions. A lesion would impair satiety and lead to obesity; a selective depletion of α-2 input or a deficit of α-2 receptor function should theoretically promote satiety. On the other hand, loss of the α-1 function would theoretically contribute to obesity. Dopamine has an action at D_2 receptors in the LH where it suppresses a feeding system. This partially accounts for amphetamine-induced anorexia and neuroleptic-induced hyperphagia. Natural overexcitation of this hypothalamic dopamine subsystem might contribute to some aspect of anorexia nervosa, whereas a functional deficit would promote obesity. Dopamine is also important in the mesolimbic projection to the nucleus accumbens and prefrontal cortex. This system is thought to be involved in some aspect of taste and nutritional reinforcement of feeding behavior (20,25,27,54).

Recent and future discoveries are bound to show a role for other neurochemicals in the control of feeding behavior. γ-Aminobutyric acid (GABA) is a neurotransmitter that is found in high concentrations in the medial hypothalamus. The concentration increases during conditions such as hypoglycemia-induced feeding. Predictably a GABA agonist increased feeding when injected in the medial hypothalamus, and a GABA antagonist blocked the effect.

Opioids

Injection of β-endorphin in the medial hypothalamus induced feeding (25,42). This may relate to the discovery that genetically obese mice and rats have higher concentrations of β-endorphin in the hypophysis and plasma than their lean littermates. Margules's group also found that naloxone given to block endogenous opioids decreased food intake in these obese animals. On this basis they postulated that dysfunction of β-endorphin secretion might produce obesity. Carr (7) finds that food deprivation potentiates the lateral hypothalamic feeding–reward system via an opioid system that involves the central gray, and Wise (65) suggests the hypothalamus may also link to an opioid reward system connected to the mesolimbic dopamine system in the midbrain (Fig. 3). Morley relates the loss of brain opioid systems to anorexia in the elderly (46).

REGULATORY PEPTIDES WITH INTEGRATIVE FUNCTIONS

Some peptides are both hormones and neurotransmitters. As such they are capable of modulating both physiological functions, and specific behaviors. The premier example is angiotensin that controls blood pressure in a variety of ways including cardiovascular effects, hormonal effects, and thirst. Angiotensin acts as a hormone in the body and a neurotransmitter in the brain. It is a neurotransmitter in a neural circuit that is intimately involved in water intake. In combination with aldosterone, brain angiotensin also controls salt appetite (for review, see refs. 13,25).

Two "energy control" peptides have been discovered. NPY is, in part, a cotransmitter with norepinephrine in the PVN. Like norepinephrine, NPY induces food intake. If the animal is given a choice of macronutrients, NPY injected in the hypothalamus will induce a strong appetite for carbohydrate. Galanin is another hypothalamic peptide that works in concert with NPY, but its neural actions are apparently geared for fat intake (38,39).

Three "satiety peptides" have been shown to suppress food intake. The already classic example is CCK (17,18,45). It promotes digestion and a feeling of stomach fullness by actions in the gastrointestinal tract. It also is a neurotransmitter in neurons that project from the vagal sensory nucleus (nucleus tractus solitarius: NTS) to the medial hypothalamus. When injected into the MH or PVN region, CCK decreased food intake in mildly deprived animals. When we injected CCK antagonists into the hypothalamus, these drugs competed with the brain's own CCK, with the result that rats overate (25). Therefore a normal function of endogenous CCK must be to prevent eating. Bombesin also serves a satiety function in the hypothalamus, as does neurotensin. The interactions between these peptides that suppress food intake is not yet known. Recent evidence suggests that CCK may work synergistically with serotonin, which would help to explain serotonergic satiety and the appetite-suppressant effect of serotonergic drugs such as d-fenfluramine (9,23,30).

CCK may promote the release of oxytocin under certain conditions, and this could cause nausea in rats. CCK satiety without evidence of nausea has also been demonstrated. Oxytocin nausea may prove important in the generation of conditioned taste aversions. The oxytocin discovery also suggests that human radiation sickness, some chemotherapy anorexia, and cancer-induced anorexia might be prevented by treatment with antagonists for the peptides that induce nausea in humans (45,60).

BRAIN STIMULATION:
ELECTRICALLY INDUCED FEEDING,
REWARD, AND PUNISHMENT

Electrodes implanted in the medial or lateral hypothalamus do exactly what one would predict. Medial stimulation inhibits feeding and lateral stimulation induces it. Medial stimulation is aversive, however, and tends to interrupt any ongoing behavior. Lateral stimulation is rewarding and can induce a number of behavior patterns including eating, drinking, gnawing, and sometimes mating. Chronic stimulation for 20 hours a day can cause so much eating it will make the rat fat. The animal will even voluntarily stimulate itself enough to become obese from self-stimulation-induced feeding (20,24,25).

Rats will turn on a stimulator 3,000 times an hour to get half-second bursts of self-stimulation in the lateral hypothalamus. The effect releases dopamine in the accumbens and is dopamine dependent. With some electrode placements, self-stimulation directly activates dopamine neurons that course through the lateral hypothalamus. Other electrodes apparently activate dopamine neurons indirectly via a descending path to the midbrain (Fig. 3). Authors variously suggest that dopamine serves an arousal, motivation, reward, or salience role in self-stimulation.

Self-stimulation, when it will induce feeding, is closely linked to feeding. The rate of self-stimulation decreases after a meal or after intragastric or intravenous glucose infusions. Injections of anorectic drugs, PPA or fenfluramine, also inhibit self-stimulation (20,24,25).

Manipulations that increase feeding cause a parallel increase in lateral hypothalamic self-stimulation. Food deprivation, diabetes, medial hypothalamic lesions, or 6-hydroxy-dopamine injections that cause hyperphagia can all augment self-stimulation. Just like feeding, self-stimulation remains augmented after the VMH lesions until the rat reaches its stable body weight plateau, and then feeding and self-stimulation return towards normal. The exception to this rule is 2DG, which increases feeding, but for some reason inhibits self-stimulation (20).

In the midhypothalamus, stimulation is rewarding, as in the far lateral region, but is also has an aversive component like the medial region. We use a test program in which rats will self-stimulate at about 300 responses/5 min, alternated with 5-minute tests of stimulation–escape when the animals voluntarily press a second lever about 10–20 times for

5-second escape from automatic stimulation. Stimulation–escape behavior usually varies inversely with self-stimulation. For example, force-feeding or the anorectic drug PPA increases stimulation–escape and decreases self-stimulation.

We believe that self-stimulation and stimulation–escape in this brain region may reflect the rewards and aversions that control food intake. Self-stimulation gives a reward something like the rewards of eating, but after too much food the dual system shifts to a greater predominance of the aversive component. This presumably punishes the animal for any additional eating. Hypothalamic stimulation gives the experimenter a way to tap into the substrate that controls the behavioral aspects of energy homeostasis.

RECORDING FROM NEURAL NETWORKS

It is possible to record from a self-stimulation electrode. When this was done in the monkey, it was discovered that single neural units near the lateral hypothalamic electrode fired when the monkey was ready to eat. If bananas were preferred that day, then the sight or taste of bananas fired the nerve. If peanuts were preferred, then peanuts fired it. The rate of neural firing was also proportional to the degree of food deprivation. Apparently these researchers were recording from the same type of reward neurons that support self-stimulation and feeding (52).

By combining neural recording with iontophoretic injection of neurochemicals, it has been possible to discover the effect of neuromodulators on glucoreceptive and insulin-receptive neurons in the rat hypothalamus. Oomura suggested that a population of VMH glucoreceptive neurons are suited to play a role in satiety, whereas lateral hypothalamic insulin-receptive neurons are hyperpolarized by the action of glucose plus insulin and thus would only fire when the animal needs to find a renewed source of food and fuel. Norepinephrine iontophoresed onto these LH neurons helped to inhibit their firing rate. This corroborated our suggestion that the ascending ventral noradrenergic bundle projects in part to the LH, where it may help to inhibit feeding and maintain a normal body weight.

It has now become possible to record from hypothalamic neurons without anesthesia in freely moving rats. Cells were discovered that decreased their firing rate when the animal tasted glucose and increased firing in response to an annoying pinch or foot shock. Such cells "learned" to respond to discriminative stimuli that signaled forthcoming glucose or shock. The role of such cells in a network controlling feeding is not yet known, but it is clear that hypothalamic neurons could be involved in the decision to eat or not eat. Some hypothalamic neurons are sensitive to circulating glucose and integrate chemosensory inputs from many parts of the brain and body. The neurons not sensitive to glucose respond best to external stimuli such as meaningful visual signals. Somehow the network combines these signals from internal, external, and secondary reinforcers in a manner that contributes to the control of operant feeding behavior and parasympathetic–sympathetic balance (22,48,52,57).

A hierarchy of local networks for energy control extends all the way from the hindbrain to the prefrontal cortex (22). The brainstem networks in the NTS and parabrachial nucleus (PBN) must be influenced by the hypothalamus because LH stimulation that elicits feeding mimics some taste effects on taste relay neurons and modulates hindbrain feeding reflexes. The hypothalamus also interacts with higher forebrain networks including the nucleus accumbens, amygdala, and prefrontal cortex (25).

LEARNED NEURAL PATTERNS AND LEARNED NEUROMODULATOR RELEASE

Only in invertebrate slugs, *Limax* and *Aplysia,* has a true computational neural network analysis been attempted (16). A mathematical model of taste processing in the garden slug has accurately predicted the existence of a slow cyclic (50-Hz) variation in neuronal excitability on which the action potentials are superimposed. This phase relationship serves to identify separate cells responding to the same signal, so that their output to a feature detector cell will summate and create a "meaningful" signal based on parallel processing followed by convergence to an output cell. In this slug, outputs are coded "go" or "no go" based on taste and learned aversions.

Scott and his colleagues used learned aversion to condition neural responses and neurotransmitter release in rats. A saccharin taste that was paired with experimentally induced nausea soon came to produce a bitter-type neural response instead of sweet-type neural pattern in the hindbrain NTS (57). It also caused a shift from dopamine increase to dopamine decrease in the forebrain accumbens (29,30). The behavioral response to this paradigm is to avoid eating that flavor. The results are interpreted to mean that the hindbrain taste nucleus codes on a safety–toxicity dimension as well as taste per se. Accumbens dopamine followed the satiety–toxicity feature and therefore may modulate withdrawal and negative reinforcement (30). Moreover, while dopamine was decreasing, accumbens acetylcholine was increasing. Therefore acetylcholine might play some role in the avoidance response, but this new hypothesis is still being tested.

Possible interactions between neuromodulatory events in different networks are starting to come to light. Serotonin is known to play some role in satiety, perhaps in combination with CCK (9); so we predicted serotonin might increase in the hypothalamus as a conditioned response to prior nausea. It did. Thus hypothalamic serotonin release was rising while accumbens dopamine was falling (21,28).

Even the same neuromodulator may change in different directions in different areas. For example, Rada and Hernandez found that when the amygdala was electrically stimulated to cause epileptic-like activity, dopamine decreased in the accumbens, but increased in the prefrontal cortex (see 28). Le Moal (*unpublished data*) suggested that the goal of psychopharmacology and psychotherapy is to adjust the interacting neurochemical influences to provide the normal balance of neuromodulators in these forebrain regions.

Modern behaviorists point out that Pavlovian conditioning is the learning of relations among events in the animal's environment (51). The study of feeding as an integrated combination of environmental and physiological events expands this view to include the learning of nutrition and toxicity. The neural basis of food acceptability based on anticipated consequences is an important adjunct to purely homeostatic considerations (8,30,55).

In summary, Pavlov conditioned salivary secretion; we have conditioned neurotransmitter secretion. In other words, neurotransmitters in the forebrain are released to modulate networks that control ingestive decision making. Dopamine in the nucleus accumbens is somehow involved in salience, locomotion, and behavior reinforcement. It is released in the nucleus accumbens during a number of feeding situations as measured by microdialysis. When a novel taste was paired with nausea, the taste became a conditioned stimulus for serotonin release in the hypothalamus and dopamine decrease in the nucleus accumbens. Theoretically this depotentiates forward locomotion and ingestion.

Microdialysis shows us that part of what the animal is learning is to release neuromodulators such as dopamine, acetylcholine, and serotonin. These classically conditioned neurotransmitters are capable of altering the animal's instrumental responses for food. As another example, a taste paired with a stomach load of caloric food became a conditioned stimulus that increased accumbens dopamine release. Self-injection of accumbens dopamine is reinforcing. Therefore it is logical to surmise that the conditioned taste will reinforce ingestive behavior by virtue of neural activity in accumbens circuits modulated by dopamine. The analysis links Pavlovian reflex conditioning to Skinnerian response conditioning with dopamine as the bridge (30). What remains is to find out exactly what dopamine is doing to increase the probability of responses. Presumably it alters neural connections in networks, such as the accumbens based on neuronal activity at the time of learning. These connections then remain as a memory that affects that animal's stimulus choices and response choices in the future.

Animals and people not only learn what to eat this way, they may also learn to medicate themselves for mental problems by using food to release neurotransmitters that have curative properties (67). For example, some depressed people might learn that serotonin released by eating is as helpful as serotonin boosted by fluoxetine (Prozac).

In addition to learned ingestive behavior and learned self-medication, one can add learned addictions. Most drugs of abuse increase extracellular dopamine in the nucleus accumbens, and most psychostimulants can increase serotonin as well. Thus drug abuse is not only euphorogenic, it may be temporarily therapeutic. Unfortunately, it is addictive by virtue of its actions in the behavior reinforcement system, which evolved for feeding and other behaviors that require learning and memory (25).

METABOLIC MEASUREMENTS ONLINE

It is usually assumed that the neural, behavioral, and metabolic abnormalities provoked by the experimenter are an exaggerated expression of normal mechanisms. Microdialysis allowed measures of extracellular neurotransmitters in freely moving rats. Recently blood glucose and basal metabolic rate have also gone "online." Campfield's group (6) finds that venous blood glucose falls and then starts to rise just before every meal in an undisturbed rat. Nicolaidis's group (47) used a computerized O_2–CO_2 chamber to find that basal metabolic rate falls before a meal. Friedman (15) suggests that it is this total metabolic signal reflecting glucose, fat, and protein utilization, probably in the liver, that signals the brain when it is time for a short-term adjustment in fuel intake, i.e., a meal. In summary, there is a new thrust in feeding research in which electrophysiological, metabolic, and neurochemical variations have been detected in animals eating spontaneously. Even receptor binding will soon be monitored in "real time" using brain imaging techniques in humans while they eat.

PRENATAL CAUSES OF OBESITY

It is well known that testosterone programs adult sexual behavior during an early "organization" phase that begins in the womb. Recently Epstein's group (13) discovered that salt deprivation or its chemical consequence, aldosterone and angiotensin, given to pregnant rats or newborns can cause a lifelong avidity for salt. The animals "remember" months later and consume excess salt "just in case it is needed," even when it is not.

Now this principle has been extended to obesity research. Jones (33) reports that food deprivation followed by refeeding, or just insulin injections, in the third trimester of pregnancy causes birth of rat pups that will grow up to be overweight. There is evidence for this in humans from World War II as well as in laboratory rats.

INDIVIDUAL DIFFERENCES

Other laboratories are showing that they can predict adult obesity based on a baby rat's choice of carbohydrates, fat, and protein in the diet. Animals from the same litter will tend to have different body weights. Self-choice of a sucrose diet predicts a heavier adult (31,39).

CONCLUSIONS

We have been very selective in an attempt to illustrate important aspects of the mechanisms for the control of body weight. We have overemphasized the hypothalamus and its inputs because this is the best studied region and one that appears capable of integrating the autonomic and somatic aspects of energy homeostasis. Some features of the model are admittedly speculative in our effort to tie together the results of several techniques: lesions, recording, neuropharmacology, electrical stimulation, and neurochemistry. Figure 3 illustrates a few of the many pathways for feeding functions. It shows that it is becoming possible to label certain anatomically defined pathways for some of their functions. The neurotransmitters are known for some of these paths. At the diagram's core can be seen the classic MH satiety and LH feeding systems. The evidence suggests that norepinephrine and NPY in the PVN is part of a CRF–ACTH–corticosterone-linked system for carbohydrate control through physiological reflexes and behavioral responses. Under other less well-studied circumstances, norepinephrine or epinephrine and dopamine can act in the LH to curb feeding. Serotonin is shown in Figure 3 as potentiating the classic PVN–MH satiety system or inhibiting an LH feeding system. Also shown is the LH self-stimulation reward system that has a close link to the reinforcement properties of food. Presumably the various pathways ascending from the hindbrain and midbrain bring information from the cranial nerves and brainstem centers to be integrated with the locally obtained information from receptors that sample hypothalamic blood.

The biggest single advance since the first edition of this chapter is the discovery of neuropeptides that influence appetite and satiety. Some of them such as NPY are colocalized, in part, in the same neurons with monoamines. Some, such as CCK, may give temporal and behavioral specificity to the monoamines when released at appropriate times. Along with new drugs to manipulate these neurochemical systems came new understanding that appetite for specific macronutrients is controlled by specific neurotransmitters. In some cases, notably serotonin, the neurotransmitter that affects diet choice is itself affected by the diet under special circumstances.

Behavioral paradigms such as learned taste preference have been used for electrophysiological and neurochemical studies of brain circuitry. It has become clear that taste is not just coded for what is in the mouth; it is coded in neural networks such as the NTS, and in neuromodulators such as dopamine on a safety–toxicity dimension that reflects past experience. The ultimate in long-term memory is the discovery that experiences in the womb can program the brain for excess salt intake or excess fat storage in adulthood.

REFERENCES

1. Blundell JE. Serotonin manipulations and the structure of feeding behavior. In: Nicolaidis S, ed. *Serotoninergic system, feeding and body weight regulation.* London: Academic Press, 1986:39–56.
2. Blundell JE, Tombros E, Rogers PJ, Latham CJ. Behavioural analysis of feeding: implications for the pharmacological manipulation of food intake in animals and man. *Prog Neuropharmacol* 1980; 4:319–26.
3. Bray GA. Hypothalamic and genetic obesity: an appraisal of the autonomic hypothesis and the endocrine hypothesis. In: Sullivan AC, Garattini S., eds. *Novel approaches and drugs for obesity.* London: John Libbey, 1985;119–37.
4. Bray GA. Genetic and hypothalamic mechanisms for obesity—finding the needle in the haystack. *Am J Clin Nutr* 1989;50:891–902.
5. Bray GA, Ricquier D, Spiegelman BM (eds). *Obesity: towards a molecular approach.* New York: Wiley-Liss, 1990.
6. Campfield LA, Smith FJ. Systemic factors in the control of food intake: evidence for patterns as signals. In: Stricker EM, ed. *Handbook of behavioral neurobiology.* New York: Plenum Press, 1990; 183–206.
7. Carr KD. Central nervous system opioid mechanisms that mediate stimulation-induced feeding in the rat. In: Schneider LH, Cooper SJ, Halmi KA, eds. *The psychobiology of human eating disorders.* New York: The New York Academy of Sciences, 1989;503–5.
8. Collier G. Operant methodologies for studying feed-

ing and drinking. In: Toates FM, Rowland NE, eds. *Feeding and drinking.* Amsterdam: Elsevier Science Publishing, 1987;37–76.

9. Cooper SJ, Dourish CT, Barber DJ. Reversal of the anorectic effect of (+)-fenfluramine in the rat by selective cholecystokinin receptor antagonist MK-329. *Br J Pharmacol* 1990;99:65–70.

10. Cooper SJ, Rusk IN, Clifton PG. Dopamine, D1 and D2 receptor subtypes, and feeding behaviour. In: Cooper SJ, Liebman JM, eds. *Neuropharmacology of appetite.* London: Oxford University Press [*in press*].

11. Deutsh JA. Food intake: gastric factors. In: Stricker EM, ed. *Handbook of behavioral neurobiology.* New York: Plenum Press, 1990;151–82.

12. Dourish CT. The role of multiple serotonin receptors in the control of feeding. In: Cooper SJ, Leibman JM, eds. *Neuropharmacology of appetite.* London: Oxford University Press [*in press*].

13. Epstein AN. The physiology of thirst. In: Pfaff DW, ed. *The physiological mechanisms of motivation.* New York: Springer-Verlag, 1982;164–214.

14. Fernstrom JD. Brain serotonin, food intake regulation, and obesity. In: Bjorntorp P, Brodoff BN, eds. *Obesity.* Philadelphia: JB Lippincott, 1992.

15. Friedman MI. Metabolic control of calorie intake. In: Friedman MI, Tordoff ME, Kare MR, eds. *Chemical senses; appetite and nutrition, vol. 4.* New York: Marcel Dekker, 1991;19–38.

16. Gelperin A, Tank DW. Odour-modulated collective network oscillations of olfactory interneurons in a terrestrial mollusc. *Nature* 1990;345:437–40.

17. Gibbs J, Smith GP. Effects of brain-gut peptides on satiety. In: Bjorntorp P, Brodoff BN, eds. *Obesity.* Philadelphia: JB Lippincott, 1992.

18. Gibbs J, Smith GP. Gut peptides and feeding behavior: the model of cholecystokinin. In: Ritter RC, Ritter S, Barnes CD, eds. *Feeding behavior neural and humoral controls.* Orlando: Academic Press, 1986; 329–52.

19. Grill HJ, Kaplan JM. Caudal brainstem participates in the distributed neural control of feeding. In: Stricker EM, ed. *Handbook of behavioral neurobiology.* New York: Plenum Press, 1990;125–49.

20. Hernandez L, Hoebel BG. Hypothalamic reward and aversion: a link between metabolism and behavior. In: Veale WL, Lederis K, ed. *Current studies of hypothalamic function, metabolism and behavior.* Basel: Karger, 1978;72–92.

21. Hernandez L, Hoebel BG. Basic mechanisms of feeding and weight regulation. In: Stunkard AJ, ed. *Obesity.* Philadelphia: WB Saunders, 1980;25–47.

22. Hernandez L, Murzi E, Schwartz DH, Hoebel BG. Neuroelectrophysiological and neurochemical approach to a hierarchical feeding organization. In: Bjorntorp P, Brodoff B, eds. *Obesity.* Philadelphia: JB Lippincott, 1992;171–83.

23. Hernandez L, Parada M, Baptista T, et al. Hypothalamic serotonin in treatments for feeding disorders and depression as studied by microdialysis. *J Clin Psychiatry* 1991;52:12(suppl)32–40.

24. Hoebel BG. Neurotransmitters in the control of feeding and its rewards: monoamines, opiates and brain-gut peptides. In: Stunkard AJ, Stellar E, eds. *Eating and its disorders.* New York: Association for Research in Nervous and Mental Disease, Raven Press, 1984;15–38.

25. Hoebel BG. Neuroscience and motivation: pathways and peptides that define motivation. In: Atkinson RC, Herrnstein RJ, Lindzey G, Luce RD, eds. *Stevens' handbook of experimental psychology.* New York: John Wiley & Sons, 1988;547–625.

26. Hoebel BG, Leibowitz SF. Brain monoamines in the regulation of self-stimulation, feeding and body weight. In: Weiner H, Hofer MA, Stunkard AJ, eds. *Brain, behavior & bodily disease.* New York: Association for Research in Nervous and Mental Disease, Raven Press, 1981;103–142.

27. Hoebel BG, Novin D, eds. *The neural basis of feeding and reward.* Brunswick, ME, Haer Institute, 1982.

28. Hoebel BG, Hernandez L, Schwartz DH, Mark GP, Hunter GA. Microdialysis studies of brain norepinephrine, serotonin and dopamine release during ingestive behavior: theoretical and clinical implications. In: Schneider LH, Cooper SJ, Halmi KA. *The psychobiology of human eating disorders: preclinical and clinical perspectives. Ann NY Acad Sci* 1989;575:171–93.

29. Hoebel BG, Hernandez L, Mark GP, et al. Brain microdialysis as a molecular approach to obesity: serotonin, dopamine, cyclic-amp. In: Bray G, Ricquier D, Spiegleman B, eds. *Obesity: towards a molecular approach.* New York: Alan R. Liss, 1990;45–61.

30. Hoebel BG, Mark GP, Hernandez L. New approaches to the neuropharmacology of appetite. In: Cooper SJ, Liebman JM, eds. *The neuropharmacology of appetite.* New York: Oxford University Press [*in press*].

31. Hoebel BG, Leibowitz SL, Hernandez L. Neurochemistry of anorexia and bulimia. In: Anderson H, ed. *The biology of feast and famine: relevance to eating disorders.* New York: Academic Press 1992; 21–45.

32. Inoue S. Animal models of obesity: hypothalamic lesions. In: Bjorntorp P, Brodoff BN, eds. *Obesity.* Philadelphia: JB Lippincott, 1992;266–278.

33. Jacobs BL, Fornal C. Activity of brain serotonergic neurons in the behaving animal. *Pharmacol Rev* 1991;43:563–578.

34. Jones AP, Dayries M. Maternal hormone manipulations and the development of obesity in rats. *Physiol Behav* 1990;47:1107–1110.

35. Kaye WH, Gwirtsman HE, Brewerton TD, George DT, Wurtman RJ. Bingeing behavior and plasma amino acids: a possible involvement of brain serotonin in bulimia nervosa. *Psychiatr Res* 1988;23:31–43.

36. Keesey RE. A set-point analysis of the regulation of body weight. In: Stunkard AJ, ed. *Obesity.* Philadelphia: WB Saunders, 1980;144–65.

37. Koob GF, Goeders NE. Neuroanatomical substrates of drug self-administration. In: Liebman JM, Cooper SJ, eds. *The neuropharmacological basis of reward.* Oxford: Oxford University Press, 1989; 214–63.

38. Leibowitz SF. Neurochemical control of macronutri-

ent intake. In: Oomura T, et al., eds. *Progress in obesity research 1990.* London: John Libbey & Co., 1991.

39. Leibowitz SF. Brain neurotransmitters and hormones in relation to eating behavior and its disorders. In Bjorntorp P, Brodoff BN, eds. *Obesity.* Philadelphia: JB Lippincott, 1992;184–205.

40. Leibowitz SF, Shor-Posner. Hypothalamic monoamine systems for control of food intake: analysis of meal patterns and macronutrient selection. In: Carruba MO, Blundell JE, eds. *Pharmacology of eating disorders: theoretical and clinical developments.* New York: Raven Press, 1986;29–50.

41. Leibowitz SF, Myers RD. The neurochemistry of ingestion: chemical stimulation of the brain and in vivo measurement of transmitter release. In: Toates FM, Rowland NE, eds. *Feeding and drinking.* Amsterdam: Elsevier Science Publishers, 1987; 271–315.

42. Margules DL, Moisset B, Lewis MJ, Shibuya H, Pert CB. Beta-endorphin is associated with overeating in genetically obese mice (ob/ob) and rats (fa/fa). *Science* 1978;202:988–991.

43. Marshall JP. Brain function: neural adaptations and recovery from injury. *Ann Rev Physiol* 1984; 35:277–308.

44. McGowan MK, Andrews KM, Grossman, SP. Effects of chronic intrahypothalamic infusion of insulin on food intake and diurnal meal patterning in the rat. *Behav Neurosci* 1990;104:371–381.

45. Moran TH, McHugh PR. Gastric mechanisms in CCK satiety. In: Dourish CT, Cooper SJ, Iversen SD, Iversen LL, eds. *Multiple cholecystokinin receptors in the CNS.* New York: Oxford University Press [in press].

46. Morley JE, Silver AJ, Miller DK, Rubenstein LZ. The anorexia of the elderly. In: Schneider LH, Cooper SJ, Halmi KA, eds. *The psychobiology of human eating disorders.* New York: Annals of the New York Academy of Sciences, 1989;50–9.

47. Nicolaids S, Even P. Metabolic action of leptogenic (anorexigenic) agents on feeding body weight. In: Carruba MO, Blundell JE, eds. *Pharmacology of eating disorders: theoretical and clinical developments.* New York: Raven Press, 1986;117–131.

48. Oomura Y, Sasaki K, Hanai K. Chemical and neuronal regulation of food intake. In: Oomura Y, Tarui S, Inoue S, Shimizu T, eds. *Progress in obesity research 1990.* London: Libbey, 1990;3–12.

49. Parada MA, Hernandez L, Puig De Parada M, Paez X, Hoebel BG. Dopamine in the lateral hypothalamus may be involved in the inhibition of locomotion related to food and water seeking. *Brain Res Bull* 1990;25:961–968.

50. Powley TL, Berthoud H. Participation of the vagus and other autonomic nerves in the control of food intake. In: Ritter RC, Ritter S, Barnes CD, eds. *Feeding behavior neural and humoral controls.* Orlando: Academic Press, 1986;67–101.

51. Rescorla RA. Pavlovian conditioning: it's not what you think it is. *Am Psychol* 1988;43:151–60.

52. Rolls ET. Neuronal activity related to the control of feeding. In: Ritter RC, Ritter S, Barnes CD, eds. *Feeding behavior neural and humoral controls.* Orlando: Academic Press, 1986;163–90.

53. Rowland NE, Carlton J. Dexfenfluramine: effects on food intake in various animal models. *Clin Neuropharmacol* 1988;2:S33–S50.

54. Schneider LH. Orosensory self-stimulation by sucrose involves brain dopaminergic mechanisms. In: Schneider LH, Cooper SJ, Halmi KA, eds. *The psychobiology of human eating disorders.* New York: Annals of the New York Academy of Sciences, 1989;307–20.

55. Sclafani A. Nutritionally based learned flavor preferences in rats. In: Capaldi ED, Powley TL, eds. *Taste experience and feeding.* Washington, DC: Amer Psychol Assoc 1990;139–156.

56. Sclafani A. Dietary obesity models. In: Bjorntorp P, Brodoff BN, eds. *Obesity.* Philadelphia: JB Lippincott, 1992;241–248.

57. Scott TR. Gustatory control of food selection. In: Stricker EM, ed. *Handbook of behavioral neurobiology.* New York: Plenum Press, 1990;243–62.

58. Steffens AB, Strubbe JH, Balkan B, Scheurink AJW. Neuroendocrine mechanisms involved in regulation of body weight, food intake and metabolism. *Neurosci Biobehav Rev* 1990;14:305–13.

59. Stricker EM. Brain neurochemistry and the control of food intake. In: Satinoff E, Teitelbaum P, eds. *Handbook of behavioral neurobiology, Volume 6: Motivation.* New York: Plenum Press, 1983;329–66.

60. Stricker EM. Homeostatic origins of ingestive behavior. In: Stricker EM, ed. *Handbook of behavioral neurobiology, Volume 10: Neurobiology of food and fluid intake.* New York: Plenum Press, 1990;45–60.

61. Teitelbaum P, Schallert T, Whishaw IQ. Sources of spontaneity in motivated behavior. In: Satinoff E, Teitelbaum P, eds. *Handbook of behavioral neurobiology: motivation, vol. 6.* New York: Plenum Press, 1983;23–65.

62. Vasselli JR, Maggio CA. Mechanisms of appetite and body-weight regulation. In: Frankle RT, Yang M-U, eds. *Obesity and weight control: the health professionals guide to understanding and treatment.* New York: Aspen Publishing, 1987;17–34.

63. Weingarten HP, Chang PE, McDonald TJ. Comparison of the metabolic and behavioral disturbances following paraventricular- and ventromedial-hypothalamic lesions. *Brain Res Bull* 1985:14;551–9.

64. Wellman PJ. A review of the physiological bases of the anoretic action of phenylpropanolamine (d,l-norepinephrine). *Neurosci Biobehav Rev* 1990; 14:339–55.

65. Wise RA. Common neural basis for brain stimulation reward, drug reward, and food reward. In: Hoebel BG, Novin D, eds. *The neural basis of feeding and reward.* Brunswick, ME: Haer Institute for Electrophysiological Research, 1982;445–54.

66. Woods SC, Porte D, Strubbe JH, Steffens AB. The relationships among body fat, feeding, and insulin. In: Ritter RC, Ritter S, Barnes CD, eds. *Feeding behavior neural and humoral controls.* Orlando: Academic Press, 1986;315–27.

67. Wurtman RJ, Wurtman JJ. Carbohydrate craving, obesity and brain serotonin. In: Nicolaidis S, ed. *Serotoninergic system, feeding and body weight regulation.* London: Academic Press, 1986;99–103.

Obesity: Theory and Therapy, Second Edition,
edited by A. J. Stunkard and T. A. Wadden.
Raven Press, Ltd., New York © 1993.

4

Pharmacological Aspects of Appetite

John E. Blundell and Clare L. Lawton

*BioPsychology Group, Department of Psychology, University of Leeds,
Leeds LS2 9JT, United Kingdom*

How easy is it for chemical agents to suppress the expression of human appetite? Can drugs be more effective than other therapies in the treatment of human obesity? Is the inhibition of feeding by drugs in animals a good predictor of the likely effectiveness of these drugs on humans? These questions are central to any consideration of the pharmacology of appetite. According to notions of a biological imperative underlying the causation of behavior, it might be supposed that the identification of a neural network regulating energy balance would provide the substrate for the actions of a large number of chemicals that could modify eating. Indeed, there are now many studies showing that chemicals suppress food consumption in rats and other experimental animals. However, one major methodological problem is how to decide when food is left uneaten by rats because of drugs intervening in processes that tend to match food intake to nutritional requirements, and when it is due to some nonspecific blockade or impediment of eating. Moreover, the existence of a biochemical substrate controlling feeding and energy balance is not a sufficient reason alone to claim that a chemical basis for drug action will automatically lead to potent and permanent pharmacological control of appetite. Drugs certainly can modify the expression of human appetite, but their actions need to be considered in relation to knowledge of appetite control in general and not simply in relation to biochemical targets. This should provide a realistic

basis for understanding drug action and for assessing potential therapeutic benefits. In turn, such an exercise could guide the thinking of regulatory authorities, the pharmaceutical industry, appetite researchers, and clinicians. Although it will involve consideration of drug research in animals, it is primarily an evaluation of the effects of drugs on the appetite response in humans.

APPETITE, DRUGS, AND OVERWEIGHT—A PROPOSAL

Appetite can be considered as a phenomenon that links biological happenings (under the skin) with environmental events (beyond the skin). Indeed, the expression of appetite can be viewed as the end product of an intimate interaction between physiology and the environment that takes place within a biopsychological system. The concept of a system (e.g., ref. 1) is important since it is clear that the expression of appetite is influenced by a variety of physiological and nonphysiological variables. The pattern of meals and the profile of motivation represents the output of the system. The diagram in Fig. 1 indicates how appetite is shaped by the principles of biological regulation and environmental adaptation. All living organisms require food (a nutritional supply) for growth and maintenance of tissues. This supply is achieved through behavior (commonly called eating). The expression of this behavior is controlled

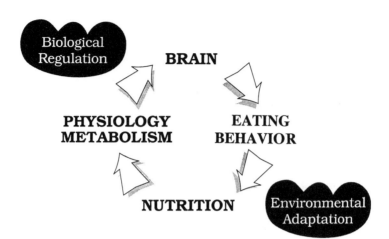

FIG. 1. Schematic indicating how the expression of appetite (eating behavior) is adjusted in the interests of biological regulation or environmental adaptation.

according to the state of the biological system. A complex system of signals operates to ensure the appropriate direction and quality of this (eating) behavior. The extension of Claude Bernard's principle of homeostasis to include behavior is often referred to as the behavioral regulation of internal states (2). However, the expression of behavior is also subject to environmental demands, and behavior is therefore adapted in the face of particular circumstances.

One issue constantly faced by research on appetite is whether food intake is predominantly influenced by psychosocial variables or by physiological events. Within any economic class within a particular culture the measured expression of appetite can be considered to be determined largely by biological drives (physiological–metabolic processes) and cognitive decisions (conscious effort).

In the case of human appetite consideration should be given to the conscious and deliberate (external) control over behavior. Human beings can decide to alter their own behavior (eating) in order to meet particular objectives. For example, a display of moral conviction (political hunger strike) or a demonstration of aesthetic achievement (dieting). In both of these cases eating is curtailed with an ensuing interruption of the nutritional supply. The regulatory properties of the system will tend to oppose this undersupply and generate a drive to eat. In the technically advanced cultures of Europe and the United States the nutritional supply may be adjusted by the environment in another way. The existence of an abundant supply of palatable, high-energy-dense food promotes overconsumption. This in turn (in an interaction with genetic susceptibility) leads to an increase in fat deposition (3). However, this oversupply of calories leading to deposition of fat does not generate a biological drive to undereat. Hence the operation of the regulatory system is not symmetrical: there is a strong defense against undernutrition and only weak response to the effects of overnutrition. Moreover, since it can be assumed that overweight people are not actually trying to eat more in order to increase their weight, their weight gain can be regarded as due to passive overconsumption. On the other hand, undereating is the result of a conscious, deliberate effort and can be regarded as an active process.

What is the significance of these issues for the drug treatment of appetite in overweight people? It may be supposed that if human beings can volitionally inhibit their own biological drives to eat, then a drug acting on a biochemical substrate could achieve a similar outcome. However, a safe drug with this sort of potency has yet to be demonstrated and is probably not a realistic objective. First, it appears that when trying to reduce their food intake, overweight people do not get any help from their fat stores, that is, fat depots do not seem to depress the biological drive to eat. Indeed, owing to their greater body cell mass, overweight people have a higher resting metabolic rate and therefore require a higher energy intake in order to achieve energy balance. Attempts to undereat in overweight people appear to provoke the same counteractive biological drive as in normal weight individuals. Indeed, it has recently been suggested that obese individuals display a defect in appetite control that is manifest as a drive to overeat (4) rather than a defect in energy expenditure. Second, many overweight people make conscious, though often unsystematic, efforts to restrict their pattern of eating. These attempts at conscious control are countered by physiologically mediated stimuli (biological drives) that thwart any intended undereating. A drug acting on the appetite control system could moderate the intensity of biological impulses, thereby making conscious control easier. In this way a drug would provide support for the self-management of appetite rather than mechanically stopping behavior. Therefore it appears that a drug will probably have to be effective in two ways, first in inhibiting and overcoming the active biological drives that oppose any form of food restriction and second, in combating the passive overeating that appears to occur casually and unintentionally in the presence of an abundant high-fat food supply.

THE BIOPSYCHOLOGICAL SYSTEM OF APPETITE CONTROL

The biopsychological system that is concerned with the expression of appetite can be conceptualized on three levels (Fig. 2): psychological events (hunger perception, cravings, hedonic sensations) and behavioral operations (meals, snacks, energy, and macro-nutrient intakes); peripheral physiology and metabolic events; and neurotransmitter and metabolic interactions in the brain. The essence of the approach advocated here is that appetite can best be understood by adopting a systems view in which the expression of appetite reflects the synchronous operation of events and processes in the three levels (5). Neural events trigger and guide behavior, but each act of behavior involves a response in the peripheral physiological system; in turn these physiological events are translated into brain neurochemical activity. This brain activity represents the strength of motivation and the willingness to feed or refrain from feeding.

Eating is a form of behavior that has a definable structure and pattern. The feeding of mammals is a discontinuous process in which periods of eating are interspersed with periods of noneating. These may be regarded as meals and intermeal intervals, an analysis that applies equally well to rats and humans (6). It is useful to distinguish between the processes of satiation and satiety. Satiation is the process that brings a period of eating (meal) to an end, while satiety refers to the inhibition of hunger and eating brought about by food consumption itself. The capacity of food to induce satiety is known as satiating efficiency (7), and this phenomenon is markedly influenced by the total energy and composition of the food consumed (8). Satiety is initiated and maintained by a series of overlapping mediating processes, which can be referred to as the satiety cascade (9). Satiation (control of meal size) and satiety (control of postmeal interval) are influenced separately by the nature and timing of physiological processes. Even before food touches the mouth, physiological signals are generated by the sight and smell of food. These events constitute the cephalic phase of appetite (10). Cephalic-phase responses are generated in many parts of the gastrointestinal tract and their function is to anticipate the ingestion of food. During and immediately after eating, afferent information provides the major control over appetite. It has been noted that "Af-

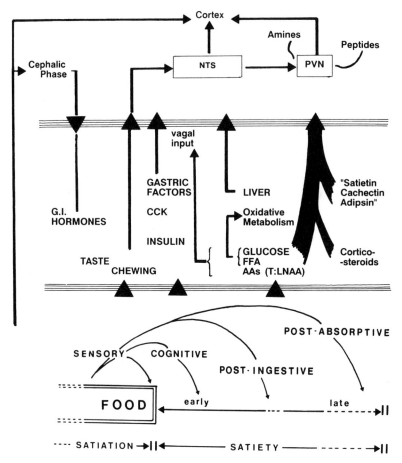

FIG. 2. Postulated relationships among three levels of the biopsychological system of appetite control. The three levels are behavioral operations (meals, snacks, energy and macronutrient intakes), peripheral physiology and metabolic events, and neurotransmitter and metabolic interactions in the brain. *AA,* amino acid; *CCK,* cholecystokinin; *FFA,* free fatty acid; *G.I.,* gastrointestinal; *NTS,* nucleus of the solitary tract; *PVN,* paraventricular nucleus; *T:LNAA,* tryptophan.

ferent information from ingested food acting in the mouth provides primarily positive feedback for eating; that from the stomach and small intestine primarily negative feedback. . . ." (11). Initially the brain is informed about the amount of food ingested and its nutrient context via afferent input. The gastrointestinal tract is equipped with specialized chemo- and mechanoreceptors that monitor physiological activity and pass information to the brain mainly via the vagus nerve (12). This afferent information constitutes one class of "satiety signals" and forms part of the postingestive control of appetite. It is usual to identify a postabsorptive phase, which arises, naturally enough, when nutrients have undergone digestion and cross the wall of the intestine to enter the circulation. These products, which accurately reflect the food that has been consumed, may be metabolized in the peripheral tissues or organs or may enter the brain directly. In either case these products constitute a further class of metabolic "satiety signals." It has been argued that the degree of oxidative metabolism of glucose and free fatty acids in the liver constitutes a significant source of information useful for the control of appetite (13). Additionally, products of digestion and agents responsible for their metabolism may reach the brain and bind to specific chemoreceptors, or influence neurotransmitter synthesis or alter some aspect of neuronal metabolism. In each case the brain is informed about some aspect of the metabolic state resulting from food consumption.

It has also been hypothesized that the blood carries specific substances that reflect the state of depletion or repletion of energy reserves and directly modulate critical brain mechanisms. These substances could include satietin (14), adipsin (15) (a more likely regulator of fat than appetite), and the sugar acids 3,4-dihydroxybutanoic acid-lactone, 2-buten-4-olide, and 2,4,5-trihydroxy pentanoic acid-lactone (16). From an evolutionary perspective it is possible to envisage that many peripheral regulators of the handling of ingested nutrients could be exploited as potential signals of food-related activities or bodily needs. One such possibility is the activation peptide of pancreatic procolipase (17).

Traditional views of the neural control of appetite have been based on opposed hunger and satiety centres in the hypothalamus. These concepts are now out of date. It may be useful to recognize distinct roles for the hindbrain—particularly the nucleus of the solitary tract (NTS) and the closely associated area postrema—and the forebrain, and to consider separate processes of registration, transcription, and integration. Changes in the gastrointestinal tract resulting from food consumption are registered in the hindbrain. This information is transcribed onto neurotransmitter pathways (amines and associated peptides) and projected to primarily hypothalamic zones where integration with neuroendocrine and metabolic activity is organized. Information arriving from the periphery via neural pathways is complemented by qualitatively different types of information, which can be detected in blood and cerebrospinal fluid (CSF). These include the polypeptides acidic fibroblast growth factor (aFGF), interleukin-1, and tumor necrosis factor (cachectin) (18), together with brain insulin. Another feature of the brain's detection system is the presence of so-called glucose-monitoring neurons (18), which are also sensitive to other nutrients. These are located at strategic sites in the hindbrain and forebrain (as well as in the periphery).

A large number of neurotransmitters, neuromodulators, pathways, and receptors are implicated in the central processing of information relevant to appetite (see Hoebel and Hernandez, *this volume*). The profile of this activity reflects the flux of physiological and biochemical transactions in the periphery and represents the pattern of behavioral events and associated motivational states.

TARGETS FOR DRUG ACTION

A consideration of the various components of the biopsychological system suggests many sites, in the brain and periphery, at which pharmacological agents could be aimed to suppress appetite. For example, in the periphery drugs could blunt positive afferent information or intensify inhibitory afferent information; agents could stimulate chemoreceptor activity in the gut or modulate gastrointestinal functioning via the network of neurotransmitters in the enteric plexus. Drugs could also mimic or substitute for proposed appetite-regulating factors in blood, alter oxidative metabolism in the liver, adjust metabolic satiety signals, change amino acid profiles, or affect steroid levels reflecting energy metabolism, which in turn influence neuronal function. Drugs affecting digestion or absorption would be expected to alter the timing and pattern of nutritional information reaching the brain. Within the brain drugs can alter appetite via a number of receptors, involving a variety of neurotransmitters and neuromodulators at a number of specific sites. This complex pattern of neurochemical activity reveals that the appetite system is vulnerable to pharmacological action, which is reflected in the large number of chemicals that have been reported to inhibit food intake (5). The probable site and mode of action of many of these chemicals can be approximately located on the diagram in Fig.

2. Despite this abundance of pharmaceutical activity, safe and effective appetite-controlling drugs have been difficult to develop.

Peripheral Action

A good deal of interest in peripheral sites of action for the suppression of appetite has focused upon peptidergic inhibition of food intake. Many peripherally administered peptides lead to an anorexic response, and good experimental evidence for a natural role exists for cholecystokinin (CCK), pancreatic glucagon, bombesin, and somatostatin (19). Recent research has now confirmed the status of CCK as a hormone mediating satiation and early phase satiety. The consumption of protein or fat stimulates the release of CCK, which activates CCK-A receptors in the pyloric region of the stomach. This signal is transmitted via vagal afferents to the NTS, from where it is relayed to the medial zones of the hypothalamus including the paraventricular nucleus (PVN) and ventromedial hypothalamus (VMH). The anorexic effect of systemically administered CCK can be blocked by vagotomy (20) and by the selective CCK-A receptor antagonist devazepide (MK-329) (21). Significantly, many reports now exist demonstrating that the CCK-A-type antagonist administered alone leads to an increase in food intake in experimental animals (22). Interestingly, trypsin inhibitors that block the inactivation of CCK produce a suppression of food intake in animals (23) and humans (24). Not surprisingly, considerable research activity has been directed toward the development of CCK analogs or peptoids with anorexic potency. Many products now exist, but their future as clinical appetite suppressants may depend upon finding ways to prevent adaptive responses in the pancreas, which appear to develop with repeated administration. The pharmacological action of glucagon in suppressing food intake is notable, but there is currently no evidence on how glucagon induces vagal afferent signals (25).

Another peptide, insulin, appears to have significant peripheral and central actions. Peripheral effects on carbohydrate metabolism are well known, but it appears that an appetite or body weight signal may be generated by CSF insulin (26).

Central Action

The influence of central neurochemical activity on the expression of appetite is complex and involves numerous interactions between different loci and different receptors, which result in shifts in the magnitude, direction, and quality of eating behavior. A good deal of evidence has been accumulated from the direct application of chemicals to the brain either via the CSF or directly into specific sites. Most agents suppress intake, but a significant number stimulate eating, sometimes in a dramatic fashion. The most frequently demonstrated action is the stimulation of feeding following activation of α-2 adrenoceptors in the PVN (27). It is also known that spontaneous feeding is associated with endogenous release of noradrenaline in the PVN and with an increase in PVN α-2 receptor density (28). In turn it appears that the PVN is a site for the long-established anorexic action of serotoninergic agents (29). The PVN also contains glucosensitive neurons and therefore may be a point of interaction for neurotransmitter activity and metabolic states reflecting energy regulation. Circulating corticosteroids have been demonstrated to influence noradrenaline receptor sensitivity, and it has been argued that noradrenaline and serotonin (5-HT) act antagonistically to influence the release of corticotropin-releasing factor (CRF). Since the PVN is also a potent anorectic drug-binding site (30), neurochemical activity in this area may serve to integrate behavioral, metabolic, and neuroendocrine responses. In more lateral areas of the hypothalamus (perifornical zone), feeding is suppressed by microinjection of agents that activate dopamine D_2 or β_2 adrenergic receptors (31). Consequently, noradrenaline, 5-HT, and dopamine produce quantitative shifts in feeding from closely related sites in the hypothalamus.

Potent feeding responses can also be obtained by microinjection of peptides to the brain. Many peptides such as insulin, CCK, calcitonin, bombesin, neurotensin, thyroid hormone releasing hormone (THRH), somatostatin, vasointestinal polypeptide (VIP), CRF, and glucagon suppress feeding after cerebroventricular administration (32). A smaller number of peptides increase food intake; this group includes β endorphin, dynorphin, neuropeptide Y (NPY), peptide YY, (PYY) and galanin. When injected into the PVN, NPY and PYY can induce 50% of daily food intake within 1 hour. The stimulation of feeding by galanin appears to be specific to the PVN and closely related sites (33). Classic research of a decade ago indicated how projections between the brainstem and hypothalamic nuclei were involved in neuroendocrine regulation (34). This pattern of projections is also important for feeding; peptides such as NPY and galanin appear to originate (in part) in adrenergic (C1, C2) or noradrenergic (A1, A2, A6) nuclei in the brainstem. In summary, peptides such as CCK, CRF, THRH, and NPY, opioids, and galanin appear to have important central roles in conjunction with noradrenaline, 5-HT, and dopamine in the organization of the expression of appetite (and energy balance more generally). These actions are generated in response to visceral and metabolic information that reflects the immediate past history of feeding and the body's nutritional status. Other neural mechanisms involving cholinergic, benzodiazepine, and γ-aminobutyric acid (GABA)ergic receptors may also be implicated at some point.

STRATEGIES FOR THE ACTION OF DRUGS ON THE APPETITE SYSTEM

It follows from the discussion above that potential drugs could be targeted on any component in the complex neural matrix that controls food intake and contributes to energy balance. In principle it may be more effective to direct attention to some components rather than others. Such strategies can be decided in part by considering the accessibility of the component and also its role in the overall system.

Preabsorptive or Postabsorptive Action

The earlier consideration of the satiety cascade drew attention to the separation of postingestive and postabsorptive processes in the mediation of satiety. The preabsorptive phase of satiety is largely dependent upon mediation by afferent stimuli arising in the upper gastrointestinal tract following food consumption. This information reaches the brain via neural pathways—especially the vagus nerve. Clearly this preabsorptive information reaches the brain earlier than the monitoring of postabsorptive information. It should be noted that the qualitative nature of the food consumed (including its nutrient composition) can be detected preabsorptively by chemoreceptors in the gastrointestinal tract as well as by monitoring of the digested products after they have been transported into the blood supply.

What is the significance of this separation of processes for drug action? It is noticeable that following a period of food consumption the intensity of satiety (inhibition of hunger, suppression of the tendency to eat) is strongest immediately after eating has stopped; then satiety gradually dissipates and hunger returns. Consequently the mechanisms subserving early phase satiety (preabsorptive stage) have a potent inhibitory action on consumption. In contrast, it appears that the postabsorptive phase of satiety (mediated by the effects of blood-borne metabolites) exerts a milder suppression over appetite. It follows therefore that effective drug action may arise from targeting preabsorptive mechanisms and by attempts to prolong the duration of action of such mechanisms beyond their normal short-lasting period. In functional terms it seems likely that the strong early postingestive inhibitory action serves to exert control over the pattern of eating and to ensure that epochs of eating are appropriately separated. The postabsorptive processes are probably much more intimately involved in the monitoring of calories and in the processes of energy balance. Any drug that acted on both pre- and postabsorptive components would be likely to give rise to a meaningful modulation of the pattern of eating and also influence physiological processes involved in energy balance.

QUALITATIVE ASPECTS OF APPETITE

A good deal of experimental work on animals has been concerned with quantitative shifts in food consumption (hypophagia). However, appetite involves qualitative aspects of eating and changes in choice of foods as well as adjustments of the overall amount. Appetite is more than a measure of the weight of food eaten. In addition, in humans appetite embraces conscious sensations including hunger, fullness, and cravings for foods together with an appreciation of the hedonic aspects of foods—pleasantness and pleasure.

Hunger

The conscious sensation of hunger is one index of motivation and reflects the strength of satiation and satiety. It is worth keeping in mind that hunger is a biologically useful sensation. It is a nagging, irritating feeling that prompts thoughts of food and reminds us that the body needs energy (35). Moreover, there is good evidence that in most cases hunger is positively related to food intake. For example, after tracking diurnal rhythms of hunger and eating it was noted that "correlation using hunger ratings and intake during the same hour of the day was r = 0.50 ($p <$ 0.02), that is, hunger ratings at the start of each hour were correlated with reported intake in the hour following each hunger rat-

ing" (36). Other researchers measuring spontaneous feeding in humans have concluded that "subjective hunger represents an intermediary step in the cause-effect sequence between gut filling and cessation of meal ingestion" (37). Consequently, the identification and management of hunger appear to be important factors underlying appetite function, and therefore they should occupy an important position in the drug treatment of overweight.

Although the neurochemical substrate underlying hunger has not been identified, it can be inferred that hunger rises and falls contingent upon the activation of neural circuitry related to food intake itself. Many chemical agents that influence energy intake in humans also modulate the sensation of hunger (Table 1). Interestingly, some drugs do not exert an equal action on hunger and food intake, and these instances tell us a good deal about the neurochemical basis of appetite control (see below).

Nutrition and Pharmacology— Macronutrient Intake

Significantly, in recent years many researchers have begun measuring the intake of macronutrients (fat, protein, carbohydrate), have considered the hedonic aspects of food (particularly sweet taste), and have taken an interest in the relationship between nutrition and pharmacology (38). The outcome has been a revelation. For example, the stimulation of feeding by PVN injections of α_2 agonists is represented primarily by an increase in carbohydrate intake (39). This action is limited to the early dark phase of the diurnal cycle when the rat's selection of carbohydrate is normally high. Administration of serotoninergic agonists (central or peripheral) during this period suppresses selection of carbohydrate. This effect gives support to a provocative hypothesis that links the dietary proportions of protein and carbohydrate consumed to brain serotonin activity by way of adjustments in plasma ratios of trypto-

TABLE 1. *Effects of pharmacological agents on human appetite*[a]

Chemical	Type of study	Hunger and food preference	Caloric intake and body weight	Reference no.
Alcohol 0.7–1.0 ml/kg oral	Lab study; 24 healthy subjects	Small ↓ hunger (n.s.)	Small ↓ food intake (n.s.)	48
Amphetamine 5–20 mg	Lab study; 16 males	↓ Hunger but great individual variability	Overall ↓ calorie intake but responses very variable	49
Aspartame 230–470 mg by capsule	Lab study; 27 healthy adults (16 men, 11 women)	No effect on premeal hunger	↓ Intake 1 hour later by 9% (men) and 14% (women)	50
Butorphanol tartrate 1 μg/kg	Lab study; 10 normal weight subjects	No effect	Doubling of food intake in 2 hours	51
CCK$_8$ 4 ng/kg/min i.v.	Lab study; 12 nonobese men	—	↓ Food intake and meal duration	52
CCK$_8$ 4 ng/kg/min i.v.	8 obese men	—	6 of 8 subjects ate less food	53
Chlorpromazine	Experimental study on 32 psychiatric patients	↑ Rating of appetite	Marked gain of body weight	54
Cyproheptadine 4 mg three times daily	Lab study; 16 thin subjects, 4 weeks	↑ Hunger	↑ Food intake, significant weight gain	55
2-Deoxy-D-glucose 50 mg/kg	Lab study; 5 men normal weight	↑ Hunger: ↑ pleasantness of sucrose	—	56
D-Fenfluramine 2 × 15 mg daily	Lab study: 8 obese women (body mass index = 38)	↓ Hunger; ↑ fullness after first meal	11–19% ↓ energy intake of second meal	57
D-Fenfluramine 2 × 15 mg daily	Clinical study; 80 obese subjects (58 carbohydrate cravers); 3 months treatment	—	Carbohydrate cravers ↓ snake intake; ↓ carbohydrate and protein intake at meals	58
Fluoxetine 60 mg daily	Lab study; healthy men, 2-week study	↓ Hunger on days 8 and 15, not on day 1	↓ Food intake on days 1 and 8, not on day 15	59
Glucagon i.v. infusion 3 mg/kg/min	Lab study; 12 normal subjects	No change	20% ↓ in test meal size	25
Insulin 1 U/kg i.v.	Lab study; 12 healthy subjects	↑ Hunger; ↑ pleasantness of sucrose	↑ Liquid drink intake	60
Isocarboxazid plus trimipramine	Double-blind clinical trial	↑ Preference for carbohydrates	↑ Body weight	61
Levodopa variable 0.2–3.0 g	Clinic; 9 anorexia nervosa patients	—	7 of 9 clear weight increases	62
Lithium	Clinical treatment	—	↑ Weight	63
Marihuana 0.35–0.5 mg/kg oral	Lab study; 24 healthy subjects	↑ Hunger	↑ Food intake especially in prefed subjects	48
Metergoline 4 mg	Lab study; male subjects	No effect	↑ Intake of sweet food	64
Methysergide 1 mg oral	Normal subjects	↑ Hunger ratings	—	65
Morphine 10 mg/70 kg s.c.	Lab study; 85 healthy subjects	Small ↓ hunger (n.s.)	—	66
Nalmefene 2.5 mg	Lab study; male subjects	—	22% ↓ in meal intake with ↓ in fat and protein	67
Naloxone 0.8 and 1.6 mg i.v.	Lab study; normal subjects	No effect	Dose-related ↓ food intake	46
Naltrexone 120 mg oral	Lab study; 8 healthy adults	Little effect	↓ Pleasantness of sucrose	45
Phentermine 15–30 mg	Lab study; six mildly overweight women	↓ Hunger with 30 mg	↓ Calorie intake	68
Phenylalanine up to 10.8 g	Lab study	Results variable	Small ↓ food intake (n.s.)	69
Phenylpropanolamine 37.5 mg	Lab study; nonobese women	Small ↓ hunger (n.s.)	Small ↓ food intake (n.s.)	70
Proteinase inhibitor Ryan/Potato II 1.5 g	Lab study; 11 healthy subjects (8 female, 3 male)	No effect at test meal	↓ Calorie intake at test meal by 17.5% (with a protein/fat preload)	24
Tricyclic antidepressants (e.g., amitryptiline)	Outpatient treatment; 100 subjects minimum, 1 month	38% ↑ appetite; 34% ↑ sweet craving	Food preference related to weight gain	71
Tryptophan 0.5, 1.0, 2.0 g	Lab study; 16 healthy subjects	Not reported	↓ Intake (2.0 g)	72

[a] This table is representative, not exhaustive. n.s., not significant; —, not measured.
CCK, cholecystokinin.

phan (serotonin precursor) to other large neutral amino acids (40). In this hypothesis specific neurotransmitter activity is the mediating link between nutrition and psychological phenomena (mood changes, food choice). Interestingly, the feeding response to NPY, like that of noradrenaline, reflects a preferential selection of carbohydrate rather than protein or fat. In contrast, the stimulation of eating by galanin is reported to be directed mainly toward fat (41). Conversely, it is believed that the anorexic action of VPDPR (Val-Pro-Asp-Pro-Arg), because of its association with fat digestion, will preferentially suppress the intake of fat (17). These findings represent a significant development in the pharmacological study of appetite control, and they have theoretical and clinical implications. Theoretically these data suggest new ways of looking at the peripheral processes of macronutrient digestion and absorption and their relationship to neurotransmitter pathways in the brain. Clinically, the development of drugs that could prevent a high intake of fat (by whatever mechanism) would have great antiobesity potential. However, it is worth keeping in mind that the measurement of nutrient intakes in animals is beset with methodological problems, while adjustments that are limited to particular portions of the light–dark cycle may have only limited clinical relevance.

Hedonic Aspects of Eating

Another dimension of appetite susceptible to pharmacological adjustment is the hedonic response to foods. One of the best known hedonic aspects of food is sweet taste. Sweetness is a potent psychobiological phenomenon that can stimulate food intake and act as a powerful reward (see Sclafani, *this volume*). Some agents have been reported to exert strong effects on the ingestion of sweet substances. For example, a number of neuroleptics suppress the intake of sweet sucrose solutions in sham feeding rats (42). The effect is brought about by D_1 antagonists such as

SCH 23390 and D_2 antagonists such as (—) – sulpiride. Since sucrose feeding increases dopamine metabolism in the hypothalamus, it appears likely that central dopamine mechanisms are necessary for a normal eating response to sweet-tasting stimuli. Using the microdialysis technique, Hoebel et al. (43) have shown that the taste of saccharine causes a release of dopamine in the nucleus accumbens.

An additional proposal is that opioid peptides are implicated in hedonic responses to foods, especially sweet tastes. For example, opioid agonists apparently enhance preferences, while the antagonist naloxone abolishes preferences for saccharine and glucose (44). Pharmacological studies in humans have thrown light upon the extent to which human appetite is influenced by the hedonic response to food (feeling of pleasure) or by sensations of hunger. It has been demonstrated that naltrexone (another opioid receptor antagonist) depresses the perceived pleasantness of a sweet solution, while having no effect on hunger (45), and that naloxone reduces food intake but does not affect hunger (46). On the other hand some 5-HT receptor agonists exert a potent suppression of hunger but have little or no effect on the hedonic response to sweetness (47). Consequently, these two aspects of human appetite —hedonics and hunger—can be pharmacologically uncoupled.

PHARMACOLOGICAL MODULATION OF HUMAN APPETITE—POTENTIAL AND POSSIBILITY

In principle a number of possible ways exist in which drugs could influence the expression of human appetite. These include the following:

1. Overall reduction in energy intake
2. Suppression of hunger/increased duration of feelings of fullness
3. Reduction of the hedonic value (perceived pleasantness) of food; decrease in

the perceived attractiveness of food stimuli

4. Intensification of the satiating efficiency of food; strengthening of satiety (early or late phase)
5. Quickening the onset of satiation (decreasing meal size)
6. Reduction of snack intake; control of the intermeal interval
7. Modulation of nutrient selection (protein, fat, carbohydrate)
8. Altered preference for particular tastes (e.g., sweet versus savoury)
9. Adjustment of the pattern of eating and the profile of motivation

There is no doubt that drugs can influence the expression of human appetite. Some examples are set out in Table 1. As in animal studies, both increases and decreases in energy intake are observed. It is possible that some drugs, prescribed for an unrelated clinical condition, may have an adverse effect on weight control by facilitating appetite (73). In other cases drugs can exert a restraining effect on the feeling of hunger and can modify the pattern of eating by reducing meal sizes and intensifying or prolonging postprandial satiety (74). As a general philosophy, it may be useful to regard potential appetite suppressant drugs not as blockers of eating but as agents that amplify and exploit the mechanisms of the natural anorexic agent—food. Presently, the most effective drugs (and also the safest) are those that enhance or intensify the satiety mechanisms induced by consumption (these may be in the periphery or in the brain).

In recent years pharmacological studies of appetite that have given attention to nutrient composition of foods or to sensory qualities have created new possibilities for researchers. Appetite is not a unitary phenomenon, and drugs that exert specific effects on key components of appetite (e.g., nutrients, hedonics, or hunger) may have the greatest clinical relevance for the treatment of appetite and/or weight disorder. Such drugs may be able to block these food cravings, which are often believed to undermine self-imposed appetite control.

Can drug-induced appetite control be used to combat obesity? Having reviewed possible mechanisms of action, pharmacological targets, and drug-induced effects, this issue continues the arguments set out at the start of this chapter. Although obesity has a clear genetic component (75), this need not imply biological inevitability, for there exists clear gene × environment interactions (3). The nature of the food supply is the most critical environmental feature. An abundance of readily available, highly palatable high-fat foods favors overconsumption and therefore promotes obesity (with varying rates of development) in those vulnerable individuals. Can drugs prevent the environment from promoting a hyperphagia response? This idea implies no particular fault in the appetite control system of obese people. Drugs that influence macronutrient intake, hedonics, or hunger or that adjust the pattern of eating should be useful. An alternative view of obesity is that fat people achieve positive energy balance because of some defect at some site/process in their appetite control system. If this is the case, then a decision is required about whether to "repair" the defect or to act upon those parts of the system that are intact and functioning normally. The search for causal physiological or metabolic abnormalities in animal genetic models of obesity continues. However, the existence of the model of cafeteria obesity, in which obesity is induced in normal animals offered a surfeit of palatable, energy-dense food, indicates a susceptibility to weight gain in the presence of appetite control systems in apparently good working order (See Sclafani, *this volume*). The same applies to humans. Why is this? It appears that the appetite control system contains within its matrix of processes strong regulatory mechanisms that guard against underconsumption (hence dieting evokes a strong compensatory response) but only rather weak mechanisms to prevent overconsumption. During the course of human evolution food scarcity has been the usual problem rather than abundance (see Brown, *this volume*). Moreover, in evolutionary terms, adult-onset obesity carries with it no biological penalty. Although the mechanisms that subserve early-phase satiety are potent suppressors of intake, in the longer term inhibition of appetite becomes much weaker and can be overridden by the presence of readily available, palatable, easily consumed foods. It is worth noting that bodily fatness does not suppress appetite; large adipose stores do not reduce the biological drive to eat. Fat people therefore need all the help they can get—pharmacological or other—to restrain the expression of their appetites. Evidence already indicates that drugs that modulate satiation *and* satiety should produce the most effective control (74). Moreover, long-term studies on the action of drugs on body weight (76) appear to indicate a two-phase process: first a period of weight suppression followed by a period of weight maintenance. This pattern is quite consistent with the idea that certain drugs (among them serotoninergic agents) have the capacity both to oppose the active biological resistance to caloric deficit and also to prevent passive overconsumption. In this way pharmacological agents can provide biological assistance to allow obese people to achieve a better management of their appetites.

REFERENCES

1. Blundell JE, Hill AJ. BioPsychological interactions underlying the study and treatment of obesity. In: Christie MJ, Mellett PG, eds. *The psychosomatic approach: contemporary practice of whole person care.* Chichester: John Wiley & Sons, 1986;115–38.
2. Richter CP. Total self-regulatory functions in animals and human beings. *Harvey Lect* 1943; 38:63–103.
3. Bouchard C. Inheritance of fat distribution and adipose tissue metabolism. In: Vague J, Bjorntorp P, Guy-Grand B, Rebuffe-Scrive M, Vague P, eds. *Metabolic complications of human obesities.* Amsterdam: Excerpta Medica, 1985;87–96.
4. Prentice AM, Black AE, Murgatroyd PR, Goldberg GR, Coward WA. Metabolism on appetite: questions of energy balance with particular reference to obesity. *J Nutr Diet* 1980;2:95–104.
5. Blundell JE. Pharmacological approaches to appetite suppression. *Trends Pharmacol Sci* 1991; 12:147–57.
6. Blundell JE. Pharmacological adjustment of the mechanisms underlying feeding and obesity. In: Stunkard AJ, ed. *Obesity.* Philadelphia: WB Saunders, 1980;182–207.
7. Kissileff HR, Gruss LP, Thornton J, Jordan HA. The satiating efficiency of foods. *Physiol Behav* 1984;32:319–32.
8. Blundell JE, Rogers PJ, Hill AJ. Evaluating the satiating power of foods: implications for acance and consumption. On: Solms J, ed. *Chemical composition and sensory properties of food and their influence on nutrition.* London: Academic Press, 1987;205–19.
9. Blundell JE, Hill AJ, Rogers PJ. Hunger and the satiety cascade—importance for food acceptance in the late 20th century. In: Thompson DMH, ed. *Food acceptability.* Amsterdam: Elsevier, 1988; 233–50.
10. Powley J. The ventromedial hypothalamic syndrome, satiety and a cephalic phase hypothesis. *Psychol Rev* 1977;84:89–126.
11. Smith GP, Greenberg D, Corp E, Gibbs J. Afferent information in the control of eating. In: Bray GA, ed. *Obesity: towards a molecular approach.* New York: Alan R Liss, 1990;63–79.
12. Mei N. Intestinal chemosensitivity. *Physiol Rev* 1985;65:211–37.
13. Friedman MI, Tordoff MG, Ramirez I. Integrated metabolic control of food intake. *Brain Res Bull* 1986;17:855–9.
14. Knoll J. Satietin: a highly potent anorexigenic substance in human serum. *Physiol Behav* 1979;23:497–502.
15. Cook KS, Spiegelman BM. Adipsin, a circulating serine protease homolog secreted by adipose tissue and sciatic nerve. *Science* 1987;237:402–4.
16. Schimizu N, Oomura Y, Sakata T. Modulation of feeding by endogenous sugar acids acting as hunger or satiety factors. *Am J Physiol* 1984;246:R542–50.
17. Erlanson-Albertsson C, Larsson A. The activation peptide of pancreatic procolipase decreases food intake in rats. *Regul Pept* 1988;22:325–31.
18. Oomura Y. Chemical and neuronal control of feeding motivation. *Physiol Behav* 1988;44:555–60.
19. Smith GP. Humoral mechanisms in the control of body weight. In: Weiner H, Baum A, eds. *Perspectives in behavioural medicine. Eating regulation and dyscontrol.* Hillsdale: Lawrence Erlbaum Assoc., 1988;59–65.
20. Smith GP, Jerome C, Norgren R. Afferent axons in abdominal vagus mediate satiety effect of cholecystokinin in rats. *Am J Physiol* 1985;249:R638–R641.
21. Dourish CT, Coughlan J, Hawley D, Clark M, Iversen SD. Blockade of CCK-induced hypophagia and prevention of morphine tolerance by the CCK antagonist L-364,718. In: Wang RY, Schoenfeld R, eds. *CCK antagonists.* New York: Alan R Liss, 1988;307–25.
22. Hewson G, Leighton GE, Hill RG, Hughes J. The cholecystokinin receptor agonist L364,718 increases food intake in the rat by attenuation of the action of endogenous cholecystokinin. *Br J Pharmacol* 1988;93:79–84.
23. McLaughlin CL, Peikin SR, Baile CA. Trypsin inhibitor effects on food intake and weight gain in Zucker rats. *Physiol Behav* 1983;31:487–91.

24. Hill AJ, Peiken SR, Ryan CA, Blundell JE. Oral administration of proteinase inhibitor II from potatoes reduces energy intake in man. *Physiol Behav* 1990;48:241–6.

25. Geary N. Pancreatic glucagon signals postprandial satiety. *Neurosci Biobehav Rev* 1990;14:323–38.

26. Woods SC, Lotter EC, McKay LD, Porte D. Chronic intracerebroventricular infusion of insulin reduces food intake and body weight of baboons. *Nature* 1979;282:503–5.

27. Leibowitz SF. Paraventricular nucleus: a primary site mediating adrenergic stimulation of feeding and drinking. *Pharmacol Biochem Behav* 1978; 8:163–75.

28. Leibowitz SF. Hypothalamic paraventricular nucleus: interaction between α_2-noradrenergic system and circulating hormones and nutrients in relation to energy balance. *Neurosci Biobehav Rev* 1988; 12:101–9.

29. Blundell JE. Serotonin and appetite. *Neuropharmacology* 1984;33:1537–52.

30. Angel I. Central receptors and recognition sites mediating the effects of monoamines and anorectic drugs on feeding behaviour. *Clin Neuropharmacol* 1990;13:361–91.

31. Leibowitz SF, Brown LL. Histochemical and pharmacological analysis of catecholaminergic projections to the perifornical hypothalamus in relation feeding inhibition. *Brain Res* 1980;201:315–45.

32. Morley JE, Levine AS, Grace M, Kneip J. Peptide YY (PY), a potent orexigenic agent. *Brain Res* 1985;341:200–3.

33. Leibowitz SF. Hypothalamic neuropeptide Y, galanin and amines: concepts of coexistence in relation to feeding behaviour. *Ann NY Acad Sci* 1989;575:221–35.

34. Sawchenko PE, Swanson LW. The organization of noradrenergic pathways from the brainstem to the paraventricular and supraoptic nuclei in the rat. *Brain Res Rev* 1982;4:275–325.

35. Blundell JE, Rogers PJ. The satiating power of food. In: *Encyclopedia of human biology,* vol 6. Orlando: Academic Press, 1991;273–733.

36. Mattes R. Hunger ratings are not a valid proxy measure of reported food intakes in humans. *Appetite* 1990;15:103–13.

37. De Castro JM, Elmore DK. Subjective hunger relationships with meal patterns in the spontaneous feeding behaviour of humans: evidence for a causal connection. *Physiol Behav* 1988;43:159–65.

38. Blundell JE. Impact of nutrition on the pharmacology of appetite—some conceptual issues. *Ann NY Acad Sci* 1990;575:163–70.

39. Leibowitz SF, Shor-Posner G. Monoamine meal patterns in the rat. In: Carruba MO, Blundell JE, eds. *Psychopharmacology of eating disorders: theoretical and clinical advances.* New York: Raven Press, 1986;29–50.

40. Wurtman RJ. Nutrients that modify brain function. *Sci Am* 1982;243:42–51.

41. Kyrkouli SE, Stanley BG, Seirafi RD, Leibowitz SF. Stimulation of feeding by galanin: anatomical localization and behavioural specificity of this peptide's effects in the brain. *Peptides* 1990;11:995–1001.

42. Schneider LH, Gibbs J, Smith GP. D-2 selective receptor antagonists suppress sucrose sham feeding in the rat. *Brain Res Bull* 1986;17:605–11.

43. Hoebel BG, Hernandez L, Schwartz DH, Mark GP, Hunter GA. Microdialysis studies of brain norepinephrine, serotonin and dopamine release during ingestive behaviour: theoretical and clinical implications. *Ann NY Acad Sci* 1989;575:171–93.

44. Marks-Kaufman R, Kanarek RB. The endogenous opioid peptides: relationship to food intake, obesity and sweet tastes. In: Walsh TB, ed. *Eating behaviour in eating disorders.* Progress in Psychiatry. Washington: American Psychiatric Press, 1989;53–68.

45. Fantino M, Hosotte J, Apelbaum M. An opioid antagonist, naltrexone, reduces preference for sucrose in humans. *Am J Physiol* 1986;251:R91–R96.

46. Trenchard E, Silverstone T. Naloxone reduces the food intake of normal human volunteers. *Appetite* 1983;4:43–50.

47. Blundell JE, Hill AJ. On the mechanism of action of dexfenfluramine: effect on alliesthesia and appetite motivation in lean and obese subjects. *Clin Neuropharmacol* 1988;11[Suppl 1]:S121–S134.

48. Hollister LE. Hunger and appetite after single doses of marihuana, alcohol and dextrophetamine. *Clin Pharmacol Ther* 1971;12:44–9.

49. Silverstone JT, Stunkard A. The anorectic effect of desamphetamine sulphate. *Br J Pharmacol Chemother* 1968;33:513–22.

50. Rogers PJ, Pleming HC, Blundell JE. Aspartame ingested without tasting inhibits hunger and food intake. *Physiol Behav* 1990;47:1239–1243.

51. Morley JE, Parker S, Levine AS. Effect of butorphanol tatrate on food and water consumption in humans. *Am J Clin Nutr* 1985;42:1175–8.

52. Kissileff HR, Pi-Sunyer FX, Thornton J, Smith GP. C-terminal octapeptide of cholecystokinin decreases food intake in man. *Am J Clin Nutr* 1981; 34:154–60.

53. Pi-Sunyer X, Kissileff HR, Thornton J, Smith GP. C-terminal octapeptide of cholecystokinin decreases food intake in obese man. *Physiol Behav* 1982;29:627–30.

54. Robinson RG, McHugh PR, Bloom FE. Chlorpromazine-induced hyperphagia in the rat. *Psychopharmacol Commun* 1975;1:37–50.

55. Silverstone T, Schuyler D. The effect of cyproheptadine on hunger, calorie intake and body weight in man. *Psychopharmacologia* 1975;40:335–40.

56. Thompson DA, Campbell RG. Hunger in humans induced by 2-deoxy-d-glucose: glucoprivic control of taste preference and food intake. *Science* 1977;198:1065–8.

57. Hill AJ, Blundell JE. Sensitivity of the appetite control system in obese subjects to nutritional and serotoninergic challenges. *Int J Obes* 1990;14:219–33.

58. Wurtman J, Wurtman R, Reynolds S, Tsay R, Chew B. Fenfluramine suppresses snack intake among carbohydrate cravers but not among non-carbohydrate cravers. *Int J Eating Disorders* 1987;6:687–99.

59. McQuirk J, Silverstone T. The effect of the 5-HT reuptake inhibitor fluoxetine on food intake and body weight in healthy male subjects. *Int J Obes* 1990;4:361–72.

60. Rodin J, Wack J, Ferrannini E, Defronzo RA. Effect of insulin and glucose on feeding behaviour. *Metabolism* 1985;34:826–31.

61. Harris B, Young J, Hughes B. Changes occurring in appetite and weight during short-term anti-depressant treatment. *Br J Psychiatry* 1984;145:645–8.

62. Johanson AJ, Knorr NJ. L-DOPA as treatment for anorexia nervosa. In: Vigersky RA, ed. *Anorexia nervosa.* New York: Raven Press, 1977;363–72.

63. Vendsborg PB, Bech P, Rafaelson OJ. Lithium treatment and weight gain. *Acta Psychiatr Scand* 1976;53:139–47.

64. Goodall E, Silverstone JT. Different effect of d-fenfluramine and metergoline on food intake in human subjects. *Appetite* 1988;11:215–28.

65. Silverstone T, Kyriakides M. Clinical pharmacology of appetite. In: Silverstone T, ed. *Drugs and appetite.* London: Academic Press, 1982;93–123.

66. Beecher HK. *Measurement of subjective responses. Quantitative effects of drugs.* New York: Oxford University Press, 1959;352–63.

67. Yeomans MR, Wright P, Malleod HA, Critchley JH. Effects of nalmathene on feeding in humans—dissociation of hunger and palatability. *Psychopharmacology* 1990;100:426–32.

68. Silverston JT. The anorectic effects of a long acting preparation of phentermine (duromine). *Psychopharmacologia* 1972;25:315–20.

69. Ryan-Harshman M, Leiter LA, Anderson GH. Phenylalanine and aspartame fail to alter feeding behaviour, mood and arousal in men. *Physiol Behav* 1987;39:247–53.

70. Caffry EW, Kissileff HR, Thornton JC. Assessment of the effects of phenylpropanolamine on appetite and food intake. *Pharmacol Biochem Behav* 1987;26:321–5.

71. Stein EM, Stein S, Linn MW. Geriatric sweet tooth. A problem with tricyclics. *J Am Geriatr Soc* 1985;33:687–92.

72. Silverstone T, Goodall E. The clinical pharmacology of appetite suppressant drugs. *Int J Obes* 1984;8[Suppl 1]:23–33.

73. Blundell JE. Systems and interactions: an approach to the pharmacology of eating and hunger. In: Stunkard AJ, Stellar E: *Eating and its disorders.* New York: Raven Press, 1984;39–65.

74. Blundell JE, Hill AJ. Serotonergic modulation of the pattern of eating and the profile of hunger-satiety in humans. *Int J Obes* 1987;11[Suppl 3]:141–53.

75. Stunkard AJ, Sorensen TIA, Hanis C, et al. An adoption study of human obesity. *N Engl J Med* 1986;314:193–8.

76. Guy-Grand B, Crepaldi G, Lefevre P, Apfelbaum M, Gries A, Turner P. International trial of long-term dexfenfluramine in obesity. *Lancet* 1989;ii:1142–5.

Obesity: Theory and Therapy, Second Edition,
edited by A. J. Stunkard and T. A. Wadden.
Raven Press, Ltd., New York © 1993.

5

Physiological Regulation of Body Energy

Implications for Obesity

Richard E. Keesey

Departments of Psychology and Nutritional Sciences, University of Wisconsin,
Madison, Wisconsin 53706

Historically, obesity has been viewed as being behavioral in origin, stemming primarily from a disordered pattern of food intake. It thus follows that behavioral therapy, with its aim of modifying existing eating habits, constitutes the most common form of treatment. However, the resistance of obesity to such treatment raises concern that its origins may, in fact, not be behavioral.

As an alternative to this behavioral perspective, the present chapter develops a thesis that the body energy of individuals, including the obese, is physiologically regulated. Evidence that body weight (or, more precisely, some associated factor for which weight serves as a useful index) is a factor regulated at a physiologically specified level or "set point" is presented and discussed. Both the adjustments in energy intake and expenditure that serve to stabilize body energy at the regulated level and the factors that influence or can alter the set point of the energy-regulating system are also considered.

PRINCIPLES OF PHYSIOLOGICAL REGULATION

A remarkable feature of complex organisms is the stability of their internal environment in the face of widely varying external conditions. Body core temperature, body fluid volume and tonicity, and blood glucose and pH, as well as numerous other physiological conditions remain at characteristic levels throughout the many changes that occur daily and seasonally in external environments. The level at which each of these physiological variables is maintained is often characteristic not just of the single organism but of its species or, sometimes, even the entire animal kingdom.

Of course, the constancy of these physiological conditions is not absolute. Rather, each factor is maintained within certain limits, with the variance around the average level ranging from less than 1% (e.g., blood pH) to more than 10% (e.g., blood glucose). Furthermore, the average value maintained can vary daily or seasonally, or can undergo systematic change over a life span.

Organisms able to achieve internal stability of this sort clearly must be capable both of monitoring their internal state continuously and of initiating whatever compensatory adjustments are necessary to hold each physiological factor close to the regulated level. In pondering what elements a physiological system capable of accomplishing this would require, some investigators look for guidance to the set-point models developed by systems engineers. To control systems engineers, a set point is an independent signal that serves as a standard or reference level for a feedback control system. As such, it "sets" the value of the variable the control system maintains. Physiologists often find set-point models helpful in thinking about the organization and workings of the complex regulatory systems with which they work. A strict translation of the formally defined features of the set-point regulators of system engineering to physiological systems is not always possible. Still, many such systems certainly behave as if they were so organized and, by providing the basis for a formal description of experimental results, by revealing gaps in our knowledge, and by generating hypotheses about the nature of the control system under study, set-point models are often helpful in guiding the systematic study of physiologically regulated variables. The body temperature regulation literature provides but one example of how the set-point concept has influenced research on physiological systems (1).

REGULATION OF BODY WEIGHT

What evidence is there that body weight is indeed regulated? Consideration of certain aspects of the body weight of humans might actually lead one to the contrary conclusion. Consider, for example, the large variations in the weight of different individuals. The mean weight of a 35-year-old American man standing 5 feet 10 inches tall is, for example, 170 lb (2), yet we could readily find men of this height weighing twice this amount. Variance this great among members of the same species is certainly not characteristic of other physiological variables in which the value of the regulated factor seldom deviates from the population mean by more than 10%, typically by even less.

Curiously, if the focus is shifted from the variance in weight between individuals to the variability in weight within an individual, a different picture emerges. In the individual case, stability of body weight can match or surpass that of most other physiologic variables. The variation of one's body weight over relatively short periods of observation (i.e., 6 to 10 weeks) is remarkably low. Average coefficients of variation over such periods are only ±0.5 to 0.6% of the mean (3–5). Cross-sectional data suggest that weight changes over still longer periods are likewise quite small. The average weight of a 60-year-old white American man is only 4 to 5 lb more than one 30 years of age (6). Even diabetic persons display coefficients of variation in body weight of only 3.7 to 4.6% over periods of 5 years (7).

However, the condition of body weight stability, while suggestive of regulation, is by itself not sufficient to establish the case for regulation. Nor for that matter does variability of an individual's weight provide a basis for dismissing regulation. The body temperature of large dinosaurs was not physiologically regulated, although it did remain stable from day to day due to the great thermal mass of these animals. At the same time the circadian and circannual fluctuations in the core temperature of mammals, as well as its elevation with infection or injury, represent changes that are physiologically regulated (8). Thus stability is not a requisite condition for regulation and variation does not indicate its absence. Rather, regulation implies the active physiological defense of a particular condition. In a system for regulating body temperature, it is through the appearance of appropriate heat loss and heat gain responses to core temperature perturbation that we know temperature is regulated at a particular level. In a system for regulating body weight, it would be through the appropriate control of both energy intake and expenditure that the regulated level or set point would be maintained. When at the specified value, intake and expenditure are in balance; but, when body weight is perturbed and displaced from this level, it is the appearance of appropriate intake and expenditure adjustments that allows us to infer that body weight is actively regulated at some specified level.

Control of Energy Flux

Traditionally, interest has focused on food intake as the key controlled factor in the process of body energy regulation. Indeed, compensatory adjustments in food intake are readily seen when the weight of an individual is displaced from his or her normally maintained level. When weight is elevated by force-feeding, for example, eating is sharply reduced (9); if lowered by caloric restriction, intake is elevated (10). Yet, it has become increasingly clear that the relative stability of body weight is not accounted for by intake alone. One telling observation is that changes in intake often fail to produce the expected changes in body weight. The weight loss produced by food restriction, for example, is almost invariably less than expected from the apparent caloric deficit; likewise, overconsumption fails to produce weight gains commensurate with the apparent caloric excess (11). In other cases, weight gains have occurred in the absence of hyperphagia (12), while weight loss can be seen without a reduction in intake (13). Failing to appreciate the contributions of energy expenditure adjustments in these circumstances, one might well question just how well body weight is regulated.

One cannot stress too strongly how important the control of energy expenditure is to the normal regulation of body weight. The view presented here is that the failure to recognize the contribution of energy expenditure has not only been a serious oversight, but that an appreciation of its role provides some of the most useful and compelling evidence for the physiological regulation of body weight.

Energy Expenditure: Primary Components

Several factors appear to have contributed to the prior neglect of energy expenditure in the assessment of systems regulating body weight. First, it has traditionally been assumed that the energy spent to fuel our essential organs and processes is essentially fixed. Resting or "basal" metabolism has been viewed as the obligatory cost of sustaining the body's vital functions. Similarly, the heat increment to a meal [the specific dynamic action of food or SDA] is often assumed to be fixed by the type and amount of ingested energy.

Consistent with such views were observations that the daily resting energy requirement of animals, ranging in size from small birds and rodents to large mammals, was a function of their "metabolic body size" or body weight raised to the $\frac{3}{4}$ (14). This relationship is depicted in Fig. 1, in which the log of the daily resting energy expenditures of various animal species is plotted as a function of the log of their body weight. The slope of this function relating log body weight and log daily expenditure is 0.75, indicating that daily energy expenditure increases at $\frac{3}{4}$ the rate of body mass as animal species increase in size.

Based upon 26 animal species for which Kleiber (14) had data, the best-fit equation for the relationship between daily resting expenditure and body weight (BW) was found to be kcal/day = 68.5 ± 1.4 BW$_{kg}^{.75}$. It follows from this equation that one can test whether or not the resting metabolism of any particular animal species conforms to the Kleiber rule simply by dividing its daily resting caloric expenditure by its body weight raised to the $\frac{3}{4}$ power and seeing how closely the number thus obtained approximates the expected value of 68.5 ± 1.4 kcal/BW$_{kg}^{.75}$. When so expressed, Kleiber found the daily resting expenditures of a 410-g guinea pig (35.1 kcal/day), of a 3-kg cat (152 kcal/day), of a 57.2-kg woman (1,368 kcal/day), and of a 600-kg cow (7,877 kcal/day) to conform closely by yielding values of 68.5, 66.7, 65.8, and 65.0 kcal/BW$_{kg}^{.75}$, respectively.

Whether or not the Kleiber equation likewise accounts for the variation in daily energy needs of different-sized members of the same species is less clear. Kleiber (14) favored the application of his rule to intraspecies com-

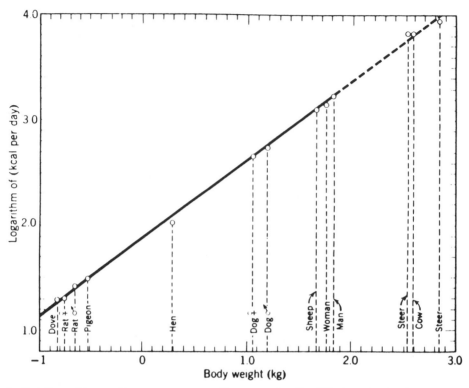

FIG. 1. Relation of log resting energy expenditure per day (kcal/day) to log body weight (kg) in different species of animals. (From Kleiber, ref. 14, with permission.)

parisons, though others suggest that within-species data are often better expressed by raising body weight to the $\frac{2}{3}$ power (15). However, the predicted differences between these two exponents are not large and the relatively small range of body weights seen within a species renders a critical choice between the two problematical. Relevant to this issue, we have found the original Kleiber formulation to provide a good account of the daily energy expenditures of different sized (but same age) rats. The total daily caloric expenditure of some 70 rats studied was, as expected, larger for heavier animals. However, as one can see in Fig. 2, dividing the daily expenditure of each rat by its body weight raised to the $\frac{3}{4}$ power effectively equalized the daily expenditure for all. Note that the average value thus obtained, indicated by the horizontal line, is 65.3 $BW_{kg}^{.75}$, a value closely approximating that predicted by Kleiber's equation based on interspecies com-

parisons. Apparently, whether comparing animals of different species or different members of the same species, daily resting energy expenditure can be approximated by the equation kcal/d = 68.5 $BW_{kg}^{.75}$.

Energy Expenditure: Facultative Components

Given the traditional views concerning both "basal metabolism" and the origins of the heat increment to a meal, and given the close relationship between daily energy expenditure and the mass of metabolically active tissue, it is none too surprising that active control of expenditure was not regarded as playing a key role in body energy regulation. However, it must be recognized that there are conditions under which the daily expenditure of body energy does not conform to these assumed rules. Evidence is emerging,

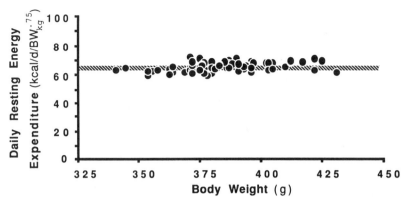

FIG. 2. Daily resting energy expenditure (kcal/day), expressed per body weight to the $\frac{3}{4}$ power ($BW_{kg}^{.75}$) of individual male rats of the same strain and age spontaneously maintaining body weights in the range of 340–430 gm. (Unpublished observations of Hirvonen and Keesey.)

for example, that the Kleiber formula, while accurately predicting an animal's resting energy expenditure at the body weight it normally maintains, fails to do so when that animal's weight is displaced from this level. For example, when food intake is restricted and weight loss occurs, resting or "basal" metabolism is lowered by an amount that significantly exceeds that expected from the loss in body size. We have observed, for example, that when the weight of rats was reduced by 14.9% through caloric restriction, their rate of resting metabolism declined by 24.6% (16). This proportionately larger decline in

resting energy expenditure than in body mass suggests that less energy is required to maintain a gram of tissue in a weight-reduced than in a normal-weight rat. To see that this is indeed the case, observe in Fig. 3 what happens to the daily resting energy expenditure of one of the 70 rats previously shown when its food intake was restricted and its weight caused to decline by about 8% (from 431–397 g). It no longer expended energy at a rate appropriate for its body size (as did the other rats at this body weight) but displayed a daily energy expenditure (kcal/day) of 43.3 $BW_{kg}^{.75}$, a level substantially below that of all the other male

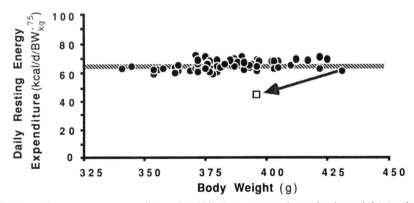

FIG. 3. Daily resting energy expenditure (kcal/day), expressed per body weight to the $\frac{3}{4}$ power ($BW_{kg}^{.75}$), of individual male rats of the same strain and age. The body weight of the largest rat in this group was reduced by 8% by restricting its intake. The arrow indicates the change in its daily resting energy expenditure associated with this weight loss. Although this rat is still one of the heavier, note that its daily energy expenditure after weight loss is lower than that of any other rat. (Unpublished observations of Hirvonen and Keesey.)

rats of this age (i.e., 65.3 $BW_{kg}^{.75}$). Comparably larger than expected reductions in resting metabolism have been reported in food-deprived men (17). Clearly, the resting (post-absorptive) metabolism of normal-weight individuals is not "basal". When weight is reduced from the level normally maintained, daily energy needs decline to levels substantially below those formerly seen and below those predicted by the Kleiber equation.

The thermogenic response to a meal likewise displays an adaptive adjustment to weight loss. In rats whose weight has been reduced, the increment in heat production normally seen following a meal can be diminished to the point of being barely detectable (18). Evidently only a portion of the normally seen increment in heat production is associated with the processing of ingested nutrients.

In the event of overconsumption and weight gain, there is, in a converse fashion, an exaggerated increase in daily resting heat production (19). Just as daily expenditure declines following weight loss, thermogenesis following weight gain is elevated significantly above that expected from the increase in tissue mass. It appears that this exaggerated heat production can be linked to the activation of a specific thermogenic effector organ, viz., the brown adipose tissue (20).

It should be evident that these adjustments in energy expenditure will dampen the effects of food intake variation on body weight and impede the displacement of body weight from the normal level; or, if weight is displaced, these expenditure adjustments will facilitate its being restored to that level. More to the point of this chapter, metabolic adjustments of this sort provide compelling evidence both for the regulation of body weight and for the existence of a physiologically preferred weight level or set point.

Energy Expenditure and the Body Weight Set Point

The preceding observations can be taken to indicate that Kleiber's empirically derived formula relating daily resting energy expenditure to body weight was derived from animals in energy stasis. As such, it accurately predicts energy expenditure when the animal is at its physiologically regulated body weight. However, as noted, metabolic adjustments occur when weight is perturbed, causing energy expenditure to increase (or decline) to a greater extent than this equation would predict. What this implies is that resting energy expenditure will be consonant with the value predicted by Kleiber's equation only when an individual is at his or her physiologically regulated body weight or set point.

As a way of illustrating this point, consider once again the daily energy expenditure of the 70 rats depicted in Fig. 2. Note that the daily energy expenditures of these different sized rats are approximately all the same when expressed relative to their body weight raised to the $\frac{3}{4}$ power. As noted, the average observed kcal/day value of $65.3 \times BW_{kg}^{.75}$ approximates the expected value. Yet, if any rat is displaced from the body weight it spontaneously maintains, its resting rate of energy expenditure will no longer conform to the expected value. As seen in Fig. 3, the daily resting energy expenditure of the rat caused to lose weight fell substantially below the level appropriate for its new body weight.

The point illustrated is that the resting energy expenditure of any individual rat is consonant with the value predicted by Kleiber's rule only when at its physiologically regulated body weight or set point. We therefore can define the body weight set point for each individual as that particular weight at which its daily resting energy expenditure is consonant with the value predicted by the Kleiber equation relating expenditure to body mass. For each individual there should be but one weight at which expenditure will be congruent with the predicted value.

It must be recognized that the weight at which this concurrence with daily expenditure is seen can and does change. It changes over the individual's life span and can be altered by dietary and/or surgical interventions. Factors capable of producing such set-point changes are discussed later in this paper. However, at any particular time in an organism's life, there is a particular body weight at which it expends energy at the "normal" or predicted rate. It is proposed that we take this weight to be that individual's set point.

IS OBESITY REGULATED?

It likewise follows from this perspective on daily energy expenditure that obesity may be the natural condition of particular individuals. Consider, for example, that the rat in Fig. 3 singled out for study was the largest in the entire group of 70. Before weight loss, this rat metabolized energy at a daily rate that was normal (i.e., appropriate to its body size). Its use of energy at a normal rate, however, was evidently dependent upon its remaining the largest rat. After only a modest weight loss, its metabolic rate declined to a level below that of all other rats. In this sense, being the heaviest member of the group was as natural for this particular rat as being of average weight was for others. That is to say, "overweight" appeared to be the natural state of this rat.

It could be argued, of course, that the rat used here to illustrate this point was not genuinely obese and that frank obesity may not fit this pattern of apparently normal regulation at a high body weight. Whether obesity is a condition in which the physiological system regulating body energy is set to be in stasis at a high level of adiposity is, however, a proposition that can be tested. The general rationale and procedures described previously for specifying the regulated body weight of an individual can also be applied to an assessment of whether or not obesity is physiologically regulated. Examining the rate of energy expenditure in obese individuals at the body weights they maintain can provide one critical piece of information on this point. Whether or not obese individuals display compensatory adjustments in energy expenditure when weight is displaced from its elevated level can provide a second.

In the section that follows, this logic is applied to an analysis of the underlying disorder in obese animals. Animal models of obesity have contributed much to the ways we conceptualize and deal with this condition in humans. Two rodent models that have played a significant role in this regard are used here to illustrate how obesity can be analyzed from a regulatory perspective. The two (dietary obesity and genetic obesity) are characterized by both increased adipocyte size and number, conditions that also characterize obese humans.

Diet-Induced Obesity

It is believed that a significant portion of obesity in modern industrialized societies can be traced to the abundant supply of tasty foods high in fat and calorically dense. Support for this notion comes from experimental studies with laboratory animals in which diets high in fat and/or sugar have been successfully employed to produce obesity (see Sclafani, *this volume*). While under certain circumstances the resulting obesity can be reversed by restoring the animals to the regular diet, at other times these changes seem to be permanent (21).

In a recent experiment (22), rats were maintained on a palatable high-fat diet for an extended time (6 months). As seen in Fig. 4, their body weights become progressively higher than those of rats fed a standard laboratory diet. After eating this diet for 6 months, these rats weighed 26% more than others fed a standard diet. Toward the end of this 6-month period, the intake of half the now obese rats and half the normal-weight control rats was restricted so as to lower their body weights from the level maintained by the rats fed either the high-fat or regular diet ad libitum (see Fig. 4).

When body composition was examined, the rats fed the high-fat diet were found to have more than double the amount of adipose tissue seen in rats fed a standard diet (145.5 versus 64.7 g, respectively). Analysis of the gonadal, retroperitoneal, and dorsal subcutaneous fat depots revealed that changes in both adipose cell size and number contributed to this increase in body fat. Average fat cell size in the high-fat-fed rats

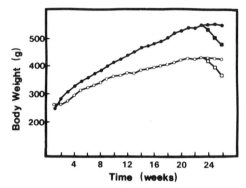

FIG. 4. Body weight of rats fed either a high-fat or conventional laboratory diet for 26 weeks. After 23 weeks, the body weight of half the high-fat fed rats and half the rats fed the control diet were reduced by restricting food intake. (Adapted from Corbett et al., ref. 22, with permission.)

increased by 61% (from 0.416 to 0.669 μg lipid/cell). The total number of adipocytes also increased significantly (from 45.38 to 66.95 × 10⁶) in these rats.

The weight adjustments that occurred when the intake of some of these rats was then restricted was also achieved largely by changes in the adipose tissue mass. The body

fat of the restricted high-fat-fed and control rats fell to 108.4 g and 32.4 g, respectively. However, the gain in adipocyte number that resulted from 6 months of ad libitum high-fat feeding was not subsequently reversed by caloric restriction. Rather, this body fat loss was achieved almost entirely by reducing the amount of lipid per adipocyte. Consistent with other reports (23), diet-induced increases in fat cell number are apparently irreversible.

Just prior to sacrifice, the resting energy expenditure of the obese and control rats was assessed, both at the spontaneously maintained body weight and at the reduced weights produced by the caloric restriction. The results of these tests are seen in Fig. 5.

Note that the resting rate of energy expenditure of the unrestricted obese rats was not elevated, but was normal for the body size ($BW_{kg}^{.75}$) they now maintained (see Fig. 5). That is, energy expenditure in these rats (kcal/day = 63.9 $BW_{kg}^{.75}$) was, as with normal weight rats (kcal/day = 64.7 $BW_{kg}^{.75}$), appropriate to body size according to the Kleiber equation. Evidently, the physiological conditions responsible for producing the elevations

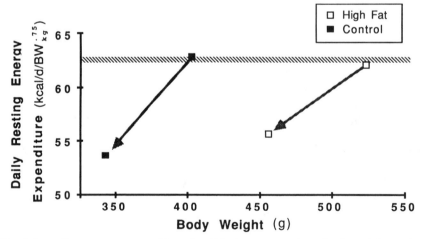

FIG. 5. The daily resting energy expenditure (kcal/day), expressed per body weight to the $\frac{3}{4}$ power ($BW_{kg}^{.75}$), of rats fed either a conventional laboratory diet or a high-fat diet for 26 weeks. At 26 weeks, the daily resting energy expenditure of the now obese rats was comparable to that of normal-weight controls (*hatched line*). Restricting food intake so as to produce the indicated weight losses caused the decline in resting expenditure shown by the arrows in both obese and normal-weight rats. (Adapted from Corbett et al, ref. 22, with permission.)

in daily energy expenditure typically seen in the initial stages of diet-induced weight gain do not persist indefinitely.

Equally interesting are the results obtained from the calorically restricted obese and control rats. The ensuing weight loss led to the expected decline in daily resting energy expenditure in the normal weight rats (from $64.7 \times BW_{kg}^{.75}$ to $55.2 \times BW_{kg}^{.75}$). And, the obese rats showed a similar adjustment to weight loss (see Fig. 5). In fact, total calories expended daily by the weight-reduced obese actually rats dropped below that of the normal weight rats (31.7 versus 32.7 kcal/day) despite the fact that the formerly obese rats still weighed 53 g more.

The findings of (a) normal rates of resting metabolism at elevated body weights, and (b) adaptive declines in resting metabolism when weight falls from these higher levels together indicate that prolonged maintenance on high-fat diets can elevate the body weight set point and thus contribute to life span changes in regulated body energy. Such a view is consistent with the observation that dietary obesity is often irreversible. It is also consistent with certain morphological and physiological changes that have been noted in animals chronically maintained on weight-promoting diets. Among these are irreversible increases in adipocyte number, which can be detected some weeks after exposure to such diets (23). Another is the pattern of change in tissue norepinephrine (NE) turnover rates following exposure to weight-promoting diets. Although initially elevated, NE turnover rates decline following continued exposure to such diets and return to near normal levels in several months (24). Whether changes in these systems simply covary with other internal adjustments crucial to elevating the level of regulation or are themselves responsible for this regulatory adjustment is not presently known.

Genetic Obesity

While genetic influence on obesity has been long assumed, the case has been greatly strengthened by recently reported observations. The results of a large-scale adoption study in Denmark and of twin studies in the United States and Sweden are noteworthy in this regard (25). The findings of the former were a high correlation of the body weight of adoptees with that of their biological parents, coupled with no significant correlation between the weight of adoptees and that of their adoptive parents. The twin studies demonstrated a very high heritability for obesity in monozygotic pairs, even when raised apart under disparate conditions.

Our understanding of the underlying basis for this genetic contribution to obesity derives in part from studies of genetically obese strains of rodents. One of the most widely studied is the Zucker rat, in which obesity is transmitted as a single Mendelian recessive gene (fafa) from the mating of two heterozygous (Fa/fa) lean rats (26).

The development of obesity in the Zucker fafa rat is facilitated both by an elevated level of energy intake and a reduced rate of expenditure. Daily energy expenditure is lower than expected (27) and expenditure on thermoregulation is blunted (28). Yet, as a weight-stable adult, both the intake and expenditure of the Zucker rat are controlled so as to sustain its obesity. Its intake of adulturated diets, for example, remains at levels sufficient to sustain the obesity (29).

The obese Zucker rat's energy expenditure deviates from that previously noted in normal weight and dietary obese rats in that it is lower than predicted on the basis of its body mass (30). Compared with lean Zucker rats (Fa?), whose daily expenditure closely approximates the rate predicted by the Kleiber equation, the daily expenditure of the obese Zucker (kcal/day = $49.5\ BW_{kg}^{.75}$) is significantly reduced. The fatty's greatly increased adipose tissue mass (which is metabolically less active than lean tissue), coupled with a lower-than-normal lean tissue mass provides at least a partial explanation for this condition.

Nevertheless, the adult Zucker fatty appropriately adjusts its daily energy expenditure in the defense of its obesity. If body weight is lowered from the elevated levels they typically maintain, obese Zucker rats display an adaptive reduction in resting energy expenditure just as do rats regulating at normal body weights (30). In order to appreciate how effective this expenditure adjustment can be in the case of the obese Zucker, consider the weight and expenditure data shown in Fig. 6. Note that the total daily caloric expenditure of the unrestricted fatty is normally 26% higher than that of lean littermates. However, with only a modest weight loss (from 623 to 583 g), the daily resting expenditure of the obese rats declines to such an extent that it is now comparable to that of unrestricted lean rats weighing only 285 g. That is, a diet-induced weight loss of only 6% essentially caused the obese Zucker's daily energy needs to decline to the level of normal-weight lean Zucker rats weighing less than half as much! Clearly, there is a strong metabolic resistance to weight loss in these obese rats. If such a mechanism operates in obese humans, the frequent claim of many unsuccessful dieters that they eat no more (or even less) than their lean friends must be given credence.

Obese Zucker rats also seem to commit the same proportion of their daily energy expenditure to somatomotor activity as do their

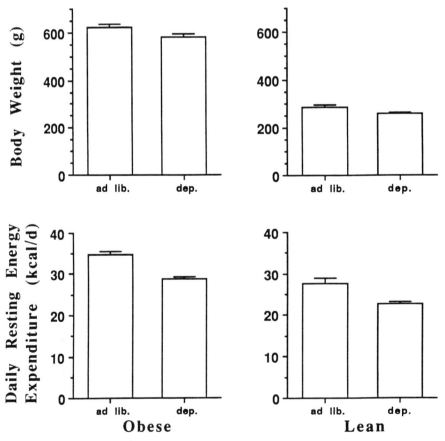

FIG. 6. Body weight (g) and daily resting energy expenditure (kcal/day) of normal weight and weight-reduced Zucker obese and lean rats. The daily resting energy expenditure of both the obese and lean rats declined following caloric restriction and weight loss. Note that the total daily resting expenditure (kcal/day) of the weight-reduced obese rats is comparable to that of lean rats, even though the obese rats still weigh more than twice as much as lean rats that ate ad libitum; *dep.,* deprived rats. (Adapted from Keesey and Corbett, ref. 30, with permission.)

lean littermates. Although it is often assumed that a reduced expenditure on activity contributes both to the development (31) and the maintenance of obesity (32,33), and though it has been reported that obese Zucker rats display less wheel running than their lean siblings, our observations (34) suggest that the maintenance of obesity in adult Zuckers is not facilitated by a reduced expenditure on activity. Measuring total energy expenditure and stabilimeter activity continuously for 5 days, we found the amount of activity, as well as its circadian pattern of occurrence, to be highly similar in the lean and obese rats. This

can be seen in Fig. 7, in which the daily pattern of both activity and of energy expenditure of lean and obese Zucker rats are displayed. An estimate of the proportion of total daily energy expenditure committed by the obese Zuckers to activity was found to be nearly identical to that estimated for leans (19.3 versus 19.7%, respectively).

In summary, a reduced rate of energy expenditure, coupled with overconsumption, predisposes developing Zucker fafa rats to the obese condition they display as adults. However, the obese adult's expenditure no longer appears to convey any energetic advantage.

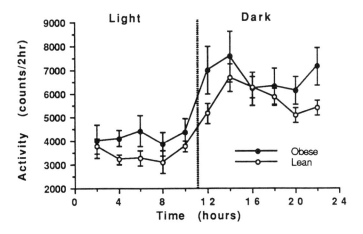

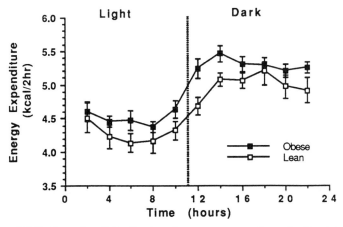

FIG. 7. Circadian distribution of activity (top) and energy expenditure (bottom) by lean and obese Zucker rats. (Adapted from Keesey et al., ref. 34, with permission.)

The daily expenditure (kcal/day) of obese Zuckers is actually higher in total amount than that of smaller lean Zuckers. The total energy they expend daily on activity is also higher, though activity-related expenditure expressed as a percentage of total daily expenditure is normal. Likewise, when energy intake is restricted, the daily expenditure of obese Zucker rats is sharply reduced, demonstrating that their elevated body weight is defended in the same way (and, apparently, as effectively) as lean rats defend a normal body weight. Thus the expenditure of Zucker fafa rats seems to be controlled in ways that favor both the achievement and the subsequent maintenance of an obese condition.

Is Human Obesity Regulated?

In both the rat models discussed above, the obesity appears to be physiologically regulated. In one, the factors seemingly responsible for causing regulation to take place at an elevated level or set point is genetically transmitted. In the other, a nutritional influence appears to be responsible for irreversibly elevating the regulatory set point. Both genetic and nutritional factors are thought to contribute to human obesity. Is it then possible that human obesity, like these two forms of animal obesity, is also a physiologically regulated condition? It should be possible to answer this question by comparing the characteristics of these obese animal models with those of human obese. Unfortunately, the observations critical to answering questions as to whether obese individuals fail to regulate energy normally, or do regulate normally but at an elevated set point, are not readily found in the clinical literature. Still, enough is known for a preliminary assessment.

It appears that obese persons, like individuals of normal weight, often maintain body weight rather stably. Of course, given the pressure exerted on obese people to lose weight, it would be surprising if their weight was not somewhat more variable. Certainly,

when they are successful in shedding weight, their subsequent tendency to regain is well documented (35).

However, neither a stable body weight, nor the tendency to restore weight to a particular level after it has been displaced, are alone sufficient to establish that obese individuals are regulating at a high set point. What is required is evidence of an active physiological defense of their obesity. It is thus interesting to note that obese individuals undergoing weight loss often display adjustments in resting metabolism consistent with their actively regulating body weight at an obese level. In one report, obese patients undergoing weight loss dropped their daily maintenance requirements by 28% (36). While the 7-day energy intake required for weight maintenance by these obese patients was initially comparable to that of normal weight control subjects (1,432 versus 1,341 kcal/m^2/day, respectively), after the obese underwent weight loss, their maintenance requirements dropped to 1,021 kcal/m^2/day. In fact, the total daily caloric requirements for the weight-reduced obese patients was actually less (2,171 kcal/day) than that of the control subjects (2,280 kcal/day) in spite of the former still weighing 60% more! Furthermore, this enhanced metabolic efficiency was not a transient effect. Three of these formerly obese individuals who were successful in maintaining a reduced body weight for as long as 4 to 6 years still displayed daily maintenance requirements of only 1,031 kcal/m^2/day.

That the reduced maintenance requirements of these obese patients following weight loss result from a lowered rate of resting metabolism is indicated by other results. Bray (37) has shown that obese patients who lost 3% of their initial body weight while dieting for 4 weeks dropped their resting rates of energy expenditure by 17%. This large a decline in metabolic rate with so modest a weight loss again suggests the active participation of physiological processes resisting weight change. Nor is this an isolated observation. Declines in the resting metabolism of dieting patients substantially in excess of that expected on the basis of tissue loss is a well-documented effect (11,17,38).

Clinical Implications

Both the human and animal observations cited above suggest that obesity can be and often is a physiologically regulated condition. When it is, the obese will maintain body weight in the same manner and, as observations suggest, as effectively as others maintain normal body weights. The animal research indicates that both genetic and nutritional factors can contribute to this condition of weight regulation at an elevated set point. Presumably, both factors contribute to human obesity as well.

It should thus be expected that an individual with a regulated form of obesity will encounter considerable natural resistance to diet-induced weight loss. Compensatory metabolic adjustments to dieting will not only diminish initial weight loss but facilitate the restoration of previously lost weight. Sustained weight reduction in formerly obese individuals will therefore require a lifelong commitment to diets providing a daily caloric intake that is not only less than satisfying, but possibly less than that consumed by individuals of normal body weight. Inasmuch as current treatment focuses primarily on the control of intake, some observers (39) have asked whether the eating and other life-style adjustments that chronic dieting entail, in conjunction with the possible nutritional inadequacies and depressed metabolism that constricted intake can produce, might not be too great a price to pay for the modest weight losses that most obese individuals are able to achieve and sustain.

This may, however, be too pessimistic a view. If obesity is indeed a physiologically regulated phenomenon, it is understandable that past treatment approaches, which have focused on dieting, have not been particularly successful. However, were ways found to adjust the level the energy-regulating system is set to maintain, physiological adjustments such as these could serve to facilitate,

rather than resist, the desired weight changes. This is to suggest that a more promising approach to the problem of obesity would be one that aimed, first, at identifying the factors responsible for setting the level at which such individuals regulate body energy and, second, at applying this knowledge to the development of procedures that would permit one to readjust this regulatory set point. To this end, the following section first reviews what is known about the central nervous mechanisms responsible for setting the regulated level of body energy and then describes several currently available means for adjusting the value the body's energy-regulating system strives to maintain.

The Hypothalamus and Regulated Body Energy

The hypothalamus plays a key role in the physiological regulation of many body factors. In some cases (e.g., thermoregulation) the hypothalamic mechanisms responsible for setting the level of the factor the system is set to maintain, as well as the agents capable of readjusting the system set point, have been identified (8). Although our understanding of the system for regulating body energy is certainly less advanced, available evidence suggests that the hypothalamus also plays a primary role in setting the regulated level of body energy. There is also evidence that one can experimentally manipulate these hypothalamic mechanisms so as to adjust the set point of this energy-regulating system.

Lesions of the lateral hypothalamus (LH) in rats produce a syndrome of aphagia and anorexia, leading to the historic designation of this hypothalamic region as a "feeding center" (40). In time, intake returns and LH-lesioned rats again ingest food in sufficient amounts to maintain body weight. More recent work (41) has shown, however, that the weight lost during the postlesion period of aphagia and anorexia is not restored upon the return of spontaneous food intake. Instead, LH-lesioned rats chronically maintain body weight at some reduced percentage of normal

(See Fig. 8). Furthermore, they clearly defend these reduced body weights when challenged. It can be seen in Fig. 9 that, just as nonlesioned rats quickly restore body weight to its proper level following a period of food restriction and weight loss, LH-lesioned rats quickly restore weight to its reduced level of postlesion maintenance (42). Also, just as nonlesioned rats restore body weight to a normal level after it has been elevated by force-feeding, so do LH-lesioned rats quickly restore weight to a reduced level after being force-fed to normal levels (43). It has also been demonstrated that lowering body weight prior to lesioning the LH not only eliminates the usual aphagia and anorexia but, in some cases, leads to a postlesion hyperphagia (41). This demonstrates that aphagia and anorexia are not direct effects of the LH lesion but should instead be viewed as behaviors appropriate to adjusting body weight to a new, lesion-produced level of regulation. Thus, if above the new (reduced) level of weight maintenance when lesioned, LH rats respond adaptively by restricting or eliminating intake; if below it, they respond by increasing their daily intake.

The general pattern of daily energy expenditure in LH-lesioned rats provides some of the strongest evidence that they are regulating body energy at a reduced set point. In an energy balance study, it was observed that the daily resting expenditure of LH rats was normal in that it was appropriate for their reduced body sizes (44). That is, their total daily resting expenditure, expressed relative to their body weight raised to the $\frac{3}{4}$ power, was indistinguishable from that of nonlesioned, normal-weight rats. As previously discussed, rats whose weight is lowered from the regulated level typically display a resting metabolic rate markedly lower than ex-

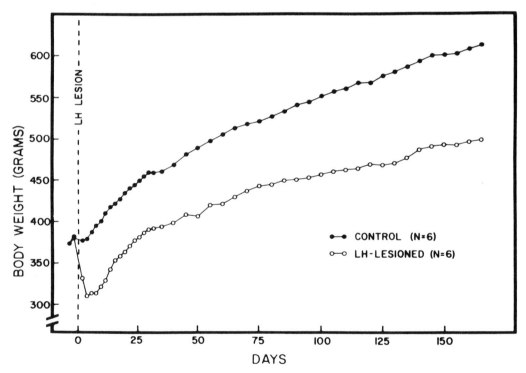

FIG. 8. Body weight of control rats and rats with lateral hypothalamic (*LH*) lesions over a 24-week period following surgery. The body weight of the lesioned rats stabilized at 86 ± 2% that of control rats from the third week postlesion until the experiment ended. (From Keesey et al., ref. 43, with permission.)

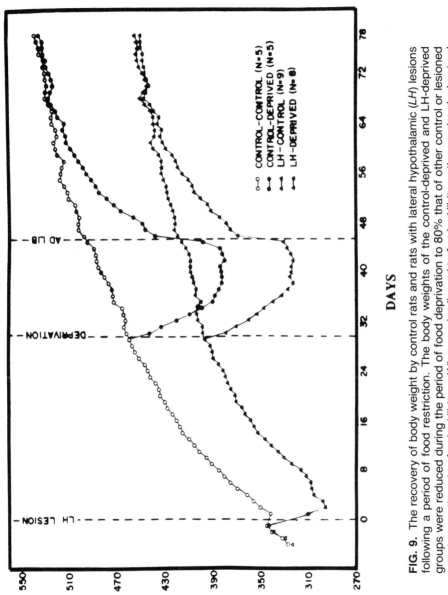

FIG. 9. The recovery of body weight by control rats and rats with lateral hypothalamic (*LH*) lesions following a period of food restriction. The body weights of the control-deprived and LH-deprived groups were reduced during the period of food deprivation to 80% that of other control or lesioned rats that continued to feed ad libitum. When again allowed to feed ad libitum, the previously deprived control and lesioned rats quickly restored their body weights to the appropriate level. (From Mitchel and Keesey, ref. 42, with permission.)

pected. Thus LH-lesioned rats do not appear to be displaced from their regulated or set-point energy level at the reduced weight they maintain; rather, they display rates of resting metabolism appropriate to the reduced tissue mass they now maintain. Displaying normal levels of daily energy flux at a reduced body weight is indicative of a reduced set point.

This conclusion has been tested in two further experiments. The rationale in each was that, if the set point for body energy has indeed been reduced, LH-lesioned rats should metabolically resist being displaced from their lower body weights in the same way that nonlesioned rats resist being displaced from normal body weights. To this end, rats maintaining stable (reduced) body weights following LH lesions were given either (a) a highly palatable liquid diet or (b) restricted amounts of the regular diet. The palatable diet produced substantial weight gain (restoring the weight of the lesioned rats to normal levels), while caloric restriction produced a further 12% weight loss. Similar weight gains or losses were produced by these procedures in nonlesioned rats.

The results of the first of these two experiments are summarized in Fig. 10. As can be seen, the LH-lesioned rats, though at reduced body weights, initially display a daily rate of energy expenditure that (when expressed relative to body weight raised to the $\frac{3}{4}$ power) is normal and virtually the same as that of normal weight rats (kcal/day = 69.4 versus 70.3 $BW_{kg}^{.75}$). However, elevating body weight to the level maintained by nonlesioned animals caused the daily expenditure of the lesioned rats to rise substantially above normal values (to 77.5 $BW_{kg}^{.75}$). Thus restoring the weight of LH-lesioned rats to normal levels caused them to become hypermetabolic, in apparently the same way that nonlesioned rats become hypermetabolic when they overeat and become obese.

In a similar fashion, lowering the body weight of LH-lesioned rats from the already reduced levels they maintain caused a sharp decline in daily expenditure from the normal level. Nonlesioned rats also displayed this adjustment in expenditure when their weight was reduced to the level the lesioned rats spontaneously maintained. The differ-

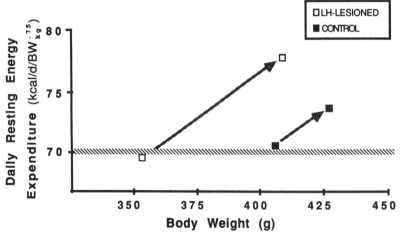

FIG. 10. Relation of daily resting energy expenditure (kcal/d/$BW_{kg}^{.75}$) to body weight (g) in control rats and rats with lateral hypothalamic (*LH*) lesions. A palatable high-fat diet was used to stimulate increased intake by half the control and half the LH-lesioned rats to produce the weight gains and daily expenditure increases indicated by the arrows. Note that when the body weight of the LH-lesioned rats was restored to that of nonlesioned rats, daily resting energy expenditure is considerably in excess of what is appropriate for that weight (*hatched line*). (From Corbett et al., ref. 16, with permission.)

ence, of course, is that the lesioned rats displayed this response only when their weight declined from an already reduced level of maintenance.

Each of the preceding observations concerning the energy expenditure of LH-lesioned rats is consistent with the view that these hypothalamic lesions cause body energy to be down-regulated. By displaying (a) a normal expenditure of energy at a reduced body weight, (b) a disproportionately lower than expected energy expenditure when their weight declines from this reduced level, and (c) a disproportionately higher than expected heat production following gain to normal body weights, rats with lesions of this hypothalamic area give every indication of regulating body energy at a reduced set point.

Natural or Experimentally Induced Changes in Regulated Body Weight

It is known that the set point for regulated body temperature can be elevated by endogenous pyrogens produced in response to bacteria, viruses, and endotoxins. Indications are that the hypothalamic mechanisms responsible for setting the level of regulated body energy can also be altered. Naturally occurring instances of adjustments in regulated body energy are seen in migratory animals and in hibernators in which the variation follows an endogenous circannual rhythm (45). Regulated body energy similarly appears to undergo gradual change over the normal life span of men and women. Dietary factors can also cause the body's regulated energy level to be altered. Earlier in this chapter, it was shown that long-term maintenance on high-fat diets can chronically elevate regulated body energy in the rat.

There are reasons to believe that some agents that characteristically cause body weight changes may exert this influence by directly altering the set point for regulated body energy. "Anorectic" drugs offer one such example. While it is generally assumed that these drugs act by suppressing appetite, certain observations are not easily reconciled with this view. Anorectic drugs are, for example, effective in suppressing food intake only until body weight drops to a certain amount. Intake then returns to essentially normal levels, although body weight remains at a reduced level. Tolerance to the anorectic agent has traditionally been offered as the explanation for its failure to continue suppressing food intake. Stunkard (46), however, offered an alternative explanation based on the proposition that anorectic drugs lower the body weight set point. Accordingly, he proposed that the initial food intake suppression these drugs cause is secondary to lowering body weight to the new (reduced) maintenance level they produce. Once at the reduced level, however, food intake is restored to levels appropriate to stable maintenance of this new weight. The observation (47) that fenfluramine in rats fails to suppress food intake if body weight has been reduced prior to the start of drug administration favors Stunkard's interpretation. It might be noted in this regard that the acute adjustments in energy intake and expenditure displayed by former smokers, followed by the stable maintenance of body weight at a higher level, has prompted others to suggest that nicotine also lowers the set point for regulated body weight (48).

The toxin TCDD (2,3,7,8-tetrachlorodibenzo-p-dioxin) also appears to cause the body weight set point to be lowered (49). Rats administered TCDD at sublethal doses not only maintain chronically reduced body weights but display an unimpaired capacity to defend this reduced weight. If challenged by changes in the caloric density of a diet, TCDD-treated rats display the same adjustments in intake as control rats. If their weight is experimentally displaced by underfeeding, they restore weight to its former level as quickly and precisely as do normal-weight rats (see Fig. 11). Also like normal rats, TCDD-treated rats stimulated to overeat a highly palatable diet deposit the excess calories as fat. As a result, the body composition of TCDD-treated rats whose weights have been restored to control levels are not nor-

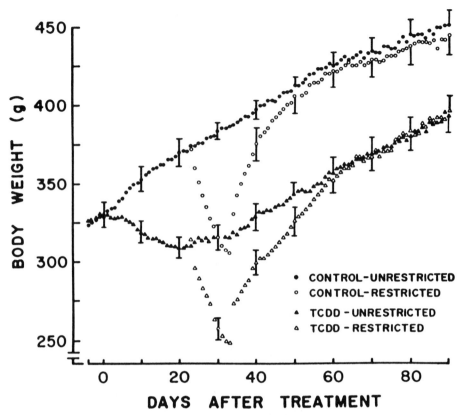

FIG. 11. Recovery of body weight in control and TCDD-treated rats following weight loss produced by food restriction. On day 0, rats were treated with a single dose of TCDD (15 μg/kg) or with vehicle alone. Food restriction began on day 23, and continued ad libitum feeding was reinstated on day 33. (From Seefeld, et al., ref. 49, with permission.)

mal; instead, such rats are obese. It thus appears that this toxin also reduces the level of body energy regulation.

At present we do not have a clear understanding of how regulated body energy is naturally readjusted. Likewise, none of the available means for lowering regulated body energy experimentally now offer a safe or acceptable means of treating obesity. What these observations do offer, however, is the promise that a safe and effective means for lowering the level at which obese individuals regulate body energy is possible. Certainly, the search for such a means should be a primary objective of future research on obesity.

CONCLUSIONS

This chapter dealt initially with the issue of how the regulation of body energy can be

demonstrated and how, by an analysis of daily energy expenditure, the level that each individual's energy-regulating system is set to maintain might be specified. On the basis of experimental studies on two animal forms of obesity, and from published observations of obese humans, the proposal was made that obesity itself may often be a physiologically regulated condition. It was noted that the general lack of success in treating obesity by means such as dieting is consistent with this proposal. Physiological resistance, in the form of energy-conserving adjustments in daily expenditure, impedes diet-induced weight loss; or, when weight loss does occur, these adjustments serve to facilitate the recovery of the lost energy. Sustained weight loss would thus require a life-long commitment by the formerly obese to daily caloric intakes substantially less than desired.

These considerations led to the proposition that a potentially more promising approach to the treatment of obesity would be one based upon a strategy of directly altering the set point of the energy-regulating system. Were it possible to lower the system set point, the physiological adjustments that act to resist weight change when the system is perturbed by dieting would instead serve to facilitate the achievement and subsequent maintenance of a lower weight.

The second part of the chapter thus initially considers the hypothalamic systems apparently responsible for setting the level at which body energy is regulated. Experiments demonstrating that regulated body energy can be chronically lowered by direct manipulation of these hypothalamic mechanisms are described. Other instances in which body energy appears to be lowered experimentally, or in which it seems to be altered as the result of naturally occurring but unspecified physiological changes, are discussed. While none of the experimental means for reducing regulated body energy now provide an acceptable means of treating obese humans, it is proposed that a better understanding of the mechanism responsible for bringing about these adjustments may well point the way to our devising a safe and effective means of achieving this goal.

REFERENCES

1. Hardy JD. The "set-point" concept in physiological temperature regulation. In: Yamamoto WAS, Brobeck JR, eds. *Physiological controls and regulations.* Philadelphia: WB Saunders, 1965;98–116.
2. Metropolitan Life Insurance Co. Metropolitan height and weight tables. *Stat Bull* 1983;64:1–9.
3. Adam JM, Bestrand TW, Edholm OG. Weight changes in young men. *J Physiol (Lond)* 1961; 156:38.
4. Khosha T, Billewicz WZ. Measurement of changes in body weight. *Br J Nutr* 1964;18:227–39.
5. Robinson MD, Watson PE. Day to day variations in body weight of young women. *Br J Nutr* 1965; 19:225–35.
6. Ten-State Nutrition Survey 1968–1970. US DHEW publication no (HSM)72-8131.
7. Goodner CJ, Ogilvie JT. Homeostasis of body weight in a diabetes clinic population. *Diabetes* 1974;23:318–26.
8. Hensel H. Displacement of set-point. In: *Thermoreception and temperature regulation.* London: Academic Press, 1981:199–218.
9. Cohn C, Joseph D. Influence of body weight and body fat on appetite of "normal" lean and obese rats. *Yale J Biol Med* 1962;34:598–607.
10. Levitsky DA. Feeding patterns of rats in response to fasts and changes in environmental conditions. *Physiol Behav* 1970;5:291–300.
11. Apfelbaum M, Bostsarron J, Lacatis D. Effect of caloric restriction and excessive intake on energy expenditure. *Am J Clin Nutr* 1971;24:1405–9.
12. Levitsky DA, Faust I, Glassman M. The ingestion of food and the recovery of body weight following fasting in the naive rat. *Physiol Behav* 1976;17:575–80.
13. Obarzanek E, Levitsky DA. Weight gain through overeating and return to normal without undereating. *Fed Proc* 1984;43:1057.
14. Kleiber M. *The fire of life: an introduction to animal energetics.* Huntington, NY: Robert E, Krieger Co., 1975.
15. Donhoffer S. Body size and metabolic rate: exponent and coefficient of the allometric equation. The role of units. *J Theor Biol* 1986;19:125–37.
16. Corbett SW, Wilterdink EJ, Keesey RE. Resting oxygen consumption in over- and underfed rats with lateral hypothalamic lesions. *Physiol Behav* 1985; 35:971–7.
17. Keys A, Brozek J, Henschel A. *The biology of human starvation.* Minneapolis: University of Minnesota Press, 1950.
18. Boyle PC, Storlien LH, Harper AE, Keesey RE. Oxygen consumption and locomotor activity during restricted feeding and realimentation. *Am J Physiol* 1981;241:R392–7.
19. Rothwell NJ, Stock MJ. Energy expenditure of 'cafeteria'-fed rats determined from measurements of energy balance and indirect calorimetry. *J Physiol* 1982;328:371–7.
20. Rothwell NJ, Stock MJ. A role for brown adipose tissue in diet-induced thermogenesis. *Nature* 1979;281:31–5.
21. Rolls BJ, Rowe EA, Turner RC. Persistent obesity in rats following a period of consumption of a mixed high energy diet. *J Physiol (Lond)* 1980;298:415–27.
22. Corbett SW, Stern JS, Keesey RE. Energy expenditure of rats with diet-induced obesity. *Am J Clin Nutr* 1986;44:173–80.
23. Faust IM, Johnson PR, Stern JS, Hirsch J. Diet-induced adipocyte number increase in adult rats: a new model of obesity. *Am J Physiol* 1978; 235:E279–86.
24. Levin BE, Triscari J, Sullivan AC. Altered sympathetic activity during development of diet induced obesity in the rat. *Am J Physiol* 1983;244:R347–55.
25. Stunkard AJ. Genes, environment and human obesity. In: Oomura Y, Tarui S, Inoue S, Shimazu T, eds. *Progress in obesity research 1990.* London: John Libby, 1991;669–74.
26. Zucker LM, Zucker TF. 'Fatty', a new mutation in the rat. *J Hered* 1961;52:275–8.
27. Planche E, Joliff M. Evolution des dépenses énergétiques chez le rat Zucker au cours de la première semaine de la vie. Effet de l'heure mesures. *Reprod Nutr Dev* 1987;27:673–9.

28. Trayhurn PL, Thurlby PL, James WPT. A defective response to cold in the obese (obob) mouse and the obese Zucker (fafa) rat. *Proc Nutr Soc* 1976; 35:133A.

29. Cruce JAF, Greenwood MRC, Johnson PR, Quartermain D. Genetic versus hypothalamic obesity; studies of intake and dietary manipulations in rats. *J Comp Physiol Psychol* 1974;87:295–301.

30. Keesey RE, Corbett SW. Adjustments in daily energy expenditure to caloric restriction and weight loss by adult obese and lean Zucker rats. *Int J Obes* 1990;14:1079–84.

31. Griffith M, Payne RR. Energy expenditure in small children of obese and non-obese parents. *Nature* 1976;260:698–700.

32. Chirico A, Stunkard AJ. Physical activity and human obesity. *N Engl J Med* 1960;263:935–40.

33. Stern JS, Johnson PR. Spontaneous activity and adipose cellularity in the genetically obese Zucker (fa/fa) rat. *Metabolism* 1977;26:371–80.

34. Keesey RE, Swiergiel AH, Corbett SW. Contribution of spontaneous activity to daily energy expenditure of adult obese and lean Zucker rats. *Physiol Behav* 1990;48:327–31.

35. Stunkard AJ, Penick SB. Behavior modification in the treatment of obesity. The problem of maintaining weight loss. *Arch Gen Psychiatry* 1979;36:801–6.

36. Leibel RL, Hirsch J. Diminished energy requirements in reduced-obese patients. *Metabolism* 1984;33:164–70.

37. Bray GA. Effect of caloric restriction on energy expenditure in obese patients. *Lancet* 1969;2:397–8.

38. Drenick EJ, Dennin HF. Energy expenditure in fasting obese men. *J Lab Clin Med* 1973;81:421–30.

39. Wooley SC, Wooley OW. Should obesity be treated at all? In: Stunkard AJ, Stellar E, eds. *Eating and its disorders.* New York: Raven Press, 1984;185–92.

40. Anand BK, Brobeck JR. Localization of a "feeding center" in the hypothalamus of the rat. *Proc Soc Exp Biol Med* 1951;77:323–4.

41. Powley TL, Keesey RE. Relationship of body weight to the lateral hypothalmic feeding syndrome. *J Comp Physiol Psychol* 1970;70:25–36.

42. Mitchel JS, Keesey RE. Defense of a lowered weight maintenance level by lateral hypothalamically lesioned rats: evidence from a restriction-refeeding regimen. *Physiol Behav* 1977;18:1121–5.

43. Keesey RE, Boyle PD, Kemnitz JW, Mitchel JS. The role of the lateral hypothalamus in determining the body weight set-point. In: Novin D, Wyrwicka W, Bray GA, eds. *Hunger: basic mechanisms and clinical implications.* New York: Raven Press, 1976;243–55.

44. Corbett SW, Keesey RE. Energy balance of rats with lateral hypothalamic lesions. *Am J Physiol* 1982;242:E273–9.

45. Mrosovsky N. *Rheostasis: the physiology of change.* New York: Oxford Press, 1990.

46. Stunkard AJ. Anorectic agents lower a body weight set point. *Life Sci* 1982;30:2043–55.

47. Levitsky DA, Strupp BJ, Lupoli J. Tolerance to anorectic drugs: pharmacological or artifactual? *Pharmacol Biochem Behav* 1981;14:661–7.

48. Schwid SR, Hirvonen MD, Keesey RE. Nicotine effects on body weight: a regulatory perspective. *Am J Clin Nutr* 1992;55:878–884.

49. Seefeld MD, Keesey RE, Peterson RF. Body weight regulation in rats treated with 2,3,7,8-tetrachlorodibenzo-p-dioxin. *Toxicol Appl Pharmacol* 1984; 76:526–36.

Obesity: Theory and Therapy, Second Edition,
edited by A. J. Stunkard and T. A. Wadden.
Published by Raven Press, Ltd., New York, 1993.

6

Energy Metabolism

Eric Ravussin and *Boyd A. Swinburn

*National Institute of Diabetes and Digestive and Kidney Diseases, National Institutes
of Health, Phoenix, Arizona 85016; °Department of Community Health,
University of Auckland, New Zealand*

Obesity is highly prevalent in the industrialized world, and the chronic diseases associated with it are the major killers in these countries. Perhaps even more importantly, alarming figures on the increasing prevalence of obesity-related diseases are emerging from many developing countries in Africa, Asia, and Latin America. In the long run, the success of prevention and/or treatment of obesity and its related diseases will depend upon basic research uncovering the etiology of energy imbalance and applied research converting that knowledge into successful population and individual strategies. This chapter will review the current knowledge of the role of energy metabolism in the etiology of obesity.

Daily energy expenditure can be divided into three major components: the resting metabolic rate, the thermic effect of food, and the energy cost of physical activity. In spite of the close correlation between resting metabolic rate and body size, recent studies have shown that at any given body size and body composition, there is considerable variance in resting metabolic rate and that part of this variance is genetically determined. Whether the decreased thermic effect of food frequently reported in the obese is the cause or the consequence of the obese state remains controversial. The recent application of the doubly labeled water method to measure energy expenditure in free-living conditions in humans will provide new insights into the role of physical activity in the pathogenesis of obesity.

A new approach for determining the most appropriate energy balance equation in humans is provided by separately considering the different nutrient balances. Since carbohydrate and protein stores are closely regulated while fat stores are not, fat balance instead of energy balance offers an improved framework for understanding the pathogenesis of obesity.

Prospective studies have recently shown that the major metabolic risk factors for weight gain are a low energy expenditure, a low rate of fat oxidation, and insulin sensitivity. These are briefly summarized and the emerging pattern of their relationships with weight gain is described. This current knowledge should lead to future studies designed to uncover the mechanisms underlying the variability in metabolic rate, fat oxidation, and fat storage. So far, in all the longitudinal studies, only part of the weight gain can be explained by decreased rates of energy expenditure and/or fat oxidation. The current methods for measuring food intake are not accurate enough to quantify the contribution of "overeating" to obesity. However, while precise measurements of energy intake and energy expenditure are important, a deeper understanding of the etiology of obesity will emerge only after the mechanisms that balance energy input with energy output are further clarified. Therefore, research into these balancing mechanisms should be given the highest priority.

ENERGY EXPENDITURE: COMPONENTS, MEASUREMENTS, AND RELEVANCE TO OBESITY

Components of Energy Expenditure

In 1973, Durnin and colleagues (1) emphasized the need to understand the basis of energy requirements in humans so that the variability in requirements between individuals and the development of obesity could be understood. Before discussing the methods used to measure energy expenditure in humans and the major determinants of energy expenditure, it is important to define the major components of daily energy expenditure (Fig. 1).

The *resting metabolic rate* (RMR) is the energy expended by a subject resting in bed in the morning in the fasting state under comfortable, ambient conditions. RMR includes the cost of maintaining the integrated systems of the body and the homeothermic temperature at rest. In most sedentary adults, RMR accounts for approximately 60 to 70% of daily energy expenditure (2,3). *Thermogenesis* can be defined as an increase in resting metabolic rate in response to stimuli such as food intake, cold or heat exposure, psychological influences like fear or stress, or as the result of administration of drugs or hormones that mimic the physiological response

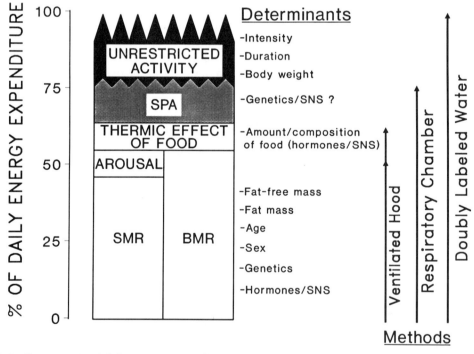

FIG. 1. Components of daily energy expenditure in humans. Daily energy expenditure can be divided into three major components: the basal metabolic rate (*BMR*) [sum of the sleeping metabolic rate (*SMR*) and the energy cost of arousal], which represents 50 to 70% of daily energy expenditure; the thermic effect of food, which represents ~10% of daily energy expenditure; and the energy cost of physical activity [sum of spontaneous physical activity (*SPA*) and unrestricted/voluntary physical activity], which represents 20 to 40% of daily energy expenditure. The major determinants of the different components of daily energy expenditure, as well as the methods to measure them, are presented. *SNS,* sympathetic nervous system.

to such stimuli. The thermic effect of food (the major form of thermogenesis) accounts for approximately 10% of the daily energy expenditure (4). Lastly, *physical activity,* the most variable component of daily energy expenditure, can account for a significant amount of calories in very active people. However, sedentary adult individuals exhibit a range of physical activity that represents only 20 to 30% of total energy expenditure.

Methods of Measuring Energy Expenditure

Many methods have been developed to measure energy expenditure. The most accurate methods involve continuous measurements of heat output (direct calorimetry) or gas exchange (indirect calorimetry) in subjects confined in metabolic chambers. Because confined subjects are unable to pursue habitual activities, several field methods have been developed to measure energy expenditure in free-living conditions. These include factorial methods, heart rate monitoring, energy intake and energy balance, and the newly developed doubly labeled water method.

Direct Calorimetry

Total heat loss from the body can be assessed by direct calorimetry. This method has been extensively applied to animal studies and in a few instances to human studies (5–7). The technique of direct calorimetry requires placing an individual in a small chamber in which all the heat released in the form of dry heat or evaporative heat is measured. Dry heat loss represents the heat dissipated by convection and radiation, whereas evaporative heat loss is related to the evaporation of water from the lungs and skin. Direct calorimeters have been useful to validate other indirect methods but have the disadvantage of being very expensive and requiring the confinement of subjects in a very small room.

Indirect Calorimetry

Under normal physiological conditions, neither oxygen nor carbon dioxide are stored within the body. The indirect method of assessing energy expenditure is therefore to measure oxygen consumption, carbon dioxide production, and nitrogen excretion. Protein oxidation is estimated on the basis of urinary nitrogen excretion. A nonprotein respiratory quotient (nonprotein $\dot{V}CO_2$/nonprotein $\dot{V}O_2$) can be calculated and the ratio between carbohydrate and lipid oxidation can be assessed (8). Knowing the amount of each energy substrate oxidized, i.e., carbohydrate, fat, and protein, it is possible to calculate the energy generated as a function of these oxidative processes. Indirect calorimetry techniques have proved useful for the study of energy expenditure and/or substrate oxidation in normal and diseased states. The earlier measurements were performed using mouthpieces or face masks and were later replaced by ventilated hood systems. The latter system has the advantage of being easily tolerated for several hours.

During the past decade, indirect calorimetry has been used in respiratory chambers (2,3,9–13). The chamber is a room large enough (12,000 to 40,000 liters) for a subject to live in comfortably for up to several days. The measurements from the chamber are accurate and are now used extensively to assess the determinants of sedentary energy expenditure in humans. Respiratory chambers enable us to measure the different components of energy expenditure, including the sleeping metabolic rate, the energy cost of arousal, the thermic effect of food, and the energy cost of spontaneous physical activity (Fig. 1). The only disadvantage is the confinement of the subjects in a small room.

Indirect Methods Used in Free-Living Conditions

Because confined subjects are unable to pursue habitual activities, several field methods have been developed to measure energy expenditure in free-living situations. These include factorial methods (14), heart rate monitoring (15), and measured metabolizable energy intake (16). The factorial method in which energy expenditure is computed from time spent in various activities and their energy costs is used most often. This method, which is very time-consuming and produces disturbances of daily routine, has been both criticized (17) and defended (18). Variations in the method occur because of differences in recording and describing activities, as well as in assigning energy costs to these activities. Comparisons of factorial methods against other field methods have provided reasonable or good agreement for groups but not for individuals (16,19–22). Recent assessment against simultaneous measurement of 24-hour energy expenditure in a respiratory chamber (23) also showed reasonable group agreement but poor agreement for individuals. The heart rate method needs an intraindividual calibration of heart rate against energy expenditure and is subject to numerous breakdowns and failures of the different systems used. Finally, very indirect assessment of energy expenditure has been developed using weight-maintenance energy intake over a period of weeks in conjunction with the determination of changes in body composition (24–26). With this technique, the best estimates have been obtained using liquid formula diets.

Doubly Labeled Water Technique

The doubly labeled water method, which was developed in animals by Lifson (27) and first used in human subjects by Schoeller and Van Santen (28), is a form of indirect calorimetry based on the differential elimination of deuterium and ^{18}oxygen from body water following a loading dose of these two stable isotopes. Since the ^{18}oxygen is in equilibrium with the water pool and the bicarbonate pool, the disappearance rates of the two isotopes measure the turnover of water (for deute-

rium) and water + carbon dioxide (for ^{18}oxygen), from which carbon dioxide production is calculated by difference. Energy expenditure is then calculated from carbon dioxide production by classical indirect calorimetric equations. The major advantage of the doubly labeled water method is that it provides an integrated measure of total carbon dioxide production over periods of 5 to 20 days and yet only requires periodic sampling of urine for measurements of deuterium and ^{18}oxygen enrichments. Subjects can be studied in the free-living state, and are not limited in their activity by wearing cumbersome monitors. A recent review by Schoeller and Field (29) of the studies using this method summarizes what we have learned to date from the doubly labeled water method. The method, which is noninvasive, has now been validated repeatedly in humans and can be used in pregnant women, infants, children, and the elderly (30–36). In conjunction with other determinations of resting or sedentary energy expenditure using indirect calorimetry, this new method represents the best and most accurate way of assessing the energy cost of physical activity in people (Fig. 1). The major problem is the high costs of the ^{18}oxygen isotope, its availability, and of the isotope ratio mass spectrometer necessary to determine the isotopic enrichment in deuterium and ^{18}oxygen.

Components of Energy Expenditure and Relevance to Obesity

Resting Metabolic Rate

The close correlation between RMR and body size has been known for many years. Although earlier investigators observed some variance in RMR among normal individuals (37), they were more concerned with defining the limits of the normal range to identify disease states such as hypo- or hyperthyroidism. At that time, RMR was essentially considered constant for a given body size and this led to the development of equations, now widely used, to predict RMR based on height and weight (38–41). More recent studies, however, have shown that at any given body size and body composition, RMR can be quite different between individuals. In a study of 130 siblings from 54 families, Bogardus et al. (42) have shown that RMR correlated best with fat-free body mass. In addition, RMR varied more between individuals than could be accounted for by differences in fat-free body mass, age, and sex, by daily fluctuations in RMR, or by methodological variability. Fat-free mass, fat mass, age, and sex are the major determinants of RMR, explaining ~80% of its variance (3,42). In their study, Bogardus et al. (42) concluded that some of the unexplained variance in RMR was explained by family membership, suggesting that RMR is at least partially genetically determined. Further support for a genetic determinant of RMR comes from studies of twins by Bouchard et al. (43). These authors showed convincingly that the RMRs of monozygotic twins were more alike than RMRs of dizygotic twins, even after adjustment for individual differences in body size and body composition.

In our search for the possible mechanisms underlying the intersubject variability in resting metabolic rate, we have recently explored the impact of gender, physical training, age, muscle metabolism, sympathetic nervous activity, and body temperature on resting metabolic rate. In a large number of Caucasian volunteers, we found that females had a lower resting metabolic rate when compared to males (~100 kcal/day less) independently of differences in fat-free mass, fat mass, and age (44). This difference can most likely be attributed to the effect of sex hormones on metabolic rate. Whether the level of physical activity is a determinant of the resting metabolic rate is still controversial. Some studies have demonstrated a relationship between the level of physical fitness and the resting metabolic rate (45,46), others have found a reduction of the resting metabolic rate during detraining (47), and still other studies could not demonstrate any relationship between

physical fitness and metabolic rate (48–50). Whether inclusion of a training program during weight therapy protects against the drop in RMR is also controversial (51–53).

Cross-sectional studies of basal metabolic rate indicate significant age-related declines (54,55). Based on a more recent longitudinal study, Keys et al. (56) estimated that the decline in basal metabolic rate was less than 1 to 2% per decade from the second to the seventh decade of life. Subsequent work (57–59) has supported Keys's conclusion that the decrease in basal metabolic rate seen in elderly people can be explained largely by decreases in lean body mass. In a recent study (60), we found a small, but significant negative impact of age on metabolic rate independently of fat-free mass, fat mass, and sex.

Recent data in studies using indirect assessment of sympathetic nervous system (SNS) activity suggest that the SNS may regulate the resting metabolic rate under eucaloric conditions (61,62). Also, resting skeletal muscle metabolism seems to be a major determinant of whole-body metabolism (63,64). Finally, we have recently reported that in males the variability in resting metabolic rate after adjusting for differences in fat-free mass, fat mass, and age was related to the variability in body temperature (65). These results indicate that body temperature may be a marker of a high or low relative metabolic rate. It is not clear whether the heat production in the body, i.e., the metabolic rate, is regulated to maintain a given "preset" temperature or whether the temperature is simply a reflection of the equilibrium between the heat-producing and heat-losing mechanisms, which are controlled by other factors.

The impact of a low resting metabolic rate as a risk factor for weight gain will be discussed later.

Thermic Effect of Food

Since Pittet's study in 1976 (66), showing a decreased thermic effect of glucose in obese compared with lean controls, studies of energy expenditure in lean and obese individuals have focused primarily on a lower thermic effect of food as a possible cause of weight gain. This seems to have occurred for two reasons: first, it was assumed that RMR was constant for a given body size and therefore would be an unlikely cause of variation in daily energy expenditure among individuals; second, studies using crude methods to assess physical activity failed to demonstrate that obese subjects were consistently less active than lean persons. Thus the thermic effect of food appeared to be the only component of daily energy expenditure that could cause variations in energy expenditure and therefore predispose individuals to obesity. Indeed, many factors influence the thermic effect of food: the test meal size and composition, the palatability of the food, and the time of the meal, as well as the subject's genetic background, age, physical fitness, and sensitivity to insulin. These influences plus the technical aspects such as the position of the subject and the duration of measurement mean that the thermic effect of food is the most difficult and the least reproducible component of daily energy expenditure to measure (3). All of these physiological and technical factors might explain the inconsistency and the variability of the thermic effect of food as reviewed by Sims (67) and D'Alessio et al. (68). Studies demonstrating a reduced thermic effect of food in obese compared with lean subjects and studies that showed no difference are listed in Table 1.

Despite the proliferation of studies on the thermic effect of food, its underlying determinants and mechanisms remain poorly understood. Repeatedly, the measured thermic effect of food has been found to be larger than what can be accounted for by the stoichiometric energy cost of nutrient absorption, transport, and storage (69). This has led to the view that the thermic effect of food can be divided into two parts: (a) an obligatory component related to the metabolic cost of processing the nutrients, and (b) a facultative component that seems to have a "cephalic phase" and a "postprandial phase" (70,71).

The relevance of the "facultative cephalic phase" of the thermic effect of food has been questioned in humans (72), but the "facultative postprandial phase" is believed to be mediated through the sympathetic nervous system (62,70).

D'Alessio et al. (68) elegantly demonstrated that in any given subject the thermic effect of food increases linearly with caloric intake but is independent of leanness and obesity. In contrast, an impressive series of studies by Segal et al. (73–75) have convincingly shown that increasing body fat is associated with a decreased thermic effect of food (see Table 1). However, studies in postobese patients after a 44 ± 5 kg weight loss (76) or in obese patients before and after weight loss (18 ± 3 kg) (77) suggest that the diminished thermic effect of food in the obese is a secondary phenomenon rather than a primary pathogenic factor in human obesity. In very innovative and elegant studies, Thörne (78) showed that the thermic effect of a meal is inversely related to blood-drained heat from the splanchnic region and therefore to the amount of abdominal adipose tissue. Furthermore, it was shown that the thermic effect of food was reduced in lean subjects during artificial abdominal insulation with blankets and heat-reflecting aluminum foil, suggesting that the postprandial dissipation of heat is of importance for the regulation of the thermic effect of food (78). Finally, a decreased thermogenic response to an oral glucose load (79) or to a mixed meal (80) has been reported in the elderly when compared with younger adults. This decreased thermic effect of food with increasing age may be related to a reduced sympathetic nervous response (81).

Despite the vast disagreement found in the literature regarding the role of an impaired thermic effect of food in the pathogenesis of obesity, one can safely state that individual differences in the thermic effect of food can only account for small differences in daily energy expenditure. This implies that a minimal weight gain will increase energy expenditure (mostly in relationship to resting metabolic rate and the energy cost of physical

TABLE 1. *Studies showing defects and no defects in thermogenesis in obesity*

Year	First author	Stimulus	No. subjects	Duration (hours)	Data expression
Defects					
1976	Pittet (66)	200 kcal, oral glucose	21	2.5	↑ RMR over baseline (%)
1976	Kaplan (159)	823 kcal, oral CHO/PRO	8	5	↑ V̇O₂ over baseline (%)
1980	Zahorska-Markiewicz (160)	1,000 kcal, mixed + exercise	24	1.5	↑ EE over RMR (%)
1981	Shetty (161)	9.8 kcal/kg ideal body weight, mixed	15	2	↑ EE over RMR
1982	Golay (162)	400 kcal, oral glucose	55	3	% of RMR
1983	Schwartz (163)	800 kcal, mixed	13	2	↑ V̇O₂ over RMR
1983	Bessard (164)	60% 24-h EE, mixed	12	5	% of RMR; % of caloric intake
1983	Ravussin (165)	20% i.v. glucose infusion	29	0.5	% of RMR
1983	Segal (166)	910 kcal, mixed	20	4	↑ V̇O₂ over RMR
1984	Segal (167)	910 kcal, mixed + graded exercise	12	6 × 1 min	↑ V̇O₂
1984	Schutz (4)	41.2 kcal/kg FFM, mixed	28	24	% of RMR; % of caloric intake
1984	Schutz (168)	400 kcal, oral glucose	62	3	% of RMR; % of caloric intake
1985	Bogardus (169)	i.v. glucose and insulin	120	4	↑ EE over RMR
1985	Swaminathan (170)	400 kcal, fat, protein, or glucose 400 kcal, mixed	22	1.5	% RMR; mean EE; ↑ EE over fasting
1985	Segal (73)	750 kcal, mixed	16	3	↑ V̇O₂ over baseline
1986	Devlin (171)	i.v. glucose and insulin	17	3.3	↑ EE over RMR (%)
1986	Golay (172)	i.v. glucose and insulin	44	2	Change in glucose oxidation & storage
1986	Zed (173)	2,390 and 1,195 kcal/day, mixed with fat supplement	16	24	↑ EE over RMR
1987	Acheson (174)	500 g dextrin maltose	12	14	↑ EE over RMR
1987	Steiniger (175)	1.2 MJ protein, 2 MJ CHO	25	10	↑ EE over RMR
1987	Segal (74)	750 kcal, mixed	16	3	↑ V̇O₂ over baseline
1987	Schutz (176)	60% of 24-h EE, mixed	12	5	↑ EE over RMR
1989	Golay (177)	100 g oral glucose	12	3	↑ EE over RMR
1989	Thörne (77)	60% of BMR, mixed	10	3	% above BMR
1989	Katzeff (178)	800 kcal, liquid meal	12	4	↑ EE over RMR
1989	Tremblay (179)	1,000 kcal, mixed	15	4	↑ EE over RMR
1989	Segal (180)	720 kcal, mixed	22	3	↑ V̇O₂ over 0 kcal meal
1990	Segal (75)	35% of 24-h RMR, mixed	22	3	↑ EE over 0 kcal meal
No defect					
1981	Felber (181)	100 g, oral glucose	36	3	Change in glucose oxidation and storage
1982	Sharief (182)	5 g glucose, sucrose/kg IBW	11	3	↑ EE over RMR
1983	Welle (183)	400 kcal, oral dextrose	24	3	↑ EE over RMR
1983	Segal (166)	910 kcal, mixed	20	4	↑ V̇O₂ over RMR
1983	Nair (184)	300 kcal, fat, protein	10	2.5	↑ EE over RMR
1983	Blaza (185)	1,050 kcal, mixed	10	24	↑ Over control
1983	Felig (186)	800 kcal, mixed	20	3	↑ EE over RMR
1984	Welle (187)	800 kcal, mixed	6	3	↑ EE over RMR
1985	Schwartz (188)	800 kcal, high carbohydrate, high fat	16	6	↑ EE over RMR; % caloric intake
1985	Ravussin (189)	i.v. insulin and glucose	15	4	Change in glucose oxidation and storage
1985	Anton-Kuchly (190)	1,340 kJ (6 egg whites and 50 g casein)	19	5	↑ V̇O₂ over baseline
1986	Owen (191)	11 kcal/kg, mixed	44	4–6	↑ EE over RMR
1986	Nair (192)	300 kcal, oral glucose	20	2.5	↑ EE over RMR
1986	Vernet (193)	Twice 3 h RMR, mixed; i.v. or NG tube	20	3 infusion 3 postinfusion	% RMR; % caloric intake
1990	Thörne (194)	60% of RMR, mixed	18	3	% above RMR
1988	D'Alessio (68)	Up to 52 kcal/kg FFM	10	8	↑ EE over RMR
1991	Scalfi (195)	(MCT) 1,270 kcal, mixed	12	6	% above RMR
		(LCT) 1,300 kcal, mixed	12	6	% above RMR

BMR, basal metabolic rate; CHO, carbohydrate; EE, energy expenditure; FFM, fat-free mass; IBW, ideal body weight; kJ, kilojoules; LCT, long chain triglycerides; MCT, medium chain triglycerides; MJ, megajoules; NG, nasogastral; RMR, resting metabolic rate.

activity) and will therefore be sufficient to offset any impairment in the thermic effect of food. Decreased thermogenesis is therefore a very unlikely explanation for significant degrees of obesity.

Physical Activity

Reduced physical activity as a cause of obesity is an obvious and attractive hypothesis. The energy expended in physical activity is quite variable, and the secular increase in obesity parallels the increase in sedentary lifestyles. However, until the very recent introduction of the doubly labeled water method to measure energy expenditure in free-living conditions (29), there has been no satisfactory method by which to assess the impact of physical activity on daily energy expenditure. Under the artificial conditions of a respiratory chamber, large differences in energy expenditure between individuals (100 to 800 kcal/day) could be attributed to differences in spontaneous physical activity (3). More importantly, in male subjects, we found that a low spontaneous activity was associated with subsequent weight gain (82). Clearly, these differences may be much larger in free-living conditions in which voluntary physical activity varies widely among individuals.

The energy cost of a given activity is proportional to body weight and therefore is higher in obese individuals, although obesity is generally associated with lower activity levels (83,84). Recently, Ferraro et al. (85) found a negative relationship between the energy expenditure of activity and the degree of obesity, implying that the higher cost of activity was more than offset by the lower activity level among obese subjects.

Figure 1 illustrates the methods by which it is possible to assess the different components of daily energy expenditure and how it is possible to differentiate unrestricted and spontaneous physical activity by combining measurements of energy expenditure using doubly labeled water and the respiratory chamber. Studies in a large number of subjects using these two methods are needed to assess physical activity and its impact on the development of obesity. Preliminary data collected in our laboratory on more than 50 Pima Indians suggest that the level of physical activity decreases with both increasing age (86) and increasing adiposity (87). Whether a low level of physical activity is the cause or the consequence of obesity cannot be derived from such cross-sectional studies.

24-Hour Sedentary Energy Expenditure

As described above, measurements in the respiratory chamber are accurate and can be used to assess the determinants of sedentary energy expenditure in humans. All of the different components of energy expenditure, except for the energy cost of free-living physical activity, can be determined in a respiratory chamber. From 1985 to 1990, we performed measurements of 24-hour energy expenditure on more than 500 healthy, nondiabetic subjects fed a weight maintenance diet for at least 3 days prior to being measured (88). Body composition was estimated by hydrostatic weighing. The physical characteristics and energy expenditure of these subjects are presented in Table 2. Analysis of covariance and single and multiple linear regression analyses were performed to assess the different determinants of energy expenditure. Fat-free mass, fat mass, age, spontaneous physical activity, and gender were all significant determinants of 24-hour energy expenditure (EE) in these sedentary conditions. The predictive equation generated from the 597 subjects is: 24EE (kcal/day) = 618 + 18.1 FFM + 10.0 FM − 1.4 age + 17 SPA + 204 for males (0 for females) where FFM (fat-free mass) and FM (fat mass) are expressed in kg and SPA (spontaneous physical activity) in percent of the 24 hours during which the subjects were in motion as measured by a radar system. The above covariates explained 89% of the variance in 24-hour energy expenditure between subjects. The relationship between 24-hour energy expenditure and fat-free mass

TABLE 2. *Physical characteristics and energy expenditure in 597 healthy subjects measured for 24 hours in a respiratory chamber after at least 3 days on a weight maintenance diet (means and ranges)*

	Men (n = 327)	Women (n = 270)
Age (y)	32 (18–81)	34 (18–85)
Body weight (kg)	93.2 (50.6–209.9)	83.6 (41.3–215.2)
Body fat (%)	25 (3–49)	36 (9–53)
24-h energy expenditure (kcal/day)	2,418 (1,584–4,225)	2,049 (1,259–3,723)
Basal metabolic rate (kcal/day)	1,903 (1,191–3,797)	1,618 (904–2,889)
Sleeping metabolic rate (kcal/day)	1,732 (1,096–3,728)	1,499 (876–3,096)

(the single most important determinant) is presented in Figure 2. In this large cohort, covering a wide range of body weights (41 to 215 kg) and body fatness (3 to 53%), 24-hour energy expenditure varied in proportion with body size from 1,259 kcal/day to 4,225 kcal/day. These results are of importance and re-emphasize the fact that obese subjects have higher metabolic rates than lean subjects, as pointed out many years ago by James et al. (89). Also, the lowest 24-hour energy expenditure was 1,259 kcal/day in one of the lightest women: this demonstrates once more that an 800-kcal/day diet is sufficient to produce energy deficit in any obese patient. These results also give little credence to energy intake studies in which no correlations or negative correlations between energy intake and body weight have been found (see below).

ENERGY BALANCE EQUATIONS

Energy stores are determined by the balance between energy intake and energy expenditure. Since living organisms must obey the first law of thermodynamics, the energy balance equation has been used to predict changes in body weight when energy intake or expenditure were changed. The classic equation of energy balance, which states that the body energy store is equal to energy intake minus energy expenditure, has provided both insights and confusion in the understanding of energy balance in humans.

Equation during Weight Maintenance

$$\text{energy intake} = \text{energy expenditure} \quad (1)$$

This equation is self-evident and quite ac-

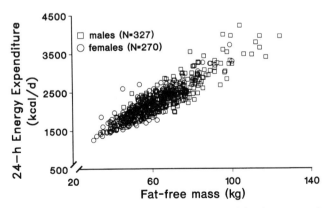

FIG. 2. Relationship between 24-hour energy expenditure and fat-free mass in 597 subjects (see Table 2 for physical characteristics). Twenty-four-hour energy expenditure was measured after at least 3 days on a weight-maintaining diet (50% carbohydrate, 30% fat, 20% protein) and fat-free body mass was assessed by underwater weighing using the Keys and Brozek formula. Fat-free body mass could explain 81% of the variance in 24-hour energy expenditure ($r^2 = 0.81$). Note that the lowest sedentary 24-hour energy expenditure is 1,259 kcal/day.

curate at weight maintenance because only limited changes in body composition are possible without changing body weight. This form of the energy balance equation has been extremely useful because of the light it has shed on the nature of reported energy intake.

Most dietary intake studies show either no correlation or a negative correlation between energy intake and body weight (90). This is in marked contrast to studies of energy expenditure in which there is a positive relationship (Fig. 2). In addition to their greater fat mass, obese individuals have a greater fat-free mass, which is the main determinant of both resting metabolic rate and 24-hour metabolic rate as measured in a respiratory chamber (2,3). One possible resolution of these conflicting observations is that the measurement of energy expenditure with the subject in a resting state or confined to a respiratory chamber introduces a significant artifact. The suggestion is that under free-living conditions, the leaner subjects would exercise much more, thereby increasing their energy expenditure beyond that of the obese subjects. Indeed, the reported level of activity under free-living conditions (90) and the energy cost of activity on a metabolic ward (85) or in free-ranging subjects (86) is lower in obese subjects. However, this reduced activity is not sufficient to bring their total energy expenditure down to the level of the lean subjects (91–93).

Recent studies involving free-living individuals have simultaneously measured energy expenditure using the doubly labeled water technique and energy intake using continuous recording of diet diaries (90,91). Under these careful conditions of food intake assessment, the obese subjects reported only one-half to two-thirds of their total energy intake compared with 80 to 100% for the lean subjects. Thus the conflict between energy intake and energy expenditure correlations with body weight is largely due to marked underreporting of food intake by overweight individuals. The true amount of food obese individuals eat to maintain body weight is not registered in their diet diaries and is prob-

ably not registered in their consciousness. This gap between the food that obese people perceive themselves eating and what they actually eat represents a major challenge for psychologists and psychiatrists interested in obesity and food intake and could be termed the "eye–mouth gap."

Static Energy Balance Equation

change in energy stores

$$= \text{energy intake} - \text{energy expenditure} \quad (2)$$

This is the most common equation used in discussions and calculations of energy balance. Intuitively, it seems valid, but Alpert (94) has elegantly demonstrated that this equation is static and mathematically unbounded; this makes it invalid for calculations on living organisms, in which energy balance is dynamic and bounded. Thus a small increase in energy intake sustained over a number of years should not lead to a large weight increase, as is often predicted (95).

Since the early studies by Von Voit in 1881 (96), several investigators (97–100) reported that overfeeding did not result in the weight gain predicted (using Eq. 2), and this gave rise to the concept of "Luxuskonsumption" or heat wasting. A more likely explanation for this discrepancy, proposed by Alpert (94), is that the static equation (Eq. 2) is inappropriate for predicting weight change following energy imbalance because it does not take into account the increasing energy expenditure with increasing weight.

Our short-term overfeeding study with measurements of energy expenditure in a respiratory chamber has shown that all the excess energy intake can be accounted for by increasing body weight and predictable increases in the different components of daily energy expenditure (101). Another consequence of using the static equation has been the search for small "defects" in energy expenditure using cross-sectional studies (such as the pursuit of an impaired thermic effect of food in obese compared with lean subjects) to explain significant obesity (95,102,103). With the dynamic energy balance equation (see below) as the underlying tenet, the search moves away from small initial defects in energy intake or expenditure toward chronic states of imbalance between the two. In this way of thinking, a "low" energy expenditure can be associated with a "high" energy intake, as shown repeatedly in genetic models of obesity in rodents.

Dynamic Energy Balance Equation

rate of change of energy stores

= rate of energy intake

$$- \text{rate of energy expenditure} \quad (3)$$

The use of "rates" in this equation introduces time dependency, thereby allowing the effect of changing energy stores (especially fat-free mass and weight) on energy expenditure to enter into the calculations (94). Thus, a small initial positive energy balance (for example from an increased energy intake or a defect in the thermic effect of food) will not lead to large weight increases over a number of years. After a short period of positive energy balance, the energy stores (fat mass and fat-free mass) will increase and cause an increase in energy expenditure (Fig. 2), which will balance the increased energy intake. The individual will then once again be in energy balance, but with a higher energy intake, a higher energy expenditure, and higher energy stores. Weight gain can therefore be viewed not only as the consequence of an initial positive energy balance but also as the mechanism by which energy balance is eventually restored. In the free-living organism, energy balance is achieved either by alterations in appetite over hours and days, or by changes in body weight (especially fat-free mass) over weeks or months. Indeed, the majority of adults maintain a fairly constant body weight over years and decades without real conscious effort, suggesting the presence of well-tuned energy balancing mechanisms. This is truly amazing when one considers

that if an average-sized man is to maintain weight over 10 years, then these mechanisms must match about 10 million kcal of food intake (intermittent and variable) with the same number of calories of energy expenditure (continuous and variable). How is one balanced against the other, and how might a chronic mismatch between the two occur? A fruitful approach to these questions has been to dissect the energy balance equation into its various nutrient balance equations.

NUTRIENT BALANCE EQUATIONS

If the origins of a positive energy balance lie in the chronic imbalance of energy intake and oxidation, then the absolute intake and oxidation rates are probably less important than the relationship between the two. An examination of each nutrient balance equation to determine if a chronic imbalance between nutrient intake and oxidation exists is only valid if each nutrient has its separate balance equation, implying separate regulation (Fig. 3). In practical terms: Is each nutrient either oxidized or stored in its own compartment (separate regulation), or does it get converted into another compartment for storage? This applies particularly to the issue of whether dietary carbohydrate is stored as fat (de novo lipogenesis), as is commonly believed. If de novo lipogenesis does not occur in humans under physiological conditions, then it would be reasonable to consider each nutrient balance equation as a separate entity.

De Novo Lipogenesis

Lipogenic enzyme activities are detectable in the liver of humans, but are 4- to 70-fold lower than in rat or bird livers (104). In vitro lipogenesis can also be demonstrated in human adipose tissue (105). Whole body net de novo lipogenesis can be readily demonstrated (as indicated by a respiratory quotient greater than 1.00) during parenteral infusions (106) or peritoneal dialysis (107). However, huge

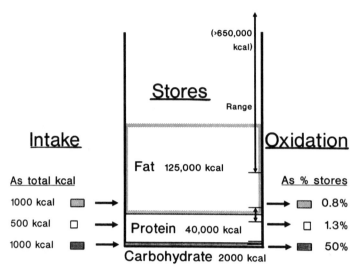

FIG. 3. The daily nutrient balance of a 70-kg (20% body fat) man in relationship to nutrient stores, macronutrient intake, and macronutrient oxidation. Each nutrient intake and oxidation on a 2,500 kcal/day diet (40% fat, 40% carbohydrate, 20% protein) is shown on the left as absolute calorie intake and on the right as a percentage of its respective nutrient store. The ranges for each of the nutrient stores are shown and are based on values for a 50-kg man (10% body fat) and a 150-kg man (50% body fat). The fat stores for a 150-kg man are more than 5 times that of a 70-kg man and extend far beyond the top of the diagram.

amounts of oral carbohydrate are needed before small amounts are converted into triglyceride. Acheson et al. (108) found that the acute ingestion of 2,000 kcal of simple sugar (500 g of dextrin maltose) resulted in only a few grams of lipid production, and even massive carbohydrate overfeeding (about 5,000 kcal, 85% carbohydrate) for several days after saturation of glycogen stores resulted in about 150 g/day of lipid synthesis (109). Clearly, none of the situations in which de novo lipogenesis has been demonstrated could be considered physiological, and indeed the respiratory quotient does not exceed 1.00 under normal conditions. Some studies of isocaloric diets rich in carbohydrates (especially simple carbohydrates) have shown an increase in triglyceride concentrations and very low-density lipoprotein (VLDL) ApoB pool size (110–112), but this is not equivalent to lipogenesis. The increase in VLDL is largely due to a decrease in the conversion of VLDL to intermediate-density lipoprotein (IDL) and low-density lipoprotein (LDL) (111–113), although those individuals who

are susceptible to carbohydrate-induced hypertriglyceridemia usually also demonstrate an increased VLDL production rate as well (111,112). In summary, de novo lipogenesis in humans should be regarded as negligible under the dietary conditions of industrialized countries.

Alcohol Balance

rate of alcohol intake

$$= \text{rate of alcohol oxidation} \quad (4)$$

There is an inconsistent relationship between reported alcohol intake and body mass index, with many studies showing a negative relationship (114,115). Indeed, under controlled conditions, alcohol does not seem to contribute its 7 kcal/g to the body's energy balance (116,117). In chronic alcohol abusers, isocaloric substitution of alcohol for carbohydrate to 50% of total calories leads to weight loss and doubling weight maintenance calories by the addition of alcohol has no significant effect on body weight (117).

This apparent "calorie wasting" of alcohol calories may be due to substrate cycling (116) oxidation via microsomal enzymes [non-adenosine triphosphate (ATP) producing], increased sympathetic tone, or enhanced ATP breakdown (117). These possibilities notwithstanding, Shelmet et al. (118) found that all of an infused load of ethanol was metabolized through oxidation and that it became the priority fuel, markedly suppressing the oxidation of fat and, to a lesser extent, carbohydrate and protein. Since the destination of alcohol is oxidation and not storage (as fat), perfect alcohol balance is achieved. Alcohol does, however, divert dietary fat away from oxidation and toward storage, as does dietary carbohydrate. Therefore a chronic imbalance between alcohol intake and oxidation cannot be a direct cause of obesity, although by contributing to overall energy balance, it may indirectly influence fat balance (Table 3). Recently, Lieber (117) reviewed the literature on alcohol and energy balance in an article entitled: "Do Alcohol Calories Count?"

Protein Balance

rate of change of protein stores

= rate of protein intake

$$- \text{ rate of protein oxidation} \quad (5)$$

Protein intake is usually about 15% of calories, and the protein stores in the body represent about one-third of the total stored calories in a 70-kg man (119). The daily protein intake amounts to a little over 1% of the total protein stores (120) (Fig. 3). The protein stores increase in size in response to such growth stimuli as growth hormone, androgens, physical training, and weight gain, but do not increase simply from increased dietary protein. Protein stores are therefore tightly controlled and, on a day-to-day basis protein balance is achieved (121). Ingested protein is used to replace stores (structural proteins, enzymes) as required and to respond to growth stimuli (if present), and the remainder is oxidized for metabolic needs. While some degree of chronic energy imbalance caused by the mismatch of protein intake and oxidation in response to growth stimuli occurs, it cannot be implicated directly as a cause of obesity, although, as with the other nonfat nutrients, it may indirectly affect the fat balance equation (Table 3).

Carbohydrate Balance

rate of change of carbohydrate stores

= rate of carbohydrate intake

$$- \text{ rate of carbohydrate oxidation} \quad (6)$$

Carbohydrate is usually the main source of dietary calories, yet the body stores of glycogen are very limited, 500 to 1,000 g on average (109). The daily intake of carbohydrate corresponds to about 50 to 100% of the carbohydrate stores compared with about 1% for protein and fat (120) (Fig. 3), so that over a

TABLE 3. *Comparison of macronutrient stores and balance in an adult man*

	Carbohydrate	Protein	Alcohol	Fat
Stores				
Stored in tissues as	Glycogen	Protein	—	Fat
Sizes of stores	Tiny	Moderate	—	Large
Daily variability in size	Large	Small	—	Small
Potential for expansion	Tiny	Moderate	—	Large
Stores regulated	Yes	Yes	—	No
Balance				
Oxidation stimulated by intake	Yes	Yes	Yes	No
Potential for long-term intake/ oxidation imbalance	No	Yes[a]	No	Yes

[a] Only under the influence of growth stimuli (hormones, exercise, increasing fat mass, drugs, etc.).

period of hours and days, the carbohydrate stores fluctuate markedly compared with those of protein and fat. However, as with protein stores, they are tightly controlled (121). Flatt (122) uses these concepts and experimental data to build a persuasive case that the organism's energy balance is sensed by fluctuations in glycogen stores, which are then translated into hunger and food intake. The hypothesis is appealing because it explains the known consequences of altering nutrient intake or exercise levels. However, the mechanisms by which the glycogen stores may be monitored is poorly understood, and it is unknown how much interindividual variations in this feedback loop relate to interindividual differences in obesity.

Nonetheless, it is established that dietary carbohydrate stimulates both glycogen storage and glucose oxidation and suppresses fat oxidation (123). That which is not stored as glycogen is oxidized (not converted to fat), and carbohydrate balance is achieved (121). Therefore, as with the other nonfat nutrients, a chronic imbalance between carbohydrate intake and oxidation cannot be the basis of weight gain because storage capacity is limited and controlled, conversion to fat is an option that only occurs under extreme conditions in humans, and oxidation is increased to match intake (Table 3).

Fat Balance

rate of change of fat stores

    = rate of fat intake

            − rate of fat oxidation   (7)

In marked contrast to the other nutrients, body fat stores are large, and fat intake has no influence on fat oxidation (121). As with protein, the daily fat intake represents less than 1% of the total energy stored as fat, but the fat stores contain about six times the energy of the protein stores (120) (Fig. 3). These fat stores are the energy buffer for the body and the slope of the relationship between energy balance and fat balance is 1 in conditions of

day-to-day small positive or negative energy balances (121): In other words, a deficit of 200 kcal of energy over 24 hours means 200 kcal comes from the fat stores, and the same holds true for an excess of 200 kcal of energy that ends up in the fat stores. Even in conditions of spontaneous overfeeding, all the excess fat intake is stored as body fat (126). Ingestion of a mixed meal is followed by an increase in carbohydrate oxidation and a decrease in fat oxidation and the addition of extra fat does not alter that mix of nutrient oxidation (124,125). So what promotes fat oxidation if it is not dietary fat intake? The amount of total body fat exerts a small, but significant, effect on fat oxidation and this promotion of fat oxidation at higher body fat levels may represent a mechanism for attenuating the rate of weight gain (127). The major influence on fat oxidation, however, is energy balance (121,127) with energy expenditure beyond current energy intake (i.e., negative energy balance) promoting fat oxidation. Table 3 summarizes the differences between the four nutrient balance equations.

From these observations it can be deduced that energy balance is virtually equivalent to fat balance and that there is room for a chronic imbalance between fat intake and fat oxidation. In fact, for body weight to change (largely dependent on changes in adipose tissue), a prerequisite is that there is an imbalance between fat intake and oxidation. This imbalance can also be measured and expressed as a chronic mismatch of the food quotient ($\approx$ratio of carbohydrate to fat intake) and the respiratory quotient ($\approx$ratio of carbohydrate to fat oxidation) (122).

Implications of the Fat Balance Equation

The static energy balance equation (Eq. 2) is a physics equation derived from the first principle of energy conservation. The dynamic equation (Eq. 3) includes the physiological dimension that changes in energy stores with time alter energy expenditure and possibly energy intake. However, both equations offer only two possible avenues for weight reduction: either increasing exercise or conscious limitation of total energy intake (i.e., restricted amount of food). Equation 7, on the other hand, represents the usual realm of human physiology and as such offers three avenues for weight reduction. The first two (increased exercise or restricted food quantity) act by increasing fat oxidation. The third avenue is simply to decrease fat intake (alteration of food quality alone).

This concept implies that a high-fat, ad libitum diet will cause weight gain, and that a low-fat, ad libitum diet will result in weight loss. A diet high in fat is consequently low in carbohydrate, and Flatt's model (122) would predict that this would lead to earlier depletion of the glycogen stores, a greater food intake (more high-fat food), and consequently a positive energy balance (128). This imbalance would persist until the adipose stores built up sufficiently to provide a greater supply of fat for oxidation. A higher percent of body fat is associated with a greater fat oxidation (127). When the higher fat oxidation matches the higher fat intake, the individual would then be in fat balance (and energy balance) but at a higher level of percent body fat, i.e., obesity. The reverse would apply if an overweight person changed to a low-fat, ad libitum diet: The reduced fat intake is not initially followed by a reduced fat oxidation. This fat imbalance burns up fat stores until the point at which the diminished fat mass, its associated lower fat oxidation, and the new reduced-fat diet are all in equilibrium once more.

Several studies have found that the reported fat intake is higher in obese compared with lean subjects (91,92,129,130). The effect of a high-fat diet is also seen in controlled studies of up to 11 weeks duration that compared an ad libitum diet composed of high-fat foods to a low-fat diet of similar palatability (131–132). The energy intake (and weight gain) is significantly greater with higher fat foods than with lower fat foods.

In summary, when one considers energy balance in humans under physiological conditions, fat is the only nutrient that can maintain a chronic imbalance between intake and oxidation and that can directly contribute fat to the adipose tissue. The other nutrients will indirectly influence adiposity by their contribution to overall energy balance and thus fat balance. The use of the fat balance equation instead of the energy balance equation offers a new framework for understanding the pathogenesis of obesity. Fat is handled differently from the other energy-providing substrates, and, quite apart from its increased caloric density, an increase in dietary fat leads to weight gain and a decrease leads to weight loss (131,132).

RISK FACTORS FOR BODY WEIGHT GAIN

An understanding of the etiology of human obesity demands longitudinal studies. Cross-sectional studies can only provide associations, whereas longitudinal studies provide predictors or risk factors. Several studies have examined these predictors in the Pima Indian population in Arizona. Obesity is extremely prevalent among the Pima, and therefore weight gain is very common in young adults, making this group well suited for longitudinal studies of various metabolic risk factors of weight gain (133).

Metabolic Rate

The *absolute* metabolic rate, expressed in kcal/day, is positively correlated with fat-free mass (Fig. 2). The relationship holds for either basal or 24-hour metabolic rate versus fat-free mass or body weight, so that obesity clearly is associated with a high *absolute* metabolic rate (88). However, the scatter about the regression line means that at any given body size some individuals have a high, a normal, or a low *relative* metabolic rate. This is illustrated in Fig. 4 with four hypothetical individuals with different *relative* and *absolute* metabolic rates. The lean (A) compared to the obese person (B) has a low *absolute* metabolic

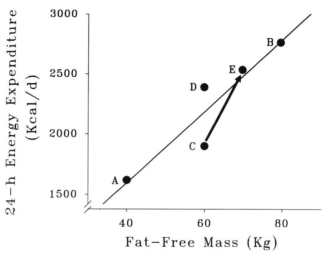

FIG. 4. Relationship between 24-hour energy expenditure and fat-free mass derived from a large population (597 subjects as described in Fig. 2 and Table 2). This figure represents values for different subjects. In terms of the *absolute* 24-hour energy expenditure, *the lean person A has a low value and the obese person B has a high value.* In terms of relative 24-hour energy expenditure, both A and B are normal. Subjects C and D are of similar body size, but subject C has a low *relative* metabolic rate and subject D has a high *relative* metabolic rate. Subject C is at the greatest risk for weight gain, but upon gaining that weight, his/her previous low *relative* metabolic rate becomes "normalized" (C to E).

rate, but both have normal *relative* metabolic rates. Individuals at points C and D have the same fat-free mass, but C has a low *relative* and D has a high *relative* metabolic rate. The question is whether the person at point C with the low *relative* metabolic rate is at higher risk of gaining weight than individuals at points A, B, or D.

Three studies have examined this question in different populations (134–136). Roberts et al. (134) measured energy expenditure by the doubly labeled water technique in 18 infants at 3 months of age and then divided them post hoc into overweight and normal weight at age 12 months. Energy expenditure (mostly activity) was, on average, 20% lower in those who became overweight at 12 months compared with those who did not become overweight. Similarly, Griffiths et al. (135) reported that a lower energy expenditure (assessed by measured energy intake and expressed per kg body weight) in 5-year-old girls correlated negatively with body mass index at adolescence. This implies that a low *relative* metabolic rate in childhood predicts adolescent obesity. From our own studies in

adult Pima Indians (136), we have found that low *relative* metabolic rates (resting and 24-hour, normalized to fat-free mass, fat mass, age, and sex) were risk factors for body weight gain. After 4 years of follow-up, the risk of gaining 10 kg was approximately 8 times greater in those subjects with the lowest RMR (lower tertile) compared with those with the highest RMR (higher tertile) (Fig. 5). In 95 subjects the rate of 24-hour energy expenditure, adjusted for fat-free mass, fat mass, age, and sex, correlated negatively with the rate of weight change (r = −0.39, $p <$ 0.001). The low *relative* metabolic rate could account for no more than 40% of the weight gain; upon gaining the weight, the metabolic rate "normalized" and, indeed, even went higher than normal (136), as illustrated in Fig. 4 (C to E).

Another important component of the 24-hour metabolic rate is the energy cost of physical activity. In a recent study in Pima Indians, we found that spontaneous physical activity, even in the confined environment of a respiratory chamber, is an important component of daily energy expenditure and is a

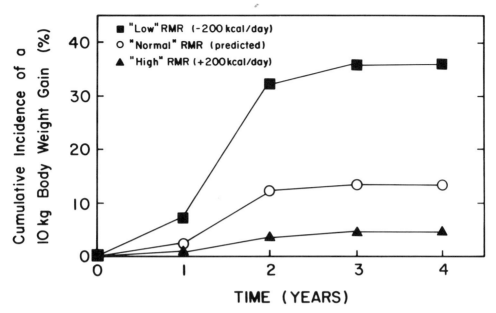

FIG. 5. Cumulative incidence of a 10-kg body weight gain for a subject with a "high" relative metabolic rate (*RMR*) (200 kcal/day above that predicted for body size and body composition) ▲, for a subject with a "normal" relative RMR (equal to that predicted) ○, and for a subject with a "low" RMR (200 kcal/day below that predicted) ■. The cumulative incidence was calculated on the basis of follow-up data obtained in 126 Pima Indians followed for more than 3 years on average (136) using a survival analysis (proportional hazard linear model). Note that subjects with a "low" metabolic rate are at approximately 8 times the risk of gaining weight as compared with those with a "high" metabolic rate.

familial trait (82). Importantly, in this study we also found that a low level of spontaneous physical activity was associated with subsequent weight gain in males, but not in females. We have also examined other metabolic predictors of weight gain, and a pattern of predictors of and responses to weight gain is beginning to emerge.

Respiratory Quotient and Low Rates of Fat Oxidation

If the composition of nutrient intake is an important factor in the genesis of obesity, as previously discussed, one might expect that the composition of nutrient oxidation would also play a role. The nonprotein respiratory quotient, which is the ratio of carbohydrate to fat oxidation, ranges from a value of about 0.80 after an overnight fast in which fat is the main oxidative substrate (137) to values close

to 1.00 after a large carbohydrate meal in which glucose is the major substrate (123). Under unusual conditions of massive carbohydrate loading (usually parenteral), respiratory quotient values can go beyond 1.00, indicating de novo lipogenesis (106–109). Apart from these effects of diet composition, the respiratory quotient is also influenced by recent energy balance (negative balance causing more fat oxidation), sex (females tending toward carbohydrate oxidation and fat storage), adiposity (higher fat mass means higher fat oxidation), and family membership, suggesting genetic determinants. However, all of these factors only explain about 40% of the variance in the 24-hour respiratory quotient as measured in a respiratory chamber (127).

In a longitudinal study in Pima Indians, we found that even after adjusting for these known effects, the 24-hour respiratory quotient showed considerable interindividual variation and predicted weight gain (127).

Those in the 90th percentile for respiratory quotient ("carbohydrate oxidizers") had a 2.5 times greater risk of gaining 5 kg or more body weight than those in the 10th percentile (127). This effect was independent of a "low" or "high" 24-hour metabolic rate. Thus "carbohydrate oxidizers" tend to conserve fat and over time gain weight faster than "fat oxidizers"; conversely, a low respiratory quotient ("exaggerated" fat oxidation) is associated with a slower weight gain.

Insulin Sensitivity

Insulin sensitivity is measured as the total glucose disposal stimulated by insulin and is the sum of carbohydrate oxidation and non-oxidative glucose disposal (mainly storage). Since higher rates of carbohydrate oxidation (as measured by the 24-hour respiratory quotient) predict weight gain, we investigated whether insulin sensitivity would also predict weight gain in Pima Indians. Subjects in the 90th percentile (most insulin sensitive) were 3 to 4 times more likely to gain 10 kg or more body weight compared with those in the 10th percentile (most insulin resistant), and this effect was more closely related to the oxidative than the nonoxidative component (138). Thus insulin sensitivity predicts weight gain, or conversely, insulin resistance is associated with significantly lower rates of weight gain.

Summary of Risk Factors for Weight Gain

These studies in the Pima population have shown that a low relative metabolic rate (24-hour metabolic rate, resting metabolic rate, and spontaneous physical activity), a high 24-hour respiratory quotient, and insulin sensitivity predict body weight gain. These metabolic factors all show the same pattern of relationships to body weight. Cross-sectionally, obesity is associated with high absolute energy expenditure, low respiratory quotient, and insulin resistance. On the contrary, in longitudinal studies and relative to body size, a low metabolic rate, a high respiratory quo-

tient, and insulin sensitivity predict weight gain. Furthermore, upon gaining that weight the original "abnormal" metabolic state becomes "normalized" (Fig. 4). Weight gain causes an increase in metabolic rate (136), a decrease in respiratory quotient (127), and a decrease in insulin sensitivity (138), which are much greater than the cross-sectional data would predict, and all counteract further weight gain. As discussed below, these changes in metabolic factors, which are not explained by the changes in body weight and composition, are the hallmark of adaptation.

ADAPTATION OF ENERGY EXPENDITURE TO OVER- AND UNDERFEEDING

Common experience suggests that obese individuals are very resistant to the weight loss effects of a hypocaloric diet, but are very susceptible to regaining the weight while eating an apparently normal diet. Is metabolic adaptation responsible for this? Conversely, does adaptation explain why an individual of normal weight does not gain weight on a hypercaloric diet as fast as predicted, but then loses it with ease? Also, do differences in these metabolic responses explain the great variation among individuals in response to the same change in energy balance?

Definition of Metabolic Adaptation

In their work on the biology of semistarvation, Keys et al. (139) stated: "It might seem entirely reasonable that the energetic processes of the body diminish in intensity as the exogenous food supply is reduced. It is reasonable, in the sense that a wise man reduces his expenditure when his income is cut." They define adaptation as "a useful adjustment to altered circumstances." A more recent definition of adaptation has been proposed in the 1985 FAO/WHO/UNU report (140) as "a process by which a new or different steady state is reached in response to a change or difference in the intake of food and nutrients." In this context, the adaptation can be genetic, metabolic, social, or behavioral.

At the practical level, however, a more quantifiable method is needed for assessing the presence and extent of adaptation. The gap between observed and predicted weight change could be used provided that the prediction is based on the dynamic energy balance equation (Eq. 3) as previously discussed. Perhaps a better method is to compare the changes predicted from cross-sectional data with those observed in longitudinal studies. For example, if the fall in resting metabolic rate associated with a 20-kg weight loss is greater than would be expected for that loss of fat-free mass and fat mass, then adaptation can be implied. The validity of this method is probably improved by comparing stable states (i.e., measurements made during weight stability before and after weight loss), by correcting for all important determinants (e.g., correcting metabolic rates for changes in fat-free mass and fat mass), and by appropriate normalization (141) (e.g., a simple division of metabolic rate by fat-free mass ignores the significant intercept between the two and can give erroneous results).

Metabolic Adaptation to Overfeeding

In 1902, Neumann (97), in his pioneering work on himself, observed that the changes in his body weight and nitrogen balance were lower than predicted in conditions of positive energy balance. He therefore proposed that in response to energy excess, the body can adapt and waste part of the excess energy intake and he termed this mechanism "Luxuskonsumption." Twenty years later, Gulick (98) performed a similar long-term experiment on himself. In the late sixties and early seventies, the studies of Miller and Mumford (99,100), on the effects of overfeeding in humans upon body weight and the energy cost of exercise, as well as the classical studies of experimental obesity on the Vermont prisoners (142,143), served to revive the interest in this area. In his 1978 review of overfeeding

studies, Garrow (144) found that in 11 of 16 studies, energy expenditure increased in response to overfeeding, whereas five other studies showed no significant thermogenesis. On the basis of his review, Garrow suggested that a possible metabolic adaptation and detectable thermogenesis occur only when the excess energy intake is over 20,000 kcal.

Unfortunately, most of these pioneering studies have been difficult to interpret since only partial measurements of energy expenditure were performed, and some of the studies were poorly controlled for food intake. In 1980, Norgan and Durnin (145) extended their previous overfeeding studies (146) and overfed six subjects for 42 days with a total energy excess of 62,000 kcal. Their metabolic rate for standard test tasks increased 10% after overfeeding, but not in relation to total body weight. The discrepancy between the weight gain and energy intake was attributed to probable errors in calculations based on the measured variables, and to the fact that the degree of physical activity was not measured. In their conclusions, the authors pointed out that "the causes for the individual differences are obscure." For these reasons, in 1985 (101), we conducted an overfeeding study for 9 days after a 13-day period of dietary equilibration. Twenty-four-hour energy expenditure was measured at the end of the baseline period and on the second and ninth day of overfeeding. Body weight increased by 3.2 kg, 56% being fat and the remainder fat-free mass. After 9 days of overfeeding, only 25% of the energy excess was dissipated as increased energy expenditure (490 kcal/day). One-third of this increase in energy expenditure was accounted for by an increase in resting metabolic rate, mostly related to the increase in fat-free mass. Another third was accounted for by the increase in the thermic effect of food in response to the increased energy intake and the remainder by an increased energy cost of physical activity at the heavier body weight. Thus all of the excess energy expenditure could be accounted for without the need to invoke a "facultative" or "adaptive" component. Clearly, in modern studies, better methods of assessing both food intake and energy expenditure over prolonged periods of time are required to be able to balance all of the energy.

The use of the doubly labeled water technique has already shed some light on the effect of overfeeding on total energy expenditure (147). Roberts et al. (147) overfed seven young lean men for 3 weeks with approximately 1,000 kcal/day excess energy intake. In response to overfeeding, 85 to 90% of the excess energy intake was deposited mostly as body fat, whereas the energy expenditure for physical activity or thermoregulation was unchanged. Only the 24-hour resting metabolic rate increased (RMR + thermic effect of food) and accounted for ~15% of the excess metabolizable energy. Therefore, all the calories were accounted for by increased energy stores and a small increase in energy expenditure. The authors concluded that regulation of food intake rather than energy expenditure is the primary determinant of energy balance in young adult men.

Whether obese individuals gain weight more easily than nonobese individuals remains an open question. In his recent review of the literature, Forbes (148) tends to imply that, in response to similar excess energy intake, obese individuals gain less weight than thin individuals because they tend to gain a larger proportion of fat.

Recently, the impressive 100-day overfeeding study on 12 pairs of monozygotic twins has elegantly highlighted the importance of genetic background to the weight gain in response to overfeeding (149). The large interpair variability in weight gain was surprising, as was the small intrapair variability in weight gain. Clearly, these results point out that human subjects have different genetic susceptibilities to environmental changes, which would lead to variable positive energy balances and variable weight gains. Under free-living conditions, both the genetic susceptibility and the extent to which the environment favors weight gain (such as the availability of fatty foods and labor-saving devices) seem to determine the magnitude of weight gain in response to spontaneous overfeeding.

Metabolic Adaptation to Underfeeding

Under the conditions of a large deficit of energy intake, does the body adapt its metabolic rate (over and beyond the predictable effects just described) to minimize the impact of negative energy imbalance on body weight? This concept of metabolic adaptation implies a drop in the metabolic rate that is dependent upon the recent history of negative energy balance and leads to a smaller reduction in body weight than would be predicted from the reduction in energy intake. Therefore an appropriate definition of adaptation to a low-calorie diet would be any decrease in energy expenditure that is more than would be expected from the decrease in fat-free mass, fat mass, and energy intake.

Three studies have indirectly assessed 24-hour energy expenditure using accurate energy intake measurements in weight-stable subjects. Leibel and Hirsch (24) studied 26 subjects in the obese state and in their reduced state. In the obese state, the subjects needed 9% more energy per surface area for weight maintenance than controls, whereas, in the reduced state, they required 24% fewer calories while still being 38 kg heavier than the controls. Weigle and colleagues (25,26) found that the energy expenditure in the reduced-obese fell below the regression line between 24-hour energy expenditure and fat-free mass, which was established in their baseline, obese state. This was related mostly to the predictable decreased energy cost of physical activity. Other studies that have used indirect calorimetry in the steady obese state and nonsteady weight-losing state have also found a fall in 24-hour energy expenditure (150–154). These studies did not all agree on the presence or the absence of adaptation to hypocaloric diets.

We have recently reviewed the impact of hypocaloric diets on total energy expenditure and its major components (155). There is general agreement among the studies that weight loss in obese subjects on hypocaloric diets causes a fall in 24-hour energy expenditure corrected for fat-free mass, the major but not the sole determinant of energy expenditure. This fall is mainly related to the nonresting metabolic rate. Possible adaptive changes to weight loss include a decrease in activity levels with weight loss, a decrease in the thermic effect of food (beyond that expected from the reduction in calories), and, under certain circumstances, a decrease in resting metabolic rate (beyond that expected for the decreased body size). Quantitative estimates of the contribution of these adaptive changes to the overall lower metabolic rate are clearly not possible, but based on our review of the current data, it seems that in obese individuals the adaptive changes are minor compared with the predictable changes. On the other hand, low-calorie diets in lean subjects seem to evoke significant adaptive changes in resting metabolic rate and probably in the energy cost of physical activity (139,155). This more dramatic response is not surprising, since the threat that a hypocaloric diet poses to survival is greater in leaner subjects.

FUTURE DIRECTIONS

Obesity has been highly prevalent in the industrialized world for many decades, and the chronic diseases associated with it are the major killers in those countries. However, the 1990 WHO report on Diet, Nutrition, and the Prevention of Chronic Diseases (156) provides alarming figures on the increasing prevalence of obesity-related diseases in many developing countries, some of which are still struggling under the burden of poorly controlled infectious diseases. Population drifts to urban centers bring abrupt changes in lifestyle. The diet tends to become enriched in fats, especially animal fats, sugar, and alcohol, with the more complex carbohydrates becoming less dominant. Smoking, inactivity, and stress also tend to increase. In this setting, obesity is a readily visible *risk*

factor for such chronic diseases as diabetes and heart disease, and cost-effective *population interventions* to prevent and decrease obesity are desperately needed. Research in this field is in its infancy and much work is yet to be done.

On the other hand, obesity in many individuals is more than just a risk factor, and is better considered a *disease* that is partly genetically determined and that demands *individual interventions.* These individuals can be identified by a family history of obesity, they often suffer from hypertension, and, more importantly, they have failed repeatedly to keep off the weight lost during diet therapy. Unfortunately, the treatment of these patients is notoriously difficult because the personal, social, and psychological habits related to food and eating are inherently resistant to changes. Even after significant weight loss, maintenance of the new lower weight is usually unsuccessful. To maintain long-term weight loss, a person is often faced with a lifelong struggle against the "adverse" westernized culture and a genetic predisposition, often with inadequate physiological tools in face of tremendous cultural obstacles.

Disappointing results in both individual and population interventions are in large part due to our incomplete understanding of the causes of obesity. Thus future successes in prevention and treatment of obesity will depend upon improvements in the basic understanding of the disease. Prospective studies examining the etiology and pathogenesis of obesity are likely to be the platform from which interventional research will develop. Several fruitful areas of research could be: a closer examination of the fat balance equation in humans such as the determinants of fat oxidation and the effects of altered fat intake; the identification of predictors of obesity and its complications; and population-based strategies for preventing and correcting obesity in obesity-prone populations. Pharmacological research that would result in the development of safe drugs for the treatment of obesity would also be of value and may result in obesity being treated in a fashion similar to "essential" hypertension (157,158). This would be of benefit to some obese individuals and would increase the perceived seriousness of obesity as a risk factor for chronic diseases. In the long run, the success of prevention and/or treatment of obesity will depend upon basic research uncovering the etiology of fat imbalance and applied research converting that knowledge into successful population and individual intervention strategies.

REFERENCES

1. Durnin JVGA, Edholm OG, Miller DS, Waterlow J. How much food does man require? *Nature* 1973;242:418.
2. Jéquier E, Schutz Y. Long-term measurements of energy expenditure in humans using a respiration chamber. *Am J Clin Nutr* 1983;38:989–98.
3. Ravussin E, Lillioja S, Anderson TE, Christin L, Bogardus C. Determinants of 24-hour energy expenditure in man: methods and results using a respiratory chamber. *J Clin Invest* 1986;78:1568–78.
4. Schutz Y, Bessard T, Jéquier E. Thermogenesis measured over a whole day in obese and non-obese women. *Am J Clin Nutr* 1984;40:542–52.
5. Benzinger TH, Kitzinger G. Gradient layer calorimetry and human calorimetry. In Hardy: *Temperature. Its measurement and control in science and industry,* vol 3. New York: Reinhold, 1963; 87–109.
6. Spinnler G, Jéquier E, Favre R, Dolivo M, Vannotti A. Human calorimeter with a new type of gradient layer. *J Appl Physiol* 1973;35:158–65.
7. Webb P. *Human calorimeters.* Westport CT: Praeger Publishers Division of Greenwood Press, Inc., 1985. (*Endocrinology and metabolism;* vol 7).
8. Jéquier E, Acheson K, Schutz Y. Assessment of energy expenditure and fuel utilization in man. *Annu Rev Nutr* 1987;7:187–208.
9. Van Es AJ, Voghy JE, Niessen C, et al. Human energy metabolism below, near and above energy equilibrium. *Br J Nutr* 1984;52:429–42.
10. Dauncey YMJ, Murgatroyd PR, Cole TJ. A human calorimeter for the direct and indirect measurement of 24 h energy expenditure. *Br J Nutr* 1978;39:557–66.
11. Dullo AG, Ismail MN, Ryall M, Meals G, Geissler CA, Miller DS. A low budget easy-to-operate room respirometer for measuring daily energy expenditure in man. *Am J Clin Nutr* 1988;48:1267–74.
12. Rumpler WV, Seale JL, Conway JM, Moe PW. Repeatability of 24-h energy expenditure in humans by indirect calorimetry. *Am J Clin Nutr* 1990;51:147–52.
13. Mingheli G, Schutz Y, Charbonnier A, Whitehead R, Jéquier E. Twenty-four hour energy expenditure and basal metabolic rate measured in a whole-body indirect calorimeter in Gambian men. *Am J Clin Nutr* 1990;51:563–70.
14. Durnin JVGA, Passemore R. *Energy work and leisure.* London: Heinemann Educational Books, 1967.
15. Bradfield RB. A technique for determination of usual daily energy expenditure in the field. *Am J Clin Nutr* 1971;24:1148–54.
16. Acheson KJ, Campbell IT, Edholm OG, Miller DS, Stock MJ. The measurement of daily energy expenditure: an evaluation of some techniques. *Am J Clin Nutr* 1980;33:1155–64.
17. Garrow JS. *Energy balance and obesity in man,* 1st ed. Amsterdam: North-Holland, 1974.
18. Durnin JVGA. Indirect calorimetry in man: a critique of practical problems. *Proc Nutr Soc* 1978;37:5–12.
19. Durnin JVGA. Determination of total daily energy expenditure in man by indirect calorimetry: assessment of the accuracy of a modern technique. *Br J Nutr* 1959;13:41–53.
20. Borel MJ, Riley RE, Snook JT. Estimation of energy expenditure and maintenance energy requirements of college-age men and women. *Am J Clin Nutr* 1984;40:1264–72.
21. Edholm OG. Energy expenditure and food intake. In: Apfelbaum M, ed. *Energy balance in man.* Paris: Masson, 1973;51–60.
22. Bradfield RB, Huntzicker PB, Fruehan GJ. Simultaneous comparison of respirometer and heart-rate telemetry techniques as measures of human energy expenditure. *Am J Clin Nutr* 1969;22:696–700.
23. Geissler CA, Dzumbira TMO, Noor MI. Validation of a field technique for the measurement of energy expenditure: factorial method versus continuous respirometry. *Am J Clin Nutr* 1986;44: 596–602.
24. Leibel RL, Hirsch J. Diminished energy requirements in reduced-obese patients. *Metabolism* 1984;33:164–70.
25. Weigle DS. Contribution of decreased body mass to diminished thermic effect of exercise in reduced-obese men. *Int J Obes* 1988;12:567–78.
26. Weigle DS, Sande KJ, Iverius PH, Monsen ER, Brunzell JD. Weight loss leads to a marked decrease in nonresting energy expenditure in ambulatory human subjects. *Metabolism* 1988;37:930–6.
27. Lifson N. Theory of use of the turnover rates of body water for measuring energy and material balance. *J Theor Biol* 1966;12:46–74.
28. Schoeller DA, van Santen E. Measurement of energy expenditure in humans by doubly labeled water method. *J Appl Physiol* 1982;53:955–9.
29. Schoeller DA, Field CR. Human energy metabolism: what have we learned from the doubly labeled water method? *Annu Rev Nutr* 1991;11:355–73.
30. Schoeller DA, Webb P. Five-day comparison of the doubly labeled water method with respiratory gas exchange. *Am J Clin Nutr* 1984;40:143–58.
31. Klein PD, James WPT, Wong WW, et al. Calorimetric validation of the doubly labelled water method for determination of energy expenditure in man. *Hum Nutr Clin Nutr* 1984;38C:95–106.
32. Coward WA, Prentice AM, Murgatroyd PR, et al. Measurement of CO_2 and water production rates in

man using ^2H, ^{18}O-labelled H_2O; comparisons between calorimeter and isotope values. In: van Es. Wageningen, AJH, ed. *Human energy metabolic: physical activity and energy expenditure measurements in epidemiological research based upon direct and indirect calorimetry.* Stichting Netherlands Instituut voor de Voeding, 1984;126–128. (*European nutrition report,* vol 5).

33. Schoeller DA, Ravussin E, Schutz Y, Acheson KJ, Baertschi P, Jéquier E. Energy expenditure by doubly labeled water: validation in humans and proposed calculation. *Am J Physiol* 1986;250: R823–R830.

34. Roberts SB, Coward WA, Schlingenseigpen KH, Nohria V, Lucas A. Comparison of the doubly labeled water ($H_2{}^{18}O$) method with indirect calorimetry and a nutrient balance study for simultaneous determination of energy expenditure, water intake, and metabolized energy intake in preterm infants. *Am J Clin Nutr* 1986;44:315–22.

35. Jones PJH, Winthrop AL, Schoeller DA, et al. Validation of doubly labeled water for assessing energy expenditure in infants. *Pediatr Res* 1987;21:242–6.

36. Ravussin E, Harper IT, Rising R, Bogardus C. Energy expenditure by doubly labeled water; validation in lean and obese subjects. *Am J Physiol* 1991;261:E402–E409.

37. Boothby WM, Sandiford I. Summary of the basal metabolism data on 8,614 subjects with special reference to the normal standards for the estimation of the basal metabolic rate. *J Biol Chem* 1922;54:783–803.

38. Harris JA, Benedict FG. *A biometric study of basal metabolism in man.* Washington, DC: The Carnegie Institute, 1919.

39. Roza AM, Shizgal HM. The Harris-Benedict equation reevaluated: resting energy requirements and the body cell mass. *Am J Clin Nutr* 1984; 40:168–82.

40. Schofield WN. Predicting basal metabolic rate, new standards and review of previous work. *Hum Nutr: Clin Nutr* 1985;39C[Suppl 1]:5–14.

41. Cunningham JJ. Body composition as a determinant of energy expenditure: a synthetic review and a proposed general prediction equation. *Am J Clin Nutr* 1991;54:963–9.

42. Bogardus C, Lillioja S, Ravussin E, et al. Familial dependence of the resting metabolic rate. *N Engl J Med* 1986;315:96–100.

43. Bouchard C, Tremblay A, Nadeau A, et al. Genetic effect in resting and exercise metabolic rates. *Metabolism* 1989;38:364–70.

44. Ferraro R, Lillioja S, Fontvieille AM, Rising R, Bogardus C, Ravussin E. Lower sedentary metabolic rate in women compared to men. *J Clin Invest* 1992;90:in press.

45. Tremblay A, Fontaine E, Poehlman ET, Mitchell D, Perron L, Bouchard C. The effect of exercise-training on resting metabolic rate in lean and moderately obese individuals. *Int J Obes* 1986; 10:511–7.

46. Poehlman ET, Melby CL, Bradylak SJ. Resting metabolic rate and postprandial thermogenesis in highly trained and untrained males. *Am J Clin Nutr* 1988;47:793–8.

47. Tremblay A, Nadeau A, Fournier G, Bouchard C. Effect of a three-day interruption of exercise-training on resting metabolic rate and glucose-induced thermogenesis in trained individuals. *Int J Obes* 1988;12:163–8.

48. Schulz LO, Nyomba BL, Alger S, Anderson TE, Ravussin E. Effect of endurance training on sedentary energy expenditure measured in a respiratory chamber. *Am J Physiol* 1991;260:E257–E261.

49. Davis JR, Tagliaferro AR, Kertzer R, Gerardo T, Nichols J, Wheeler J. Variations in dietary-induced thermogenesis and body fatness with aerobic capacity. *Eur J Appl Physiol* 1983;50:319–29.

50. Hill JO, Sparling PB, Shields TW, Heller PA. Effects of exercise and food restriction on body composition and metabolic rate in obese women. *Am J Clin Nutr* 1987;46:522–630.

51. Stern JS, Schutz C, Mole P, et al. Effect of caloric restriction and exercise on basal metabolism and thyroid hormone. *Aliment Nutr Metab* 1980;1:361.

52. Lennon D, Nagle F, Stratment F, Shrago E, Dennis S. Diet and exercise training effects on resting metabolic rate. *Int J Obes* 1985;9:39–47.

53. Donahoe CP Jr, Daria HL, Kirschenbaum DS, Keesey RE. Metabolic consequences of dieting and exercise in the treatment of obesity. *J Consult Clin Psychol* 1984;52:827–86.

54. Boothby WM, Berkson J, Dunn HL. Studies of the energy of metabolism of normal individuals: a standard for basal metabolism with a nomogram for clinical application. *Am J Physiol* 1936; 116:468–84.

55. Shock NW, Yiengst MJ. Age changes in basal respiratory measurements and metabolism in males. *J Gerontol* 1955;10:31–40.

56. Keys A, Taylor HL, Grande F. Basal metabolism and age of adult man. *Metabolism* 1987; 22:5979–87.

57. Calloway DH, Zanni E. Energy requirements and energy expenditure of elderly men. *Am J Clin Nutr* 1980;33:2088–92.

58. Tzankoff SP, Norris AH. Effect of muscle mass decrease on age-related BMR changes. *J Appl Physiol* 1977;43:1001–6.

59. Cohn SH, Vartzky D, Yasumura S, et al. Compartmental body composition based on total-body nitrogen, potassium, and calcium. *Am J Physiol* 1980;239:E524–E530.

60. Vaughan L, Zurlo F, Ravussin E. Aging and energy expenditure. *Am J Clin Nutr* 1991;53:821–5.

61. Saad MF, Alger SA, Zurlo F, Young JB, Bogardus C, Ravussin E. Ethnic differences in sympathetic nervous system-mediated energy expenditure. *Am J Physiol* 1991;261:E789–E794.

62. Schwartz RS, Jaeger LF, Veith RC. Effect of clonidine on the thermic effect of feeding in humans. *Am J Physiol* 1988;254:R90–R94.

63. Zurlo F, Larson K, Bogardus C, Ravussin E. Skeletal muscle metabolism is a major determinant of resting energy expenditure. *J Clin Invest* 1990;86:1423–7.

64. Kirkwood SP, Zurlo F, Larson K, Ravussin E. Muscle mitochondrial morphology body composition, and energy expenditure in sedentary individuals. *Am J Physiol* 1991;260:E89–E94.

65. Rising R, Keys A, Ravussin E, Bogardus C. Concomitant inter-individual variation in body temperature and metabolic rate. *Am J Physiol* 1992;in press.

66. Pittet Ph, Chappuis Ph, Acheson K, de Techtermann F, Jéquier E. Thermic effect of glucose in obese subjects studied by direct and indirect calorimetry. *Br J Nutr* 1976;35:281–92.

67. Sims EA. Energy balance in human beings: the problems of plenitude. *Vitam Horm* 1986; 43:1–101.

68. D'Allessio DA, Kavle EC, Mozzoli MA, et al. Thermic effect of food in lean and obese men. *J Clin Invest* 1988;81:1781–9.

69. Flatt JP. Biochemistry of energy expenditure. In: Bray G, ed. *Recent advances in obesity research II.* London: John Libbey, 1978;211–228.

70. Acheson KJ, Ravussin E, Wahren J, Jéquier E. Obligatory and facultative thermogenesis. *J Clin Invest* 1984;70:1570–780.

71. LeBlanc J, Cabanac M. Cephalic postprandial thermogenesis in human subjects. *Physiol Behavior* 1989;46:479–82.

72. Hill JO, DiGirolamo M, Heymsfield SB. Thermic effect of food after ingested versus tube delivered meals. *Am J Physiol* 1985;248:E370–E374.

73. Segal KR, Gutin B, Nyman AM, Pi-Sunyer FX. Thermic effect of food at rest, during exercise, and after exercise in lean and obese men of similar body weight. *J Clin Invest* 1985;76:1107–12.

74. Segal KR, Gutin B, Albu J, Pi-Sunyer FX. Thermic effects of food and exercise in lean and obese men of similar lean body mass. *Am J Physiol* 1987;252:E110–E117.

75. Segal KR, Eda A, Blando L, Pi-Sunyer FX. Comparison of thermic effects of constant and relative caloric loads in lean and obese men. *Am J Clin Nutr* 1990;51:14–21.

76. Thörne A, Naslund I, Wahren J. Meal-induced thermogenesis in previously obese patients. *Clin Physiol* 1990;10:99–109.

77. Thörne A, Hallberg D, Wahren J. Meal-induced thermogenesis in obese patients before and after weight reduction. *Clin Physiol* 1989;9:481–98.

78. Thörne A. Diet-induced thermogenesis. An experimental study in healthy and obese individuals. Review article: 145 refs. *Acta Chir Scand [Suppl]* 1990;558:6–59.

79. Golay A, Schutz Y, Broquet C, Moeri R, Felber JP, Jéquier E. Decreased thermogenic response to an oral glucose load in older subjects. *J Am Geriatr Soc* 1983;31:144–8.

80. Thörne A, Wahren J. Diminished meal-induced thermogenesis in elderly man. *Clin Physiol* 1990;10:427–37.

81. Schwartz RS, Jaeger LF, Veith RC. The thermic effect of feeding on older men: the importance of the sympathetic nervous system *Metabolism* 1990;39:733–7.

82. Zurlo F, Ferraro R, Fontvieille AM, Rising R, Bogardus C, Ravussin E. Spontaneous physical activity and obesity: cross-sectional and longitudinal studies in Pima Indians. *Am J Physiol* 1992; in press.

83. Bullen BA, Reed RB, Mayer J. Physical activity of obese and non-obese adolescent girls, appraised by motion pictures sampling. *Am J Clin Nutr* 1964;14:211–23.

84. Chirico AM, Stunkard AJ. Physical activity and human obesity. *N Engl J Med* 1960;263:935–40.

85. Ferraro R, Boyce VL, Swinburn B, DeGregorio M, Ravussin E. Energy cost of physical activity on a metabolic ward in relationship to obesity. *Am J Clin Nutr* 1991;53:1368–71.

86. Rising R, Harper I, Ferraro R, Fontvieille AM, Ravussin E. Effect of age on free-living energy expenditure in Pima Indians. *FASEB J* 1991;F:A555.

87. Ravussin E, Harper I, Rising R, Ferraro R, Fontvieille AM. Human obesity is associated with lower levels of physical activity: results from doubly labelled water and gas exchanges. *FASEB J* 1991;5:554A.

88. Ravussin E, Zurlo F, Ferraro R, Bogardus C. Energy expenditure in man: determinants and risk factors for body weight gain. In: *Recent advances in obesity research.* London: John Libbey, 175–182.

89. James WPT, Bailes J, Davies HL, Dauncey MJ. Elevated metabolic rates in obesity. *Lancet* 1978;1:1122–5.

90. Romieu I, Willett WC, Stampfer MJ, et al. Energy intake and other determinants of relative weight. *Am J Clin Nutr* 1988;47:406–12.

91. Prentice AM, Black AE, Coward WA, et al. High levels of energy expenditure in obese women. *Br Med J* 1986;292:983–7.

92. Bandini LG, Schoeller DA, Cyr H, Dietz WH. Validity of reported energy intake in obese and non-obese adolescents. *Am J Clin Nutr* 1990;52:421–5.

93. Mertz W, Tsui JC, Judd JT, et al. What are people really eating? The relation between energy derived from estimated diet records and intake determined to maintain body weight. *Am J Clin Nutr* 1991;54:291–5.

94. Alpert S. Growth, thermogenesis, and hyperphagia. *Am J Clin Nutr* 1990;52:784–92.

95. [Anonymous]. Exercise and energy balance. *Lancet* 1988;1:392–4.

96. Von Voit C. Physiology of general metabolism and nutrition. In: Hermann L, ed. *Handbook of physiology,* vol 6, part 1. Leipzig: FCW Vogel, 1881;1–566.

97. Neumann RO. Experimentelle Beitraege zur Lehre von dem taeglichen Nahrungsbedarf des Menschen unter besonderer Beruecksichtigung der notwendigen Eiweissmenge. *Arch Hyg* 1902;XLV:1–87.

98. Gulick A. A study of weight regulation in the adult human body during over-nutrition. *Am J Physiol* 1922;60:371–95.

99. Miller DS, Mumford P. Gluttony. I. An experimental study of overeating low- or high-protein diets. *Am J Clin Nutr* 1967;20:1212–22.

100. Miller DS, Mumford P, Stock MJ. Gluttony. II. Thermogenesis in overeating man. *Am J Clin Nutr* 1967;20:1223–9.

101. Ravussin E, Schutz Y, Acheson KJ, Dusmet M, Bourquin L, Jéquier E. Short-term, mixed diet overfeeding in man: no evidence for "luxuskonsumption." *Am J Physiol* 1985;249:E470–E477.

102. Leibel RL. Is obesity due to a heritable difference in "set-point" for adiposity. *West J Med* 1990; 153:429–31.

103. Willett WC, Stampfer MJ. Total energy intake: implications for epidemiologic analyses. *Am J Epidemiol* 1986;124:17–27.

104. Zelewski M, Swierczynki J. Comparative studies on lipogenic enzyme activities in the liver of human and some animal species. *Comp Biochem Physiol* 1990;95:469–72.

105. Chascione C, Elwyn DH, Davila M, Gil KM, Askanazi J, Kinney JM. Effect of carbohydrate intake on de novo lipogenesis in human adipose tissue. *Am J Physiol* 1987;253:E664–E669.

106. Just B, Messing B, Darmaun B, Rongier M, Carmillo E. Comparison of substrate utilization by indirect calorimetry during cyclic and continuous total parenteral nutrition. *Am J Clin Nutr* 1990;51:107–11.

107. Manji S, Shikora S, McMahon M, Blackburn GL, Bistrian BR. Peritoneal dialysis for acute renal failure: overfeeding resulting from dextrose absorbed during dialysis. *Crit Care Med* 1990;18:29–31.

108. Acheson KJ, Schutz Y, Bessard T, Flatt JP, Jéquier E. Carbohydrate metabolism and de novo lipogenesis in human obesity. *Am J Clin Nutr* 1987;45:78–85.

109. Acheson KJ, Schutz Y, Bessard T, Anantharaman K, Flatt JP, Jéquier E. Glycogen storage capacity and de novo lipogenesis during massive carbohydrate overfeeding in man. *Am J Clin Nutr* 1988;48:240–7.

110. Coulston AM, Hollenbeck CB, Swislocki ALM, Chen YDI, Reavan GM. Deleterious effects of high-carbohydrate, sucrose-containing diets in patients with non-insulin dependent diabetes mellitus. *Am J Med* 1987;82:213–20.

111. Reaven GM, Hill DB, Gross RC, Farqhuar JW. Kinetics of triglyceride turnover of very low density lipoproteins of human plasma. *J Clin Invest* 1965;44:1826–33.

112. Quarfordt SH, Frank A, Shames DM, Berman M, Steinberg D. Very low density lipoprotein triglyceride transport in type IV hyperlipoproteinemia and the effects of carbohydrate rich diets. *J Clin Invest* 1970;49:2281–97.

113. Abbott WGH, Swinburn BA, Ruotolo G, et al. Effect of a high-carbohydrate, low-saturated-fat diet on apolipoprotein B and triglyceride metabolism in Pima Indians. *J Clin Invest* 1990;86:642–50.

114. Hellerstedt WL, Jeffery RW, Murray DM. The association between alcohol intake and adiposity in the general population. *Am J Epidemiol* 1990; 132:594–611.

115. Colditz GA, Giovannucci E, Rimm EB, et al. Alcohol intake in relation to diet and obesity in women and men. *Am J Clin Nutr* 1991;54:49–55.

116. Lands WEM, Zakhari S. The case of the missing calories. *Am J Clin Nutr* 1991;54:47–48.

117. Lieber CS. Perspectives: do alcohol calories count? *Am J Clin Nutr* 1991;54:976–82.

118. Shelmet JJ, Reichard GA, Skutches CL, Hoeldtke RD, Owen OE, Boden G. Ethanol causes acute inhibition of carbohydrate, fat, and protein oxidation

119. Snyder WS, Cook MJ, Nasset ES, Karhausen LR, Howells GP, Tipton IH. Report of the task group on reference man. The International Commission on Radiological Protection, no. 23. New York: Pergamon Press, 1974.

120. Bray GA. Treatment for obesity: a nutrient balance/nutrient partition approach. *Nutr Rev* 1991;49:33–45.

121. Abbott WGH, Howard BV, Christin L, et al. Short-term energy balance: relationship with protein, carbohydrate, and fat balances. *Am J Physiol* 1988;255:E332–E337.

122. Flatt JP. Importance of nutrient balance in body weight regulation. *Diabetes Metab Rev* 1988; 6:571–81.

123. Felber JP, Ferrannini E, Golay A, et al. Role of lipid oxidation in pathogenesis of insulin resistance of obesity and type II diabetes. *Diabetes* 1987;36:1341–50.

124. Flatt JP, Ravussin E, Acheson KJ, Jéquier E. Effects of dietary fat on postprandial substrate oxidation and on carbohydrate and fat balance. *J Clin Invest* 1985;76:1019–24.

125. Schutz Y, Flatt JP, Jéquier E. Failure of dietary fat intake to promote fat oxidation: a factor favoring the development of obesity. *Am J Clin Nutr* 1989;50:307–14.

126. Rising R, Alger S, Boyce V, et al. Food intake measured by an automated food-selection system: relationship to energy expenditure. *Am J Clin Nutr* 1992;55:343–349.

127. Zurlo F, Lillioja S, Esposito-Del Puente A, et al. Low ratio of fat to carbohydrate oxidation as a predictor of weight gain: study of 24-h RQ. *Am J Physiol* 1990;259:E650–E657.

128. Salmon DMW, Flatt JP. Effect of dietary fat content on the incidence of obesity among ad libitum fed mice. *Int J Obes* 1985;9:443–9.

129. Dreon DM, Frey-Hewitt B, Ellsworth N, Williams PT, Terry RB, Wood PD. Dietary fat:carbohydrate ratio and obesity in middle-aged men. *Am J Clin Nutr* 1988;47:995–1000.

130. Tremblay A, Ploure G, Déspres JP, Bouchard C. Impact of dietary fat content and fat oxidation on energy intake in humans. *Am J Clin Nutr* 1989;49:799–805.

131. Kendall A, Levitsky DA, Strupp BJ, Lissner L. Weight loss on a low fat diet: consequence of the imprecision of the control of food intake in humans. *Am J Clin Nutr* 1991;53:1124–9.

132. Lissner L, Levitsky DA. Dietary fat and the regulation of energy intake in human subjects. *Am J Clin Nutr* 1987;46:886–92.

133. Knowler WC, Pettitt DJ, Saad MF, et al. Obesity in Pima Indians: its magnitude and relationship with diabetes. *Am J Clin Nutr* 1991;53:1543S–1551S.

134. Roberts SB, Savage J, Coward WA, Chew B, Lucas A. Energy expenditure and intake in infants born to lean and overweight mothers. *N Engl J Med* 1988;318:461–6.

135. Griffiths M, Payne PR, Stunkard AJ, Rivers JPW, Cox M. Metabolic rate and physical development

and insulin resistance. *J Clin Invest* 1988; 81:1137–45.

in children at risk of obesity. *Lancet* 1990; 336:76–7.

136. Ravussin E, Lillioja S, Knowler WC, et al. Reduced rate of energy expenditure as a risk factor for body weight gain. *N Engl J Med* 1988;318:467–72.

137. McNeil G, Bruce AC, Ralph A, James WPT. Interindividual differences in fasting nutrient oxidation and the influence of diet composition. *Int J Obes* 1988;12:445–63.

138. Swinburn BA, Nyomba BL, Saad MF, et al. Insulin resistance associated with lower rates of weight gain in Pima Indians. *J Clin Invest* 1991;88:168–73.

139. Keys A, Brozek J, Henschel A, Mickelsen O, Taylor HL. *The biology of human starvation,* vol 1. Minneapolis: University of Minnesota Press, 1950.

140. Food and Agriculture Organization/World Health Organization/United Nations University. *Energy and protein requirements.* WHO Technical Report Series no 724. Geneva: WHO, 1985.

141. Ravussin E, Bogardus C. Relationship of genetics, age, and physical fitness to daily energy expenditure and fuel utilization. *Am J Clin Nutr* 1989;49:968–75.

142. Sims EAH. Experimental obesity, dietary induced thermogenesis and their clinical implications. *Clin Endocrinol* 1976;5:377–95.

143. Goldman RF, Haisman MF, Bynum G, Horton ES, Sims EAH. Experimental obesity in man: metabolic rate in relation to dietary intake. In: Bray GA, ed., *Obesity in perspective.* Washington, DC: U.S. Government Printing Office, 1975;165–86.

144. Garrow JS. The regulation of energy expenditure in man. In: Bray GA, ed., *Recent advances in obesity research,* vol 2. London: Newman, 1978; 200–10.

145. Norgan NG, Durnin JVGA. The effect of 6 weeks of overfeeding on the body weight, body composition, and energy metabolism of young men. *Am J Clin Nutr* 1980;33:978–88.

146. Durnin JVGA, Norgan N. Overfeeding. *J Physiol* 1969;202:106P.

147. Roberts SB, Young VR, Fuss P, et al. Energy expenditure and subsequent nutrient intakes in overfed young men. *Am J Physiol* 1990;259[Pt 2]:R461–R469.

148. Forbes GB. Do obese individuals gain weight more easily than non-obese individuals? *Am J Clin Nutr* 1990;52:224–7.

149. Bouchard C, Tremblay A, Després JP, et al. The response to long-term overfeeding in identical twins. *N Engl J Med* 1990;322:1477–82.

150. Ravussin E, Burnand B, Schutz Y, Jéquier E. Energy expenditure before and during energy restriction in obese patients. *Am J Clin Nutr* 1985;41:753–9.

151. Garby L, Kurzer MS, Lammert O, Nielsen E. Effect of 12 weeks' light-moderate underfeeding on 24-hour energy expenditure in normal male and female subjects. *Eur J Clin Nutr* 1988;42:295–300.

152. Apfelbaum M, Bostsarron J, Lacatis D. Effect of caloric restriction and excessive caloric intake on energy expenditure. *Am J Clin Nutr* 1971;24: 1404–9.

153. de Groot LCGM, van Es AJH, Van Raaij JMA, Vogt JE, Hautvast JGAJ. Energy metabolism of overweight women 1 mo and 1 y after an 8-wk slimming period. *Am J Clin Nutr* 1990;51:578–83.

154. Bessard T, Schutz Y, Jéquier E. Energy expenditure and postprandial thermogenesis in obese women before and after weight loss. *Am J Clin Nutr* 1983;38:680–93.

155. Ravussin E, Swinburn BA. Effect of caloric restriction and weight loss on energy expenditure. In: Wadden TA, Van Itallie TB, eds. *Treatment of the seriously obese patient.* New York: Guilford Press, 1992:163–189.

156. World Health Organization. *Diet, nutrition, and the prevention of chronic diseases.* Report of a WHO Study Group, Series 797. Geneva: World Health Organization, 1990.

157. Bray GA. Barriers to the treatment of obesity. *Ann Intern Med* 1991;115:152–3.

158. Ravussin E, Bogardus C. A brief overview of human energy metabolism and its relationship to essential obesity. *Am J Clin Nutr* 1992;55: 242S–245S.

159. Kaplan M, Leveille GA. Calorigenic response in obese and non-obese women. *Am J Clin Nutr* 1976; 29:1108–13.

160. Zahorska-Markiewicz B. Thermic effect of food and exercise in obesity. *Eur J Appl Physiol* 1980;44:231–5.

161. Shetty PS, Jung RT, James WPT, Barrand BA. Postprandial thermogenesis in obesity. *Clin Sci* 1981;60:519–25.

162. Golay A, Schutz Y, Meyer HV, et al. Glucose induced thermogenesis in nondiabetic and diabetic obese subjects. *Diabetes* 1982;31:1023–8.

163. Schwartz RS, Halter JB, Bierman EL. Reduced thermic effect of feeding in obesity: role of norepinephrine. *Metabolism* 1983;32:114–7.

164. Bessard T, Schutz Y, Jéquier E. Energy expenditure and postprandial thermogenesis in obese women before and after weight loss. *Am J Clin Nutr* 1983;38:680–93.

165. Ravussin E, Bogardus C, Schwartz RS, et al. Thermic effect of infused glucose and insulin in man: decreased response with increased insulin resistance in obesity and non-insulin dependent diabetes mellitus. *J Clin Invest* 1983;72:893–902.

166. Segal KR, Gutin B. Thermic effect of food and exercise in lean and obese women. *Metabolism* 1983;32:581–9.

167. Segal KR, Presta E, Gutin B. Thermic effect of food during graded exercise in normal weight and obese men. *Am J Clin Nutr* 1984;40:995–1000.

168. Schutz Y, Golay A, Felber JP, Jéquier E. Decreased glucose-induced thermogenesis after weight loss in obese subjects: a predisposing factor for relapse of obesity. *Am J Clin Nutr* 1984;39:380–7.

169. Bogardus C, Lillioja S, Mott D, Zawadzki J, Young A, Abbott W. Evidence for reduced thermic effect of insulin and glucose infusions in Pima Indians. *J Clin Invest* 1985;75:1264–9.

170. Swaminathan R, King RFGJ, Holmfield J, Siwek RA, Baker M, Wales JK. Thermic effect of feeding carbohydrate, fat, protein, and mixed meal in lean and obese subjects. *Am J Clin Nutr* 1985; 42:177–81.

171. Devlin JT, Horton ES. Potentiation of the thermic

effect of insulin by exercise: differences between lean, obese, and non-insulin dependent diabetic men. *Am J Clin Nutr* 1986;43:884–90.

172. Golay A, Schutz Y, Felber JP, DeFronzo RA, Jéquier E. Lack of thermogenic response to glucose/insulin infusion in diabetic obese subjects. *Int J Obes* 1986;10:107–16.

173. Zed CL, James WPT. Dietary thermogenesis in obesity: fat feeding at different energy intakes. *Int J Obes* 1986;10:375–90.

174. Acheson KJ, Schutz Y, Bessard T, Flatt JP, Jéquier E. Carbohydrate metabolism and de novo lipogenesis in human obesity. *Am J Clin Nutr* 1987;45:78–85.

175. Steiniger J, Karst H, Noack R, Steglich HD. Diet-induced thermogenesis in man: thermic effects of single protein and carbohydrate test meals in lean and obese subjects. *Ann Nutr Metab* 1987; 31:117–125.

176. Schutz Y, Bessard T, Jéquier E. Exercise and postprandial thermogenesis in obese women before and after weight loss. *Am J Clin Nutr* 1987;45:1424–32.

177. Golay A, Schutz Y, Felber JP, Jallut D, Jéquier E. Blunted glucose-induced thermogenesis in "overweight" patients: a factor contributing to relapse of obesity. *Int J Obes* 1989;13:767–75.

178. Katzeff HL, Danforth E Jr. Decreased thermic effect of a mixed meal during overnutrition in human obesity. *Am J Clin Nutr* 1989;50:915–21.

179. Tremblay A, Sauve L, Déspres JP, Nadeau A, Theriault G, Bouchard C. Metabolic characteristics of post-obese individuals. *Int J Obes* 1989; 13:356–66.

180. Segal KR, Lacayanga I, Dunaif A, Gutin B, Pi-Sunyer FX. Impact of body fat mass and percent fat on metabolic rate and thermogenesis in men. *Am J Physiol* 1989;256:E573–E579.

181. Felber JP, Meyer HV, Curchod B, et al. Glucose storage and oxidation in different degrees of human obesity measured by continuous indirect calorimetry. *Diabetologia* 1981;20:39–44.

182. Sharief NN, Macdonald I. Differences in dietary-induced thermogenesis with various carbohydrates in normal and overweight men. *Am J Clin Nutr* 1982;35:267–72.

183. Welle SL, Campbell RG. Normal thermic effect of glucose in obese women. *Am J Clin Nutr* 1983;37:87–92.

184. Nair KS, Haliday D, Garrow JS. Thermic response to isoenergetic protein, carbohydrate or fat meals in lean and obese subjects. *Clin Sci* 1983; 65:307–12.

185. Blaza S, Garrow JS. Thermogenic response to temperature, exercise and food stimuli in lean and obese women, studied by 24 h direct calorimetry. *Br J Nutr* 1983;49:171–80.

186. Felig P, Cunningham J, Levitt M, Hendler R, Nadel E. Energy expenditure in obesity in fasting and postprandial state. *Am J Physiol* 1983;244: E45–E51.

187. Welle SL. Metabolic responses to a meal during rest and low-intensity exercise. *Am J Clin Nutr* 1984;40:990–4.

188. Schwartz RS, Ravussin E, Massari M, O'Connell M, Robbins DC. The thermic effect of carbohydrate versus fat feeding in man. *Metabolism* 1985;34:285–93.

189. Ravussin E, Acheson KJ, Vernet O, Danforth E, Jéquier E. Evidence that insulin resistance is responsible for the decreased thermic effect of glucose in human obesity. *J Clin Invest* 1985; 76:1268–73.

190. Anton-Kuchly B, Laval M, Choukroun ML, Manciet G, Roger P, Varene P. Postprandial thermogenesis and hormonal release in lean obese subjects. *J Physiol (Paris)* 1985;80:321–9.

191. Owen OE, Kavle EE, Owen RS, et al. A reappraisal of caloric requirements in healthy women. *Am J Clin Nutr* 1986;44:1–9.

192. Nair KS, Webster J, Garrow JS. Effect of impaired glucose tolerance and type II diabetes on resting metabolic rate and thermic response to a glucose meal in obese subjects. *Metabolism* 1986;35:640–4.

193. Vernet O, Christin L, Schutz Y, Danforth E Jr, Jéquier E. Enteral versus parenteral nutrition: comparison of energy metabolism in lean and moderately obese women. *Am J Clin Nutr* 1986; 43:194–209.

194. Thörne A, Näslund I, Wahren J. Meal-induced thermogenesis in previously obese patients. *Clin Physiol* 1990;10:99–109.

195. Scalfi L, Coltorti A, Contaldo F. Postprandial thermogenesis in lean and obese subjects after meals supplemented with medium-chain and long-chain triglycerides. *Am J Clin Nutr* 1991;53:1130–3.

Obesity: Theory and Therapy, Second Edition,
edited by A. J. Stunkard and T. A. Wadden.
Raven Press, Ltd., New York © 1993.

7

Dietary Obesity

Anthony Sclafani

*Department of Psychology, Brooklyn College of the City University of New York,
Brooklyn, New York 11210*

Obesity results from an imbalance in energy intake and energy expenditure. While there are many possible causes for this imbalance, the availability of energy-rich foods is a prerequisite for the development of obesity. In addition to being a precondition, the availability of certain foods may actually promote overeating and obesity. Although the evidence from human studies is circumstantial and controversial, research with laboratory animals documents the causal link between diet and obesity. Of the many different animal models of obesity (genetic, traumatic, environmental), the various forms of dietary-induced obesity in rats and mice have been among the most extensively investigated during the past decade. Research on dietary obesity has advanced from demonstrating the particular diet formulations that promote overeating and overweight in animals, to identifying the critical variables involved, to elucidating the behavioral and metabolic processes responsible for diet-induced obesity.

Dietary obesity is the subject of several recent reviews that can be consulted for comprehensive accounts of the literature (1–8). The present chapter reviews recent developments and focuses on the role of diet flavor, palatability, and postingestive metabolic effects in promoting overeating and adiposity.

BASIC CONCEPTS

Control Diets

Diet-induced changes in food intake, body weight, and adiposity in rats are typically eval-uated in reference to control groups fed a commercial chow or semisynthetic diet high in carbohydrate (starch) and low in fat. When given ad libitum access to such control diets, adult rats may accumulate up to 20 to 30% body fat, which some investigators consider excessive (9). That is, compared to animals fed restricted amounts of food, rats fed chow ad libitum are not only fatter, but have decreased longevity, reduced fertility, and greater susceptibility to disease (9,10). The limited activity levels allowed by standard laboratory caging also foster weight gain; rats housed in running-wheel cages or exercised on treadmills maintain lower body weights than do rats housed in standard cages (11,12). Thus the control animals used to assess dietary obesity—sedentary, chow-fed rats—arguably represent a form of mild obesity.

Experimental Diets

Many different diets have been investigated for their obesity-promoting effects. The most commonly used diets are high in either fat or sugar and are presented as a single food (*composite* diet method). Some studies have also fed animals composite diets that are high in both fat and sugar. Another approach is the *diet option* method, in which the animal is fed a separate source of fat and/or carbohydrate in addition to a nutritionally complete diet. There are advantages to both methods. With composite diets, the influence of variations in the concentration and/or types of nutrients on food intake and adiposity can be evaluated since the diet composition is fixed by the experimenter. In the diet option method, on the other hand, the animal selects the amount and proportion of fat or carbohydrate it prefers. Even greater choice is available with *cafeteria diets,* which consist of an assortment of different food items. The foods typically include "supermarket" foods (11) such as cookies, cheese, marshmallows, and peanut butter, although in some experiments actual "left-overs" from a cafeteria are used.

Overeating, Overweight, and Obesity

Dietary-induced obesity is usually associated with overeating and overweight, but these effects can be dissociated, that is, small increases in percent body fat can occur without elevation of body weight, and overweight and obesity can occur in the absence of increased caloric intake. Obesity without hyperphagia is possible because changes in the nutrient composition or form of the diet can alter the efficiency of food utilization and thus increase the amount of body fat stored per calorie consumed. It could be argued that any level of food intake that leads to excess fat disposition represents a form of hyperphagia, but usually overeating is defined as caloric intakes exceeding control levels (13).

Diet Palatability

When overeating does occur, it is often attributed to the *palatability* of the diet. The concept of palatability and its role in dietary-induced overeating have been critically re-evaluated in recent years (4–6,14–17). Palatability, which literally means "pleasing to the palate or taste," was originally thought to be determined solely by the flavor of food, i.e., by its taste, aroma, texture, and temperature (18). Many investigators now consider palatability not to be an invariant property of the food's flavor but a dynamic one that changes as the animal associates the flavor with the gastrointestinal and metabolic effects of the food. For example, the rat's innate preference for sweet taste can be turned

into an aversion if the taste is associated with nausea (19). Conversely, under certain conditions the innate aversion to bitter taste can be changed to a preference if the taste is associated with the nutritive actions of food (20). According to this view, food palatability is determined by innate reactions to flavor and learned responses based on the food's postingestive actions.

In the past, diets that promoted overeating were described as palatable; overeating, in turn, was "explained" by the palatability of the diet. In order to avoid this circular reasoning, it is necessary as a first step to measure palatability independently of the hyperphagic response. A number of different techniques are available to measure food palatability in animals (5,17). One simple procedure is to assess the relative palatability of different foods using a two-choice preference test. Although there may be exceptions, in general, if diet A is preferred to diet B in long-term choice tests then it can be assumed that A is more palatable than B. While food preferences are often not evaluated in dietary obesity studies, many of the foods used in these experiments are known to be palatable, e.g., high-fat diets are generally preferred to low-fat control diets. Nevertheless, not all preferred foods are overconsumed, and Ramirez (21) has reported one case in which rats consumed more of an unpreferred diet than of a preferred diet. Thus there is a less than perfect correlation between food palatability and dietary-induced overeating.

Even when a diet is preferred and overconsumed it is not necessarily the case that palatability is driving the hyperphagia (16). As illustrated in Fig. 1, hyperphagia may result directly from the food's palatable flavor (Fig. 1A) or it may be unrelated to palatability and result instead from the food's postingestive metabolic effects (Fig. 1B). (These postingestive actions may or may not be the same as those that condition food palatability.) A third alternative is that both palatability and postingestive factors contribute to the hyperphagic response (Fig. 1C). A further complexity is that palatability may influence the postingestive disposition of nutrients via ce-

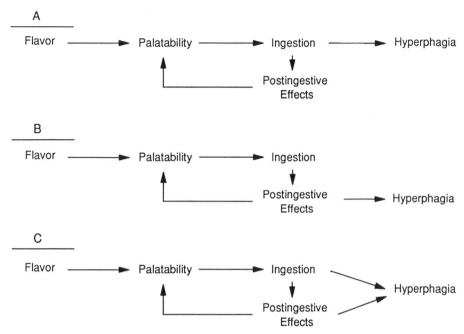

FIG. 1. Schematic representation of the possible causal relationships between palatability and hyperphagia. See text for details.

phalic-phase digestive responses. For example, sweet taste triggers a cephalic-phase insulin release that may have metabolic consequences that promote overeating and obesity, although this remains to be established (22).

Palatability can also indirectly influence caloric consumption by affecting food choice. Animals given a choice of foods may select a particular food because of its preferred flavor but overeat that food because of its postingestive metabolic effects. In many dietary obesity experiments choice is not a factor since the animals are given only one food. In the real world, however, food choice is a significant aspect of feeding behavior and may be an important determinant of long-term energy balance.

HIGH-FAT DIETS

High-fat diets have long been used to produce obesity in laboratory animals. Compared with controls fed a low-fat diet ($\approx 10\%$ fat by calories), rats and mice fed high-fat composite diets gain more weight and deposit more body fat, sometimes to the point of extreme obesity (23–27). Caloric intake is often, but not always, increased by high-fat diets (24–27). The degree of overeating, overweight, and obesity is influenced by the concentration and type of fat included in the diet. Weight gains tend to be proportional to fat concentration and are greater with solid fats (vegetable shortening, lard) than with liquid fats (oils), and with fats containing long-chain rather than short-chain triglycerides (28–31). The carbohydrate content of the high-fat diet also appears to be an important factor; greater weight gains are obtained with high-fat diets with a moderate carbohydrate content than with high-fat diets with a low carbohydrate content (32).

Hyperphagia and obesity can also be produced by offering rats a separate fat source as an option to a chow diet. For example, rats fed corn oil as an option consumed more calories and gained more weight than rats fed only chow (33). Even greater hyperphagia and obesity were produced by presenting the fat option as a 35% oil–water emulsion or as pure vegetable shortening; with these options the rats selected 58 to 68% of total calories as fat (33). Moderate obesity has also been reported in rats allowed to self-select their diet from separate sources of fat, protein, and carbohydrate. In one study, female rats self-selected a diet consisting of 50% fat and gained twice as much weight as did controls fed a low-fat chow diet (34).

As discussed in detail elsewhere, the obesity response to high-fat diets is influenced by many nondietary factors (2,35). In particular, the obesity produced by such diets is affected by the age, strain, and sex of the animal as well as its level of activity. Even when these variables are kept constant, there can be considerable individual differences in weight gains produced by high-fat diets. In a given group of animals maintained on a high-fat diet, some rats may gain more than twice as much weight as controls whereas other rats may gain no more than controls (36). Several metabolic and neural differences have been identified between obesity-prone and obesity-resistant rats, but much remains to be learned about the behavioral and physiological factors that predispose animals towards dietary obesity (36–38).

Fat Palatability and Metabolism

The postingestive metabolic consequences of high-fat diets promote adiposity, as evidenced by the findings that such diets can produce obesity even in the absence of hyperphagia. The increased feed efficiency observed with high-fat diets is attributed to the fact that dietary fat requires less energy to be converted into body fat than do dietary carbohydrate and protein (39,40). It has also been suggested that high-fat diets promote overeating because the conversion of dietary fat to body fat reduces its availability for oxidation (4). According to this hypothesis, high-fat foods are less satiating than low-fat foods because of their greater metabolic diversion to adipose tissue. Flatt (41) has argued that dietary fat intake and fat oxidation, unlike carbohydrate intake and oxidation, are not tightly regulated. Consequently excess fat consumption produces less of an inhibitory effect on subsequent food intake than does excess carbohydrate consumption.

In addition to metabolic effects, the palatability of high-fat diets has been implicated as a contributing factor in overeating and obesity. Several studies demonstrate that rats prefer high-fat to low-fat foods in choice tests (42,43; but see ref. 44). This preference is due in part to the orosensory qualities (flavor) of high-fat diets because rats also prefer foods made greasy or oily with the addition of noncaloric petrolatum or mineral oil (42). The rat's attraction to the flavor of fat begins at an early age. In a study by Ackroff et al. (45), 15-day-old rat pups displayed more ingestive responses to intraoral infusions of corn oil and mineral oil emulsions than to water infusions. The fact that the rat pups, with no prior experience with food other than mother's milk, responded to the oil infusions during the first minutes of exposure, and responded equally to the nutritive and nonnutritive oils, suggested that their attraction to oily flavors may have an innate basis (45). This hypothesis is further suggested by ingestive responses elicited by oil emulsions in adult rats with no prior experience with oils. Separate groups of adult rats given brief daily "taste" tests with corn oil or mineral oil emulsions consumed similar amounts, and increased their intakes of both oils by identical amounts when food deprived (45). Since the mineral oil provides no nutritive benefit, these data indicate that orosensory properties of oil are sufficient to stimulate ingestion.

Other findings demonstrate that the preference for high-fat foods is conditioned by postingestive nutritive effects. Hamilton (42) reported that rats, when given the choice between a 30% fat diet and a 30% petrolatum diet, initially consumed similar amounts of the two diets, but over the course of several days developed a strong preference for the fat-rich diet. Similarly, with repeated testing, food-deprived rats acquire a preference for corn oil over mineral oil emulsions (45). Rats will also learn to prefer an arbitrary flavor (e.g., cherry) that is added to a corn oil emulsion over a flavor (e.g., grape) presented in water (46,47). Lucas and Sclafani (48) further demonstrated that preferences can be conditioned by pairing the consumption of flavored water with intragastric infusions of a corn oil emulsion.

If metabolic factors condition fat appetite, then altering the postingestive disposition of dietary fat should modify the animal's intake and preference for high-fat diets. This prediction is supported by results obtained with the drug tetrahydrolipostatin (THL), a lipase inhibitor that blocks the digestion of fat (49). Rats fed a self-selection diet (separate sources of fat, carbohydrate, and protein) consumed 66% of their calories as fat and rapidly gained weight. The addition of THL to the fat source caused the rats to reduce their percent fat intake to 32% of total calories and blocked further weight gain. Other rats given the choice of two fat sources, one with and one without THL, learned to prefer the drug-free diet. It is possible that the THL–fat diet produced aversive postingestive effects but this seems unlikely because the rats continued to eat the diet if it was the only fat source available. Rather, it appears that THL, by inhibiting fat digestion, reduced the attractiveness of the THL–fat diet.

The above findings suggest that rats prefer high-fat to low-fat diets because of an unlearned attraction to the flavor of fat and a learned attraction to flavors associated with the postingestive nutritive effects of fat. These findings, however, do not establish whether or not the overeating of high-fat diets is driven by diet palatability. As mentioned above, it is conceivable that palatability influences diet choice but that caloric intake is determined solely by the diet's postingestive metabolic effects. Some evidence that flavor and palatability can influence the feeding response to high-fat diets is provided by a study by Lucas and Sclafani (50), which examined the hyperphagic effects of fat and sugar mixtures. Rats fed, as an option to chow, a 35% corn oil emulsion containing 8% sucrose con-

sumed more fat and total calories and gained more weight than did rats fed the oil emulsion without sugar. The hyperphagic response to the fat–sugar mixture was due at least in part to its sweet taste, because adding saccharin to the corn oil emulsion was also observed to increase fat and total caloric intake. Two-choice tests confirmed that the saccharin-sweetened emulsion was preferred to the unsweetened emulsion. At least in some circumstances, therefore, the flavor of high-fat diets can influence caloric intake and weight gain.

HIGH CARBOHYDRATE DIETS

Dietary sugar, like dietary fat, has been the subject of extensive research with regard to its obesity-promoting potential (3,5). Several studies report that, as compared with starch-based diets, high-sucrose composite diets increase body weight and fat, often in the absence of hyperphagia (51–54). The adiposity obtained with these high-sugar diets is typically rather modest compared with that produced by high-fat diets. However, Oscai et al. (55) obtained comparably high levels of obesity in rats fed a high-sucrose diet (55% kcal as sucrose) or high-fat diet (40% kcal as fat) for 63 weeks postweaning. The caloric intakes of the high-sugar and high-fat groups were also similar and *less* than that of the chow-fed controls. In contrast to these results, other studies report little or no change in body weight and adiposity in rats fed high-sugar composite diets (56–58). Analyses of the various studies have not identified any single factor that explains why high-sugar composite diets produce obesity in some experiments but not others (3,5). Differences in age, sex, and strain of animals and in diet composition and exposure time may all contribute to the variable results reported in the literature.

In contrast to the inconsistent effects obtained with high-sugar composite diets, obesity is reliably produced by feeding rats a concentrated sugar solution as an option to a standard chow diet; sugars producing this effect include sucrose, glucose, and fructose (3,5). In most, but not all cases, the obesity is associated with overeating and overweight. Typically, rats offered chow and a 32% sucrose solution take 60% of their calories as sugar and increase their total energy intake by about 20% as compared with controls fed only chow. As the rats decrease their chow consumption in response to their high sugar intake, this necessarily reduces their protein intake, which, according to one hypothesis, leads to a nutritional imbalance that contributes to the overfeeding response (59). This view is contradicted, however, by results obtained with rats fed a macronutrient self-selection diet (separate sources of fat, protein, and starch) (34). When given access to a 32% sucrose solution, the rats fed the self-selection diet consumed as much sucrose and increased their total caloric intake as much as or more than rats fed the sucrose solution and a composite diet. The self-selecting rats responded to their high sugar intake by decreasing their fat and starch intakes but not their protein intake, indicating that a protein deficit is not necessary for sucrose-induced overeating.

Rather than diet choice, diet hydration has proved to be a critical factor in sugar-induced obesity. This is indicated by the findings that rats overeat and gain weight when fed chow and a sugar solution but show little or no increase in energy intake or body weight when the sugar is offered as dry powder (60,61). Thus the differential effectiveness of sugar solution diets and high-sugar composite diets in producing overeating and obesity may be due in large part to the presence and absence, respectively, of water in the two type of diets. Ramirez (62), in fact, reported that adding water to a high-sucrose composite diet significantly increased caloric intake and body weight gain. Why rats consume more when fed carbohydrates in hydrated form than in dry form is not fully understood. Palatability may be one factor because sugar solutions and wet mash diets are preferred to powdered sugar and dry diets in choice tests (5). Hydra-

tion also facilitates carbohydrate digestion and absorption, which may produce metabolic effects that stimulate caloric consumption, e.g., enhanced insulin response (5).

Although most attention has focused on sugars, they are not the only carbohydrates that promote hyperphagia and obesity. Recent studies demonstrate that rats fed solutions of partially hydrolyzed starch (e.g., 32% Polycose) increase their caloric intake, body weight, and body fat as much as do rats fed sucrose or glucose solutions (60,63). Like sucrose, Polycose has minimal effects when fed in powdered form either in a composite diet or as an option to chow (60,64). Even unprocessed starch increases food intake and weight gain when presented in a hydrated form (e.g., as a gel or mash), although its effects are less than those produced by sugars and hydrolyzed starches (62,65). A particularly interesting case of starch-induced obesity was reported by Rogers and Blundell (66); they observed that rats fed white bread in addition to chow overate and rapidly gained weight compared with control rats fed only chow.

Taken together, these results support the conclusion of a 1986 Sugars Task Force Report (67) that "sugars do not have a unique role in the etiology of obesity." That is, the animal data show that (a) sugars do not always promote obesity (e.g., when presented in dry form); (b) nonsugar carbohydrates (e.g., starch, hydrolyzed starch, bread) may produce obesity; and (c) noncarbohydrates (i.e., fat) also promote obesity. Nevertheless, while not having a unique role, sugars along with complex carbohydrates can, under certain conditions, stimulate overeating and obesity in animals and may have similar effects in humans as well.

Carbohydrate Palatability and Metabolism

The sweet taste of sugar has figured prominently in discussions of sugar-induced overeating and obesity. Rats, like many other species, are very attracted to sweet taste, and this would seem to be an obvious explanation for their hyperphagic response to sugar solutions (5). This assumption has been challenged, however, and some studies suggest that post-ingestive nutritional factors are more important than sweet taste in determining long-term energy balance (4,68,69).

The initial reports that rats fed chow and hydrolyzed starch solutions overate as much as or more than rats fed chow and sugar solutions also appeared to argue against taste as an important factor in sugar-induced obesity (60,63). However, subsequent research revealed that rats, unlike humans, taste starch-derived polysaccharides and find them very attractive. In fact, at low concentrations Polycose solutions are preferred to sucrose, maltose, glucose, and fructose solutions, and at high concentrations are second only to sucrose in preference (17,70). In light of these results, the overeating response to polysaccharide solutions cannot be taken as evidence against taste as a contributing factor in carbohydrate-induced obesity. Conceivably, rats may overeat sugar solutions because of their palatable sweet taste and Polycose solutions because of their palatable "polysaccharide" taste.

To investigate the role of taste and postingestive events in carbohydrate appetite, Sclafani and coworkers (71,72) used an "electronic esophagus" preparation. With this preparation rats were fitted with chronic intragastric (IG) catheters and were automatically infused with a carbohydrate solution (CS) or water as they drank (by mouth) water containing arbitrary cue flavors; flavored water and chow were available 23 hours a day. On alternate days, the rats had one flavored water (the CS+, e.g., cherry) paired with IG infusions of Polycose, and another flavored water (the CS−, e.g., grape) paired with IG water infusions. In subsequent two-choice tests the rats displayed a strong preference ($\approx$90%) for the CS+ flavor over the CS− flavor. They also strongly preferred the CS+-flavored water to plain water, which is notable because naive rats prefer plain water. Comparable effects were obtained with rats

given bitter- or sour-tasting water paired with IG Polycose infusions (20). Thus rats will acquire preferences for otherwise unpreferred flavors when the flavors are associated with the postingestive effects of carbohydrates; sweet or polysaccharide taste is not essential for carbohydrate appetite.

In addition to conditioning flavor preferences, the IG Polycose infusions also increased total daily caloric intake (72). In one study rats consumed 16% more calories on days when they consumed flavored water paired with IG Polycose compared with the baseline condition, when only plain water and chow were available. These findings demonstrate that in the absence of carbohydrate taste, the postingestive consequences of carbohydrate solutions are sufficient to produce mild hyperphagia. However, even greater overeating was observed when saccharin was added to the CS+ flavor. The rats doubled their CS+ intake (and therefore their IG Polycose intake) when it was sweetened with saccharin, and increased their total caloric intake to 37% above baseline level. Taken together, these findings indicate that postingestive actions of carbohydrate solutions are sufficient to promote overeating, but that sweet taste can enhance the hyperphagic response. Note that these data are based on only a few days of testing and it remains to be determined if, with prolonged testing, IG carbohydrate feeding will result in overeating and obesity.

Using a different procedure, Ramirez (73) reported that sweet taste can produce long-term effects on caloric intake and body weight. In his experiment, the addition of saccharin to a dilute, high-starch diet (80% water, 20% solids) increased food intake and weight gain over several weeks. A comparable effect was not obtained with a less dilute version of the diet (60% water, 40% solids), which was overconsumed even in its unsweetened form. Although the sweetened form of the dilute diet was preferred to the unsweetened form, other findings suggested that the palatability of the sweet diet may not have been solely responsible for the feeding-stimulatory effect of saccharin. In particular, Ramirez (73) observed that the addition of saccharin to the dilute diet increased food intake only after a 1-week delay, and that prior experience with saccharin solutions blocked this effect. This finding contrasts with the results of the intragastric feeding study (72) cited above in which saccharin produced an immediate increase in caloric intake in animals that had prior experience with a saccharin solution. The reason for this discrepancy is not certain, and additional research is needed to clarify the effects of flavor manipulations on long-term energy intake.

CAFETERIA DIETS

Although direct comparisons are lacking, the hyperphagia and obesity produced by cafeteria diets containing many different "supermarket" foods are generally greater than that obtained with the high-fat and high-sugar diets described above. Furthermore, cafeteria diets can produce obesity in strains of rats that fail to become obese when fed high-fat or high-sugar diets (74). The effectiveness of cafeteria diets and their resemblance to the complex diets of humans have made the cafeteria obesity model particularly attractive. The complexity of cafeteria diets, however, has its drawbacks such as the difficulty of obtaining accurate intake measures. Thus the use of the cafeteria diet has been a source of controversy particularly with regard to studies of feed efficiency and diet-induced thermogenesis when accurate intake measures are essential (75,76).

Several factors are implicated in the hyperphagia- and obesity-promoting effects of cafeteria diets. First, many of the food items included in the diets are high in fat and/or sugar and have a relatively high water content, all of which, as discussed above, may produce postingestive effects that promote overeating and obesity. Second, in addition to its nutritional composition, the palatability of the cafeteria diet has long been assumed to contribute to the exaggerated hyperphagic response

(11). The diet includes highly preferred foods as evidenced by the fact that rats eat very little chow when given access to supermarket foods (11,66,77,78). In addition, meal pattern analysis reveals that rats eat larger meals at faster rates when eating supermarket foods (i.e., bread, chocolate) than when eating chow, which suggests that these supermarket foods are highly palatable (66). Nevertheless, the role of palatability in cafeteria diet-induced overeating remains a controversial and largely untested issue (4). As previously mentioned, the fact that a food is preferred and overconsumed does not necessarily mean that palatability, rather than postingestive metabolic effects, is driving the overconsumption.

A third aspect of cafeteria diets, and the one that has received the most research attention, is the variety of foods available. Variety in the diet may enhance food consumption in different ways (79). Individual animals have specific food preferences and thus increasing the number of food items in the diet would increase the probability that all animals had preferred foods available. These individual preferences may be based on the foods' sensory characteristics and/or on their nutritional composition, that is, some animals may preferentially overeat high-fat foods and others high-sugar foods. The availability of different foods may also promote overeating by counteracting the effect of monotony or "sensory-specific" satiety (80). Experiments demonstrate that rats, like people, consume larger meals when given multiple foods than when offered a single food (77). Furthermore, when given continuous access to a varied diet (chow plus two or three supermarket foods), rats eat more total calories and gain more weight than when fed chow alone or chow plus one supermarket food (66,77). A variety effect was also reported with an "isocafeteria" diet consisting of 12 powdered and pelleted rodent chows containing differing flavoring agents and macronutrient compositions, i.e., percent fat, protein, carbohydrate varied from 22 to 32%, 4 to 16%, and 53 to 75%, respectively (81). Rats fed the isocafeteria diet consumed 46% more calories and gained 83% more weight than did rats fed a single chow diet. On the other hand, Naim et al. (82) observed that rats fed three nutritionally identical foods that differed only in flavor failed to overeat or gain weight relative to rats fed a single diet. They concluded that flavor variety alone is not sufficient to promote overeating. This issue requires further investigation because it is possible that the diets used by Naim et al. (82) were not sufficiently different in flavor and palatability to produce a variety effect.

CONCLUSIONS

Dietary factors can have a major impact on daily caloric intake, body weight, and adiposity, as documented by the many different animal models of dietary obesity that have been reported in recent years. A variety of dietary manipulations, including changes in the fat, carbohydrate, and/or water content of the diet and changes in diet flavor and variety, can lead to overeating and obesity. The magnitude of the response is influenced by age, sex, and strain of animals as well as housing conditions. As discussed elsewhere (83), dietary manipulations that promote obesity in normal animals can also exaggerate the adiposity of animals with preexisting obesity such as hypothalamic obese and genetically obese rodents.

As illustrated in Fig. 2, dietary factors can influence food intake and adiposity via several different paths. The nutrient composition, physical form, and flavor elements in the diet determine its orosensory effects (path 1a), which, in turn, determine the initial palatability of the diet (path 1b). Dietary palatability is then modulated by the postingestive actions of foods (path 2). Thus a food that is not particularly good tasting at first may become highly preferred as the animal associates its flavor with its nutritive effects. Food palatability may have direct and indirect effects on total caloric intake. Palatability determines diet selection (path 3a) and thus can promote the intake of foods that have metabolic effects that promote obesity. In some cases, improving palatability by adding a preferred flavor to the food can stimulate overconsumption (path 3b) and thereby increase fat deposition (path 4). Palatability factors may also influence postingestive metabolic events via cephalic-phase digestive responses, e.g., insulin release (path 5). Food may also have postingestive effects that promote overeating independent of changes in palatability (path 6). As mentioned above, high-fat diets may stimulate overeating because the conversion of dietary fat to body fat reduces the energy available for oxidation. The postingestive actions of some diets can also promote obesity even in the absence of overt hyperphagia (path 7). The increased efficiency of utilization of dietary fat, and in some cases dietary sugar, can also increase the deposition of body fat when overeating does occur (paths 4 and 7).

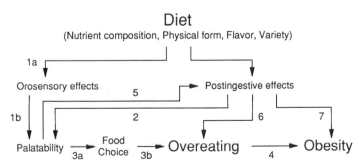

FIG. 2. Schematic representation of the multiple ways that dietary factors can influence food intake and adiposity. See text for details.

Given the multiplicity of ways that food can promote overeating and obesity, the prevalence of obesity in human societies in which palatable and energy-rich foods are widely available is not surprising. The challenge is to develop diets that satisfy the palate without stimulating excess consumption or fat deposition. A greater understanding of the complex relationships among diet composition, ingestive behavior, and metabolism is essential if this goal is to be achieved.

ACKNOWLEDGMENTS

The preparation of this chapter was supported by a grant from the National Institute of Diabetes and Digestive and Kidney Diseases (DK-31135). The author thanks Dr. Karen Ackroff for her helpful comments on this paper.

REFERENCES

1. Blundell JE. Nutritional manipulations for altering food intake: towards a causal model of experimental obesity. *Ann NY Acad Sci* 1987;449:144–55.
2. Kanarek RB, Orthen-Gambill N. Dietary-induced obesity in experimental animals. In: Beynen AC, West CE, eds. *Use of animal models for research in human nutrition.* Basel: Karger, 1988;83–110.
3. Ramirez I. When does sucrose increase appetite and adiposity? *Appetite* 1987;9:1–19.
4. Ramirez I, Tordoff MG, Friedman MI. Dietary hyperphagia and obesity: what causes them? *Physiol Behav* 1989;45:163–8.
5. Sclafani A. Carbohydrate taste, appetite, and obesity: an overview. *Neurosci Biobehav Rev* 1987; 11:131–153.
6. Sclafani A. Dietary-induced overeating. *Ann NY Acad Sci* 1989;575:281–9.
7. Sclafani A. Diet-induced obesity in rodents. In: Oomura Y, Tarui S, Inoue S, et al., eds. *Progress in obesity research, 1990.* London: John Libbey & Co, 1991;441–4.
8. Sclafani A. Dietary-obesity models. In: Bjorntorp P, Brodoff B, eds. *Obesity.* Philadelphia: JB Lippincott, 1992;241–248.
9. Berg BN. Nutrition and longevity in the rat. I. Food intake in relation to size, health and fertility. *J Nutr* 1960;71:242–54.
10. Berg BN, Simms HS. Nutrition and longevity in the rat. II. Longevity and onset of disease with different levels of food intake. *J Nutr* 1960;71:255–63.
11. Sclafani A, Springer D. Dietary obesity in adult rats: similarities to hypothalamic and human obesity syndromes. *Physiol Behav* 1976;17:461–71.

12. Applegate EA, Upton DE, Stern JS. Food intake, body composition and blood lipids following treadmill exercise in male and female rats. *Physiol Behav* 1982;28:917–20.
13. Slattery JM, Potter RM. Hyperphagia: a necessary precondition to obesity? *Appetite* 1985;6:113–42.
14. Grill HJ, Berridge KC. Taste reactivity as a measure of the neural control of palatability. In: Sprague JM, Epstein AN, eds. *Progress in psychobiology and physiological psychology.* New York: Academic Press, 1985;1–61.
15. Le Magnen J. Palatability: concept, terminology, and mechanisms. In: Boakes RA, Popplewell DA, Burton MJ, eds. *Eating habits.* Chichester: John Wiley & Sons, 1987;131–54.
16. Ramirez I. What do we mean when we say "palatable food?" *Appetite* 1990;14:159–61.
17. Sclafani A. The hedonics of sugar and starch. In: Bolles RC, ed. *The hedonics of taste.* Hillsdale, NJ: Erlbaum Associates, 1991;59–87.
18. Young PT. *Motivation and emotion.* New York: John Wiley & Sons, 1961.
19. Berridge KC, Grill HJ, Norgren R. Relation of consummatory responses and preabsorptive insulin release to palatability and learned taste aversions. *J Comp Physiol Psychol* 1981;95:363–82.
20. Sclafani A. Conditioned food preferences. *Bull Psychon Soc* 1991;29:256–60.
21. Ramirez I. Overeating, overweight and obesity induced by an unpreferred diet. *Physiol Behav* 1988;43:501–6.
22. Powley TL, Berthoud HR. Diet and cephalic phase insulin responses. *Am J Clin Nutr* 1985;42: 991–1002.
23. Mickelsen O, Takahashi S, Craig C. Experimental obesity: I. Production of obesity in rats by feeding high-fat diets. *J Nutr* 1955;57:541–54.
24. Schemmel R, Mickelsen O, Gill JL. Dietary obesity in rats: body weight and body fat accretion in seven strains of rats. *J Nutr* 1970;100:1041–48.
25. Schemmel R, Mickelsen O, Fisher L. Body composition and fat depot weights of rats as influenced by ration fed dams during lactation and that fed rats after weaning. *J Nutr* 1973;103:477–87.
26. Jen K-LC, Greenwood MRC, Brasel JA. Sex differences in the effects of high-fat feeding on behavior and carcass composition. *Physiol Behav* 1981; 27:161–6.
27. Oscai LB, Brown MM, Miller WC. Effect of dietary fat on food intake, growth and body composition in rats. *Growth* 1984;48:415–24.
28. Bray GA, Lee M, Bray TL. Weight gain of rats fed medium-chain triglycerides is less than rats fed longchain triglycerides. *Int J Obes* 1980;4:27–32.
29. Barboriak JJ, Krehl WA, Cowgill GR, et al. Influence of high-fat diets on growth and development of obesity in the albino rat. *J Nutr* 1958;64:241–9.
30. Fenton PF, Carr C. The nutrition of the mouse: responses of four strains to diets differing in fat content. *J Nutr* 1951;45:225–34.
31. Schemmel R. Physiological considerations of lipid storage and utilization. *Am Zool* 1976;16:661–70.
32. Ramirez I, Friedman MI. Dietary hyperphagia in rats: role of fat, carbohydrate, and energy content. *Physiol Behav* 1990;47:1157–63.

33. Lucas F, Ackroff K, Sclafani A. Dietary fat induced hyperphagia in rats as a function of fat type and physical form. *Physiol Behav* 1989;45:937–46.

34. Ackroff K, Sclafani A. Sucrose-induced hyperphagia and obesity in rats fed a macronutrient self-selection diet. *Physiol Behav* 1988;44:181–87.

35. Sclafani A. Dietary obesity. In: Stunkard AJ, ed. *Obesity.* Philadelphia: WB Saunders, 1980;166–81.

36. Chang S, Graham B, Yakubu F, et al. Metabolic differences between obesity-prone and obesity-resistant rats. *Am J Physiol* 1990;259:R1103–R1110.

37. Berthoud HR. Cephalic phase insulin response as a predictor of body weight gain and obesity induced by a palatable cafeteria diet. *J Obes Weight Reg* 1985;4:120–8.

38. Levin BE, Sullivan AC. Glucose-induced norepinephrine levels and obesity resistance. *Am J Physiol* 1987;253:R475–R481.

39. Schemmel R, Mickelsen O. Influence of diet, strain, age and sex on fat depot mass and body composition of the nutritionally obese rat. In: Vague J, Boyer J, eds. *The regulation of the adipose tissue.* New York: Elsevier, 1974;238–53.

40. Wood JD, Reid JT. The influence of dietary fat on fat metabolism and body fat deposition in meal-feeding and nibbling rats. *Br J Nutr* 1975;34:15–24.

41. Flatt JP. Dietary fat, carbohydrate balance and weight maintenance: effects of exercise. *Am J Clin Nutr* 1987;45:296–306.

42. Hamilton CL. Rat's preference for high fat diets. *J Comp Physiol Psychol* 1964;58:459–60.

43. Rockwood GA, Bhathena SJ. High-fat-diet preference in developing and adult rats. *Physiol Behav* 1990;48:79–82.

44. Naim M, Brand JG, Kare MR. The preference-aversion behavior of rats for nutritionally controlled diets containing oil or fat. *Physiol Behav* 1987;39:285–90.

45. Ackroff K, Vigorito M, Sclafani A. Fat appetite in rats: the response of infant and adult rats to nutritive and nonnutritive oil emulsions. *Appetite* 1990;15:171–88.

46. Elizalde G, Sclafani A. Fat appetite in rats: flavor preferences conditioned by nutritive and non-nutritive oil emulsions. *Appetite* 1990;15:189–97.

47. Mehiel R, Bolles RC. Learned flavor preferences based on calories are independent of initial hedonic value. *Anim Learn Behav* 1988;16:383–7.

48. Lucas F, Sclafani A. Flavor preferences conditioned by intragastric fat infusions in rats. *Physiol Behav* 1989;46:403–12.

49. Ackroff K, Sclafani A. Inhibiting fat digestion with tetrahydrolipostatin alters macronutrient selection in rats. *Proc Eastern Psychol Assoc Meeting* 1990; 61:48.

50. Lucas F, Sclafani A. Hyperphagia in rats produced by a mixture of fat and sugar. *Physiol Behav* 1990;47:51–5.

51. Allen RJL, Leahy JS. Some effects of dietary dextrose, fructose, liquid glucose and sucrose in the adult male rat. *Br J Nutr* 1966;20:339–47.

52. Hallfrisch J, Lazar F, Jorgensen C, et al. Insulin and glucose responses in rats fed sucrose or starch. *Am J Clin Nutr* 1979;32:787–93.

53. Marshall MW, Womack M, Hildebrand HH, et al.

Effects of types and levels of carbohydrates and proteins on carcass composition of adult rats. *Proc Soc Exp Biol Med* 1969;132:227–32.

54. Reiser S, Hallfrisch J. Insulin sensitivity and adipose tissue weight of rats fed starch or sucrose diets ad libitum or in meals. *J Nutr* 1977;107:147–55.

55. Oscai LB, Miller WC, Arnall DA. Effects of dietary sugar and of dietary fat on food intake and body fat content in rats. *Growth* 1987;51:64–73.

56. Dulloo AG, Eisa OA, Miller DS, et al. A comparative study of the effects of white sugar, unrefined sugar and starch on the efficiency of food utilization and thermogenesis. *Am J Clin Nutr* 1985;42:214–9.

57. McCusker RH, Deaver OE Jr, Berdanier CD. Effect of sucrose or starch feeding on the hepatic mitochondrial activity of BHE and Wistar rats. *J Nutr* 1983;113:1327–34.

58. Lakshmann FL, Howe JC, Schuster EM, et al. Response of two strains of rats to a high-protein diet containing sucrose or cornstarch. *Proc Soc Exp Biol Med* 1981;167:224–32.

59. Kratz CM, Levitsky DA. Dietary obesity: differential effects with self-selection and composite dietary feeding techniques. *Physiol Behav* 1979;22:245–9.

60. Sclafani A. Carbohydrate-induced hyperphagia and obesity in the rat: effects of saccharide type, form, and taste. *Neurosci Biobehav Rev* 1987;11:155–62.

61. Kanarek RB, Orthen-Gambill N. Differential effects of sucrose, fructose, and glucose on carbohydrate-induced obesity in rats. *J Nutr* 1982;112:1546–54.

62. Ramirez I. Feeding a liquid diet increases energy intake, weight gain and body fat in rats. *J Nutr* 1987;117:2127–34.

63. Sclafani A, Xenakis S. Sucrose and polysaccharide induced obesity in the rat. *Physiol Behav* 1984; 32:169–74.

64. Sclafani A, Xenakis S. Influence of diet form on the hyperphagia-promoting effect of polysaccharide in rats. *Life Sci* 1984;34:1253–9.

65. Sclafani A, Vigorito M, Pfeiffer CL. Starch-induced overeating and overweight in rats: influence of starch type and form. *Physiol Behav* 1988; 42:409–15.

66. Rogers PJ, Blundell JE. Meal patterns and food selection during the development of obesity in rats fed a cafeteria diet. *Neurosci Biobehav Rev* 1984; 8:441–53.

67. Glinsmann WH, Irausquin H, Park YK. Evaluation of health aspects of sugars contained in carbohydrate sweeteners: report of Sugars Task Force, 1986. *J Nutr* 1986;116[Suppl 11]:S1–S216.

68. Castonguay TW, Hirsch E, Collier G. Palatability of sugar solutions and dietary selection? *Physiol Behav* 1981;27:7–12.

69. Hill W, Castonguay TW, Collier GH. Taste or diet balancing? *Physiol Behav* 1980;24:765–67.

70. Sclafani A, Mann S. Carbohydrate taste preferences in rats: glucose, sucrose, maltose, fructose and Polycose compared. *Physiol Behav* 1987;40:563–8.

71. Sclafani A, Nissenbaum JW. Robust conditioned flavor preference produced by intragastric starch infusions in rats. *Am J Physiol* 1988;255:R672–R675.

72. Elizalde G, Sclafani A. Flavor preferences conditioned by intragastric Polycose: a detailed analysis

using an electronic esophagus preparation. *Physiol Behav* 1990;47:63–77.

73. Ramirez I. Stimulation of energy intake and growth by saccharin in rats. *J Nutr* 1990;120:123–33.

74. Fisler JS, Lupien JR, Wood RD, et al. Brown fat thermogenesis in a rat model of dietary obesity. *Am J Physiol* 1987;253:R756–R762.

75. Rothwell NJ, Stock MJ. The cafeteria diet as a tool for studies of thermogenesis. *J Nutr* 1988; 118:925–8.

76. Moore BJ. The cafeteria diet—an inappropriate tool for studies of thermogenesis. *J Nutr* 1987; 117:227–31.

77. Rolls BJ, Van Duijvenvoorde PM, Rowe EA. Variety in the diet enhances intake in a meal and contributes to the development of obesity in the rat. *Physiol Behav* 1983;31:21–7.

78. Prats E, Monfar J, Castella R, et al. Energy intake of rats fed a cafeteria diet. *Physiol Behav* 1989; 45:263–72.

79. Rolls BJ. How variety and palatability can stimulate appetite. *Nutr Bull* 1979;5:78–86.

80. Rolls BJ. Sensory-specific satiety. *Nutr Rev* 1986; 44:93–101.

81. Louis-Sylvestre J, Giachetti I, Le Magnen J. Sensory versus dietary factors in cafeteria-induced overweight. *Physiol Behav* 1984;32:901–5.

82. Naim M, Brand JC, Kare MR, et al. Energy intake, weight gain and fat deposition in rats fed flavored, nutritionally controlled diets in a multichoice ("cafeteria") design. *J Nutr* 1985;115:1447–58.

83. Sclafani A. Animal models of obesity: classification and characterization. *Int J Obes* 1984;8:491–508.

Obesity: Theory and Therapy, Second Edition,
edited by A. J. Stunkard and T. A. Wadden.
Raven Press, Ltd., New York © 1993.

8

Genetics and Human Obesity

Joanne M. Meyer and *Albert J. Stunkard

*Department of Human Genetics, Medical College of Virginia, Virginia Commonwealth
University, Richmond, Virginia 23298; *Department of Psychiatry, University
of Pennsylvania, Philadelphia, Pennsylvania 19104-2648*

In no other field in the recent past has our knowledge of obesity increased more rapidly than in the field of genetics. In the previous edition of this volume, the chapter on obesity dealt largely with how genetic factors *might* influence variation in human obesity. The present chapter provides concrete examples of how genetic factors *do* influence human obesity.

Studies of genetic factors in human obesity start with one well-established fact—human obesity is a familial disorder. For many years it was unclear why obesity runs in families, and proponents of both genetic and environmental causes turned to animal studies to support their opposing views. These studies provided support for each view. Thus, among rodents, genetic forms of obesity have long been recognized, as have been environmental forms (produced by highly palatable diets) (see Sclafani, *this volume*). Very recently, however, studies of humans—of families, adoptees, and twins—have begun to clarify and quantify the roles of genes and environment in *human* obesity.

Underlying these studies has been a general assumption regarding the role of genes and environment: they are not antagonists and neither acts alone to determine a clinical outcome. Such outcomes are determined instead by the combination of a genetic vulnerability and an adverse environment. This combination is diagrammed in Fig. 1, in which the small inner circle represents those persons who are genetically predisposed to a disorder. The wedge represents adverse environmental conditions to which these individuals may be exposed. The model indicates that only those genetically predisposed persons who are exposed to adverse environmental conditions develop disorders such as obesity.

GENES AND ENVIRONMENT: EVIDENCE FROM RELATIVES

Studying obesity in related pairs of individuals provides insight into the relative sizes of the inner "genetic" circle and the "environmental" wedge in Fig. 1. Specifically, data from pairs of related individuals permit us to partition the variance into its genetic and environmental components. This partitioning of the variance forms the basis of all family, adoption, and twin studies. The only difference between these three study designs is in the nature of the data.

In nuclear *family studies,* parent/offspring and sibling data have helped to identify the extent to which obesity is familial in nature. Unfortunately, since parents and their offspring, as well as sibling pairs, often share environments (such as dietary habits) in addition to one-half of their genes, it is impossible to determine whether the familial aggregation for obesity is due to shared genes or shared environments. For this reason, family studies involving only parents and their off-

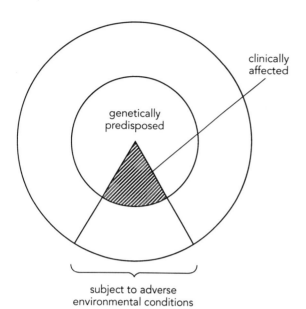

clinically
affected

genetically
predisposed

subject to adverse
environmental conditions

FIG. 1. Model for the interaction between genetic vulnerability and environmental challenge. See text for further information.

spring or sibling pairs are not fully genetically informative. Nonetheless, results from family studies provide a useful starting point for the investigation of obesity and help to generate hypotheses that can be tested with other types of data.

Adoption studies overcome some of the difficulties encountered in family studies. These investigations make use of data from adoptees and from their biologic and adoptive parents. Since adoptees do not share a "family environment" with their biologic parents, any similarity between parents and offspring reflects only genes that they share. In contrast, the similarity between adoptees and their adoptive parents reflects only the environment that they share or have shared in the past. Both types of information permit assessment of the genetic *and* family environmental contributions to obesity. As a result, adoption studies provide information above and beyond that gained in family studies.

Studies of *identical and fraternal twins* are the third type that can be used to estimate genetic and environmental contributions to human obesity. The classical twin study uses the fact that identical, or monozygotic (MZ), twins share all of their genes as well as all of the early rearing environment. Fraternal or

dizygotic (DZ) twins, in contrast, share on the average only one-half of their genes and all features of the early rearing environment. By comparing the similarity of MZ twins to DZ twins, one can assess the relative contribution of genes and environment to a trait or disorder.

In summary, family, adoption, and twin studies are all useful means of investigating genetic and environmental influences on obesity. However, since each mode of inquiry is limited in some respect, it is most productive to consider results from all types of studies.

FAMILY STUDIES

Most family studies of obesity have used the body mass index (BMI; weight (kg)/ height (m^2) as a proxy for body fat. This measure has the advantage of making it possible to collect data on height and weight from large numbers of relatives, but the disadvantage of not really measuring body fat. Methods that do measure body fat, such as underwater weighing, are so cumbersome as to be impractical for most studies. It is therefore noteworthy that Bouchard and his colleagues (2) have conducted a study of 1,698 members of 409 families that determined body fat (and fat free mass) by underwater weighing. In addition, these investigators, as well as others (see review in Mueller (21)) have used skinfold thicknesses to assess subcutaneous fat distribution.

To assess the extent of similarity for obesity in relatives, most studies begin by computing an intraclass or Pearson product moment correlation for the phenotype among family members. This correlation coefficient is an index of the percent of total variation for obesity that is shared by the relatives. If similarity between parent and child or between siblings were solely due to the additive effect of a large number of genetic loci, the maximum expected correlation for these pairs of relatives would be 0.50, reflecting the fact that they share one-half of their genes. Correlations below 0.50 indicate that environmental factors not shared with other family members and unique to the individual also influence his/her obesity. These *unique* environmental impacts reduce familial similarity, and thus reduce the correlation coefficient.

An estimate of the extent to which additive genetic effects contribute to the overall variance of a phenotype (its *heritability*) can be obtained by dividing a parent/offspring or sibling correlation by 0.5 (the amount of shared genes). Table 1 shows parent/offspring and sibling correlations for BMI described in recent reports. These figures indicate that parents and their offspring correlate approximately 0.20–0.30 for BMI, while the sibling correlations are somewhat higher. Thus, rough heritability estimates range from 0.40 to 0.60—suggesting that genes are responsible for approximately one-half of the total phenotypic variation in obesity.

It should be noted that calculating heritability in this manner involves at least three assumptions:

1. *Only* genes contribute to the relatives' similarity. As noted previously, relatives may also share environments that increase their similarity in body composition. Family data alone provide no way of assessing the importance of these environmental effects.
2. There are no *age-specific genetic effects* on obesity; in other words, the same genes influence obesity across the life span.
3. There are no *gender-specific* effects; the same genes influence obesity in men and

TABLE 1. *Familial correlations for body mass index*

Study	Relative pair	No.	r
Khoury et al., 1983 (13)	Mother/child	186	0.23
	Father/child	150	0.29
	Siblings	77	0.35
Heller et al., 1984 (9)	Father/son	1057	0.27
	Father/daughter	954	0.23
	Mother/son	1063	0.23
	Mother/daughter	1133	0.21
	Brother/brother	331	0.27
Longini et al., 1984 (16)	Father/child	842	0.27
	Mother/child	842	0.25
	Siblings	445	0.36
Zonta et al., 1987 (38)	Father/child	317	0.31
	Mother/child	317	0.37
Bouchard et al., 1988 (2)	Parent/offspring	1239	0.23
	Siblings	370	0.26
Perusse et al., 1987 (22)	Parent/child	7102	0.20
	Siblings	3372	0.31
Price et al., 1990 (27)	Parent/offspring	3076	0.18
	Siblings	2602	0.22
Moll et al., 1991 (20)	Parent/offspring	920	0.22
	Siblings	332	0.35

women. These assumptions can be tested empirically and will be discussed in subsequent sections of the chapter.

The method we have described for estimating heritability is useful for generating an approximate measure of genetic variation in human obesity when data are available from pairs of relatives with the same degree of relationship (such as parent/child or sibling pairs). However, when data are available from several types of relatives, this method loses much of its appeal since it is unable to use all of the information about similarity among relatives. In order to use this information, more rigorous model-fitting methods have been developed. Such model-fitting partitions similarity among relatives into genetic and environmental effects, and uses methods such as weighted least squares or maximum likelihood to estimate those parameters that best explain the observed data. Province and Rao (28) and Longini et al. (16) have applied these methods to family data on BMI and have obtained heritability estimates ranging from 0.32 to 0.51, and 0.31 to 0.37, respectively.

The most ambitious study to use model fitting to estimate genetic influences on different measures of obesity was carried out by Bouchard et al. (2) on 1,698 individuals in the Quebec Study. These individuals were related in many ways: parents and offspring, full siblings, MZ and DZ twins, adoptive siblings, adoptive parents and adoptees, spouses, first-degree cousins, and uncle/aunt–nephew/niece pairs. The investigators' model assessed the extent to which (a) additive genetic factors, (b) environmental transmission from parents to offspring, and (c) special environments (of related siblings, and MZ and DZ twins) each contribute to familial similarity. Total transmissible variances for BMI, subcutaneous fat (skinfold thicknesses), percent body fat, fat mass and fat-free mass were comparable, ranging from 40 to 60%. However, the genetic variance for these obesity indices differed, ranging from 5% for BMI and subcutaneous fat to 25% for fat mass, fat-free mass, and percentage body

fat. These results are important since they highlight a possible familial but not genetic transmission of obesity, as well as differential genetic contributions to the various obesity indices.

ADOPTION STUDIES

Early adoption studies had yielded conflicting reports of the relative importance of genetic and environmental influences on obesity. None of them, however, had contained information about the biologic parents of the adoptees. The first "full adoption study" (which included information about the biologic parents), resolved the conflict (32,36). This study made use of the Danish Adoption Register, which had previously provided useful assessment of genetic influences on schizophrenia and alcoholism. Information was obtained about the heights and weights of 3,580 adoptees who were living in Copenhagen and whose average age at the time of the study was 42 years. BMI of the adoptees was calculated and a sample of 804 men and women was selected to represent four critical weight classes: the thinnest 4%, the fattest 4%, the next fattest 4%, and 4% at the median. Data on the heights and weights of both biologic and adoptive parents, siblings, and half-siblings were then collected and compared with those of the adoptees. Original analyses of these data showed that the weight class of the adoptees was strongly related to the BMI of the biologic parents and not at all related to the BMI of the adoptive parents. Genetic influences were clearly present; early family environmental influences were not. More recent analyses of the Danish adoption data by Sorensen et al. (33) have quantified these genetic effects. As seen in Fig. 2A, biologic parent/offspring correlations ranged from 0.11 to 0.15, while the correlation for full siblings was 0.23. Together, these correlations suggest a heritability for BMI of 20 to 40%—values quite comparable to those found in family studies (with the exception of the heritability estimates of Bouchard et al. (2)). Not shown in Fig. 2A are the correlations between adop-

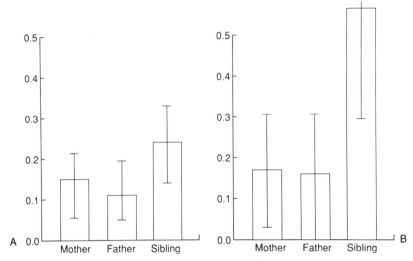

FIG. 2. A: The correlation coefficients relating adoptees' BMI with that of their biologic mother and siblings when the adoptees were adult (mean age 42). **B:** The correlation coefficients relating the BMI of the adoptees to the same types of relatives when the adoptees were in school (ages 7–13).

tive parents and adult adoptees. These were very close to zero, confirming the results of the earlier analyses that the family environment shared by parents and children had no apparent effect on the BMI of adoptees *when they were adults.* A question remained, though: "Did the early family environment have an effect on the adoptees *while they were still living with their adoptive parents?*"

To answer that question, Sorensen et al. (34) obtained yearly measurements of height and weight from school records of 289 adoptees from ages 7 through 13. During these years the BMI of the adoptees showed a weak correlation with that of their adoptive mothers, ($r = 0.10$, $p < 0.05$) and did not correlate at all with that of their adoptive fathers. It appears as if the early family environment provided by the adoptive mother had a small effect on the BMI of the adoptees while they were living together, but this effect had vanished by the time the adoptees reached middle age.

The data on the adoptees as children were also used to compute correlations with their biologic parents. These parent/offspring correlations, shown in Fig. 2B, indicate that parent/offspring similarity is as great in childhood as it is in later life. Genetic determi-

nants of the BMI appear to be fully expressed early in life.

Another complete adoption study (which included biologic parents) confirmed the major findings of the Danish study. In the Iowa study, Price et al. (25) found that the BMI of 357 young adult adoptees was correlated with that of their biologic but not their adoptive parents. The BMI of the female adoptees was highly correlated with that of their biologic mothers ($r = 0.40$, $p < 0.001$), and less highly with that of their biologic fathers ($r = 0.18$, $p < 0.05$). The correlations between the BMI of sons and their biologic parents were positive, but did not reach statistical significance. In contrast to the significant biologic parent/offspring correlations, adoptive parent/offspring correlations were negligible and nonsignificant. Thus, both the Danish and the Iowa adoption results showed a substantial biologic parent/offspring correlation and a negligible adoptive parent/offspring correlation.

TWIN STUDIES

Twin studies have been used for nearly a century in the attempt to separate genetic from environmental influences on human traits. As mentioned previously, these studies are based on the fact that MZ twins are genetically identical while DZ twins, like siblings, share on average no more than half their genes. The expected genetic correlations for MZ and DZ twins are thus 1.0 and 0.5, respectively. If the rearing environments of the two types of twins is similar, any difference in the similarity of MZ and DZ twin pairs should be due to genetic factors.

Twin studies have suggested that there is a strong genetic influence on human obesity. For example, one large twin study (35) compared the BMI of 1,974 MZ and 2,097 DZ male veteran twin pairs from the National Academy of Science/National Research Council (NAS/NRC) Twin Registry. Information about height and weight was obtained by measurement when the twins were about 20 years old and by questionnaire 25 years later. As befits army inductees, most were of normal weight at age 20 and only 1.8% were more than 30% overweight. Twenty-five years later, 8.3% were more than 30% overweight.

At age 20, the correlation of the BMI of the MZ pairs was 0.81, and that of the DZ pairs was 0.42. Twenty-five years later, the corresponding correlations had fallen to 0.67 and 0.24, but the difference between them remained approximately the same. Heritability of the BMI, estimated as twice the difference between the intraclass correlations of MZ and DZ twins, was thus 0.78 and 0.84 at ages 20 and 45, respectively. These values are very high and probably overestimate the genetic contribution to the body mass index. Nevertheless, they can be used for a more conservative estimate—comparison of the heritability of the BMI with that of the many disorders that have been studied by the twin method. Table 2 shows that obesity outranks several other disorders that have been studied by the twin method.

The study of the NAS/NRC twins revealed that the BMI resulted from different types of genetic variance at ages 20 and 45. When the intraclass correlation of MZ twins is approximately twice that of DZ twins, the genetic

TABLE 2. *Heritability estimates of a variety of medical conditions obtained through twin studies*

Condition	Study	Heritability
Obesity (age 20)	Stunkard et al., 1986 (35)	0.77
Obesity (age 45)	Stunkard et al., 1986 (35)	0.84
Schizophrenia	Kendler, 1983 (12)	0.68
Hypertension	Harvald and Hauge, 1965 (7)	0.57
Alcoholism	Hrubec and Omenn, 1981 (11)	0.57
Cirrhosis of the liver	Hrubec and Omenn, 1981 (11)	0.53
Epilepsy	Hauge et al., 1968 (8)	0.50
Coronary artery disease	Berg, 1981 (1)	0.49
Breast cancer	Holm, 1981 (10)	0.45

From Zonta et al., ref. 38, with permission.

variance is of the additive type, the result of small effects of a number of genes. When the correlation of MZ twins is more than twice that of the DZ twins, however, the variance is nonadditive, the result of interaction at the same genetic locus (dominance) or between alleles at different genetic loci (epistasis). By these criteria the NAS/NRC twins showed only additive genetic variance at age 20 (0.81 versus 0.42) and nonadditive variance at age 45 (0.67 versus 0.24). Furthermore, the presence of nonadditive variance at age 45 means the heritability estimate (0.84) is too high.

Recently, Meyer (19) has reported results from a large twin study that investigated the issue of genetic dominance. She used model-fitting techniques to estimate additive genetic, dominant genetic, and specific environmental variance components for BMI in 5,588 pairs of like-sex and unlike-sex twins from the Virginia and American Association of Retired Persons adult twin registries. Total genetic variance was again high—69% for men and 75% for women. Among men, however, dominant effects accounted for 50% of the variance, while among women genetic dominance did not play a role; additive variance accounted for all of the genetic influence. These results confirmed the indication of nonadditive variance among men in the NAS/NRC twin data at age 45, and also pointed to significant gender differences in the genetic control of BMI.

An assumption of the twin method is that the rearing environment affects the two types of twins (MZ and DZ) equally, the "equal environments assumption." If this were not the case, and MZ twins shared a "special twin environment," their increased similarity might incorrectly be attributed to genetic effects. One way of obviating this problem is to study MZ twin pairs in which the twins were reared apart and whose rearing environment could therefore not have increased their similarity. Such a study, carried out with 93 twin pairs from the Swedish Adoption/Twin Study of Aging (35), indicated that earlier twin studies had overestimated the influence of genetic factors only slightly. Thus the most direct estimate of heritability, the intraclass correlation coefficient of the BMI of MZ twins reared apart, was 0.70 for men and 0.66 for women.

Data on 673 other pairs of Swedish twins, representing MZ pairs reared together and DZ pairs reared apart and together, were further analyzed by model-fitting methods (37). These analyses confirmed the finding of adoption studies that the early family environment had no effect on the BMI of adults, nor did the age at separation or the degree of separation. These analyses also confirmed the presence of the nonadditive genetic variance among older persons that had been suggested by the NAS/NRC and the AARP twin studies. Figure 3 shows that at least half of the genetic variance is of the nonadditive type.

Results very similar to those from the Swedish twin study have been reported from two studies of an English sample of 34 MZ twins reared apart and a comparable sample of MZ twins reared together (17,24). The intraclass correlation coefficient for body mass index of the separated twin pairs was not significantly different from that of the twin pairs that had been reared together. Additionally, one of the studies found that the degree of similarity of the rearing environment of those MZ twins who had been reared apart had no apparent effect on the similarity of their BMI (24).

Another assumption of the twin method, as with the methods used for the analysis of family and adoption data, is that genes and environment act *independently* of each other. This assumption may be violated by a genotype × environment interaction, which occurs when genotypes respond differentially to

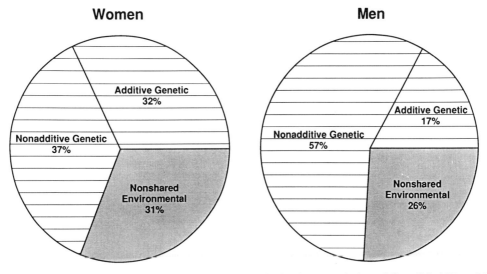

FIG. 3. Genetic and environmental contributions to the body mass index of Swedish MZ and DZ twins, reared together and reared apart. There was no evidence of a contribution of the childhood rearing environment, "shared" by parents and offspring. (From Stunkard et al., ref. 37, with permission).

the *same* environmental factors. This type of differential response has sometimes been termed genetic sensitivity to the environment, and has been found to play a significant role in plants and animals (18).

Striking evidence of a genotype × environment interaction was obtained by the long-term feeding studies of Bouchard and colleagues (3). After a 2-week baseline period, 12 pairs of young adult male MZ twins of normal weight received a diet containing 1,000 kcal a day in excess of their energy requirements for a period of 84 days. Subjects gained an average of 8.1 kg during this time, with a wide range of responses—from 4.3 to 13.3 kg. Despite this wide range *between* pairs, gains of members of each twin pair were quite similar, the intraclass correlation coefficient for weight gain being 0.55 ($p < 0.05$). Of perhaps greater importance was the fact that

increases in body fat showed even higher correlations between members of a twin pair. For abdominal visceral fat, the fat that is believed to confer the major health risk, for example, the correlation between members of a twin pair was 0.72 ($p < 0.01$), as shown in Fig. 4.

A finding that appears to represent genotype × environment interaction was made by Sonne-Holm and Sorenson (31) in their large-scale study of obesity in young male Danish draftees. For 17 years, from 1943 to 1960, the percentage of draftees who were severely obese remained constant at 0.01%. However, in the next 12 years, during a time when there was no change in mean levels of body weight, there was a marked increase in the prevalence of severe obesity to 0.07% by 1972. The most reasonable explanation for this striking increase in such a short period of

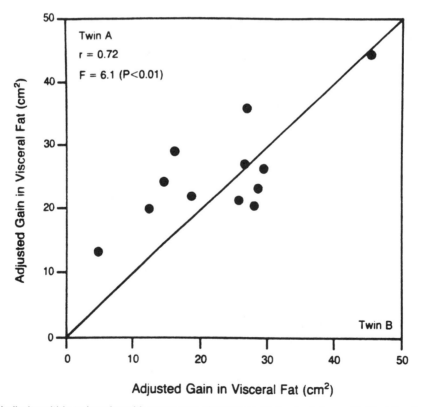

FIG. 4. Similarity within twin pairs with respect to changes in abdominal visceral fat in 12 pairs of male MZ twins in response to 100 days of overfeeding, after adjustment for gain in fat mass. (From Bouchard et al., ref. 3, with permission.)

time was an increase in the standard of living that affected a small number of genetically predisposed persons. We do not know which aspects of the standard of living had this effect, but attractive candidates are the increase in highly palatable foods and labor-saving devices.

AGE-SPECIFIC GENETIC EFFECTS

As noted above, twin studies have limitations. They do, however, have one important advantage: *there are no age differences in the relatives being studied.* This advantage is important because heritability estimates from twin studies are not affected by age-specific genetic effects. Age-specific genetic effects are genetic influences that operate at one age but not at another. Two twin studies and one adoption study suggest that these effects are important.

The study of male twins from the NAS/NRC Registry estimated that genetic factors influencing BMI at 20 years of age correlated 0.69 with genetic factors influencing BMI 25 years later (35). Thus, between the ages 20 and 45, new genetic effects influencing the BMI were presumedly expressed. Fabsitz et al. (6) extended this longitudinal study of the NAS/NRC Registry by a third measurement, and found further support for these results. They noted that there were two independent genetic contributions to the BMI—one expressed at or before age 20, and a second expressed between the ages of 20 and 48. Moreover, they showed that the "tracking" of BMI over time was due predominantly to the persistence of the "young adult" genetic effect into the later years. Environmental effects unique to the individual, in contrast, contributed relatively little to the tracking.

A recent longitudinal study of 245 adoptive and nonadoptive families by Cardon and Fulker (4) suggests that new genetic effects are not only expressed *during* adulthood, but also during childhood and *between* childhood and adulthood. By fitting a series of developmental models to data from adoptive

and nonadoptive children (followed from birth to age 9), the investigators concluded that new genetic effects were expressed throughout childhood, and the impact of these genes persisted over time. In contrast, environmental effects not shared by family members were occasion specific, and not transmitted from one age to the next. When data from biological parents were included in the analyses and an adult heritability of 0.6 was assumed, the investigators found significant correlations between the genetic influences on childhood and adult BMI. Their estimates of these genetic correlations averaged 0.50 over all childhood ages, suggesting that approximately 50% of the genetic variation in childhood BMI is due to the same genes that affect adult BMI.

Cardon and Fulker (4) also investigated genetic contributions to "adiposity rebound" —the rapid growth in body fat that occurs between ages 4 and 7 and that has recently been shown to predict obesity in adult life. About 40% of the variance in adiposity rebound is attributable to genetic factors; the home environment shared by siblings made no appreciable contribution.

Results from these longitudinal analyses have important implications for the interpretation of heritability estimates. They suggest that heritability estimates obtained from siblings or parents and their offspring reflect only the *common set* of genes that influences obesity during the ages that are being considered. They do not reflect the impact of age-specific genetic effects, and for this reason, they may well underestimate total heritability of obesity at any given point in time. These provocative results point to a pressing need for more longitudinal studies to understand changes and continuity in the genetic control of obesity over the life span.

ARE THERE MAJOR GENE EFFECTS ON OBESITY?

Thus far, we have considered obesity as a multifactorial trait, that is, the result of many genetic and environmental factors, acting additively or interactively. However, there is increasing evidence from human and animal studies that single genetic loci or specific chromosomal segments may have a marked effect on obesity (15,30). Statistical evidence for major gene effects on human obesity has been found in two ways, through either commingling or segregation analyses.

A commingling analysis does not require data from related individuals, but analyzes the distribution of a continuous measure (such as BMI) to determine whether the distribution can best be described by a single underlying normal distribution or by multiple underlying normal distributions. If there is a major gene affecting the phenotype, multimodality should be found. Three commingling analyses have already found evidence for mixtures of two or three normal distributions of BMI (20,23,26).

In contrast to commingling analyses, complex segregation analyses require information about family members (5,14). In this approach family data are analyzed and phenotypic variation is decomposed into components due to the effects of a major gene, effects due to additive effects of several genes, and effects due to environmental factors. In addition, common environmental factors, shared by all nuclear family members or by spouses or siblings only, may also be included in the model. Three large segregation analyses of BMI have already been reported (20,27,29). Despite differences in ascertainment of the subjects and in their age range, the results of these studies are remarkably similar. In all three, there was strong support for a single recessive major gene influencing obesity and accounting for 20 to 35% of the total variance. In addition, all three studies found significant polygenic effects, contributing from 20 to 42% of the variance. One study (20) found that the environment shared by spouses accounted for 12% of the variance in adults, while the environment shared by siblings accounted for 10% of the variance in children.

The promising results of the segregation analyses suggest that linkage studies seeking a major gene for obesity may prove fruitful. However, the segregation analyses leave many unanswered questions. For example, how does the action of age-dependent genetic effects influence the outcome of a segregation analysis on data from persons of differing ages? It may be possible to circumvent these potentially confounding effects by confining analyses to data on persons from comparable age groups. However, the cost would be a serious limitation of the conclusions that could be drawn. Similarly, how do genotype × environment interactions affect the outcome of a segregation analysis? Simulation studies are required to determine whether such effects could lead to erroneous conclusions about the presence of a major gene. Finally, it must be remembered that so far these analyses have been conducted on BMI data; the results may not be applicable to other indices of obesity, such as skinfold thicknesses or fat mass.

CLINICAL IMPLICATIONS

It seems fitting to close this chapter with some remarks about the clinical implications of the new genetic findings. The flood of these new findings has been accompanied by interpretations that go far beyond the data and ascribe a power to genetic influences so great as to call into question any efforts as treatment. "If obesity is genetic," the reasoning goes, "there isn't much that can be done about it."

These views are far wide of the mark. It is important to remember the message of Fig. 1: obesity arises from combination between a genetic vulnerability and an unfavorable environment. This message is particularly well conveyed by a study that shows the importance of the environment in determining human obesity. It consisted of a bivariate analysis of the BMI of the MZ twins in the NAS/NRC Register described earlier (23).

Figure 5 shows the bivariate distributions of the BMI of MZ twins at age 20 on the left and at age 45 on the right. Each distribution is oriented with the upper tail facing the reader so that the overweight portion is

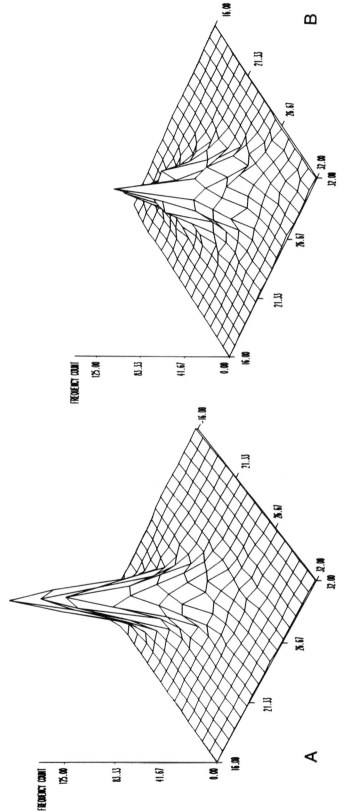

FIG. 5. Bivariate analysis of the distribution of body mass index of MZ twins at age 20 and at age 45. **A:** MZ twins at induction. **B:** MZ twins at followup. See text for further explanation. (From Price and Stunkard, ref. 23, with permission).

clearly visible. The correlation in BMI of the twins is shown by the clustering of scores along the main diagonal. This clustering is high in the normal weight range and falls dramatically as body weight increases. The figure shows that there are few obese twin pairs who show a high correlation in BMI. This impression is confirmed by the intraclass correlation coefficients of the members of the three component distributions that comprise the overall skewed distribution of the BMI in this population. Thus, at age 45, the value for members of the normal weight distribution was 0.77 and it fell to 0.35 for members of the (20%) overweight distribution and to 0.20 for members of the obese (40% overweight) distribution. This is precisely the pattern that would be found if MZ twins in the obese range were more sensitive to environmental influences than were twins in the normal weight range. Thus, while the concordance for overweight in the twins is high, the correlation in extent of overweight is low.

We interpret these findings to mean that genetic influences largely determine whether a person *can* become obese, but it is the environment that determines whether such a person *does* become obese, and the extent of that obesity. This interpretation provides no grounds for therapeutic nihilism. It is difficult for many obese people to control their weight. But this difficulty may be largely of environmental origin and one of the strongest forms of environmental influence is treatment.

REFERENCES

1. Berg K. Twin research in coronary heart disease. In: Gedda L, Parisi P, Nance WE (eds). *Twin research: III. Epidemiological and clinical studies.* New York: Alan R. Liss, 1981.
2. Bouchard C, Perusse L, Leblanc C, Tremblay A, Theriault G. Inheritance of the amount and distribution of human body fat. *Int J Obes* 1988; 12:205–15.
3. Bouchard C, Tremblay A, Despres J, et al. The response to long-term overfeeding in identical twins. *N Engl J Med* 1990;322:1477–82.
4. Cardon LR, Fulker DW. Genetic influences on body fat from birth to age 9. *Genet Epidemiol [in press].*
5. Elston RC, Stewart J. A general model for the ge-
netic analyses of pedigree data. *Hum Hered* 1971;21:523–42.
6. Fabsitz RR, Carmelli D, Hewitt JK. Evidence for independent genetic influences on obesity in middle age. *Int J Obes [in press].*
7. Harvald B, Hauge M. Heredity factors elucidated by twin studies. In: Neel JV (ed): *Genetics and the epidemiology of chronic diseases.* 1965. DHEW publication no (PHS) 1163.
8. Hauge M, Harvald B, Fischer M. The Danish twin register. *Acta Genet Med Gemellol* 1968;17:315–32.
9. Heller R, Garrison RJ, Havlik RJ, Feinleib M, Padgett S. Family resemblances in height and relative weight in the Framingham Heart Study. *Int J Obes* 1984;8:39–405.
10. Holm NV. Studies of cancer etiology in the Danish twin population: I. Breast cancer. In: Gedda L, Parisi P, Nance WE (eds): *Twin research: III. Epidemiological and clinical studies.* New York: Alan R. Liss, 1981.
11. Hrubec Z, Omenn GS. Evidence of genetic predisposition to alcoholic cirrhosis and psychosis: twin concordances for alcoholism and its biological end points by zygosity among male veterans. *Alcoholism* 1981;15:207–15.
12. Kendler KS. Overview: A current perspective on twin studies of schizophrenia. *Am J Psychiatry* 1983;140:1413–1425.
13. Khoury P, Morrison JA, Laskarzewski PM, Glueck CJ. Parent/offspring and sibling body mass index associations during and after sharing common household environments: the Princeton School District Family Study. *Metabolism* 1983;32:82–9.
14. Lalouel JM, Rao DC, Morton NE, Elston RC. A unified model for complex segregation analysis. *Am J Hum Genet* 1983;35:816–26.
15. Ledbetter D. Deletion of chromosome 15 as a cause of the Prader-Willi syndrome. *N Engl J Med* 1981;304:325–9.
16. Longini IM, Higgins MW, Hinton PC. Genetic and environmental sources of familial aggregation of body mass in Tecumseh, Michigan. *Hum Biol* 1984;56:733–57.
17. MacDonald A, Stunkard AJ. Body mass indexes of British separated twins. *N Engl J Med* 1990; 322:1530.
18. Mather K, Jinks JL. *Biometrical genetics,* 2nd ed. London: Chapman and Hall Ltd., 1986.
19. Meyer JM. Sex limitation and genotype × environment interaction. In: Neale MC, Cardon LR, eds. *Methodology for genetic studies of twins and families.* Dordrecht, Netherlands: Kluwer Academic Publishers, 1992;211–230.
20. Moll PP, Burns TL, Lauer RM. The genetic and environmental sources of body mass index variability: the Muscatine Ponderosity Family Study. *Am J Hum Genet* 1991;49:1243–55.
21. Mueller WH. The genetics of size and shape in children and adults. In: Falkner F, Tanner JM, eds. *Human growth—a comprehensive treatise.* New York: Plenum, 1986;145–68.
22. Perusse L, Leblanc C, Tremblay A, et al. Familial aggregation in physical fitness, coronary heart disease risk factors, and pulmonary function measurements. *Prev Med* 1987;16:607–615.

23. Price RA, Stunkard AJ. Commingling analysis of obesity in twins. *Hum Hered* 1989;39:121–35.

24. Price RA, Gottesman II. Body fat in identical twins reared apart: roles for genes and environment. *Behav Genet* 1991;21:1–7.

25. Price RA, Cadoret RJ, Stunkard AJ, Troughton E. Genetic contributions to human fatness: an adoption study. *Am J Psychiatry* 1987;144:1003–8.

26. Price RA, Sorensen TIA, Stunkard AJ. Component distributions of body mass index defining moderate and extreme overweight in Danish women and men. *Am J Epidemiol* 1989;130:193–201.

27. Price RA, Ness R, Laskarzewski P. Common major gene inheritance of extreme overweight. *Hum Biol* 1990;62:747–65.

28. Province MA, Rao DC. Path analysis of family resemblance with temporal trends: applications to height, weight and Quetelet index in Northeastern Brazil. *Am J Hum Genet* 1985;37:178–92.

29. Province MA, Arnqvist P, Keller J, Higgins M, Rao DC. Strong evidence for a major gene for obesity in the large, unselected, total Community Health Study of Tecumseh. *Am J Hum Genet* 1990; 47[Suppl]:A143.

30. Rajput-Williams JR, Wallis SC, Yarnell J, et al. Variation of apolipoprotein-B gene is associated with obesity, high blood cholesterol levels, and increased risk of coronary heart disease. Lancet 1988;31:1442–6.

31. Sonne-Holm S, Sorensen TIA. Post-war course of the prevalence of extreme overweight among Danish young men. *J Chron Dis* 1977;30:351–8.

32. Sorensen TIA, Price RA, Stunkard AJ, Schulsinger F. Genetics of obesity in adult adoptees and their biological siblings. *Br Med J* 1989;298:87–90.

33. Sorensen TIA, Holst C, Stunkard AJ, Skovgaard. Correlations of body mass index of adult adoptees and their biological and adoptive relatives. *Int J Obes* 1992;16(3):227–236.

34. Sorensen TIA, Holst C, Stunkard AJ. Childhood body mass index—genetic and environmental influences assessed in a longitudinal adoption study. *Int J Obes* [*in press*].

35. Stunkard AJ, Foch TT, Hrubec Z. A twin study of human obesity. *JAMA* 1986;256:52–4.

36. Stunkard AJ, Sorensen TIA, Hanis C, et al. An adoption study of human obesity. *N Engl J Med* 1986;314:193–8.

37. Stunkard AJ, Harris JR, Pedersen NL, McClearn GE. The body-mass index of twins who have been reared apart. *N Engl J Med* 1990;322:1483–7.

38. Zonta LA, Jayakar SD, Bosisio M, Galante A, Pennetti V. Genetic analysis of human obesity in an Italian sample. *Hum Hered* 1987;37:129–39.

Obesity: Theory and Therapy, Second Edition,
edited by A. J. Stunkard and T. A. Wadden.
Raven Press, Ltd., New York © 1993.

9

Restrained Eating

Karl M. Pirke and Reinhold G. Laessle

*Center of Psychobiological and Psychosomatic Research, Department of
Psychoendocrinology, University of Trier, D5500 Trier, Federal Republic of Germany*

During the past decade the concept of restrained eating has generated fruitful research that has greatly advanced the understanding of human eating behavior. Restrained eating refers to the tendency to restrict food intake consciously in order to prevent weight gain or to promote weight loss. The theory has currently received particular attention. Dieting and other efforts to control body weight have become increasingly popular in western societies (1,2). Even the majority of 12-year-old schoolgirls believe themselves to be overweight (3). Disturbances like binge eating and clinical eating disorders such as bulimia nervosa have also become increasingly prevalent in young women within the past 10 years (4,5).

HISTORICAL ROOTS OF THE RESTRAINT CONCEPT

Historically, the basic hypotheses of the restraint concept have their roots in Schachter's (6,7) and Nisbett's (8) theories of obesity. Schachter's "externality" theory proposed that the eating behavior of normal weight people was largely governed by internal physiological cues, such as gastric contractions or the sensations of hunger and satiety, whereas obese people are extremely susceptible to external cues, such as the sight and taste of food, or the time of day. In the early seventies, when the theory that obesity arose from disordered eating was at its peak, Nis-

bett (8) proposed a "set-point" model of obesity, which tried to explain why the behavioral responsiveness of obese and normal weight people might differ. Nisbett's model assumed that each person had a biologically determined, homostatically defended individual weight, or set point, and that overweight people have higher than average set points. Nisbett argued that the set point is mainly determined by the number of fat cells, which does not change during adulthood, but depends on genetic endowment and early nutritional experience. He further argued that many obese people try to suppress their weight below their set points because social pressures force people to slimness. People may be overweight by social and statistical standards, yet underweight and starving according to biological criteria. Several striking behavioral parallels between obese and hungry individuals seem to support the hypothesis. Both groups share heightened externality, emotional lability, and decreased activity levels. Nisbett (8) concluded from these observations that the behavioral characteristics (e.g., externality) of obese people are not the cause of their overweight, but the consequence of biological deprivation due to their dieting attempts.

RESTRAINT AND DISINHIBITION

Stimulated by these considerations, Herman and Mack (9) developed the concept of dietary restraint, which proposed that the purported differences in eating behavior between obese and nonobese persons were actually due to more frequent dieting in obese persons. Furthermore, they predicted the same differences when normal weight people who restrain their eating are compared with unrestrained eaters. In their first experiment they divided normal weight female college students by questionnaire into two groups of persons with low and high "restraint." In the study, which was labeled a taste test, the amount of ice cream consumed either after a milk-shake preload or after no preload was measured. In the preload condition, unrestrained eaters ate less during the subsequent ice cream taste test. Restrained eaters, however, behaved paradoxically: they ate more after having consumed a preload. This behavior has been termed *counterregulation,* and has been explained by the disinhibition of cognitive control in the restrained eaters, because they had already exceeded their normally allowed food intake by consuming the preload. The counterregulation effect in restrained eaters, classified according to their scores on the Restraint Scale, was replicated in several studies using preloads (10).

Further investigations revealed that counterregulation was triggered by beliefs about the caloric content of the preload rather than by its actual energetic value (11,12). Even an anticipated preload produced the same effect of overeating as an actual preload (13). In addition to preloads, other factors that allowed disinhibition of dietary control in restrained eaters were the consumption of alcohol or the induction of negative emotional states. Restrained eaters significantly increase their consumption when in a dysphoric or depressed mood or when anxious, whereas unrestrained eaters ate less under these conditions.

In their so-called *boundary* model, Herman and Polivy (14) have summarized their concept for the control of eating. They propose essentially that biological needs lead to food intake within a certain range. Hunger keeps the consumption above a minimum

and satiety keeps it below a maximum. The area between the "boundaries" of hunger and satiety is called the *zone of biological indifference.* Herman and Polivy claim that within this range psychological factors have their greatest impact on the regulation of eating. The model proposes that the control of food intake in restrained and unrestrained eaters differs. First, it is postulated that dieters have a wider zone of biological indifference than nondieters. The hunger boundary is lower and the satiety boundary is higher. Thus greater food deprivation is necessary for restrained eaters to report hunger and satiety boundaries, indicating their maximum desired consumption. Herman and Polivy (14) suggested that once restrained eaters have transgressed the self-imposed diet boundary, they will (over)eat until they reach the satiety boundary. This boundary model incorporates the central assumptions of the restraint concept, but its account of disordered eating patterns is purely descriptive, and not explanatory (15). In particular, the psychophysiological processes that could mediate between restrained eating and the development of disordered eating such as binge eating are not specified. Furthermore, no reference to obesity has been made.

Recent research on restrained eating is reviewed below, focusing on four areas: (a) the measurement of dietary restraint, (b) cognitive restraint and eating behavior in everyday life, (c) biological correlates of restrained eating, and (d) theoretical considerations of the link between restrained eating and binge eating.

MEASUREMENT OF DIETARY RESTRAINT

At present, three scales are available for the psychometric assessment of restrained eating: the Restraint Scale (RS) of Herman and Polivy in its latest version of Heatherton et al., (16); the Three Factor Eating Questionnaire (TFEQ) of Stunkard and Messick (17); and the Dutch Eating Behavior Questionnaire (DEBQ) of Van Strien et al. (18).

Most of the laboratory research on restrained eating was conducted with the RS, which successfully predicted the eating behavior of restrained eaters. However, the RS has been criticized on both conceptual and psychometric grounds (15). Several studies have identified two underlying factors of the RS, concern for dieting and weight fluctuation (19–21). This poses the question of construct validity of the RS, since it seems that it measures not only dietary restraint, as was intended, but also the different construct of weight fluctuations. This might be one reason why there is a significant correlation between the restraint scores of the RS and percentage overweight (22,23), because weight fluctuation is common among obese persons (24). Therefore, in obese people, high scores on the RS do not necessarily reflect high dietary restraint, but the extent of overweight. Based on these considerations, the application of the RS in obese populations is problematic (15,20). Indeed, empirical investigations using the RS to predict the behavior of the obese have failed (25). Another major problem of the RS is that the scale does not differentiate between food restriction and disinhibition of control over eating (17). This might be the reason why the RS does not predict actual food restriction in everyday life. This point has been made by Laessle et al. (26), who found no correlation (r = −0.04) between the RS and the average daily food intake of young normal weight women.

The two more recently developed restraint scales attempted to avoid the problems of the RS and were more empirically derived. The DEBQ contains three-factor analytically constructed subscales: (a) restrained, (b) emotional, and (c) external eating behaviour (18). Although the reliability of the scales in terms of internal consistency has been found satisfactory and the restraint scales of the DEBQ seem predictive of daily caloric intake (27,28), it has had only limited application. The TFEQ has also been derived from factor analysis and at present is the most widely used psychometric tool in research on restrained eating. The TFEQ was explicitly designed to assess different aspects of eating. Its three factors were (a) cognitive restraint, (b) disinhibition, and (c) hunger. The factor structure of the TFEQ has been replicated independently (29), and the reliability of the scales both in terms of internal consistency and test–retest reliability is high (30,31). The validity of the TFEQ restraint scale is well substantiated with respect to eating behavior (26). In a sample of 60 healthy young women of normal weight, the cognitive restraint score of the TFEQ was significantly correlated (r = −0.46; p < 0.0001) with mean daily caloric intake. When dividing the 60 subjects into high-restraint and low-restraint groups on the basis of a median-split on the cognitive restraint scale, the high-restraint group consumed about 400 kcal/day less than the low-restraint group. There is also support for the validity of the disinhibition scale (32). Stunkard and Messick (17) review several studies giving evidence that the phenomenon of counterregulation in restrained eaters is better explained by the disinhibition factor than by the restraint factor. However, the theoretical status of the disinhibition scale remains somewhat unclear, since disinhibition by definition requires prior inhibition. Empirical data show that subjects with low cognitive restraint may obtain high scores on the disinhibition scale (33). Although Stunkard and Messick (17) assume that behavior reported on the disinhibition factor by unrestrained eaters may reflect satisfaction of desire, there still exist problems of construct validity.

The relationship between the three available measures of restraint was investigated by relating the scales to self-reported mean caloric intake per day and to other measures associated with disordered eating behavior, figure consciousness, and weight fluctuation (26). The correlation between the RS and the cognitive restraint factor of the TFEQ was 0.35 (p < 0.01), and that between the RS and the restraint factor of the DEBQ was 0.59 (p < 0.0001). The TFEQ and the DEBQ restraint scales correlated at 0.66 (p < 0.0001). A factor analytic approach was used to explore the construct validity of the three restraint measures. One would expect that measures operationalizing different constructs would constitute different factors. The analysis revealed three meaningful factors, which are depicted in Table 1. Obviously, the three measures of restraint assess different components of the restraint construct. One component of restraint involves motivational variables that lead to restrained eating. These include concerns about shape and weight and a resulting drive to be thin in order to comply with current sociocultural standards for female beauty. These features were represented by the Eating Disorders Inventory (EDI) subscales Drive for Thinness and by the BSQ, which showed high loadings on factor 1 (which includes the RS) but also substantial loadings on factor 3 (which includes the TFEQ-R and the DEBQ-R). Therefore, the RS, the TFEQ-R, and the DEBQ-R seem to be closely related to these motivational variables. Consequently, if one is interested in studying subjects in whom these features form an integral part of their (more or less successful) restraint, all three scales seem to be appropriate measurement tools. This might be particularly important for research

on the specificity of the psychopathology of eating disorders, given that concerns about shape and weight are fundamental characteristics of bulimia nervosa (34).

The second component of restraint involves overeating or disinhibited eating as well as weight fluctuation (the latter probably being due to a large variability of intake). The RS (when the total score is used) includes both these aspects (16). Therefore, if the counterregulating behavior in the laboratory is used as a model for bulimic attacks, the restraint construct as measured by the RS seems to be useful for the experimental investigation of conditions under which overeating may occur.

The third aspect of restraint is the actual restriction of food intake in everyday life. Apart from the empirically demonstrated association of food restriction with the occurrence of bulimic attacks, caloric restriction per se has other consequences at the biological level. This has been shown in patients with bulimia, who were found to be biologically adapted to starvation despite being of normal weight, as a result of their restriction of food intake "between" bulimic episodes (35). Other biological alterations in patients, such as reduced sympathetic activity or disturbances of menstrual cycle function, have also been shown to be the consequence of dieting behavior and not of bulimic attacks (see ref. 36 for an overview). Therefore, if dietary restraint is used as a construct to investigate biological or psychobiological consequences of restricted food intake and altered eating patterns in everyday life, both the TFEQ-R and the DEBQ-R seem to be appropriate tools for identifying subjects at risk.

COGNITIVE RESTRAINT

Clinical Groups

Whereas the RS of Herman and Polivy has nearly exclusively been used to select normal subjects for laboratory research, the TFEQ has been applied to assess the degree of re-

TABLE 1. *Varimax rotated factor matrix of restraint scales and related measures*

	Factor loadings[a]		
	1	2	3
Restraint Scale	.56	.59	
TFEQ (cognitive restraint)			.78
DEBQ (restraint)			.77
TFEQ-disinhibition	.70		
Caloric intake per day			−.83
Body mass index (BMI)		.78	
Maximum BMI		.93	
Difference minimal/ maximal BMI		.68	
EDI-bulimia	.73		
EDI-body dissatisfaction	.78		
EDI-drive for thinness	.72		.47
BSQ	.77		.42

[a] Only loadings greater than .40 are given. EDI, Eating Disorder Inventory (81); BSQ, Body Shape Questionnaire (82).

straint and disinhibition in various clinical populations. Recently, Stunkard and Wadden (30) reviewed this research with regard to obesity, smoking cessation, bulimia, depression, and cancer treatment. They concluded that cognitive restraint scores appeared to be able to predict treatment outcome in obesity and might also be helpful for monitoring progress in treatment. High disinhibition scores predicted weight gain after giving up smoking.

Eating Patterns in Everyday Life

Only a few studies have investigated the actual eating behavior of restrained and unrestrained eaters in normal life. Using the 24-hour dietary recall method, two studies found a significant negative correlation between the restraint scale of the DEBQ and calorie intake (27,28). Restrained eaters particularly reduced their intake of fat and sugar (27).

Laessle et al. (37) estimated calorie intake and macronutrient composition by means of 7-day nutritional protocols in a sample of 60 normal weight young women who were divided into restrained and unrestrained eaters by median split on the cognitive restraint factor of the TFEQ. The restrained group had a significantly lower daily caloric intake (1,956 kcal) than the unrestrained group (2,338 kcal), although both groups were still within the range recommended for young women by the German Nutritional Board. An analysis of the variability of intake showed that the restrained eaters had a significantly lower minimal daily consumption during the 7-day period (1,274 kcal) than the unrestrained group (1,701 kcal). Differences were also found with respect to macronutrient composition. Restrained eaters showed a higher portion of protein intake. Further qualitative differences were suggested by a retrospective assessment of food preferences over the last 3 months. Restrained eaters less frequently ate "high carbohydrate–high calorie," "fat–car-

bohydrate combination," and "fat–protein combination" food, whereas "high-protein" food was more frequently consumed.

Tuschl et al. (38) replicated these results with respect to caloric intake. In a more detailed analysis of qualitative differences, they found that restrained eaters had a strong tendency to avoid fatty products such as oil, mayonnaise, butter, and high-fat dairy products. A large percentage of the restrained eaters consumed artificial sweeteners and other calorie-reduced foodstuff.

Similar conclusions can also be drawn from the data of a large-scale study of over 45,000 participants of a computer-aided weight reduction program (31). High cognitive restraint was correlated with lower daily caloric intake. Independently of restraint, high disinhibition was associated with increased caloric consumption. The more restrained subjects showed an increased protein and carbohydrate intake, whereas their fat intake was lower.

BIOLOGICAL CORRELATES OF RESTRAINED EATING
Energy Expenditure

In the study of Laessle et al. (37), the caloric intake of a group of female restrained eaters was significantly smaller than that of unrestrained eaters. This was surprising, since the group of restrained eaters had a significantly greater body mass index and a greater body weight. Some doubts can be expressed with regard to the validity of data derived from food diaries, as was demonstrated by studies of obese women who reported a far smaller energy intake than their energy expenditure measured by the doubly labeled water method (39,40). We therefore conducted a study on energy intake and energy expenditure in restrained and unrestrained eaters (41). Eleven young women scored less than 3 on the cognitive restraint factor of the TFEQ (17) and were classified as unrestrained eaters, while 12 women who scored greater than 10 were classified as restrained eaters. The data on food intake corresponded well with the measured average daily energy expenditure (EE) as determined over a 2-week period by the doubly labeled water method (Table 2). Body weight and body composition (lean body mass and fat) did not change during the observation period in either group.

The restrained group was slightly but significantly heavier than the unrestrained group [body mass index (BMI) 21.1 ± 1.3 versus 20.0 ± 1.3 kg/m²]. When energy expenditure was corrected for height, weight, and body composition, the difference between restrained and unrestrained eaters became even greater: restrained eaters expended on the average 620 kcal less than the unrestrained eaters. The same difference was found for the reported food intake after adjustment for height and body composition. We can therefore assume that the energy intake data obtained from the food diaries of restrained and unrestrained eaters are correct. It appears unlikely that differences in activity level and smoking cause the differences in energy expenditure since heavy exercisers and smokers were excluded from the study.

Additional measurements of the resting metabolic rate and of diet-induced thermogenesis are required to determine why energy expenditure is different between the two groups. The difference in energy expenditure could be either genetic or the consequence of behavior. Considering the second possibility first, restrained eaters frequently diet and experience major weight fluctuations. Whether frequent dieting in humans influences energy expenditure remains unclear, since some studies have found reduced EE in weight-cycling persons (42), while more recent ones have not (43).

It is also unclear whether permanently restrained eating can alter energy expenditure in humans. On the other hand, it is well known that major interindividual differences in food efficiency exist. It was demonstrated by Ravussin et al. (44) that high food efficiency predisposes for obesity. We can therefore speculate that restrained eaters would have a higher body weight and might even become obese as a consequence of their high food efficiency, if they would not permanently restrain their food intake.

We have conducted metabolic and endocrine studies in restrained and unrestrained eaters and compared these findings with results obtained in voluntarily starving healthy subjects (45,46), low-weight anorectics, and intermittently dieting bulimic patients (47–50). In contrast to starving and dieting subjects, restrained eaters had normal blood glucose levels. Ketone bodies in blood, especially β-hydroxybutyric acid, which rapidly becomes elevated in states of negative energy balance, was normal. The fact that restrained eaters were not actually dieting was further emphasized by the fact that triiodothyronine concentrations in plasma were normal and that cortisol and growth hormone levels, which become elevated when the need for increased gluconeogenesis arises in a state of reduced carbohydrate intake, were normal. The above-mentioned hormones and metabolites were measured over an 8-hour period during the night, when no food was consumed. The only abnormality observed

TABLE 2. *Energy intake and energy expenditure in restrained and unrestrained eaters (mean ± SD)[a]*

	Unrestrained (n = 11)	Restrained (n = 12)	p <
Food intake according to diaries (kcal/24 h)	2,300 ± 237	2,057 ± 334	0.03
Energy expenditure, doubly labeled water (kcal/24 h)	2,350 ± 289	2,090 ± 312	0.02

[a] Values are not corrected for height, weight, and body composition.

was significantly reduced insulin values, which was probably simply a consequence of the low caloric intake in restrained eaters. No difference was found between restrained and unrestrained eaters in glucose and insulin values after a standardized carbohydrate-rich test meal, indicating that insulin sensitivity was not altered in restrained eaters. When plasma norepinephrine was measured before and after the test meal, both restrained and unrestrained eaters showed a significant increase. However, norepinephrine values were significantly lower in restrained eaters at all points in time (45). Table 3 summarizes the metabolic and endocrine observations in restrained eaters and compares them with the findings in starving healthy subjects and anorectic and bulimic patients. From these data we can conclude that restrained eaters were not dieting while participating in our study. This point is confirmed by the fact that body weight and body composition did not change during the studies reported here. The cause of the reduced norepinephrine secretion after a test meal remains unclear. There may, however, exist consequences for the energy metabolism since norepinephrine plays a major role in regulating diet-induced thermogenesis. We may therefore speculate that there is a link between the low norepinephrine and the reduced energy expenditure described above.

The Menstrual Cycle in Restrained and Unrestrained Eaters

The menstrual cycle in restrained and unrestrained eaters was studied by sampling blood and collecting urine daily throughout one menstrual cycle (51). Estradiol and progesterone were measured in blood, and their metabolites estrone-3-glucoronide and pregnanediol-glucoronide were measured in urine. Subjects with a history of menstrual cycle disturbances, drug or alcohol abuse, and psychiatric or other severe diseases were excluded. Women who had undergone a weight-reducing diet during the past 4 months and/or taken part in any kind of endurance training were also excluded. The classification of restrained and unrestrained was done as described for the other studies. All subjects were between 18 and 24 years old. Again, restrained eaters were slightly heavier (62 ± 6 versus 59 ± 6 kg) and had a higher BMI (21.7 ± 1.4 versus 20.7 ± 1.2 kg/m^2). The food intake was again significantly lower in the restrained eaters ($1,661 \pm 396$ versus $2,170 \pm 521$ kcal/day). The menstrual cycle was significantly shorter (24 ± 3 versus 31 ± 4 days) in the restrained group, which was caused by a shorter luteal phase (9 ± 4 versus 13 ± 3 days) (Table 4).

Among the 13 unrestrained eaters only 2 had a disturbed luteal phase, as judged from plasma and urine gonadal steroids. This is a normal finding since Soules et al. (52) estimated the incidence of luteal phase defects in women as 20%. In the restrained group only two of nine women had normal cycles; one had an anovulatory cycle and six had luteal phase defects. The difference between restrained and unrestrained eaters was significant. This means that fertility in restrained eaters is severely disturbed. Luteal phase de-

TABLE 3. *Metabolic and endocrine findings in restrained eaters (RE), unrestrained eaters (UR), starving healthy subjects (ST), and anorexia nervosa (AN), and bulimia nervosa (BU) subjects[a]*

	RE	UR	ST	AN	BU
Blood glucose	n	n	−	−	−
β-Hydroxybutyric acid	n	n	+	+	+n
Triiodothyronine	n	n	−	−	−
Cortisol	n	n	+	+	+n
Growth hormone	n	n	+	+	+n
Insulin (fasting)	−	n	−	−	−
Norepinephrine	−	n	−	−	−

[a] n, normal; −, decreased; +, enhanced.

TABLE 4. *Comparison of physical and menstrual cycle characteristics in restrained and unrestrained eaters (mean ± SD)*

	Restrained (n = 9)	Unrestrained (n = 13)	p <
Age (years)	22.0 ± 0.9	22.2 ± 1.5	ns
Age of menarche	13.7 ± 1.0	13.3 ± 1.0	ns
BMI (kg/m^2)	21.7 ± 1.4	20.7 ± 1.2	ns
Caloric intake (kcal/24 h)	1,724 ± 396	2,170 ± 521	0.02
Cycle length (days)	24 ± 3	31 ± 4	0.01
Luteal phase (days)	8 ± 3	12 ± 3	0.02
Progesterone, longitudinal mean (luteal phase) (mmol/L)	18 ± 14	35 ± 17	0.05

BMI, body mass index.

fects greatly reduce the chances of becoming pregnant (52).

The question arises whether there is a correlation between reduced energy expenditure and luteal phase defects in restrained eaters. Webb (53) has shown that energy expenditure is higher in the luteal phase as a consequence of elevated progesterone levels and the elevated body temperature caused by the gestagen. Reduced progesterone secretion and a shorter period of elevated plasma progesterone may therefore contribute to the low energy need in restrained eaters. However, it appears unlikely that this could explain the entire difference of about 600 kcal/24 h. There is, however, evidence that low energy intake can cause menstrual cycle disturbances under conditions of stable body weight. Warren (54) observed menstrual disturbances in ballet dancers as a consequence of low caloric intake even when body weight was stable. Similar observations were made in endurance athletes (36,55,56). All these studies indicate that female athletes with menstrual cycle disturbances had lower caloric intake but not necessarily lower body weight than athletes with normal cycles. We might speculate that there is a common mechanism behind the menstrual cycle disturbances in restrained eaters, ballet dancers, and athletes. They keep their body weight below their "natural" body weight by cognitive control of their caloric intake. They are able —by virtue of a low energy metabolism—to keep their body weight constant with a rela-

tively low caloric intake. One of the mechanisms to spare energy is to stop reproductive function, as mentioned above.

DIETARY RESTRAINT AND BINGE EATING

On the basis of laboratory research on the counterregulation effect and the boundary model for the regulation of eating, a causal link has been suggested between dietary restraint and the development of episodes of overeating and of bulimic episodes as they occur in patients with the diagnosis of a clinical eating disorder such as bulimia nervosa (57,58).

Converging experimental and clinical evidence seemed to support the proposed connection. In particular, the overeating of restrained eaters in the laboratory has been interpreted as an experimental analog of bulimic attacks (57,59). Further evidence comes from a semistarvation experiment (60), in which for a 6-month period the volunteers had to reduce their food intake to approximately half the former amount. During this time most of the participants experienced bouts of overeating, which persisted even after they had regained their preexperimental weight. Data from studies of normal populations revealed that dietary restraint and measures of "bulimic" tendencies were significantly positively correlated (23,61–64). Similarly, patients with bulimia nervosa have high scores on measures of dietary restraint (65–67). About 80% of these patients had attempted to lose weight by dieting prior to the onset of binge eating (68). Clinical observations also suggest that bulimic episodes are commonly precipitated by conditions similar to laboratory disinhibitions such as consuming a small amount of a "forbidden" food, emotional stress, or dysphoric mood states (59,69,70).

Based on the available data on the actual eating patterns of restrained eaters, a number of mediating mechanisms between dietary restraint and disturbances of the psychophysiological regulation of food intake have been considered in a recent theoretical contribution by Tuschl (41). When eating binges are conceptualized in terms of oversized meals, and under the conditions that food is available ad libitum and conscious control of food has broken down (after disinhibition), an oversized meal may theoretically result from two simultaneous processes: an extremely enhanced motivation to eat and a severely impaired satiation process. Several effects of restrained eating disturbing the control of food intake can be postulated in this way. Restrained eaters show a dissociation between food selection and food preferences in a sense that not the liked, but only the "allowed" foods are selected. This may not only cause psychological frustration and deprivation (10), but could also enhance the attractiveness of the "forbidden fruits" by nutritional preference conditioning (71). As a consequence, the microstructure of eating changes. Eating rate is accelerated and chewing activity is decreased (72), resulting in large and long meals. Furthermore, a lack of the feeling of satisfaction that is normally induced by eating occurs (73). Because restrained eaters are likely to stop eating not in response to satiety, but because they have reached a cognitively set limit, it can be postulated that conditioned satiety signals are subsequently extinguished. The high temporal variability in intake such as skipping meals may further weaken the originally learned contingencies.

If overeating occurs more frequently, causing meals to be terminated only by gastric distension, the calibration of sensory cues by the postingestional consequences of food will no longer be possible. In addition, large but poorly satiating meals may favor the development of a "belly bulimia," in which fullness is a conditioned stimulus for the continuation of eating (74). Uncoupling the sensory characteristics of food from its calorie content, as occurs when using artificial sweeteners and calorie-reduced foodstuffs, may lead to paradoxical effects on the feeling of hunger and satiety (75,76) and to overcompensation for caloric dilution (77,78).

The proposed considerations provide a heuristic synthesis of psychobiological aspects relating dieting and binge eating. Several points, however, still require clarification. Obviously, qualitative differences exist between the simple oversized meals caused by restrained eating and the eating binges seen in patients with clinical eating disorders (10). In particular, the psychosocial context of binging is often characterized by severe emotional disturbances. In connection with poorly developed skills for managing stressful situations, binging might be viewed as an inadequate coping strategy for these patients. This may be the best way of distinguishing the functional significance of overeating between bulimics and disinhibited restrained eaters.

The most important question is still: why do some restrained eaters develop the symptom of binge eating, whereas the majority do not? Obviously the restrained eaters, who are selected by the available psychometric tools, do not represent a homogenous population with regard to their actual eating patterns and possibly with regard to their biological endowment. A group of restrained eaters manages to maintain a body weight lower than their previous weight and may therefore be labeled as successful dieters. This group did not show counterregulation in the laboratory (79). Thus dietary restraint appears to involve various cognitive and behavioral strategies in order to restrict overall food intake. Some of these strategies may be more apt to promote disturbances of intake regulation, whereas others may allow more successful weight control. This point has recently been made by Westenhöfer (80), who suggested that dietary restraint should be differentiated into two sets of behaviors and cognitions, "rigid control" and "flexible control." He operationalized these constructs with two empirically derived subscales from the cognitive restraint factor of the TFEQ. Preliminary correlational data support the hypothesis that "rigid restraint" is more likely to be associated with disturbances of eating such as binging than is "flexible control."

REFERENCES

1. Westenhoefer J, Pudel V. Einstellungen der deutschen Bevölkerung zum Essen. *Ernahrungsumschau* 1990;37:311–6.
2. Blair AJ, Booth DA, Lewis VJ, Wainwright CJ. The relative success of official and informal weight reduction techniques: retrospective correlational evidence. *Psychol Health* 1989;3:195–206.
3. Wardle J, Beales S. Restraint, body image and food attitudes in children from 12 to 18 years. *Appetite* 1986;7:209–17.
4. Cooper PJ, Fairburn CG. Binge-eating and self-induced vomiting in the community. A preliminary study. *Br J Psychiatry* 1983;142:139–44.
5. Fairburn CG, Beglin S. Studies of the epidemiology of bulimia nervosa. *Am J Psychiatry* 1990; 147:401–8.
6. Schachter S. Obesity and eating. *Science* 1968; 161:751–6.
7. Schachter S. Some extraordinary facts about obese humans and rats. *Am Psychol* 1971;26:129–44.
8. Nisbett RE. Hunger, obesity, and the ventromedial hypothalamus. *Psychol Rev* 1972;79:433–53.
9. Herman CP, Mack D. Restrained and unrestrained eating. *J Pers* 1975;43:647–60.
10. Herman CP, Polivy J. Restraint and excess in dieters and bulimics. In: Pirke KM, Vandereycken W, Ploog D, eds. *The psychobiology of bulimia nervosa.* Berlin: Springer-Verlag, 1988;33–41.
11. Polivy J. Perceptions of calories and regulation of intake in restrained and unrestrained subjects. *Addict Behav* 1976;1:237–43.
12. Woody EZ, Costanzo PR, Liefer H, Conger J. The effects of task and caloric perceptions on the eating behaviour of restrained and unrestrained subjects. *Cognitive Ther Res* 1981;5:381–90.
13. Ruderman AJ, Belzer LJ, Halperin A. Restraint, anticipated consumption, and overeating. *J Abnor Psychol* 1985;94:547–55.
14. Herman CP, Polivy J. A boundary model for the regulation of eating. In: Stunkard AJ, Stellar E, eds. *Eating and its disorders.* New York: Raven Press, 1984;141–56.
15. Ruderman AJ. Dietary restraint: a theoretical and empirical review. *Psychol Bull* 1986;99:247–62.
16. Heatherton TF, Herman CP, Polivy J, King GA, McGree ST. The (mis)measurement of restraint: an analysis of conceptual and psychometric issues. *J Ab Psychol* 1988;97:19–28.
17. Stunkard AJ, Messick S. The three-factor eating questionnaire to measure dietary restraint, disinhibition and hunger. *J Psychosom Res* 1985;29:71–83.
18. Van Strien T, Frijters JER, Bergers GPA, Defares PB. The Dutch Eating Behaviour Questionnaire (DEBQ) for assessment of restrained, emotional and external eating behaviour. *Int J Eating Disord* 1986;5:295–315.
19. Blanchard F, Frost RO. Two factors of restraint: concern for dieting and weight fluctuation. *Behav Res Ther* 1983;21:259–67.
20. Drewnowski A, Riskey D, Desor AJ. Measures of restraint: separating dieting from overweight. *Appetite* 1982;3:282.
21. Ruderman AJ. The restraint scale: a psychometric investigation. *Behav Res Ther* 1983;21:258–83.
22. Lowe MR. Dietary concern, weight fluctuation and weight status: further explorations of the restraint scale. *Behav Res Ther* 1984;22:243–8.
23. Wardle J. Dietary restraint and binge eating. *Behav Anal Modification* 1990;4:201–9.
24. Bray G. *The obese patient.* Philadelphia: WB Saunders, 1976.
25. Ruderman AJ, Christensen HC. Restraint theory and its applicability to overweight individuals. *J Abnorm Psychol* 1983;92:210–5.
26. Laessle RG, Tuschl RJ, Kotthaus BC, Pirke KM. A comparison of the validity of three scales for the assessment of dietary restraint. *J Abnorm Psychol* 1989;98:504–7.
27. Van Strien T, Frijters JER, van Staveren WA, Defares PB, Deurenberg P. The predictive validity of the dutch restrained eating scale. *Int J Eating Disord* 1986;5:747–55.
28. Wardle J, Beales S. Restraint and food intake: an experimental study of the eating patterns in the laboratory and in normal life. *Behav Res Ther* 1987;25:179–85.
29. Deleted in proof.
30. Stunkard AJ, Wadden TA. Restrained eating and human obesity. *Nutr Rev* 1990;48:78–86.
31. Pudel V, Westenhöfer J. Vier-Jahreszeiten-Kur. Eine rechnergestützte Strategie zur Beeinflussung des Ernährungsverhaltens und zur Gewichtsreduktion. Forschungsbericht zur Entwicklung und Evaluation. Göttingen: Ernährungspsychologische Forschungsstelle der Universität, 1989.
32. Westenhoefer J, Pudel V, Maus N. Some restrictions on dietary restraint. *Appetite* 1990;14:137–41.
33. Pudel V, Westenhöfer J. Fragebogen zum Eßverhalten: Handanweisung. Göttingen: Hogrefe, 1989.
34. Fairburn CG, Garner DM. The diagnosis of bulimia nervosa. *Int J Eating Disord* 1986;5:403–19.
35. Pirke KM, Pahl J, Schweiger U, Warnhoff M. Metabolic and endocrine indices of starvation in bulimia:

a comparison with anorexia nervosa. *Psychiatr Res* 1985;15:33–9.

36. Schweiger U, Laessle R, Schweiger U, Herrmann F, Riedel W, Pirke KM (1988b) Caloric intake, stress and menstrual function in athletes. *Fertility and Sterility* 49:447–450.

37. Laessle RG, Tuschl RJ, Kotthaus BC, Pirke KM. Behavioural and biological correlates of dietary restraint in normal life. *Appetite* 1989;12:83–94.

38. Tuschl RJ, Laessle RG, Platte P, Pirke KM. Differences in food choice frequencies between restrained and unrestrained eaters. *Appetite* 1990;14:9–13.

39. Prentice AM, Black AE, Coward WA, et al. High levels of energy expenditure in obese women. *Br Med J* 1986;292:983–7.

40. Platte P, Pirke KM, Trimborn P, Fichter MM. Physical activity, total energy expenditure and food intake in grossly obese and normal weight women. *Br J Nutr* (in press).

41. Tuschl RJ, Platte P, Laessle RG, Stichler W, Pirke KM. Energy expenditure and everyday eating behavior in healthy young women. *Am J Clin Nutr* 1990;52:81–86.

42. Steen SN, Opplinger RA, Brownell KD. Metabolic effects of repeated weight loss and regain in adolescent wrestlers. *JAMA* 1988;260:47–50.

43. Melby C, Schmidt WD, Corrigan D. Resting metabolic rate in weight cycling collegiate wrestlers. 1990;52:409–414.

44. Ravussin E, Lillioja S, Knowler WC, et al. Reduced rates of energy expenditure as a risk factor for body weight gain. *N Engl J Med* 1988;318:467–72.

45. Pirke KM, Tuschl RJ, Spyra B, et al. Endocrine findings in restraint eaters. *Physiol Behav* 1990; 47:903–6.

46. Fichter MM, Pirke KM. Psychobiology of human starvation. In: Remschmidt H, Schmidt MH, eds. *Child and youth psychiatry.* European Perspectives 1990;13–29.

47. Doerr P, Fichter MM, Pirke KM, Lund R. Relationship between gain and hypothalamic pituitary adrenal function in patients with anorexia nervosa. *J Steroid Biochem* 1980;13:529–37.

48. Heufelder A, Warnhoff M, Pirke KM. Platelet alpha-2-adrenoceptor and adenylate cyclase in patients with anorexia and bulimia. *J Clin Endocrinol Metab* 1985;61:1053–60.

49. Schweiger U, Warnhoff M, Pahl J, Pirke KM. Effects of carbohydrate and protein meals on plasma large neutral amino acids, glucose, and insulin plasma levels of anorectic patients. *Metabolism* 1986;35:938–43.

50. Schreiber W, Schweiger U, Werner D, et al. Circadian patterns of large neutral amino acids, glucose, insulin, and food intake in anorexia nervosa and bulimia nervosa. *Metabolism* 1991;40:503–7.

51. Schweiger U, Tuschl RJ, Platte P, Brooks A, Laessle RG, Pirke KM. Everyday eating behaviour and menstrual function in young women. *Fertil Steril* 1991;771–775.

52. Soules MR. Luteal-phase deficiency: the most common abnormality of the menstrual cycle? In: Pirke KM, Wuttke W, Schweiger U, eds. *The menstrual cycle and its disorders.* Berlin: Springer-Verlag, 1989;97–109.

53. Webb P. 24-Hour energy expenditure and the menstrual cycle. *Am J Clin Nutr* 1986;44:614–9.

54. Warren MP. Reproductive function in the ballet dancer. In: Pirke KM, Wuttke W, Schweiger U, eds. *The menstrual cycle and its disorders.* 1989;161–70.

55. Nelson. Diet and bone status in amenorrhoic athletes. *Am J Clin Nutr* 1986;43:910–6.

56. Deuster PA, Kyle SB, Moser PB, Vigersky RA, Singh A, Schoomaker EB. Nutritional intake and status of highly trained amenorrhoic and eumenorrhoic women runners. *Fertility and Sterility* 1986;46:636–643.

57. Deleted in proof.

58. Wardle J. Compulsive eating and dietary restraint. *Br J Clin Psychol* 1987;26:47–55.

59. Wardle J, Beinart H. Binge eating: a theoretical review. *Br J Clin Psychol* 1981;20:97–109.

60. Keys A, Brozek J, Henschel A, Mickelsen O, Taylor HL. *The biology of human starvation.* Minneapolis: University of Minnesota Press, 1950.

61. Ruderman AJ. Restraint, obesity, and bulimia. *Behav Res Ther* 1985;23:151–6.

62. Hawkins RC, Clement PF. Development and construct validation of a self-report measure of binge eating tendencies. *Addict Behav* 1980;5:219–26.

63. Ruderman AJ, Grace PS. Restraint, bulimia, and psychopathology. *Addict Behav* 1987;12:249–55.

64. Greenberg BR, Harvey PD. The prediction of binge eating over time. *Addict Behav* 1986;11:383–8.

65. Johnson WG, Corrigan SA, Crusco AH, Schlundt DG. Restraint among bulimic women. *Addict Behav* 1986;11:351–4.

66. Lindholm L, Wilson GT. Body image assessment in patients with bulimia nervosa and normal controls. *Int J Eating Disord* 1988;7:527–39.

67. Laessle RG, Tuschl RJ, Waadt S, Pirke KM. The specific psychopathology of bulimia nervosa: a comparison with restrained and unrestrained (normal) eaters. *J Consult Clin Psychol* 1989;57:772–5.

68. Mitchell YE, Hatsulnami D, Pyle RL, Eckert ED. The bulimia syndrome. *Comprehensive Psychiatry* 1986;17:165–170.

69. Johnson C, Larson R. Bulimia: an analysis of moods and behaviour. *Psychosom Med* 1982;44:341–51.

70. Davis R, Freeman R, Solyom L. Mood and food: an analysis of bulimic episodes. *J Psychiatr Res* 1985;19:331–5.

71. Booth DA. Hunger and satiety as conditioned reflexes. In: Weiner H, Hofer MA, Stunkard AJ, eds. *Brain, behaviour, and bodily disease.* New York: Raven Press. 1981;143–60.

72. Bellisle F, Lucas F, Amrani R, LeMagnen J. Deprivation, palatability, and the microstructure of meals in human subjects. *Appetite* 1984;5:85–94.

73. Spiegel T, Jordan HA. Effects of simultaneous oral-intragastric ingestion on meal patterns and satiety in humans. *J Comp Physiol Psychol* 1978;92:133–41.

74. Booth DA. Culturally corralled into food abuse: the eating disorders as physiologically reinforced excessive appetites. In: Pirke KM, Vandereycken W, Ploog D, eds. *The psychobiology of bulimia nervosa.* Berlin: Springer-Verlag, 1988;18–32.

75. Blundell JE, Hill AJ. Paradoxical effects of an intense sweetener (aspartame) on appetite. *Lancet* 1986;i:1092–3.

76. Rogers PJ, Carlyle J, Hill AJ, Blundell JE. Uncoupling sweet taste and calories: comparison of the effects of glucose and three intense sweeteners on hunger and food intake. *Physiol Behav* 1988; 43:547–52.

77. Mattes RD, Pierce CD, Friedman MI. Daily caloric intake of normal-weight adults: response to changes in dietary energy density of a luncheon meal. *Am J Clin Nutr* 1988;48:214–9.

78. Louis-Sylvestre J, Tournier A, Verger P, Chabert M, Delorme P, Hossenhopp J. Learned caloric adjustment of human intake. *Appetite* 1989;12:95–103.

79. Lowe MR, Kleifield EI. Cognitive restraint, weight suppression, and the regulation of eating. *Appetite* 1988;10:159–68.

80. Westenhoefer J. Dietary restraint and disinhibition: is restraint a homogeneous construct? *Appetite* 1991;16:45–55.

81. Garner DM, Olmsted MP, Polivy J. Development and validation of a multidimensional eating disorder inventory for anorexia nervosa and bulimia. *Int J Eating Disord* 1983;2:15–34.

82. Cooper PJ, Taylor MJ, Cooper Z, Fairburn CG. The development and validation of the Body Shape Questionnaire. *Int J Eating Disord* 1987;6:485–94.

Obesity: Theory and Therapy, Second Edition,
edited by A. J. Stunkard and T. A. Wadden.
Raven Press, Ltd., New York © 1993.

10

Psychosocial Consequences of Obesity and Dieting

Research and Clinical Findings

Thomas A. Wadden and *Albert J. Stunkard

Department of Psychology, Syracuse University, Syracuse, New York 13244; °Department of Psychiatry, University of Pennsylvania, Philadelphia, Pennsylvania 19104-2648

Recent research has transformed our understanding of human obesity. For many years obesity has been viewed as a disorder with strong behavioral determinants—psychopathology manifested as overeating. The obese were believed to overeat in response to negative feelings including frustration, sadness, or insecurity, and food was seen as providing comfort in the absence of other sources of solace. They were frequently portrayed as having problems with food because of their inability to establish satisfactory interpersonal relationships. As one author noted, obesity is a "particular way of handling one's difficulty in human relationships and, even more, one's poor relationship with oneself" (1).

This view has changed 180 degrees in direction. When psychopathology is observed in obese individuals, it is now seen as a consequence rather than a cause—a consequence of the prejudice and discrimination to which the overweight are subjected. This view informs the present chapter, which reviews the psychological status of obese individuals as described in the research literature, and as we have observed it in our clinical practice. We will also examine the topic of binge eating in the obese, as well as the effects on mood of dieting and cycles of weight loss and regain.

RESEARCH FINDINGS

Obese individuals in America and other industrialized nations suffer significant prejudice and discrimination (2,3). Daily, when looking at television programs and magazines, they are reminded that "thin is in" and "fat is not where it's at." Contemptuous attitudes are expressed in jokes heard on the street and on late night talk shows, as well as in the nation's respected news weeklies. Thus the author of a recent "My Turn" column in *Newsweek* wrote, "This information (about genetic determinants of obesity) should be withheld from the fat multitudes because the obese will latch onto any excuse for failing to lose weight. . . Face it Chubbo, when was the last time you were force-fed" (4).

Such prejudice has been observed in children as young as 6 years of age, who described silhouettes of an overweight child as "lazy, dirty, stupid, ugly, cheats, and lies" (5). When shown black and white line drawings of an obese child and children with various handicaps, including missing hands and facial disfigurement, both children and adults rated the obese child as the one they least wished to play with (6–8). Regrettably, overweight individuals display this same prejudice (5–7). In a similar study, college students were asked to rate various categories of persons as to their suitability as a marriage partner (9). Embezzlers, cocaine users, shoplifters, and blind persons were all rated as more suitable partners than were the obese.

Sadly, health-care professionals appear to share this prejudice. Physicians consider their obese patients to be "weak-willed, ugly and awkward" (10). Patients are fully aware of such attitudes. In a recent study, 80% of persons who underwent surgery for their obesity reported that they had "been treated disrespectfully by the medical profession because of my weight" (11) (see Table 1).

Weight-related prejudice is often accompanied by discrimination. Two studies found lower acceptance rates into prestigious colleges among obese as compared with nonobese students, despite comparable scholastic performance in the two groups (12,13). In a different setting, the work place, Roe and Eichwort (14) reported that 16% of employers would not hire obese individuals under any conditions, and an additional 44% would hire them only under special circumstances. A 1974 study of executives, when salaries were much lower, revealed that only 9% of those who earned $25,000 to $50,000 were more than 10 pounds overweight, whereas 39% of those earning $10,000 to $20,000 were similarly overweight (15). The authors calculated that each pound of fat cost an executive $1,000 per year. The police, armed forces, fire departments, and airlines will not hire significantly obese individuals and reprimand or discharge persons who fail to maintain a weight deemed acceptable to the employer (2). Furthermore, the full extent of job-related discrimination against the obese is underestimated because of employers' reluctance to acknowledge what is, in many cases, unlawful behavior.

Discrimination extends to a variety of social interactions. Landlords, for example, are less likely to rent properties to overweight individuals (16). In marrying, almost twice as many obese women fall as rise in social class (17,18). In virtually every aspect of life, the overweight are reminded that they live in a society that hates fat.

Psychopathology and Obesity

In view of the prejudice and discrimination to which they are subjected, overweight persons could be expected to show higher levels of depression and other psychological disturbance. It would seem impossible to maintain a positive self-image in a society which so scorns them. Studies of this topic, however, have yielded some surprising findings.

Population Studies

Population studies have generally failed to find significant differences between obese and nonobese persons in psychological status (as measured by self-report inventories) (2,3). Moore and colleagues (19) examined 1,660 people in midtown Manhattan and found that obese individuals scored significantly higher than nonobese persons on three of nine measures of psychological functioning

TABLE 1. *Responses of morbidly obese patients to questions concerning their weight and psychosocial functioning*

Response	Always	Usually	Sometimes	Never
At work, people talk behind my back and have a negative attitude toward me related to my weight	80.7	10.5	3.5	5.3
I feel that my weight has negatively affected whether or not I have been hired for a job	67.3	20.4	10.2	2.2
I do not like to be seen in public	66.7	17.5	14.0	1.8
I feel that I have been treated disrespectfully by the medical profession because of my weight	45.5	32.7	16.4	5.5

—immaturity, suspiciousness, and rigidity. Differences between groups on these measures were so small, however, as to be judged clinically insignificant. Stewart and Brook (20) similarly observed only small differences between obese and nonobese subjects in their study of 5,817 persons. In this investigation, however, obese individuals were found to be significantly *less* depressed and anxious than were their nonobese counterparts. Results of two British studies (21,22) and five European investigations (23–27) confirm the impression that there are few significant differences in psychological status between obese and nonobese persons in the general population.

Among children as well as among adults, the obese do not stand out psychologically. Our research team has conducted four studies of children and adolescents that found no significant differences between obese and nonobese subjects in self-esteem and measures of dysphoria (28–31). Sallade (32) similarly observed that obese and nonobese children did not differ significantly on measures of personality function. Obese children were found to have slightly lower self-esteem, but their scores fell well within normal limits.

Studies of Clinical Samples

In contrast to population data, studies of overweight persons seeking weight reduction suggest that emotional disturbance is common in the obese. Numerous studies have used the Minnesota Multiphasic Personality Inventory (MMPI) (33) to assess psychological status. Ten such investigations found at least mild levels of depression, as defined by a T score of 60 (1 standard deviation above the mean), and several observed mild to moderate elevations on scales measuring hypochondriasis, hysteria, and impulsivity (i.e., psychopathic deviancy) (34–43). We have observed comparable findings in patients whom we have treated for marked obesity by very-low-calorie diet and behavior therapy (44). Thus clinicians can anticipate that a sig-

nificant minority of persons seeking treatment for their obesity will experience significant psychological distress that may require treatment by psychotherapy or other means.

Three Caveats

Three points should be considered in interpreting the above studies. First, findings of psychopathology in some overweight individuals have little bearing on the popular notion of an obese personality type. According to this view, obese individuals may appear jolly and carefree in social interactions, but suffer from feelings of inferiority, are passive-dependent, and have a deep need to be loved (44). Although some obese individuals display these characteristics, so do nonobese persons (45). Moreover, efforts to identify an obese personality type have yielded precisely the opposite finding; there is remarkable diversity of personality types among the overweight. Three studies that used cluster analysis document this diversity (47–49). From three to ten personality subtypes were identified in these studies, subtypes varied between investigations, and one-third of subjects did not fit any of the subtypes. There can be little doubt of the heterogeneity of personality in obese individuals (3).

The second point is that most studies of psychopathology failed to include appropriate control groups (2,3). This omission is critical because most people seeking treatment, regardless of the specific disorder, report psychological distress. This finding was demonstrated by analysis of the MMPI scores of 18,328 women who underwent general medical or surgical procedures at the Mayo Clinic (50). Mean scores for this sample on the hypochondriasis, depression, and hysteria scales were 61, 60, and 62, respectively, scores that reach the criterion for psychopathology in the above studies of obese patients. In addition, approximately 15% of patients in the Mayo Clinic study scored 70 or higher on each of these scales. This score is

2 standard deviations above the mean and indicates clinically significant psychopathology. These findings suggest that, although some obese individuals display emotional disturbance, their psychological status as a group does not differ significantly from that of other clinic patients. Carefully controlled studies using either the MMPI (43,51) or other measures (52,53) of psychological status support this view.

The third point is that even if obese persons showed greater psychopathology than their nonobese peers, this finding would not prove that psychological disturbance causes overeating and weight gain, as is frequently asserted. Studies of this kind are unable to differentiate between factors that may be a consequence rather than a cause of obesity. Thus prejudice and discrimination may be responsible for the depression observed in some persons, rather than depression causing obesity (2,3).

Ultimately, the contribution of psychological factors to the development of obesity can be assessed only by longitudinal studies. Ideally, subjects should be measured on a variety of psychosocial dimensions prior to the onset of their obesity. One such study was recently completed, and it found that psychological factors were of negligible importance in the determination of body fat. Klesges et al. (54) assessed 132 obese and nonobese children, 3 to 5 years of age, annually for 3 years. They found that initial body fat was the best predictor of increases in fat over this period. Only one of the several psychosocial variables studied, physical self-esteem, was consistently related to the development of obesity, and even it was related only during the first 2 years and accounted for less than 5% of the variance in changes in body fat. At no time during the study were such variables as general self-esteem or maternal and parental regard associated with changes in body fat.

Further studies of this nature and of longer duration are needed to determine finally the contribution of psychopathology to human obesity. Children should be followed through adolescence, a time at which the prevalence of obesity increases markedly.

Psychological Disturbance Specific to the Obese

Findings of generally normal psychological function in the obese are a tribute to their resilient spirit, given the prejudice and discrimination that they endure. Despite these encouraging findings, obesity appears to be associated with a number of weight-specific problems that may adversely affect the quality of life, even if they are not so severe as to result in clinically significant complications (2,3). Moreover, most psychological inventories do not assess weight-related difficulties, which could well go undetected.

The importance of weight-related difficulties is supported by findings of two studies of adolescent girls (30,31). In neither study did obese girls score significantly higher in dysphoria (anxiety and/or depression) than did their nonobese classmates. The obese girls, however, reported significantly greater dissatisfaction with, and worry about, their weight and shape. Klesges (55) has reported similar results in college students. Even if such concerns do not result in clinically significant levels of depression, they must adversely affect an individual's quality of life.

Feelings of guilt and shame over their inability to control their weight (56) are likely to diminish the self-esteem of obese persons in some areas of functioning, even if not sufficiently to affect global self-esteem. Perhaps the greatest benefit of group treatment of obesity (as compared with individual therapy) is that it allows patients to share such feelings and to realize that they are not alone with them.

Body Image Disparagement

Although weight dissatisfaction is so common among adolescent girls as to approach a "normative discontent" (57), it is more severe in obese girls. Many feel that their bodies are "ugly and despicable and that others view them with hostility and contempt" (58). As Stunkard and Mendelson (58) have written, "it makes no difference whether the person be also talented, wealthy, or intelligent; his weight is his only concern, and he sees the whole world in terms of his weight."

The problem of body image disparagement occurs most commonly in young Caucasian women of upper-middle socioeconomic status, in whom the prevalence of obesity is very low (i.e., 5%) and the sanctions against it very high (18). Within this population, the disturbance is most severe in persons who have been obese since childhood, who have a generalized neurotic disturbance, and whose parents disparaged them for their weight. The disturbance appears to result from an internalization of parental and peer criticism, and it persists even in the absence of continued derogation. Adolescence appears to be the period of greatest risk for development of the problem (59,60).

Weight-specific psychological complications of obesity are less severe in persons of lower socioeconomic status (19). One reason may be that obesity is common in the lower class and thus is more readily accepted. Racial differences in preferred body type may also affect psychological responses. African Americans and Mexican Americans, for example, do not appear to value thinness to the same extent as Caucasians (61,62), a finding that may explain their high prevalence of obesity and low prevalence of eating disorders (63).

Binge Eating in the Obese

Binge eating as a distinct pattern of eating was first described by Stunkard in 1959, together with the loss of control that accompanied it and the expression of remorse that followed (64,65). Interest in binge eating was limited thereafter until 1979, when Russell (66) published his landmark study on "Bu-

limia Nervosa: An Ominous Variant of Anorexia Nervosa." The key features of this disorder were those described in the earlier reports—binge eating accompanied by loss of control and later remorse—with one important addition. Russell added the criterion of vomiting or other forms of purging. Russell's paper was followed by a flood of research on anorectic patients who binged and purged and soon afterwards on patients of normal weight who had never been anorectic but displayed remorse and purging after bingeing.

Binge Eating Disorder

During the past 10 years there has been a revival of interest in binge eating by obese persons (67–71). This interest culminated in a multicenter trial by Spitzer and colleagues (70), which led to the proposal of a new diagnostic category—"binge eating disorder," the features of which are shown in Table 2.

TABLE 2. *Diagnostic criteria for binge eating disorder*

A. Recurrent episodes of binge eating, an episode being characterized by the following:
  1. Eating, in a discrete period of time (e.g., in any 2-hour period), an amount of food that is definitely larger than most people would eat during a similar period of time
  2. A sense of lack of control during the episodes (e.g., a feeling that one cannot stop eating or control what or how much one is eating)
B. During most binge episodes, at least three of the following behavioral indicators of loss of control:
  1. Eating much more rapidly than usual
  2. Eating until feeling uncomfortably full
  3. Eating large amounts of food when not feeling physically hungry
  4. Eating large amounts of food throughout the day with no planned mealtimes
  5. Eating alone because of being embarrassed by how much one is eating
  6. Feeling disgusted with oneself, depressed, or feeling very guilty after overeating
  7. Eating large amounts of food because one is upset, anxious, lonely, depressed, or bored
C. The binge eating occurs, on average, at least twice a week for a 6-month period
D. Marked distress regarding binge eating
E. Does not currently meet the criteria for bulimia nervosa or abuse medication (e.g., diet pills) in an attempt to avoid weight gain

It is difficult to define what constitutes an eating binge, but the two proposed criteria provide a reasonable first approximation. They are "eating in a discrete period of time more food than most people would eat," combined with a report of lack of control during the binge. Whatever refinements in the diagnosis may occur in the future, the definition of binge eating disorder has had the valuable result of characterizing a group of distinctively different obese persons.

Prevalence

An important consequence of the delineation of this disorder was the discovery that it is a surprisingly prevalent problem. Thus recent studies indicate that from 25 to 45% of persons entering treatment programs for obesity suffer from binge eating and that in some special groups, such as Overeaters Anonymous, the figure may rise as high as 70% (67–70). Community studies of binge eating are in their infancy, but suggest a prevalence of about 2% (70).

Differences between Bingers and Nonbingers

Investigations conducted over the past 5 years have revealed several consistent differences between obese bingers and nonbingers. Binge eaters tend to be heavier than nonbingers, as shown by Telch et al. (72) (Fig. 1). In addition, they tend to be somewhat younger than nonbingers (73).

Psychological Status

The most consistent difference between bingers and nonbingers is that binge eaters report significantly greater psychological distress (on standard measures of psychopathology) and have a higher lifetime prevalence of psychiatric illness (particularly affective disorders) (74–77). In a recent study, for example, we (78) observed that binge eaters scored a mean of 14.7 (SD = 5.4) on the Beck Depression Inventory (79), as compared with 9.6 (SD = 6.2) for nonbingers, values very similar to those reported by Marcus et al. (76). (A score of 17 suggests the possibility of clinically significant depression.) In addition to higher levels of depression, binge eaters also report greater dietary disinhibition (76), as well as lower self-efficacy with regard to dieting (69,76).

The relationship between depression and binge eating is not well understood. The positive effects of antidepressant medications (including desipramine and fluoxetine) on both

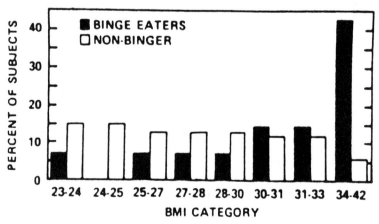

FIG. 1. The percentage of the total number of subjects in the sample meeting the full DSM-III criteria for bulimia (obese binge eaters) is shown for each of eight body mass index (BMI) categories. Those not meeting the DSM-III category for bulimia are also shown. (From Spitzer et al., ref. 70, with permission.)

mood and bingeing (in persons with bulimia nervosa) suggest that abnormalities in the same neurotransmitter(s) may underlie both disorders (80–83). Binge eating, however, may occur in the absence of significant depression but may itself induce depression through effects such as lowering self-esteem or causing weight gain. Clearly, further research is needed to determine the relationship between these two events.

Response to Treatment

Binge eaters and nonbinge eaters may also differ in their response to weight reduction therapy. Two studies found differences and one did not. Marcus et al. (76) reported a significantly higher rate of attrition in binge eaters, whereas Keefe et al. (68) found that bingers lost significantly less weight than nonbingers at the end of a 9-week program and at a 6-month follow-up. Both of these results were obtained in programs that used a conventional reducing diet. By contrast, we found no significant differences in weight loss or attrition between bingers and nonbingers who consumed a very-low-calorie diet (78).

Psychological Effects of Dieting and Weight Loss

A question frequently posed about binge eating is its relationship to dieting and weight loss. Histories obtained from persons with bulimia nervosa indicate that their first binge usually occurred while they were dieting (84). The classic Minnesota study of prolonged dietary deprivation in average weight men found marked overeating when the dietary restriction was terminated (85). The relationships, however, among weight, dieting, and binge eating in the obese are far from firmly established. Berkowitz (personal communication), for example, observed binge eating in obese adolescent girls despite their never having dieted. Careful longitudinal, as well as retrospective studies, are needed to untangle the relationships among these events.

Dieting, Weight Loss, and Mood

Regardless of the precise relationships between binge eating and dieting, there can be no denying our nation's current epidemic of weight-loss efforts. At any given time, approximately 25% of men and 50% of women report that they are trying to lose weight (86). They spend approximately $35 billion yearly on these efforts (87).

The beneficial effects of weight loss are well documented and include reductions in blood pressure, blood lipids, and insulin requirements in type II diabetics (see chapters by Sjöström and VanItallie in this volume). The effects of dieting and weight loss on psychological status are less clear, however. Stunkard and Rush (88) reviewed seven studies published between 1951 and 1973, all of which reported adverse emotional reactions to dieting. By contrast, Wing and colleagues (89) reviewed ten studies published between 1969 and 1983 and found that dieting was associated with no worsening or even with improvement in mood. The major difference between the early and later reports was the introduction of group behavioral treatment in the later investigations. Both group and behavioral interventions appear to provide patients greater social support than does individual psychodynamic therapy, which was used extensively in the 1950s and 60s. In addition, behavioral treatment of obesity incorporates elements of cognitive therapy such as those used in the treatment of depression (90). Thus psychological responses to dieting appear to be at least partially determined by the characteristics of the therapy employed.

There are, however, methodological differences between the earlier and later studies that may further explain the disparate findings. In an extensive review, Smoller et al. (91) reported that when mood was assessed concurrently and by objective psychometric instruments [e.g., Beck Depression Inventory (79), State-Trait Anxiety Inventory (92)], no change or improvement in mood was noted in all reports. By contrast, open-ended assessment, typically retrospective and by psychiatric interview, consistently revealed adverse changes in mood. The importance of method of assessment was dramatically illustrated when both objective, concurrent, and (later) subjective, retrospective assessments were used with the same group of patients. The objective tests documented improvements in mood whereas the later open-ended assessment noted adverse changes (93).

Frequency of assessment also influences outcome. Studies that limited assessment simply to before and after treatment uniformly found benign changes (91). Among studies that assessed mood more frequently, benign and adverse changes were reported with approximately equal frequency. More frequent assessment may measure the stresses of dieting, such as restricting food intake and avoiding social, food-related situations. By comparison, assessments limited to before and after treatment may capture the benefits of weight loss rather than the stress of dieting. At the end of treatment, patients may overlook the difficulties encountered in losing weight in favor of the pride that they feel in their improved appearance and health.

Weight Regain and Mood

There have been few systematic investigations of the effects on psychological status of regaining weight, lost through either supervised or unsupervised efforts. It is hard to imagine, however, that the effects are anything but negative. Regaining weight is an important issue, given its likelihood in the vast majority of obese individuals who diet (94,95). Two studies are informative.

Brownell and Stunkard (96) found that patients' scores on the Beck Depression Inventory (79) decreased as they lost weight during 6 months of treatment. Depression levels rose, however, as patients regained weight during a 1-year follow-up. The percentage increases during this time in weight and depression were comparable.

Wadden and colleagues (97) assessed the psychological effects of weight regain as part

of a 3-year follow-up evaluation of patients treated by very-low-calorie diet alone, behavior therapy combined with a 1,200 kcal/day diet, or the combination of very-low-calorie diet and behavior therapy (i.e., combined treatment). Patients who received either behavior therapy alone or combined with very-low-calorie diet displayed significant reductions in depression at the end of treatment and at the 1-year follow-up. At the 3-year follow-up, at which time patients had regained a majority of their weight loss, depression scores increased so that they were no longer significantly different from baseline. Interestingly, patients who received the very-low-calorie diet alone showed no significant change in depression during treatment or follow-up.

In this study, the effect of weight regain on physical and psychological health was assessed in 36 patients selected from the three conditions. As may be seen in Table 3, weight regain clearly had a very negative effect on satisfaction with appearance, self-esteem, self-confidence, happiness, and physical health.

CLINICAL FINDINGS

Research findings on the psychological status of obese individuals lag behind our clini-

TABLE 3. *Effect of weight regain on subjects' physical and psychological status at 3-year follow-up evaluation (N = 36)[a]*

Variable	M	SD
Satisfaction with appearance	6.39	0.92
Self-esteem	5.97	1.13
Self-confidence	5.95	1.14
General level of happiness	5.66	0.99
Physical health	5.61	1.24
Recreational activities	5.36	1.12
Job performance	5.21	0.87
Social activities	5.18	1.04
Outlook on the future	5.17	1.02
Relationship with spouse/partner	5.03	1.47
Sex life	4.97	1.48
Relationship with family members	4.61	0.72

[a] 1, very positive effect; 4, no effect; 5, slightly negative effect; 6, moderately negative effect; 7, very negative effect.

cal knowledge in many instances. In this section, we discuss the clinical impressions we have gained during several years of treating obese persons. This discussion includes a consideration of the psychological functioning of the obese and of the psychosocial effects of dieting and weight loss. We note that our findings are based primarily upon the treatment of women. Prior to therapy, our typical patient is 40 years of age, weighs 105 kg, and has been on five major diets that resulted in a combined weight loss of about 55 kg (98).

Personality and Psychopathology

In any group of ten patients receiving treatment, we usually observe several persons who are outgoing, socially skilled, and productive group members. They participate constructively in sessions, providing comfort and useful suggestions to other patients. One or two other individuals frequently are shy and reserved, but can contribute appropriately when asked to do so. These persons comprise the basis for a constructive group experience.

Personality Disorders

Groups often include, however, one or two individuals with a personality disorder (99). Those with borderline personality are frequently popular during the early stages of treatment. They disclose intimate thoughts and feelings about themselves and develop engaging relationships with group members. Over time, however, they often flood the group with reports of their troubled personal relationships and difficulties coping with life's demands. In addition, they tend to be emotionally labile in meetings and develop intense positive and/or negative feelings toward staff and other group participants. The behavior of such persons, if not controlled, can have a very negative effect on group morale and functioning.

Persons with a passive–aggressive personality style have a different effect on group dynamics. They are likely to drain the group's energy by their constant complaints that they are not "getting anything out of treatment" and that none of the suggestions offered by group members or the therapist is helpful. Such persons were first identified in traditional group psychotherapy, where they achieved recognition as "help-rejecting complainers."

Thus, consistent with the research literature, our obese clinic patients display a wide range of personality styles. The great majority of individuals display normal psychological functioning, but there clearly are exceptions.

Relationship to Obesity

It is tempting to speculate that the patient's obesity is dynamically related to the personality disturbance. Thus the borderline patient may eat to fill "profound feelings of emptiness" or binge in response to overwhelming impulses, which may also be associated with sexual promiscuity, self-mutilation, and the abuse of alcohol and other drugs. The passive–aggressive individual may overeat as an expression of anger and defiance and the resulting obesity may silently communicate "don't try to get too close to me." Obesity in persons with low self-esteem may be an outward expression of their negative opinion of themselves.

Research, rather than speculation, is needed to clarify the relationship between obesity and personality dysfunction. At present, in the absence of definitive data, we think that the relationship between obesity and personality disorders may well be coincidental. The personality disorders noted above are also found in individuals of average weight and may be independent of weight status. Regardless of the etiological relationship, however, it is important that persons with psychological disturbance receive appropriate care, which may differ from that required for the management of their obesity. In many cases, they need adjunctive psychotherapy.

Life Stressors

We have found that untoward life events significantly affect patients' psychosocial functioning and their ability to control their weight. During a 1-year treatment program, it is common for at least one member of a group of ten to experience a death in the family and another to face significant work-related or financial problems. Such occurrences are associated with anxiety, depression, and other adverse emotions, as they are in persons of average weight. In obese individuals, such experiences may result in patients' leaving therapy and/or gaining weight, as they lose control of their customary efforts to manage their weight (100).

Practitioners should be prepared to support patients during such difficult times. In many instances, two or three brief meetings are sufficient to help the individual cope with the problems and may be all that is required. When improvement is not seen within a few weeks, the practitioner should consider referring the individual for psychotherapy.

Psychosocial Effects of Dieting

The majority of our patients report mild apprehension prior to beginning a weight control program (56). Many worry that they will not be able to adhere to the diet prescribed or to lose as much weight as other group members. In addition, the thought of undertaking yet another diet often recalls previous weight-loss efforts, many of which were successful in the short-term only to end in weight regain a year or more after treatment. From this perspective, the proposed diet holds the unwelcome possibility of yet more failure and further loss of self-esteem. We address these fears with patients in both individual and group meetings (as discussed in the chapter by Wadden in this volume).

Early Dieting

Following this anxious start, a majority of patients report after the first 2 to 3 weeks of dieting that they feel happier and more self-confident (56). These verbal reports are confirmed by patients' increased attention to their dress and appearance and often by more active social calendars. The rapidity with which these changes occur is surprising, because they do so before patients have lost enough weight to be noticeable to others. For many, the improved mood simply reflects relief that they have been able to diet successfully, a demonstration of self-control that brings hope of long-term weight management. Binge eaters, in particular, frequently report with pride that, as a result of being provided a structured meal plan, they have stopped bingeing for the first time in weeks, if not months.

Treatment sessions reinforce patients' optimism and resolve during this early period (56). Many report that the group gives them greater strength and tenacity than they have ever experienced while dieting alone. The group is also a source of support and suggestions for the one or two individuals (out of a group of ten) who have difficulty "getting started" on the diet and are understandably discouraged. Brief individual meetings and telephone contacts between weekly meetings frequently help such individuals by providing greater structure and identifying impediments to adherence.

Later Dieting

A significant minority of patients enjoy a very smooth course of dieting during the 20 to 25 weeks of initial treatment. They report few adherence problems, lose weight regularly, and are often heard remarking that "I haven't felt this good in years."

A majority of patients, by contrast, have a generally favorable course of treatment but report that adherence to the diet and program of lifestyle change gets tougher after the first 10 or so weeks. Complaints about keeping diet and exercise diaries increase over time, as do frustration and annoyance associated with failure to lose weight, despite reportedly good adherence. Most of these individuals, however, maintain their efforts, continue to lose weight and, overall, are satisfied with their progress.

Most groups contain one or two individuals (out of ten) who, as treatment progresses, become discouraged by their slow weight loss or inability to control binge eating (or related difficulties). Despite efforts by the group and therapist to support them, these persons frequently appear to "give up" at some point, convinced that their efforts are futile. This resignation frequently is associated with increased feelings of hopelessness and despair, which, in turn, lead to marked overeating and perpetuation of a vicious cycle (101). We encourage these individuals to remain in group treatment but also arrange individual care to meet their additional needs.

Family Members

It is of note that the dieting fatigue (102) that befalls most patients in the later phases of treatment is also experienced by family members and treatment providers. Patients report that their spouses and children frequently ask: "When is this diet going to be over?" or "When will things return to normal around here?" Family members apparently tire of having to modify their own eating and exercise habits to support the dieter's weight control efforts.

Treatment providers (like patients) become frustrated by patients' failures to lose weight, particularly when several weeks have passed and providers have worked overtime to provide extra support (56). Not only does the honeymoon period of the first 5 to 10 weeks come to an end but, as a result of their increasing frustration, one or two patients (in a group of ten) may discontinue treatment or at least consider such action. These patients have difficulty maintaining self-esteem at such times, and their treatment providers experience difficulty maintaining professional esteem (56).

Psychosocial Effects of Weight Loss

The great majority of our patients report that they are extremely pleased with their weight losses. Specifically, they delight in the opportunity to wear more stylish clothes, to feel like a "normal person" when looking around a crowded room, and to resume recreational and other activities that previously brought them enjoyment. Feelings of self-pride are common, as are compliments from family, friends, and coworkers. Younger patients frequently report improved social life, the desire for which compelled them to lose weight. Thus most persons respond to significant weight loss with pleasure, if not elation. Problems do occasionally arise, however, that diminish a patient's overall satisfaction or, in some cases, turn weight loss into a frightening experience.

Unwanted Attention

One or two group members frequently report that they are uncomfortable with the increased attention that they receive as a result of weight loss. Those who are shy are not accustomed to being the focus of attention or having others comment on their new shape or appearance. They experience questions about their diet as intrusive.

More assertive patients frequently experience annoyance or anger in response to compliments about their weight loss. One of our patients reported that "Everyone at work wants to talk to me now that I've lost a hundred pounds. I feel like telling some of them to get lost. Don't they realize that I'm the same person now that I was a hundred pounds ago. How superficial can they be? It's insulting."

Sexuality

Most participants volunteer that after weight loss they feel more sexually attractive and are happier with their sex lives. A majority report increased libido well before they have achieved their full weight loss. We have encountered a handful of persons, however, for whom weight loss was associated with marked distress about dating and sexuality. In some cases, patients stopped losing weight or experienced severe anxiety when they reached a body weight that was previously associated with a serious trauma (i.e., rape, sexual abuse, relationship difficulty) (103). Others did not report feeling sexually vulnerable but noted that they did not "feel like themselves" or felt uncomfortable with their bodies. Some such patients regained weight while still in treatment. Further investigation of the problems precipitated by weight loss is needed to determine their prevalence (which is quite low in our experience) and how to respond to them.

Relationships

The psychosocial changes that obese individuals experience with weight loss may affect their relationships with family, friends, and coworkers. Thus, for example, a previously obese women who has lost 25 kg, now wears a size 10 dress, and feels good about herself may ask her husband to go to more movies and parties. She may also initiate sex more frequently.

While a majority of the husbands of whom we are aware are pleased by such activities, some are not. Their wives' new interests (and often assertiveness) challenge the status quo with which the men have become comfortable. In such cases, partners must redefine and renegotiate their relationships, and they may require professional assistance to do so (104). Failure to establish a new relationship, which meets the formerly obese individual's needs (which are frequently more salient after weight loss) may result in marital discord and even divorce. Termination of an unsatisfactory marriage, however, may well be considered a positive rather than a negative outcome of treatment (105,106).

Relationships at work may also require redefinition following weight loss. Several of our patients have reported that their obesity had limited their advancement at work, in terms of increased pay and/or promotion to positions of greater responsibility. With weight loss, they felt empowered to demand raises or other signs of recognition. A minor-

ity successfully negotiated these issues with their bosses. Most, however, were told that their weight had nothing to do with their salary or level of responsibility and so they could affect no redress.

Psychosocial Effects of Weight Regain

The psychosocial consequences of regaining lost weight are entirely negative in our experience. Patients routinely report that they feel disappointed if not disgusted with themselves and ashamed to meet with their health professionals and friends who helped them to lose weight. The more times the patient has lost and regained weight, the greater the burden of shame and failure the individual carries. Unfortunately, repeated gaining of lost weight makes the individual less likely to seek treatment, feeling that he or she does not deserve it or that "nothing will help anyway."

Practitioners, including ourselves, are also upset by weight regain. Regrettably, practitioners too often defend against their feelings of frustration and disappointment by blaming patients in subtle, as well as not so subtle ways. It is not uncommon to hear colleagues remark in the face of a patient's weight regain, that "I guess she wasn't ready to be thin" or "Apparently, he didn't really want to be thin." The implicit messages contained in such statements include that the patient: 1) has a psychological need to remain obese; 2) cannot tolerate being good to himself or herself; or 3) lacks the desire and willpower to work at weight control. In many cases, the patient is thought to be unaware (i.e., unconscious motivation) of the factors purportedly contributing to weight regain.

Unfortunately, scientists and practitioners are also unaware of the factors associated with weight regain. These factors include, however, genetic, physiological, behavioral, and cultural influences, to name only a few. To treat this problem as if it were solely a psychological issue serves only to blame patients for our poor long-term results.

The growing recognition that obesity, in many persons, is a chronic condition requiring long-term care makes it imperative that practitioners concern themselves with their patients' self-esteem. Only by limiting their patients' experiences of shame and guilt concerning their weight can practitioners hope to create a trusting relationship to which patients can repeatedly return for the help they need. Years after treatment, many of our patients identify such a relationship as the most important and lasting aspect of their care.

REFERENCES

1. Becker BJ. The obese patient in psychoanalysis. *Am J Psychother* 1960;14:322–7.
2. Wadden TA, Stunkard AJ. The psychological and social complications of obesity. *Ann Intern Med* 1985;103:1062–7.
3. Stunkard AJ, Wadden TA. Psychological aspects of severe obesity. *Am J Clin Nutr* 1992;55:524S–32S.
4. Hecht K. Oh, come on fatties. *Newsweek* 1990, Sep 3:8.
5. Staffieri JR. A study of social stereotype of body image in children. *J Pers Soc Psychol* 1967; 7:101–4.
6. Goodman N, Dornbusch SM, Richardson SA, Hastorf AH. Variant reactions to physical disabilities. *Am Sociol Rev* 1963;28:429–35.
7. Maddox GL, Back K, Liederman V. Overweight as social deviance and disability. *J Health Soc Behav* 1968;9:287–98.
8. Richardson SA, Goodman N, Hastorf AH, Dornbusch SM. Cultural uniformity in reaction to physical disabilities. *Am Sociol Rev* 1961;26:241–7.
9. Venes AM, Krupka LR, Gerard RJ: Overweight/obese patients: an overview. *Practitioner* 1982; 226:1102–9.
10. Maddox GL, Liederman V: Overweight as a social disability with medical implications. *J Med Educ* 1969;44:214–20.
11. Rand CSW, Macgregor AMC. Morbidly obese patients' perceptions of social discrimination before and after surgery for obesity. *South Med J* 1990;83:1390–5.
12. Canning H, Mayer J: Obesity: its possible effects on college admissions. *N Engl J Med* 1966; 275:1172–4.
13. Pargaman D. The incidence of obesity among college students. *J Sch Health* 1969;29:621–5.
14. Roe DA, Eickwort KR. Relationships between obesity and associated health factors with unemployment among low-income women. *J Am Med Wom Assoc* 1976;31:193–4, 198–9, 203–4.
15. Fat execs get slimmer paychecks. *Industry Week* 1974;180:21–4.
16. Karris L: Prejudice against obese renters. *J Social Psychol* 1977;101:159–60.
17. Goldblatt PB, Moore ME, Stunkard AJ. Social factors in obesity. *JAMA* 1965;192:1039–44.
18. Soball J, Stunkard AJ. Socioeconomic status and obesity: a review of the literature. *Psychol Bull* 1989;105:260–75.
19. Moore ME, Stunkard AJ, Srole L. Obesity, social class and mental illness. *JAMA* 1962;181:962–6.
20. Stewart AL, Brook RH. Effects of being overweight. *Am J Public Health* 1983;73:171–8.
21. Crisp AH, McGuiness B. Jolly fat: relation between obesity and psychoneurosis in general population. *Br Med J* 1976;3:7–9.
22. Silverstone JT. Psychosocial aspects of obesity. *Proc R Soc Med* 1968;61:371–5.
23. Floderus B. Psycho-social factors in relation to coronary heart disease and associated risk factors. *Nord Hyg Tidskr* 1974;Suppl 6.
24. Hallstrom T, Noppa H. Obesity in women in relation to mental illness, social factors and personality traits. *J Psychosom Res* 1981;25:75–82.
25. Hallberg L, Hogdahl A-M, Nilsson L, Rybo G. Fetma hos kvinnor: sociala data, symptom och fynd. *Lakartidn* 1966;63:621.
26. Kittel F, Rustin RM, Dramaix M, DeBacker G, Kornitzer M: Psychosocio-biological correlates of moderate overweight in an industrial population. *J Psychosom Res* 1978;22:145.
27. Larsson B: *Obesity: a population study of men, with special reference to the development and consequences for the health.* [Dissertation]. Gotab, Kungalv, Sweden: University of Goteborg, 1978.
28. Kaplan KK, Wadden TA: Childhood obesity and self-esteem. *J Pediatr* 1986;109:367–70.
29. Wadden TA, Foster GD, Brownell KD, Finley B: Self-concept in obese and normal weight children. *J Consult Clin Psychol* 1984;52:1104–5.
30. Wadden TA, Brown G, Foster GD, Linowitz JR. Salience of weight related worries in adolescent males and females. *Int J Eating Disorders* 1991;10:407–14.
31. Wadden TA, Foster GD, Stunkard AJ, Linowitz JR. Dissatisfaction with weight and figure in obese girls: discontent but not depression. *Int J Obes* 1989;13:89–97.
32. Sallade J. A comparison of the psychological adjustment of obese vs. nonobese children. *J Psychosom Res* 1973;17:89–96.
33. Hathaway SR, McKinnley JC. *Minnesota Multiphasic Personality Inventory.* Minneapolis: University of Minnesota, 1982.
34. Johnson SF, Swenson WM, Gastineau CF. Personality characteristics in obesity: relation of MMPI profile and age of onset of obesity to success in weight reduction. *Am J Clin Nutr* 1976;29:626–32.
35. Kollar EJ, Atkinson RM, Albin DL. The effectiveness of fasting in the treatment of superobesity. *Psychosomatics* 1968;10:125–35.
36. Lauer JB, Wampler RS, Lantz JB, Romine CJ. Psychosocial aspects of extremely obese women joining a diet group. *Int J Obes* 1979;3:153–61.
37. Leon GR, Eckert ED, Teed D, Buchwald H. Changes in body image and other psychological factors after intestinal bypass surgery for massive obesity. *J Behav Med* 1979;2:39–55.
38. McCall RJ. MMPI factors that differentiate reme-

diably from irremediably obese women. *J Commun Psychol* 1973;1:34–6.

39. Pomerantz AS, Greenberg S, Blackburn GL. MMPI profiles of obese men and women. *Psychol Rep* 1977;41:731–4.

40. Rosen LW, Aniskiewicz AS. Psychosocial functioning of two groups of morbidly obese patients. *Int J Obes* 1983;7:53–9.

41. Solow C, Silberfarb PM, Swift K. Psychosocial effects of intestinal bypass surgery for severe obesity. *N Engl J Med* 1974;290:300–4.

42. Svanum S, Lantz JB, Lauer JB, Wampler RS, Madura JA. Correspondence of the MMPI and the MMPI-168 with intestinal bypass surgery patients. *J Clin Psychol* 1981;37:137–41.

43. Webb WW, Phares R, Abram HS, Meixel SA, Scott HW, Gerdes JT. Jejunoileal bypass procedures in morbid obesity: preoperative psychological findings. *J Clin Psychol* 1976;32:82–5.

44. Wadden TA, Stunkard AJ, Brownell KD, Day SC. Treatment of obesity by behavior therapy and very-low-calorie diet: a pilot investigation. *J Consult Clin Psychol* 1984;52:692–4.

45. McReynolds WT. Toward a psychology of obesity: review of research on the role of personality and level of adjustments. *Int J Eating Disorders* 1982;2:37–57.

46. O'Neil PM, Jarrell MP. Psychological aspects of obesity and dieting. In: Wadden TA, VanItallie TB, eds. *Treatment of the seriously obese patient.* New York: Guilford Press, 1992;252–270.

47. Barrash J, Rodriguez EM, Scott DH, Mason EE, Sines JO. The utility of MMPI subtypes for the prediction of weight loss after bariatric surgery. *Int J Obes* 1987;11:115–28.

48. Blankenmeyer BC, Smylie KD, Price PC, Costillo RM, McFee AS, Fuller DS. A replicated 5 cluster MMPI typology of morbidly obese female candidates for gastric surgery. *Int J Obes* 1990; 14:235–47.

49. Duckro PN, Leavitt JN, Beal DG, Chang AF. Psychological status among female candidates for surgical treatment. *Int J Obes* 1983;7:477–86.

50. Swenson WM, Pearson JS, Osborne D. *An MMPI source book.* Minneapolis: University of Minnesota Press, 1973.

51. Crumpton E, Wine DB, Groot H. MMPI profiles of obese men and six other diagnostic categories. *Psychol Rep* 1966;19:1110–5.

52. Holland J, Masling J, Copley D. Mental illness in lower class normal, obese and hyperobese women. *Psychosom Med* 1970;32:351–7.

53. Mendelson N, Weinberg N, Stunkard AJ. Obesity in men: a clinical study of twenty-five cases. *Ann Intern Med* 1961;54:660–71.

54. Klesges RC. Relationship between psychological factors and body fat in preschool children: a longitudinal investigation. *J Consult Clin Psychol* [in press].

55. Klesges RC. Personality and obesity: global versus specific measures? *Behav Assess* 1984;6:347–56.

56. Wadden TA, Foster GD. Behavioral assessment and treatment of markedly obese patients. In: Wadden TA, Van Itallie TB, eds. *Treatment of the seriously obese patient.* New York: Guilford Press, 1992;290–330.

57. Rodin J, Silberstein L, Streigel-Moore R. Women and weight: a normative discontent. In: Soneregger TB, ed. *Psychology and gender: Nebraska symposium on motivation.* Lincoln, NE: University of Nebraska Press, 1988;257–307.

58. Stunkard AJ, Mendelson M. Disturbances in body image of some obese persons. *J Am Diet Assoc* 1961;38:328–31.

59. Stunkard AJ, Mendelson M. Obesity and the body image: I. Characteristics of disturbances in the body image of some obese persons. *Am J Psychiatry* 1967;123:1296–300.

60. Stunkard AJ, Burt V. Obesity and the body image: II. Age at onset of disturbances in the body image. *Am J Psychiatry* 1967;123:1443–7.

61. Wadden TA, Stunkard AJ, Rich L, Rubin CJ, Sweidel G, McKinney S. Obesity in black adolescent girls: a controlled clinical trial of treatment by diet, behavior modification, and parental support. *Pediatrics* 1990;85:345–51.

62. Stern MP, Pugh JA, Gaskill SP, et al. Knowledge, attitudes, and behavior related to obesity and dieting in Mexican Americans and Anglos: the San Antonio heart study. *Am J Epidemiol* 1982; 115:917–27.

63. Andersen AE, Hay A. Racial and socioeconomic influences in anorexia nervosa and bulimia. *Int J Eating Disorders* 1985;4:479–87.

64. Stunkard AJ. Eating patterns and obesity. *Psychiatr Q* 1959;33:284–95.

65. Stunkard AJ. *The pain of obesity.* Palo Alto: Bull Publishing, 1976.

66. Russell G. Bulimia nervosa: an ominous variant of anorexia nervosa. *Psychol Med* 1979;9:429–48.

67. Gormally J, Black S, Daston S, Rardin D. The assessment of binge eating severity among obese persons. *Addict Behav* 1982;7:47–55.

68. Keefe PH, Wyshogrod D, Weinberger E, Agras WS. Binge eating and outcome of behavioral treatment of obesity: a preliminary report. *Behav Res Ther* 1984;22:319–22.

69. Marcus MD, Wing RR, Lamparski DM: Binge eating and dietary restraint in obese patients. *Addict Behav* 1985;10:163–68.

70. Spitzer RL, Devlin M, Walsh BT, et al. Binge eating disorder: a multisite field trial of the diagnostic criteria. *Int J Eating Disorders* 1992;11:191–204.

71. Telch CF, Agras WS, Rossiter E, Wilfley D, Kenardy J. Group cognitive-behavioral treatment for the non-purging bulimic: an initial evaluation. *J Consult Clin Psychol* 1990;58:629–35.

72. Telch CF, Agras WS, Rossiter EM. Binge eating with increasing adiposity. *Int J Eating Disorders* 1988;7:115–9.

73. Lowe MR, Caputo GC. Binge eating in obesity: toward the specification of predictors. *Int J Eating Disorders* 1991;10:49–55.

74. Hudson JI, Pope HG, Wurtman J, Yurgelun-Todd D, Mark S, Rosenthal NE. Bulimia in obese individuals. Relationship to normal-weight bulimia. *J Nerv Ment Dis* 1988;176:144–52.

75. Kolotkin RL, Revis ES, Kirkley BG, Janick L. Binge eating in obesity: associated MMPI characteristics. *J Consult Clin Psychol* 1987;55:872–6.

76. Marcus MD, Wing RR, Hopkins J. Obese binge eaters: affect, cognitions, and response to behav-

ioral weight control. *J Consult Clin Psychol* 1988;56:433–9.

77. Marcus MD, Wing RR, Ewing L, Kern E, Gooding W, McDermott M. Psychiatric disorders among obese binge eaters. *Int J Eating Disorders* 1990;9:69–77.

78. Wadden TA, Foster GD, Letizia KA. Response of obese binge eaters to treatment by behavior therapy combined with very low calorie diet. *J Consult Clin Psychol* [*in press*].

79. Beck AT, Ward CH, Mendelson M, Mock J, Erbaugh J. An inventory for measuring depression. *Arch Gen Psychiatry* 1961;4:561–71.

80. Hsu LKG. *Eating disorders.* New York: Guilford Press, 1990.

81. Walsh BT, Hadigan CM, Devlin MJ, Gladis M, Roose SP. Long-term outcome of antidepressant treatment for bulimia nervosa. *Am J Psychiatry* 1991;148:1206–12.

82. Agras WS, Rossiter EM, Arnow B, et al. Pharmacologic and cognitive-behavioral treatment for bulimia nervosa: a controlled comparison. *Am J Psychiatry* 1992;149:82–7.

83. Levy AB, Dixon KN, Stern SL. How are depression and bulimia related? *Am J Psychiatry* 1989;146:162–9.

84. Polivy J, Herman CP. Dieting and binging: a causal analysis. *Am Psychol* 1985;40:193–201.

85. Keys A, Brozek J, Henschel A, Mickelsen F, Taylor HL. *The biology of human starvation.* Minneapolis: University of Minnesota Press, 1950.

86. National Center for Health Statistics. Provisional data from the Health Promotion and Disease Prevention Supplement to the National Health Interview Survey: United States, Jan–Mar 1985. *Advancedata* 1985;Nov 2–5.

87. Marketdata Enterprises. *The U.S. weight loss and diet control market.* Lynbrook, NY: Marketdata Enterprises, March, 1989.

88. Stunkard AJ, Rush J. Dieting and depression reexamined: a critical review of untoward responses during weight reduction for obesity. *Ann Intern Med* 1974;81:526–33.

89. Wing RR, Epstein LH, Marcus MD, Kupfer DJ: Mood changes in behavioral weight loss programs. *J Psychosom Res* 1984;28:189–96.

90. Beck AT, Rush AJ, Shaw BF, Emery G. *Cognitive therapy of depression.* New York: Guilford Press, 1979.

91. Smoller JW, Wadden TA, Stunkard AJ. Dieting and depression: a critical review. *J Psychosom Res* 1987;31:429–40.

92. Spielberger CD, Gorsuch RL, Lushene R. *The State-Trait Anxiety Inventory.* Palo Alto, CA: Consulting Psychologists Press, 1983.

93. Wadden TA, Stunkard AJ, Smoller JW. Dieting and depression: a methodological study. *J Consult Clin Psychol* 1986;54:869–71.

94. Kramer FM, Jeffery RW, Forster JL, Snell MK: Long-term follow-up of behavioral treatment for obesity: patterns of weight regain among men and women. *Int J Obes* 1989;13:123–36.

95. Wadden TA, Bartlett SJ. Very low calorie diets: an overview and appraisal. In: Wadden TA, VanItallie TB, eds. *Treatment of the seriously obese patient.* New York: Guilford Press, 1992;44–79.

96. Brownell KD, Stunkard AJ. Couples training, pharmacotherapy, and behavior therapy in the treatment of obesity. *Arch Gen Psychiatry* 1981; 38:1233–9.

97. Wadden TA, Stunkard AJ, Liebschutz J. Three-year follow-up of the treatment of obesity by very low calorie diet, behavior therapy and their combination. *J Consult Clin Psychol* 1988;56:925–8.

98. Wadden TA, Bartlett SJ, Letizia KA, Foster GD, Stunkard AJ, Conill A. Relationship of dieting history to resting metabolic rate, body composition, eating behavior and subsequent weight loss. *Am J Clin Nutr* [*in press*].

99. American Psychiatric Association. *Diagnostic and statistical manual of mental disorders,* 3rd ed, revised. Washington, DC: American Psychiatric Association, 1987.

100. Wadden TA, Letizia KA. Predictors of attrition and weight loss in patients treated by moderate and severe caloric restriction. In: Wadden TA, VanItallie TB, eds. *Treatment of the seriously obese patient.* New York: Guilford Press, 1992;383–410.

101. Brownell KD, Marlatt GA, Lichtenstein E, Wilson GT. Understanding and preventing relapse. *Am Psychol* 1986;41:765–82.

102. LaPorte DJ, Stunkard AJ. Predicting attrition and adherence to a very low calorie diet: a prospective investigation of the Eating Inventory. *Int J Obes* 1990;14:197–206.

103. Felitti VJ: Long-term medical consequences of incest, rape and molestation. *South Med J* 1991;84:328–31.

104. Stuart RB, Jacobson B. *Weight, sex and marriage.* New York: WW Norton, 1987.

105. Rand CSW, Kuldau JM, Robbins L. Surgery for obesity and marriage quality. *JAMA* 1982; 247:1419–22.

106. Rand CSW, Kowalski K, Kuldau JM. Characteristics of marital improvement following obesity surgery. *Psychosomatics* 1984;25:221–6.

Obesity: Theory and Therapy, Second Edition,
edited by A. J. Stunkard and T. A. Wadden.
Raven Press, Ltd., New York © 1993.

11

Cultural Perspectives on the Etiology and Treatment of Obesity

Peter J. Brown

Department of Anthropology, Emory University, Atlanta, Georgia 30322

Culturally patterned behaviors and beliefs play an important role in the etiology of human obesity and therefore have practical implications for its prevention and treatment. This chapter uses an anthropological perspective to examine the relationship between culture and obesity; the approach is both evolutionary and cross-culturally comparative. Such a perspective can add to our understanding of obesity in the broadest contexts of history and human behavior. This chapter has two goals: to examine the biocultural evolution of the genes and behaviors that cause obesity, and to identify cultural beliefs and behaviors that may predispose individuals to the condition. The first goal concerns etiology. The second goal is relevant to the treatment or prevention of obesity in different social and ethnic groups.

The etiology of obesity is complex. It is generally recognized that excess adiposity is caused by the interaction of genetic diatheses or predispositions that operate in the context of necessary "environmental" conditions. This chapter uses the anthropological concept of *culture* in preference to the undifferentiated idea of environment. Environment has too often been left undefined—relegated to a residual, nongenetic category that is idiosyncratic to individuals. In recent years, the evidence for the existence of genes that enable individuals to store energy reserves in the form of fat has been increasingly impressive; those individuals with "fat phenotypes" are likely to develop adult obesity (1–6). These genes, and the metabolic processes of fat deposition they induce, are very old; they are part of our species' evolutionary heritage dating back at least twenty thousand years and probably more.

On the other hand, the environmental/cultural conditions necessary for a high prevalence of obesity are quite new. Throughout most of human history, obesity was neither a common health problem nor a realistic possibility for most people. This is because humans have been regularly subjected to food shortages in the process of their biological and cultural evolution. These food shortages, which continue to plague humanity, have been powerful agents of natural selection for both genes and cultural traits. It is only in the context of relative affluence and constant food surpluses that obesity and overweight have become such widespread and intractable health problems.

Both genes and cultural practices are involved in the etiology of obesity, although not necessarily with equal influence. While cultural influences may be less important than genes in a statistical sense, they are more important in terms of the treatment and prevention of obesity. This is simply for the reason that cultural predispositions to obesity are changeable. As such, culture is the key to prevention: the existing beliefs and practices of populations at greatest risk for obesity must be understood if appropriate and effective health intervention are to be designed. Culture plays a role not only in diet and exercise patterns, but also in the perception of health problems, and the pattern of health-seeking behavior by individuals. Most importantly, an understanding of the cultural beliefs and practices of patient populations, particularly those from minority ethnic groups, is important for establishing effective cross-cultural communication between patients and their health-care providers. Research from medical anthropology suggests that there are practical clinical benefits to such cultural sensitivity.

This chapter is organized in three parts: it begins with a consideration of the epidemiological distribution of obesity and the basic concept of culture; next, it reviews the evidence for the biocultural evolution of predispositions to obesity; finally, it applies the cultural perspective to understanding variations in a patient's explanatory models for obesity and the symbolic meanings of obesity that may have relevance to programs for prevention or treatment. Cultural factors in five groups with elevated risk for obesity (i.e., Hispanic Americans, African Americans, Native Americans, and Pacific Islanders) are summarized.

BASIC CONCEPTS: CULTURE AND THE DESCRIPTIVE EPIDEMIOLOGY OF OBESITY

The concept of culture is intimately related to the concepts of social class and ethnicity, which are, in turn, key factors in the epidemiological distribution of obesity. Descriptive epidemiology involves analysis of the distribution of disease in regard to the variables of time, place, and person. The descriptive epidemiology of obesity, therefore, is a necessary prerequisite for developing a cultural perspective on culture.

Culture and the Case Definition of Obesity

The first step in describing the social epidemiology of obesity is the development of a case definition. The definitions of obesity and overweight have been the subject of substantial medical debate, in part because they must be based upon inferred definitions of normality or "ideal" body proportions. In this regard, it is important to remember that culture defines normalcy. Although obesity refers to excessive fat deposits, the most common measurement is not of fat tissue directly, but of an indirect surrogate measure based upon stature and total body weight (7). There are practical reasons for this situation, including the lack of reliable technology for the direct measurement of fat in a clinical setting. Nevertheless, the scientific debates about the definition of obesity appear to contain a cultural component.

The social and cultural history of height and weight standards in the United States, and the historical changes in the moral meaning of different body types, has been the subject of two recent books by Schwartz (8) and Seid (9). Until recently, the task of defining both obesity and ideal weights has been the domain of the life insurance industry. Insurance tables of "ideal" weight were not based on a random population sample nor did they consider the effects of aging. From 1943 to 1980 definitions of "ideal weights" for height for women were consistently lowered, while those for men remained approximately the same (10). The debate following the 1983 upward revision of ideal weights for women, based on new mortality statistics collected by the insurance industry, revealed that many experts saw the revision as "backsliding." In other words, definitions of ideal and normal body size reflected cultural and cosmetic standards, as well as medical issues. In contemporary American and western European societies, the cosmetic ideal of body size for women is thinner than the medical ideal.

A critically important dimension to the definition of obesity involves the distribution of fat around the body trunk or on the limbs. Truncal body fat is closely correlated with serious chronic diseases like cardiovascular disease, while peripheral body fat in the hips and limbs does not carry similar medical risks.

Because of this important distinction, measures of fat distribution like the waist-to-hip ratio (WHR), wherein a lower WHR indicates lower risk of serious medical consequences, have been suggested as a more useful measure of obesity. In fact, Bjorntorp (11) has argued that only abdominal obesity should be distinguished as obesity, and that peripheral accumulation of fat receive less emphasis in the same way that muscle enlargement, large ears, or large feet are not distinguished by medical terminology either (11). Given the cultural emphasis on body weight in American society, it is not likely that the definition of medical obesity will be changed in this way, despite its powerful medical logic.

Epidemiology of Obesity: Time, Place, and Person

The distribution of obesity can be considered in regard to time, place, and person. Like most diseases, obesity exhibits a nonrandom historical and social distribution; any theory of the etiology of obesity must account for those distributions.

From an anthropological or archaeological view of time, the current "epidemic" of overweight and obesity is very recent. For 99% of history since the appearance of the genus *Homo,* the exclusive cultural pattern for humans was one of hunting and gathering. Today, this original human life style is rare and limited to marginal ecological zones, but a few such groups have been the subject of intensive cultural and biological investigation. One important finding has been that there are *no* reported cases of obesity among people following a hunting and gathering way of life. Such food foragers do not store surplus food and, in general, demonstrate an egalitarian distribution of food brought into camp. In contrast, Paleolithic "Venus" figurines, some (but not all) of which demonstrate marked obesity, are not in agreement with the observation of no obesity in contemporary hunter gatherers. The production of these figurines is limited to a narrow prehistoric time frame (Gravettian Period, 27,000 to 19,000 BC) in Europe, during the coldest part of the last glaciation; Brown has suggested that these exceptional artifacts were produced by an extinct and unique form of food-foraging social organization based on megafauna hunting and permanent settlements (12). With this important exception, obesity was essentially nonexistent until after the invention of farming some 10,000 years ago, and more specifically until after the Industrial Revolution (8).

Obesity has become a serious and widespread health problem in only certain kinds of societies—those characterized by economic modernization, affluence, food surplus, and social stratification. Numerous studies of traditional societies undergoing the process of economic modernization demonstrate rapid increases in the prevalence of obesity (13–17). Trowell and Burkitt's volume of 15 case studies (18) of epidemiological change in modernizing societies concludes that obesity is the first of the "diseases of civilization" to appear.

In regard, to the epidemiological question of *place,* obesity appears to be most common in certain kinds of societies rather than in societies located in particular geographic zones (19). The highest reported prevalence of obesity is on the Micronesian island of Nauru; the age-standardized prevalence of adult obesity is 84.7% of males and 92.8% of females (20); the inhabitants of Nauru are extremely wealthy because of valuable mineral deposits on the island. In Europe, there are higher prevalences of obesity in southern European countries than northern ones, and within those samples the risk of obesity is higher in rural than urban areas (21). Within the United States, a country with a high overall prevalence of overweight and obesity (22), the behavioral risk factor surveys coordinated by the Centers for Disease Control indicate that states in the northern part of the Midwest have the highest prevalence of obesity, with Wisconsin characterized by the most elevated prevalence (23). In contrast, it should be remembered that certain ecological zones appear to be more prone to severe food shortages. One example is the prehistoric southwestern United States, where, according to Minnis (24), impressive Pueblo societies expanded during a period of uncharacteristic good weather and could not be maintained when the regular pattern of low rainfall resumed.

The epidemiological question of *person*—what social groupings are most at risk for obesity—is most important. There are three facts about this social distribution that are particularly cogent: (a) a gender difference in the total percent and site distribution of body fat, as well as the prevalence of obesity; (b) the concentration of obesity in certain ethnic groups; and (c) a powerful and complex relationship between social class and obesity.

The greatest degree of sexual dimorphism in humans is in the site of distribution of fat tissue; women have much more peripheral body fat in the legs and hips (25). This pattern of gender differences appears to be universal since it is found in contemporary hunting and gathering groups like the !Kung San, as well as in complex industrial countries (26). This gender dimorphism has evolutionary roots, as described below.

The relationship between the risk of obesity and social class has received substantial research attention. Social class is a powerful predictor of the prevalence of obesity in both modernizing and affluent societies, although the direction of the association varies with the type of society. This relationship is the subject of a comprehensive review by Sobal and Stunkard (27) that cites more than 100 separate studies. In developing countries, there is a strong and consistent positive association of social class and obesity for men, women, and children; correspondingly, there is an inverse correlation between social class and protein-calorie malnutrition (28). This is a logical and expected pattern in that socially dominant groups with better access to strategic resources should have better nutrition and better health.

In heterogeneous and affluent societies like the United States, there is a strong inverse correlation of social class and obesity for females (29–32). The association of obesity and social class among women in affluent societies is not constant through the life cycle. Garn and Clark (33) have demonstrated a pattern of reversal in which economically advantaged girls are initially fatter than their poor counterparts, but as adults they show less overweight and obesity. The inverse correlation of obesity and social class for females in affluent societies is extremely strong and carries with it important socially symbolic associations.

In the United States, ethnic groups with elevated rates of obesity include: African Americans (particularly in the rural south) (34), Southwestern Native Americans (34a), Hispanic Americans and Puerto Ricans (35), Gypsies (36), and Pacific Islanders (20). The high prevalence of obesity in ethnic groups probably reflects the interaction of genes, social class, and culture; it is a difficult task to disentangle the relative effects of these factors.

The Concept of Culture

The concept of culture has relevance to the descriptive epidemiology of obesity. From an anthropological perspective, culture plays a fundamental role in causing the social epidemiological distribution of obesity. Culture refers to the learned patterns of behavior and belief characteristic of a social group. A cultural system of thought and behavior may be shared by an isolated tribe or, in a complex society, an ethnic group or social class. Culture includes directly observable material aspects, like diet or productive economy, as well as important ideological components, such as aesthetic standards of ideal body type; the relationship of the material aspects of culture to the etiology of obesity may be directly demonstrated while the relationship of ideological components and obesity remains more speculative.

Cultural behaviors and beliefs are learned in childhood and they are often deeply held and seldom questioned by adults who pass this "obvious" knowledge and habits to their offspring. As such, cultural beliefs and values are largely unconscious factors in the motivation of individual behaviors. Cultural beliefs define "what is normal" and therefore constrain the choices of behaviors available to an individual.

The concept of culture is clearly related to social categories like social class and ethnicity. Social groups can be characterized by cultural beliefs and practices. It is not membership in a lower social class *per se* that causes higher rates of morbidity and mortality from infectious disease, but rather elements of the overall culture that characterize that group, e.g., levels of nutrition, hygienic conditions, crowding, or access to health care. As such, it is appropriate to think of a culture of social class. For members of the lower social class, anthropologists have shown that their cultural beliefs and practices function as adaptations to conditions of economic deprivation (37).

Ethnicity refers to the cultural commonalities of members of a group who claim reference to common origins and who operate in the context of a wider social system. Social scientists sometimes differentiate between behavioral ethnics and ideological ethnics. The first category refers to people living within urban ethnic enclaves, often distinguished by language, whose diet and daily life is shaped by the ethnic culture. Ideological ethnics are generally indistinguishable from members of the dominant society in overall behavior, but their ethnicity is a primary part of personal identity.

In terms of overall human history, culture represents *Homo sapiens'* primary mechanism of evolutionary adaptation. In fact, culture is the primary reason for the evolutionary success of humans because of its distinct advantages of greater speed and flexibility over genetic evolution (38). Anthropologists believe that the thousands of cultural variations in the world today are all derived from the original human life style of hunting and gathering; this was the exclusive cultural pattern from two million years ago until about ten thousand years ago. It can be convinc-

ingly argued that contemporary human biology was largely shaped by this prehistoric past, and that modern chronic diseases are the result of a discordance between our paleolithic biology and the modern culture of affluence (39).

One useful way of thinking about culture in relation to obesity is a cultural-materialist model developed by Harris (40). This model divides culture into three interrelated levels: (a) the productive economy, including the technology and population size the economy allows and requires; (b) the social organization, including kinship and marriage patterns, politics, and status differentiation; and (c) the ideology or belief system, including both sacred and secular ideas, beliefs, and values. In this model, each level is contingent upon the preceding one, and the entire cultural system is constrained by the local ecological setting. Ideology is probably the most important part of culture, in part because it rationalizes and reinforces the economy and social structure, but also because it allows people to make sense of their world and to share their common worldview through symbols. Cultural ideologies include systems of medical beliefs and practices.

A culture is an integrated system, so that a change in one part causes changes on the other levels. The materialist model indicates that the direction of causal change is from the bottom layer upward; an economic change, like the invention of agriculture or the industrial revolution, had drastic implications for population size, social organization, and associated beliefs. On the other hand, most people *within* a society tend to explain things from the top down, that is, the ideology is used to explain customs and social patterns. Cultural beliefs, however, are not necessary predictors of actual behavior.

Brown has shown that all three of these levels of a cultural system play a role in the etiology of obesity (26). The productive economy must produce a food surplus that is distributed through the social system. Both the productive economy and the social system had adaptive functions in the context of food shortages, particularly for the privileged classes. The way in which cultural beliefs can function as predisposing factors in the etiology of obesity is discussed below.

THE ETIOLOGY OF OBESITY: BIOCULTURAL EVOLUTION

A theory about the etiology of obesity must be able to account for the epidemiological distribution of the condition in terms of history and its relationship to gender, economic modernization, and social class. The basic biological mechanisms of genetics, adipose cell functioning, the pharmacology of satiety, and energy metabolism should be considered as proximate causes of obesity because these metabolic functions are themselves the result of evolution.

Human biology and behavior can be understood in the context of two distinct but interacting processes of evolution. Biological evolution involves changes in the frequency of particular genes over time, primarily because of the action of natural selection on individuals. Cultural evolution involves historical changes in the configurations of cultural systems, especially their economies. The anthropological record has many examples of genetic and cultural evolution enhancing each other in a pattern that may be called biocultural evolution or coevolution (41).

In the case of obesity, Stunkard (42) has described models of the possible interaction of genes and environment, whether they are additive, or whether genes affect sensitivity to environmental stimuli or exposure to the environment. The application of any of these models needs to wait until there is a better understanding of "environmental" factors; genetic studies suggest that in an additive model, the role of environment is rather small. The significant progress in recent years in clarifying the genetic contribution to obesity has, to a significant degree, highlighted our ignorance about the role of culture or environment. Both genes and cultural traits that today predispose individuals to obesity are the result of the operation of natural selection through food shortages.

Genetic Evolution and Food Scarcity

Food shortages have been so common in human prehistory and history that they could be considered an inevitable fact of life for most people. As such, they have been a powerful force in both biological and cultural evolution.

A cross-cultural ethnographic survey by Whiting (43) of 118 nonindustrial societies (with hunting and gathering, pastoral, horticultural, and agricultural economies) found some form of food shortages for *all* of the societies in the sample. Shortages occur annually or even more frequently in roughly half of the societies, and every 2 to 3 years in an additional 24%. Whiting described the shortage as "severe" (i.e., including starvation deaths) in 29% of the societies sampled. Seasonal availability of food results in a seasonal cycle of weight loss and weight gain in both hunting and gathering and agricultural societies, although the fluctuation is substantially greater among agriculturalists (44,45). The threat of food shortages and hunger plagues a large proportion of the world's population today, including an estimated 20 million Americans (46).

Since food shortages were ubiquitous for humans under natural conditions, selection favored individuals who could effectively store calories in times of surplus. For most societies, such fat stores would be called on at least every 2 to 3 years. Malnutrition from food shortages has a synergistic affect on infectious disease mortality, as well as decreasing birth weights and rates of child growth (47). Females with greater energy reserves in fat would have a selective advantage over their lean counterparts in withstanding the stress of food shortage, not only for themselves, but for their fetuses or nursing children. Humans have evolved to "save up" food energy for the inevitability of food shortages through the synthesis and storage of fat.

Females have been selected for more peripheral body fat that is usually mobilized after being endocrine-primed during later pregnancy and lactation (48). In addition, a minimal level of female fatness increases reproductive success because of its association with regular cycling as well as earlier menarche (49).

In this evolutionary context the usual range of human metabolic variation must have produced many individuals with a predisposition to become obese, yet they would never have the opportunity to do so. Furthermore, in this context there could be little or no natural selection against such a tendency. Selection could not provide for the eventuality of continuous surplus because it had simply never existed.

Genetic selection would have been particularly intense in certain historical-ecological contexts affecting small populations; such conditions may act as evolutionary "bottlenecks" combining natural selection and founder effect. Wendorf (50) has described the severe ecological conditions faced by the Paleoindian ancestors of southwestern Native American groups during their long migration along the Beringia ice corridor as an example of such a bottleneck. Other migration episodes, for example in Polynesia, may have operated in a similar way.

In the modern context, genes that predispose for obesity might be maintained within ethnic groups because of the widespread social practice of endogamy, or marriage within the group; in the United States, marriage partner correlations for ethnic minorities are extremely high (51). This social practice may concentrate the genetic predispositions to obesity in particular subpopulations. Similarly, preliminary data suggest a pattern of "assortative mating" by social class as well as body type (particularly stature), which may also be related to the genetic etiology of obesity. Genetic admixture with American Indian groups of the Southwest has been suggested as a cause of elevated non-insulin-dependent diabetes mellitus (NIDDM) and obesity rates among Mexican Americans (52).

Obesity and Cultural Evolution

Cultural evolution refers to systematic changes in social pattern of behavior and belief over time. As the population of human groups expands, their productive economies, institutions, and beliefs must accommodate that expansion. Such historical changes are relevant for understanding the possibility of obesity in regard to social class.

Approximately 12,000 years ago, some human groups shifted from a food-foraging economy to one based on agriculture; this economic transformation allowed for the evolution of complex civilizations. Archaeologists believe that the new agricultural economy was something that people were "forced" to adopt because of ecological pressures from population growth and food scarcities, or from military coercion (53). There is little doubt from the archeological record that the beginning of agriculture was associated with nutritional stress, poor health, and diminished stature (54,55).

The beginning of agriculture is also linked to the emergence of social stratification, a system of inequality that had clear advantages to the health and reproductive success of the ruling class. This continuing pattern of social inequality, particularly the fact that lower classes suffer a greater risk of experiencing hunger, still plays a critical role in the distribution of obesity. The evolution of social stratification meant that in the context of a relative food shortage, the poor would experience hunger first and therefore serve to insulate upper classes from food scarcity. Endemic hunger exists even in the most affluent societies, where it is caused not by poor production but by inequitable distribution.

The invention of agriculture, and particularly industrial agriculture, allowed for the production of a reliable surplus of food. At the same time, the evolution of a global market system allows societies to overcome any local food production shortages, if that society has sufficient political and economic power. On the other hand, the energy-intensive (and energy-inefficient) industrial agriculture system produces large surpluses of food that are generally not used to eliminate hunger. Instead, the pattern has been to transform foods in processes that most often add calories, fat, and salt. For example, "extra" grain is fed to cattle to increase the proportion of fat in their meat. Similarly, potatoes are transformed into french fries and potato chips in a process that reduces the original vegetable to a vehicle for fat and salt.

Technological changes associated with cultural evolution exclusively reduce the energy requirements of human labor. General cultural evolution has meant the harnessing of greater amounts of energy through technology. For example, traveling in a car saves energy for the passengers, but it also spends energy in the form of fossil fuel. In this regard, the statistical association of television watching and obesity in children (56) is the result of lower activity levels. Television also carries strong and sometimes contradictory symbolic messages about eating and ideal body types (57). In affluent cultures with television, physical exercise has become a commodity; people must burn energy through daily workouts rather than through daily work.

Cultural evolution has also affected patterns of human reproduction and infant feeding that may play a role in the higher elevation of obesity in females. In traditional societies, pregnancy and lactation represent serious and continuing energy demands on women. One cultural solution to this problem has been the custom of "fattening huts" for elite pubescent girls in traditional West Africa, particularly among the Annang, Efik, and Ibibio of Nigeria (58–60) as well as parts of Oceania (61). A girl spent up to 2 years in seclusion, during which she was well fed and not allowed to work; at the end of this rite of passage girls publicly display symbols of womanhood and marriageability, particularly fatness, which is a primary criterion of feminine beauty. In a detailed description of this cultural practice in contemporary Nigeria, Brink (58) emphasizes that the fattening hut is a conspicuous display of wealth by elites, who alone had the economic resources to par-

ticipate in this custom. [Similarly, fatter brides demand significantly higher bridewealth payments among the Kipsigis of Kenya (62).] The health benefit of this custom is that elite women start heavy energy demands of their reproductive careers with an energy surplus in the form of peripheral fat. Poorer women in traditional societies correspondingly suffer greater risk of protein-energy malnutrition.

On the other hand, the fact that women in economically developed societies have fewer pregnancies and are less likely to breast-feed means that they also have less opportunity to mobilize peripheral fat stores and suffer greater risk of obesity. The inverse correlation between social class and bottle feeding in the United States in this way contributes to the inverse relation of social class and obesity.

Cultural Beliefs as Predispositions to Obesity

The behavioral aspects of culture that allow for obesity have corresponding ideological or symbolic components. Fatness is symbolically linked to psychological dimensions such as "self-worth" and sexuality in many societies of the world, but the nature of that symbolic association is not constant. In mainstream US culture, obesity is socially stigmatized (63,64), but for most cultures of the world, fatness is viewed as a welcome sign of health and prosperity (65). In preindustrial societies, in contrast, thinness is stigmatized as a symptom of starvation [as among the !Kung San of Botswana (66)] or as a sign of AIDS in contemporary central Africa. Among middle and upper class women in the United States, thinness represents the moral success of self-control over one's body (57,60).

For women, fatness may also be a symbol of maternity and nurturance. In traditional societies in which women attain status primarily through motherhood, this symbolic association increases the cultural acceptability of obesity. A fat woman, symbolically, is well taken care of, and she in turn takes good care of her children. The cultural ideal of thinness in developed societies, in contrast, is found in societies in which motherhood is not the primary means of status attainment for women. This transformation is a modern historical one, and anthropologists have described the coinciding cultural changes in ecology, domestic gender relations, and cultural ideals of body type (61); in rural Spain, this change in the ideal social and physical image of women is described as moving from the Virgin Mary to the "modern woman" (67), while for Africa, Powdermaker has described the change in the role of women from that of mother to that of mate (68). Culturally defined standards of the body beautiful vary between societies and across historical epochs. In a preliminary cross-cultural survey using the Human Relation Area File data, Brown (26) found that 81% of the societies for which there were sufficient data rated "plumpness" or being "filled out" as an attribute of beauty in females; this was particularly the case for the desirability of fat deposits on the hips and legs. For example, among Havasupai of the American Southwest, if a girl at puberty is thin, a fat woman "stands" (places her foot) on the girl's back so that she will become attractively plump: in this society, fat legs and arms are considered essential to beauty (69). Among the Amhara of the Horn of Africa, thin hips are called "dog hips" in a typical insult (70). In cross-cultural research it appears that for the men, the body ideal has most often been bigness, but not necessarily fatness (26,60).

American ideals of thinness occur in a setting in which it is easy to become fat, and the preference for plumpness occurs in settings in which it is easy to remain lean. In context, both standards require the investment of individual effort and economic resources.

CULTURAL FACTORS IN THE PREVENTION AND TREATMENT OF OBESITY

There are effective ways of using the cultural perspective for improving programs for community prevention or individual treatment of obesity. The most important practical suggestion from medical anthropology is that health-care providers try to understand the "native's" point of view about health problems. Poor communication can result from assuming that the patient (or community) share a common set of interpretations about the meaning of symptoms. In the context of medical care, it is effective for the clinician to be able to elicit the patient's "explanatory model" of illness (71). A patient's explanatory model refers to the logical framework with which he or she makes sense of symptoms, interprets medical advice, and makes decisions about seeking care. While lay explanatory models show some individual variations, most research indicates that ethnicity is an extremely important factor. In the clinical context, Kleinman and colleagues (72) have shown that a patient's explanatory model can be learned through a few additional questions asked while taking a patient's history; these questions are listed in Table 1. The primary advantage of asking these questions is to provide a context in which the patient articulates her own point of view. Incongruities between the patient's explanatory model and the view of the health-care provider can then be acknowledged and addressed in a culturally sensitive manner.

It is not safe to assume that health-care providers and their obese or overweight pa-

TABLE 1. *Questions for eliciting a patient's explanatory model*

---

1. What do you think has caused your problem?
2. Why do you think it started when it did?
3. What do you think your sickness does to you? How does it work?
4. How bad (severe) do you think your illness is? Do you think it will last a long time, or will it be better soon, in your opinion?
5. What kind of treatment would you like to have?
6. What are the most important results you hope to get from treatment?
7. What are the chief problems your illness has caused you?
8. What do you fear most about your sickness?

Adapted from Kleinman et al., ref. 71, with permission.

tients share the same ideas about the symbolic meaning of fatness. Among the poor or in ethnic groups with high prevalences of obesity, weight loss may be viewed as a serious symptom of illness or it may be associated with decreased sexual attractiveness for women. Therefore, patients may experience subtle cultural pressures to regain weight. Similarly, physical exercise may be viewed as culturally inappropriate if people think of exercise as requiring the conspicuous consumption of sports products or as an activity only for the young; both of these images appear to be encouraged by the television media. For the urban poor, outdoor exercise may be dangerous.

Culture and Community Interventions

It is important to take account of existing cultural beliefs in the design and implementation of health promotion projects. In an obesity prevention campaign in a Zulu community outside of Durban (73), one health education poster depicted an obese woman and an overloaded truck with a flat tire, with a caption "Both carry too much weight." Another poster shows a slender woman easily sweeping under a table next to an obese woman who is using the table for support; it has the caption "Who do you prefer to look like?" The intended message of these posters was misinterpreted by the community because of a cultural connection between obesity and social status. The woman in the first poster was perceived to be rich and happy, since she was not only fat but had a truck overflowing with her possessions. The second poster was perceived as a scene of an affluent mistress directing her underfed servant.

Health interventions must be culturally acceptable, and in this regard we cannot assume that people place the highest priority on their health. The idea of reducing risk factors for the prevention of later chronic diseases may not be an effective strategy for populations that do not feel empowered because they live in a risky and dangerous world.

Cultural Characteristics of Ethnic Groups at Risk for Obesity

Ethnicity is an important variable both in regard to the distribution of obesity and the types of explanatory models used to explain illness. The topic of ethnicity brings with it the danger of stereotyping, the mistaken notion that all members of a group are alike. Variations in the length of time that persons have been away from their country of origin, their socioeconomic status, and language spoken at home all make cultural stereotyping a dangerous enterprise. Nevertheless, it may be valuable to describe the *range* of variation in behaviors and beliefs among ethnic groups in the United States with high prevalences of obesity. It is important to remember that these ethnic groups are heterogeneous and that upwardly mobile ethnics more closely resemble mainstream American culture in attitudes about obesity and ideal body shape.

It is first necessary, however, to consider some of the cultural behaviors and beliefs about obesity that are characteristic of the dominant white culture. Ritenbaugh (74) has persuasively argued that dominant American social beliefs about obesity are summarized in three "facts" that are, in fact, largely mythological: obesity is always bad for your health; obesity is simply due to overeating and underexercising; and anyone who wants to be can be slim. The idea that anyone can be slim is an important assumption in the social stigmatization of overweight as well as the commercialization of the weight-loss industry.

In dominant American society, overweight and obesity are viewed as obvious symbols of an individual's moral failings in self control. Conversely, slenderness (especially for women) signifies that the individual's self-control over the power of food and the temporary conquest of the body's tendency to gain weight are in decline. Both exercise classes and "dieting" foods are commodities, and the dominant ideology is that some approximation of the "perfect body" can be acquired, given sufficient physical and financial investment (75). In fact, a slender body, like a tan, is viewed as a marker of the leisure time and expendable income of rich "beautiful people." In this way the cultural stigmatization of overweight and obesity plays a central role in the etiology of eating disorders of anorexia nervosa and bulimia. Members of ethnic minorities do not share these cultural beliefs with members of the white majority, although ethnics with higher socioeconomic status are often indistinguishable in beliefs from the dominant culture.

Hispanic Americans

There has been substantial research on social and cultural factors related to obesity among Hispanic Americans, the second largest ethnic minority in the United States (76). The Centers for Disease Control survey of this category of diverse ethnic subgroups (Mexican Americans, Puerto Ricans, Cuban Americans) reported generally high prevalences of overweight and obesity (36). The subgroup with the highest prevalence was Mexican-American women. This group, according to Ritenbaugh (10), has coined a new ethnomedical term *gordura mala* (bad fatness) because the original term *gordura* continues to have positive cultural connotations of health and prosperity. Among Mexican Americans, Hazuda and colleagues (77) have shown that cultural identity has a stronger effect, one that is independent of social class, in relation to the prevalence of obesity. In other words, the more individual behavior and identity was shaped by ethnic identity, the greater the risk of obesity, regardless of social class. Stern and colleagues (78) have hypothesized that the primary mechanism by which ethnic cultural beliefs affect obesity is through the concept of fatalism; this group does not believe that everyone can be slim nor are its members optimistic about the prospects of successful dieting.

Massara's ethnographic study of the cultural meanings of weight in a Puerto Rican community in Philadelphia (79) documents the positive associations and lack of social stigma of obesity. For women, weight gain after marriage is a positive reflection on her husband as a good provider and upon the woman as wife, cook, and mother. While some degree of plumpness in women is a marker of sexual attractiveness, weight gain after marriage reflects a woman's marital fidelity, since it is not proper for a mother to be too concerned with her physical appearance. As such, weight loss is socially discouraged. The widespread concept of fatalism also plays a role in making attempts at weight loss appear futile. Massara argues that obese women gain more freedom and latitude in their activities outside the home. She has also presented quantitative evidence (80) suggesting significant differences in ideal body preferences between this ethnic community and mainstream American culture. Body types that are considered obese by biomedical standards are judged as "not too heavy" by Puerto Ricans, for whom the folk definition of obese is 82% heavier than the medical ideal weight for height. The threat of health problems caused by obesity is not a powerful source of motivation for weight loss in this group.

African Americans

Epidemiological studies over the past three decades have indicated that African American women have a great risk of overweight and obesity (81). The ratio of the prevalence of obesity for African American as compared with white women is nearly 2:1, even when controlling for social class. As in the general population, there is an inverse correlation of obesity and social class for women in this ethnic group. Collectively, African Americans appear to have a more relaxed attitude toward weight and weight gain than people in the dominant society. For example, Gillum (34) reports ethnic differences in the definition of overweight for African Americans compared to biomedical standards; less than half of the obese African American women in one sample classified themselves as being much overweight (82). Styles (83) argues that African American women view plumpness and bigness as signs of health, prosperity, and a "job well done" especially in the highly valued domestic arena of cooking and eating. For adolescent girls, low self-esteem is not correlated with obesity in African Americans as it is in whites (84). The symbolic dimension of food sharing among ghetto households has been described by anthropologists (37).

In a low-income housing project in Atlanta, Georgia, a sociological interviewer was asked by a group of obese black women, "Don't you know how hard it is to keep this weight *on?*" Their views of the advantages of a large body included being given respect and reduced chances of being bothered by young "toughs" in the neighborhood. For such women, fatness was part of their positive self-identity and the perceived risk of a food shortage—not for the society as a whole but for the immediate family—may be very important, especially if the lack of food was personally experienced in the past.

Native Americans

There is a great deal of cultural diversity among Native American groups in the United States, but in general they tend to be poor, rural, medically underserved, and marked by elevated rates of obesity. The Pima Indians of central Arizona have the highest reported rates of obesity (and associated chronic diseases) in the United States. Over one-half of all young adults in this group exceed the 90th percentile of weight/height standards (34a), and there is convincing evidence that this predisposition is largely genetic (85). Such elevated prevalences of obesity in Native Americans is a historically recent phenomenon. For both the Pima and Navajo, obesity was extremely rare 40 years ago, and in the latter group obesity was absent in children of traditional families but elevated among children of the acculturated (86). The increase of obesity has largely been laid at the feet of modernization, particularly

dietary changes in the use of lard and soft drinks. For example, among the Hualapai of Arizona the higher energy intake of obese women over lean women can be attributed almost entirely to greater consumption of nonalcoholic and alcoholic beverages (87). In this group, and in many other Native American groups, obesity does not carry negative social connotations. For example, Weidman reports that the Oklahoma Cherokee have an "obese body image," which includes the idea that for successful men the stomach should overhang one's belt (88).

Pacific Islanders

Obesity tends to be a serious problem among Pacific Islanders both in their native countries and as immigrants to the United States. According to Collins and colleagues (20), the prevalence of obesity is highest among Polynesians (44% male, 72% female) and Micronesians (54% male, 68% female) and significantly lower among Melanesians. Samoans, a Polynesian group, are the most numerous ethnic group from the Pacific islands currently residing in the United States. Samoans who migrate and become acculturated are at elevated risk of obesity and related chronic diseases. The health consequences of migration in this population have been the subject of intensive study by biological anthropologists (89). The traditional cultural values of this group in particular idealize fatness as a sign of social power and prosperity (90). Food has great social and symbolic importance in these cultures. In fact, Fitzgerald reports that traditional Cook Islanders made no ethnomedical connections between food and health (91). In many migrant populations, obesity has lost its traditional positive associations and is viewed negatively, but adult body size is also viewed as unchangeable and inevitable.

Improving Cross-Cultural Communication

Health-care workers attempting to prevent or treat obesity in an ethnic group, either in the clinic or community setting, can benefit from being aware of the range of health beliefs and practices of that group. Similarly, it can be valuable for health-care workers to recognize the cultural bases of some of their own beliefs about health conditions, especially stigmatizing ones like obesity. Berlin and Fowkes (92) suggest the mnemonic *LEARN* (Table 2) to improve communication in the clinical setting. The first suggestion is the most important—to *listen* to a patient's perception of the problem, possibly by eliciting the "explanatory model" with the questions in Table 1. Research on patient satisfaction with health-care consultations indicates that active verbal interaction, particularly time spent listening to the patient, is the strongest indicator of success (93). After the health-care provider explains his or her view of the problem in clear language, it is important to acknowledge possible differences between the patient's and provider's views so that the patient's ideas are considered with respect; the health-care worker recommends a plan of action since compliance is ultimately a decision of the patient. Better communication brings better compliance. If contrasting views of the health problem are uncovered, then a culturally acceptable treatment needs to be negotiated. Mutual respect, coming from both sides of a cultural boundary, is more likely to yield a treatment plan that is acceptable to both the patient and health-care worker.

The goal of improved communication should not be limited to interactions with patients from ethnic minorities. The cultural beliefs of members of dominant American so-ciety may predispose them to be concerned about their weight and to try to lose weight even when it is not medically advisable. Similarly, the same set of cultural beliefs may cause significant psychological distress and a feeling of a lack of self-worth when weight is regained after dieting. On the other hand, the current configuration of American cultural beliefs about the symbolic meaning of fat probably functions to prevent a significant amount of overweight and obesity in the population as a whole.

ACKNOWLEDGMENTS

I wish to thank Vicki Condit for her helpful bibliographic assistance and suggestions on the organization of the chapter. Thanks also to Melvin Konner for his many insights on this topic. This chapter was written at the School of American Research, Santa Fe, New Mexico, where I have been supported by a grant from the National Endowment for the Humanities.

REFERENCES

1. Bouchard C, Tremblay A, Despres J, et al. The response of long-term overfeeding in identical twins. *N Engl J Med* 1990;322:1477–82.
2. Price RA, Cadoret FJ, Stunkard AJ, Troughton E. Genetic contributions to human fatness: an adoption study. *Am J Psychiatry* 1987;144:1003–8.
3. Ravussin E, Lillioja S, Knowler WC, et al. Reduced rate of energy expenditure as a risk factor for body-weight gain. *N Engl J Med* 1988;318:467–72.
4. Stunkard AJ, Foch TT, Zdenek H. A twin study of human obesity. *JAMA* 1986;256:51–4.
5. Stunkard AJ, Sorenson TIA, Hanis C, et al. An adoption study of obesity. *N Engl J Med* 1986;314:193–8.
6. Stunkard AJ, Harris JR, Pedersen NL, McClearn G. The body-mass index of twins who have been reared apart. *N Engl J Med* 1990;322:1483–7.
7. Bray GA. Overweight is risking fate: definition, classification, prevalence and risks. *Ann NY Acad Sci* 1987;499:14–28.
8. Schwartz H. *Never satisfied: a cultural history of diets, fantasies, and fat.* New York: Free Press, 1986.
9. Seid RP. *Never too thin: why women are at war with their bodies.* New York: Prentice Hall, 1989.
10. Ritenbaugh C. Obesity as a culture-bound syndrome. *Cult Med Psychiatry.* 1982;6:347–61.
11. Bjorntorp P. How should obesity be defined? *J Intern Med* 1990;227:147–9.

TABLE 2. *LEARN: a guideline for improved communication*

L	*Listen* with sympathy and understanding to the patient's perception of the problem.
E	*Explain* your perceptions of the problem.
A	*Acknowledge* and discuss differences and similarities.
R	*Recommend* treatment.
N	*Negotiate* an agreement.

Adapted from Berlin and Fowkes, ref. 92, with permission.

12. Brown PJ. The biocultural evolution of obesity. In: Bjorntorp P, Brodoff B, eds. *Comprehensive textbook on obesity.* New York: JB Lippincott, 1992.
13. Page LB, Damon A, Moellering RC. Antecedents of cardiovascular disease in six Solomon Islands societies. *Circulation* 1974;49:1132–46.
14. Zimmet P. Epidemiology of diabetes and its microvascular manifestations in Pacific populations: the medical effects of social progress. *Diabetes Care* 1979;2:144–53.
15. West K. Diabetes in American Indians. *Adv Metabol Disorders* 1978;9:29–48.
16. Christakis G. The prevalence of adult obesity. In: Bray G, ed. *Obesity in perspective,* vol 2. Bethesda: Fogarty International Center Series on Preventive Medicine, 1975;209–13.
17. Phillips M, Kubisch D. Lifestyle diseases of aborigines. *Med J Aust* 1985;143:218–224.
18. Trowell HC, Burkitt DP. *Western diseases: their emergence and prevention.* Cambridge, MA: Harvard University Press, 1981.
19. Baba S, Zimmet P, eds. *World data book on obesity.* New York: Elsevier Science Publishers, 1990.
20. Collins V, Dowse G, Zimmet P. Prevalence of obesity in Pacific and Indian Ocean populations. In: Baba S, Zimmet P, eds. *World data book on obesity,* New York: Elsevier Science Publishers, 1990.
21. Kluthe R, Schubert A. Obesity in Europe. *Ann Intern Med* 1985;103:1037–42.
22. Gurney M, Gornstein J. The global prevalence of obesity—an initial view of available data. *World Health Stat Q* 1988;41:251–4.
23. Lantz P, Remington PL. Obesity in Wisconsin. *Wisconsin Med J* 1990 (April):172–6. See also: Centers for Disease Control. Prevalence of overweight—behavioral risk factor surveillance system, 1987. *MMWR* 1989;38:421–3.
24. Minnis PE. *Social adaptation to food stress: a prehistoric southwestern example.* Chicago: University of Chicago Press, 1985.
25. Kissebah AH, Freedman DS, Peiris AN. Health risks of obesity. *Med Clin North Am* 1989; 73:111–138.
26. Brown PJ. Culture and the evolution of obesity. *Hum Nature* 1991;2:31–57.
27. Sobal J, Stunkard AJ. Socioeconomic status and obesity: a review of the literature. *Psychol Bull* 1989;105:260–75.
28. Arteaga P, Dos Santos JE, Dutra de Oliveira JE. Obesity among schoolchildren of different socioeconomic levels in a developing country. *Int J Obes* 1982;6:291–7.
29. Goldblatt PB, Moore ME, Stunkard AJ. Social factors in obesity. *JAMA* 1965;192:1039–44.
30. Burnight RG, Marden PG. Social correlates of weight in an aging population. *Milbank Mem Fund Q* 1967;45:75–92.
31. Rolland-Cachera MF, Bellisle F. No correlation between adiposity and food intake: why are working class children fatter? *Am J Clin Nutr* 1986; 44:779–87.
32. Sobal J. Obesity and socioeconomic status: a framework for examining relationships between physical and social variables. *Med Anthropol* 1991;13:231–48.
33. Garn SM, Clark DC. Trends in fatness and the origin of obesity. *Pediatrics* 1976;57:443–56.
34. Gillum RF. Overweight and obesity in black women. *J Natl Med Assoc* 1987;79:865–71.
34a. Knowler WC, Pettitt DJ, Savage PJ, Bennett PH. Diabetes incidence in Pima Indians: contribution of obesity and parental diabetes. *Am J Epidemiol* 1981;113:144–56.
35. Centers for Disease Control. Prevalence of overweight for hispanics—United States, 1982–1984. *MMWR* 1989;38:838–42.
36. Thomas JD, Douchette MM, Thomas DC, Stoeckle JD. Disease, lifestyle and consanguinity in 58 American Gypsies. *Lancet* 1987;2:377–79.
37. Valentine B. *Hustling and other hard work: lifestyles of the ghetto,* New York: Free Press. 1980.
38. Brown PJ. Cultural and genetic adaptations to malaria: problems of comparison. *Hum Biol* 1986; 14:311–32.
39. Eaton SB, Shostak M, Konner M. *The paleolithic prescription.* New York: Harper and Row, 1988.
40. Harris M. *The nature of cultural things.* New York: Random House, 1964.
41. Durham WH. *Coevolution: genes, culture and human diversity.* Palo Alto: Stanford University Press, 1991.
42. Stunkard AJ. Some perspectives on human obesity: its causes. *Bull NY Acad Med* 1988;64:902–23.
43. Whiting MG. *A cross-cultural nutrition survey* [dissertation]. Harvard School of Public Health. Cambridge, MA. 1958.
44. Wilmsen E. Seasonal effects of dietary intake in the Kalahari San. *Fed Proc* 1978;37:65–71.
45. Hunter JM. Seasonal hunger in a part of the West African savanna: a survey of body weights in Nangodi, North-East Ghana. *Trans Inst Br Geographers* 1967;41:167–85.
46. Physician Task Force on Hunger in America. *Hunger in America: the growing epidemic.* Boston: Harvard School of Public Health, 1985.
47. Stein Z, Susser M. The Dutch famine, 1944–1945, and the reproductive process. *Pediatr Res* 1975;9:70–6.
48. Huss-Ashmore R. Fat and fertility: demographic implications of differential fat storage. *Yearbook Phys Anthropol* 1980;23:65–91.
49. Frisch RE. Body fat, menarche, fitness and fertility. *Hum Reprod* 1987;2:521–33.
50. Wendorf M. Diabetes, the ice free corridor, and paleoindian settlement in North America. *Am J Phys Anthropol* 1989;79:503–20.
51. Carlson EA. *Human genetics.* Lexington, MA: DC Heath, 1984.
52. Gardner LI, Stern MP, Haffner SM, et al. Prevalence of diabetes in Mexican Americans. *Diabetes* 1984;33:86–92.
53. Wenke RJ. *Patterns in prehistory.* New York: Oxford University Press, 1980.
54. Cohen MN, Armelagos GJ, eds. *Paleopathology at the origins of agriculture.* New York: Academic Press, 1984.
55. Cohen MN. *Health and the rise of civilization.* New Haven: Yale University Press, 1989.
56. Dietz WH. You are what you eat—what you eat is what you are. *J Adolesc Health Care* 1990;11:76–81.

57. Nichter M, Nichter M. Hype and weight. *Med Anthropol* 1991;13:249–84.

58. Brink PJ. The fattening room among the Annang of Nigeria. *Med Anthropol* 1989;12:131–43.

59. Malcom LW. Note on the seclusion of girls among the Efik at Old Calabar. *Man* 1925;25:113–4.

60. Cassidy C. The good body: when big is better. *Med Anthropol* 1991;13:181–214.

61. Marshall DS. Sexual behavior on Mangaia. In: Marshall D, Suggs RE, eds. *Human sexual behavior: variations in the ethnographic spectrum.* New York: Basic Books, 1971.

62. Borgerhoff Mulder M. Kipsigis bridewealth payments. In: Betzig L, Borgerhoff Mulder M, Turke P, eds. *Human reproductive behavior.* Cambridge: Cambridge University Press, 1988.

63. Allon N. The stigma of obesity in everyday life. In: Wolman BJ, ed. *Psychological aspects of obesity: a handbook.* New York: Van Nostrand Reinhold Company, 1981:130–74.

64. Cahnman WJ. The stigma of obesity. *Sociol Q* 1968;9:294–7.

65. Furnham A, Alibhai N. Cross-cultural differences in the perception of female body shapes. *Psychol Med* 1983;13:829–37.

66. Lee R. *The !Kung San: men, women, and work in a foraging society,* Cambridge: Harvard University Press, 1979.

67. Collier J. From Mary to modern woman: the material basis of marianismo and its transformation in a spanish village. *Am Ethnol* 1986;13:100–7.

68. Powdermaker H. An anthropological approach to the problem of obesity. *Bull NY Acad Sci* 1960;36:286–95.

69. Smithson CL. *The Havasupai woman.* Salt Lake City: University of Utah Press, 1958.

70. Messing SD. *The highland plateau Amhara of Ethiopia* [dissertation, Anthropology] University of Pennsylvania, 1957.

71. Kleinman A, Eisenberg L, Good B. Culture, illness and care. *Ann Intern Med* 1978;88:251–8.

72. Harwood A, ed. *Ethnicity and medical care.* Cambridge: Harvard University Press, 1981.

73. Gampel B. The "Hilltops" community. In: Kark SL, Steuart GE, eds. *Practice of social medicine.* London: E and S Livingstone, 1962:292–308.

74. Ritenbaugh C. Body size and shape: a dialogue of culture and biology. *Med Anthropol* 1991;13:173–80.

75. Glassner B. *Bodies: why we look the way we do.* New York: GP Putnam's Sons, 1988.

76. Ross CE, Mirowsky J. The social epidemiology of overweight: a substantive and methodological investigation. *J Health Soc Behav* 1983;24:288–98.

77. Hazuda HP, Haffner SM, Stern MP, Eifler CW. Effects of acculturation and socioeconomic status on obesity and diabetes in Mexican Americans. *Am J Epidemiol* 1988;128:1289–301.

78. Stern M, Pugh J, Gaskill S, Hazuda H. Knowledge, attitudes and behavior related to obesity and dieting in Mexican Americans and Anglos: the San Antonio heart study. *Am J Epidemiol* 1982;115:917–27.

79. Massara EB. *Que gordita! a study of weight among women in a Puerto Rican community.* New York: AMS Press, 1989.

80. Massara EB, Obesity and cultural weight evaluations. *Appetite* 1980;1:291–8.

81. Kumanyika S. Obesity in black women. *Epidemiol Rev* 1987;9:31–50.

82. McGee M, Hale H. Social factors and obesity among black women. *Free Inquiry* 1980;8:83–7.

83. Styles MH. Soul, black women and food. In: Kaplan JR, ed. *A woman's conflict: the special relationship between women and food.* Englewood Cliffs, NJ: Prentice Hall, 1980:161–76.

84. Kaplan KM, Wadden TA. Childhood obesity and self-esteem. *J Pediatr* 1986;109:367–70.

85. Knowler W, Pettit D, Bennett P, Williams R. Diabetes mellitus in the Pima Indians: genetic and evolutionary considerations. *Am J Phys Anthropol* 1983;62:107–14.

86. Garb JL, Garb JR, Stunkard AJ. Social factors and obesity in Navajo Indian children. In: Howard A, ed. *Recent advances in obesity research.* London: Newman, 1975:37–9.

87. Teufel NI, Dufour DL. Patterns of food use and nutrient intake of obese and non-obese Hualapai Indian women of Arizona. *J Am Diet Assoc* 1990;90:1229–35.

88. Wiedman DW. *Diabetes mellitus and Oklahoma Native Americans: a case study of culture change in Oklahoma Cherokee* [dissertation, Anthropology]. University of Oklahoma, 1979.

89. Baker PT, Hanna JM, Baker TS, eds. *The changing Samoans: behavior and health in transition.* New York: Oxford University Press, 1986.

90. Fitzpatrick-Nietchmann J. Pacific islanders—migration and health. *West J Med* 1983;139:44–9.

91. Fitzgerald TK. Dietary change among Cook Islanders in New Zealand. *Soc Sci Information* 1980;19:805–32.

92. Berlin EO, Fowkes WC. A teaching framework for cross-cultural health care. *West J Med* 1983;139:130–4.

93. Brown PJ, Ballard B. Culture, ethnicity, and behavior and the practice of medicine. In: Stoudemire A, ed. *Human behavior: an introduction for medical students.* New York: Lippincott, 1990.

Therapy

Obesity: Theory and Therapy, Second Edition,
edited by A. J. Stunkard and T. A. Wadden.
Raven Press, Ltd., New York © 1993.

12

The Treatment of Obesity

An Overview

Thomas A. Wadden

Department of Psychology, Syracuse University, Syracuse, New York 13244

These are tough times for overweight Americans. They are aware from newspaper and television reports that obesity is a serious health problem and that they should "lose those extra pounds"—and yet, many are troubled by a spate of recent reports suggesting that most weight-loss efforts are ultimately ineffective and may be associated with serious health complications.

Concerns about the ill effects of obesity were reawakened by publication of the Nurses Health Study, which found that women 30% or more overweight experienced three times the risk of death from coronary heart disease as did women of average weight (1). Even those as little as 5% overweight experienced an increased risk of complications. An editorial accompanying the publication noted that "any remaining confidence that some degree of obesity is safe is likely to be replaced by deep concern" (p. 928) (2).

Just as some individuals may have resolved to lose weight, Congressman Wyden of Oregon initiated hearings on "Deception and Fraud in the Diet Industry," which charged that many of America's commercial weight-loss programs engaged in false and misleading advertising (3). Not only could most companies not provide data to support claims of successful weight control, but former clients from some programs testified that they had been seriously harmed by treatment.

The Congressional hearings, as well as Oprah Winfrey's disclosure in late 1990 that she had regained the bulk of her highly publicized weight loss in less than 2 years, led the media to call for a moratorium on dieting (4). This proposal appeared prudent to many in light of subsequent findings that persons with a history of weight fluctuation, presumably from dieting, had a higher risk of health complications than did persons who were comparably obese but maintained a more stable weight (5).

Thus the nation's dieters, as well as its obesity experts, are uncertain about how to proceed. When weight reduction is undertaken, it is likely to be with greater forethought and caution than were exercised only 2 years earlier. This change of attitude, coupled with recent findings on the maintenance of weight loss, could well lead to better long-term results.

This chapter provides an overview of current treatments for mild and moderate obesity (which are defined as 5 to 39% and 40 to 99% over ideal weight, respectively) (6). It examines the goals of weight reduction (which are now significantly more conservative than a decade ago), the short- and long-term results of treatment, and methods to facilitate maintenance of weight loss. The treatment of severe obesity (100% or more overweight) is discussed in the chapter by Mason in this volume.

INITIAL EVALUATION AND GOALS OF TREATMENT

Initial Evaluation

Stunkard has described in this volume the goals of the initial evaluation. As he notes, the evaluation provides the practitioner with an opportunity to learn about the patient's current psychosocial functioning, explore the individual's understanding of his or her weight problem, and determine why the patient has sought treatment. In addition, careful inquiry may reveal the extent to which biological factors contribute to the patient's obesity, as well as provide important information concerning eating, exercise, and dietary habits, which will be used to plan treatment (7).

The initial evaluation, as Stunkard has indicated, should also include a physical examination and laboratory tests to assess the presence of any health complications or contraindications to specific weight reduction therapies such as very-low-calorie diets or surgery. Body fat distribution should also be assessed because of findings that fat carried in the upper body (specifically the viscera) poses far greater health complications than fat carried in the lower body (8,9) (see the chapter by Sjöström).

Goals of Treatment

The initial evaluation should conclude with a summary of the practitioner's findings and a discussion of the desirability and goals of treatment. Frequently, these two latter issues are not addressed. While it might appear that all overweight persons should reduce, there may be exceptions. It may, for example, be difficult to make a compelling case for treatment in a 60-year-old woman with lower body obesity who is 15 kg overweight but otherwise in excellent health. Weight loss might improve her appearance and self-esteem, but these benefits could be offset by the frustration and despair which are likely to occur if weight is regained. Thus the practi-

tioner and patient should discuss at length the possible benefits and liabilities of treatment and, in some cases, may elect a goal of weight stability rather than weight loss.

Persons with clear health complications of their obesity should be encouraged to reduce in most cases. Exhortation, rather than encouragement, may be required with men because of their relative comfort with obesity, as discussed by Stunkard in this volume. With women, by contrast, the objective is to select a reasonable goal weight, which may differ significantly from that required to obtain ideal weight (10). Thus a 40-year-old woman who stands 165 cm (65 inches) and weighs 100 kg (220 lb) might seek treatment to lose 45 kg (100 lb), a loss that would bring her to approximately ideal weight. A loss of this size is highly unlikely, however, in light of information that both her mother and maternal grandmother were significantly overweight and that the patient has not weighed 55 kg (121 lb) since she was 12 years old.

Selecting a Goal Weight

Selection of a reasonable goal weight can be facilitated by a careful review of the patient's weight history. Our clinical experience suggests that, as a general rule, the goal weight should be no lower than the patient's lowest weight since age 21 that was maintained for at least 1 year (11). Thus a reasonable goal for the woman described above might be 75 kg (165 lb), since that was her lowest weight as an adult. Moreover, the practitioner might suggest that the patient attempt initially to reduce her weight by 10% (10 kg). A loss of this magnitude, in many cases, may be sufficient to improve (or control) medical complications including hypertension, diabetes, and hypercholesterolemia (12,13). The practitioner should emphasize that control of medical complications and increased mobility are perhaps the principal goals of therapy and can be achieved without the patient's looking like a fashion model.

It is critical that patient and practitioner

explicitly discuss the patient's desired weight loss and the rapidity with which it is anticipated. In the absence of such discussion, patients frequently adhere to their implicit and often unrealistic goals and become demoralized when they fail to reach them (7).

Psychosocial Goals

Patient and practitioner should also discuss in detail the psychosocial benefits the patient anticipates from treatment (7). Many obese individuals seek weight loss as a means to another goal such as securing an intimate relationship or a new job, in addition to "just feeling better." The likelihood that these desired benefits will result from weight loss should be assessed because, in most cases, psychosocial changes do not readily occur. Weight loss may be a necessary condition for such changes but rarely is it sufficient. The patient and practitioner can discuss the additional steps that may be required to achieve the desired goals.

TREATMENT: AN OVERVIEW

Figure 1 provides an overview of current treatments for obesity (10). This conceptual model integrates elements of previous classifications based on body weight [such as Stunkard's (6) and Garrow (13)], with features of a stepped-care approach, and efforts to identify a patient's specific treatment needs. As a general rule, the heavier the individual, the more aggressive and intensive the therapy recommended. Thus persons needing to lose only 2 to 5 kg may benefit from a self-help approach that requires minimal intervention (and cost), while those 50 or more kg overweight may be candidates for a very-low-calorie diet or surgical therapy.

The author believes that all significantly overweight individuals should receive an initial trial of therapy by a conventional 1,000 to 1,500 kcal/day diet combined with a program of life style modification. Such treatment is provided to more than a million peo-

ple weekly by commercial programs such as Weight Watchers. Alternatively, more intensive (and costly) versions of the same approach are frequently offered at university and hospital clinics and are likely to be associated with better results. If the patient has already received an adequate trial of such therapy, then the next intervention recommended by the stepped-care model can be considered.

Preparing Patients for Treatment

In selecting treatment, the practitioner should review the patient's previous weight loss efforts to determine which approaches have been tried, which worked, and what the patient liked or disliked about specific interventions (7). Patients frequently have negative expectations of treatment based upon previous experiences. Thus it is critical that the proposed therapy be differentiated from previous approaches and that it offer new hope to the patient.

The practitioner should briefly describe a typical course of the treatment selected and spell out the behaviors (such as exercising and keeping a diet diary) that will be expected of the patient. Benefits of treatment, including the rate of weight loss and expected health improvements, should also be reviewed. Such preparation helps patients to set realistic goals and facilitates their active participation in therapy.

Taylor and Stunkard discuss in this volume the results of community, work-site, and self-help approaches for the treatment of mild obesity, as shown in step 1 of the stepped-care approach (Fig. 1). Mason's chapter describes the surgical treatment of severely obese individuals (i.e., step 5) and Silverstone's chapter the use of pharmacotherapy, which is a topic of renewed interest because of promising findings with serotonergic drugs, including dexfenfluramine (14) and fluoxetine (15). The remainder of this chapter examines the treatment of mild obesity by a 1,000 to 1,500 kcal/day diet com-

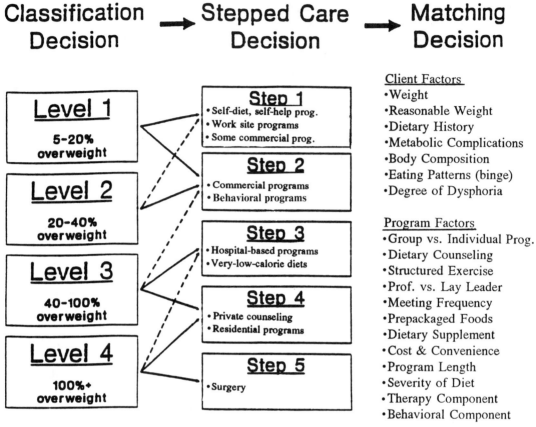

FIG. 1. A conceptual scheme showing the three-stage process in selecting a treatment for an individual. The first step, the Classification Decision, divides individuals according to percent overweight into four levels. The level dictates which of the five steps would be reasonable in a second stage, the Stepped-Care Decision. This indicates that the least intensive, costly, and risky approach will be used from among the alternative treatments. The third stage, the Matching Decision, is used to make the final selection of a program, and is based on a combination of client and program variables. The dashed lines with arrows between the Classification and Stepped-Care stages show the lowest level of treatment that may be beneficial, but more intensive treatment is usually necessary for people at the specified weight level. (From ref. 10, with permission.)

bined with behavior therapy (i.e., step 2) and the management of moderate obesity by very-low-calorie diet (i.e., step 3). We will not review the option of residential treatment (i.e., step 4) because there are few published data in this area (16).

TREATMENT OF MILD OBESITY: BEHAVIORAL THERAPY

The behavioral treatment of obesity was inaugurated in the late 1960s with Richard Stuart's (17) case report of the highly successful treatment of eight individuals. Stuart's patients lost an average of 18 kg, a loss the size of which was achieved by fewer than 5% of persons who received conventional dietary therapy, as described by Stunkard (18) less than a decade earlier. Stuart's report led to the publication of hundreds of studies on the efficacy of behavioral treatment and to the widespread adoption of this approach in research and commercial programs alike (19,20).

Assumptions and Characteristics of Treatment

The behavioral approach was founded upon Stuart's (17) belief that "only two common characteristics have been observed in obese persons: a tendency to overeat and a tendency to underexercise." This statement clearly represents a gross oversimplification of the etiology of obesity and fails to acknowledge important differences among individuals in their basal energy expenditure (21), fat cell morphology (22), body fat distribution (8), and other characteristics that may be genetically determined (23). Nevertheless, the vast majority of treatments for obesity are designed primarily to modify energy intake, energy expenditure, or both. As such, Stuart and those who followed developed a technology to modify eating and exercise systematically. This approach may help patients to manage their weight even if they do not have abnormal eating habits (24), which many obese individuals apparently do not (19).

Behavioral treatment makes extensive use of the functional analysis of behavior (19,20,24,25). Eating and exercise habits are analyzed to determine their covariation with other events including times, places, emotions, thoughts, and other persons. Problem behaviors are identified and efforts are then made to modify the events associated with them or to find alternative behaviors. Thus individuals who eat high fat/high sugar foods (i.e., cakes, ice cream, etc.) when they feel sad or lonely might be asked to keep a record of their thoughts at such times. This homework assignment might reveal that they fear they will not find an intimate relationship and will live alone for the rest of their lives. Cognitive restructuring (26) could be used to challenge these irrational assumptions and plans made to engage in other behaviors when such individuals find themselves eating in response to dysphoria.

The behavioral approach has several other distinguishing features (7). First, it is goal oriented. The objectives of therapy are clearly defined and are specified in terms that can be easily measured. This is true whether the goal is walking after dinner three times a week for 20 minutes at a time, decreasing the number of self-critical statements, or limiting breakfast to 275 calories.

Second, treatment seeks to change behavior per se. Thus it differs from dynamically oriented therapy, which is more likely to explore unconscious drives thought to control eating or to examine the meaning and origin of overeating (27).

Third, behavioral treatment is process oriented. It is more than identifying behaviors that patients should adopt; it provides a method of learning (24). When the desired behavior is not acquired, it is broken into smaller pieces in an effort to shape the patient's acquisition. When after repeated efforts a patient fails to acquire what appears to be a fairly simple behavior, treatment may examine issues more similar to those addressed by dynamically oriented therapy. This step, however, is taken only when more direct methods of behavior change are not successful (7,24).

Components of Treatment

There is a tendency for behavioral treatment to be delivered as a package (28). This is because in most clinics, therapy is usually delivered in groups of 8 to 12 persons, and it is difficult to provide each patient the attention required to complete a rigorous functional analysis of behavior. Consistent with practice, we will provide a brief description of the primary components of the behavioral package. The reader is referred to other publications in which these components and the mechanics of treatment have been described in greater detail (6,19,24,25).

Self-Monitoring

Self-monitoring—observing and recording one's behavior—is the cornerstone of behavioral treatment (19,24,25). In the initial weeks of treatment, patients are asked to record daily the types and amounts of food that they eat and their caloric value. This practice helps to identify problem foods and hidden sources of calories, and facilitates adherence to a reduced calorie diet (of 1,000 to 1,500 kcal/day). Record keeping is expanded over time to include information on exercise habits, as well as times, places, and feelings associated with eating. In the later stages of treatment, patients attempt to identify high-risk situations that are associated with dietary lapses and record their thoughts and feelings in response to such occurrences. Patients discuss in weekly group treatment sessions their success in completing the homework assignments and receive feedback from the staff and group members on methods of handling any problems. Self-monitoring is considered by patients and practitioners to be one of the most important components of treatment and has been shown to correlate significantly with both short- and long-term weight losses (29).

Problem Solving

Training in problem-solving skills provides patients a systematic method of correcting the difficulties they discover by self-monitoring. As applied to weight control, patients are taught to: (a) identify and clearly define the weight-related difficulty; (b) generate possible solutions for handling the problem; (c) evaluate the possible solutions and select one; (d) plan and implement the behavior; (e) evaluate the outcome; and, (f) if the intervention is not successful, reevaluate the problem and select another solution (30,31). Patients are taught to view overeating, weight gain, or nonadherence to the behavioral program as cues to engage in problem solving (24).

Nutrition Education

Early behavioral treatment provided minimal dietary counseling (20). Patients were told to eat 1,000 to 1,500 kcal/day of whatever foods they wished, given the prevailing belief that a calorie of fat was no different from a calorie of protein or carbohydrate. Current behavioral interventions, however, stress the importance of a well balanced, low-fat diet (25). The change is attributable to findings that the consumption of high-fat diets contributes to cardiovascular disease, as well as to findings that the body uses approximately 25% more energy to metabolize carbohydrate than fat (32,33) (as also discussed by Ravussin and Swinburn in this volume). Thus a person will gain more weight eating fat than in consuming the same number of calories as carbohydrate. Both animals (33) and humans (34) maintain a lower body weight when allowed ad libitum consumption of a low-fat as compared with high-fat diet. Dwyer and Lu have provided an excellent summary in this volume of the components of a healthy reducing diet.

Slowing the Rate of Eating

A host of techniques has been developed to help patients slow their rate of eating in order to improve satiety and thus be satisfied with less food (19,24,25). These include putting utensils down between bites, pausing during the meal, and chewing food thoroughly before swallowing. A recent study of subjects who participated in a behavioral weight-loss program showed that those who slowed their rate of eating, as measured under laboratory conditions, lost significantly more weight than subjects who failed to slow their rate of intake (35). Patients report other benefits of slowing their eating, which include increased enjoyment of the flavor and texture of food and greater feelings of self-control.

Stimulus Control

Stimulus control techniques are designed to limit the individual's exposure to food and thus prevent incidental eating (19,24,25). The procedures can be divided into five broad categories: (a) shopping prudently to keep problem foods out of the home; (b) storing foods properly; (c) leaving food on the plate; (d) limiting the times, places, and activities associated with eating; and (e) planning for social situations involving food. The contribution of these techniques to the outcome of treatment has not been clearly established, but they continue to be included because of their intuitive appeal (24).

Cognitive Restructuring

Cognitive therapy is now routinely included in the treatment of obesity and is designed to help dieters overcome self-defeating thoughts, which undermine weight control efforts. Such thoughts might include: (a) the impossibility of weight loss (e.g., "I'll never be able to lose this weight"); (b) unrealistic goals (e.g., "I'll never eat ice cream again"); or (c) self-disparaging statements (e.g., "I'm pathetic. What a failure. I'll always be fat"). Methods developed by Beck (26) and Mahoney and Mahoney (36) are used to help patients develop coping-oriented, rational responses to their negativistic beliefs. Despite its success in the treatment of depression and other mood disorders, little research has been conducted on the use of cognitive therapy with obese individuals (37).

Exercise

Increased physical activity is perhaps the single best correlate of long-term weight control (29,38,39) (as discussed in a later section on weight maintenance). Given this finding, it is perhaps surprising that exercise increases short-term weight losses only minimally, if at all (40). This is because exercise expends far fewer calories than people commonly assume. Jogging 10 miles, for example, is unlikely in most persons to burn more than 1,500 calories, or slightly less than one-half of a pound of fat. The most important message to convey to overweight individuals, as discussed by Grillo, Brownell, and Stunkard in this volume, is that exercise need not be punishing to be of benefit. Thus modest increases in daily life style activity have been shown to be of greater long-term benefit to weight control than have more traditional aerobic programs (41). In addition, even modest physical activity is associated with significant reductions in the risk of cardiovascular disease (42).

Mechanics of Treatment

Group Treatment

As practiced in university and hospital clinics, the treatment embodying the principles noted above is usually delivered in groups of 6 to 20 persons. Group treatment is not only more cost-effective than individual therapy but may also produce larger weight losses. A recent study reported that persons in a randomized clinical trial who requested individual therapy but were assigned to group treatment nevertheless achieved significantly greater weight losses than did persons who requested individual therapy and received it (43). The benefits of group treatment may derive not only from the support that patients clearly provide one another but also from a healthy dose of competition (44). Thus patients may push themselves to keep up with what they perceive as the group norm.

Individual treatment of obesity is perhaps most appropriately used as an adjunct to group therapy with persons who have special treatment needs (as well as with persons who object to group care). Such treatment is not equivalent to psychotherapy, however; it should remain behaviorally oriented, focusing on weight control issues. More traditionally oriented psychotherapy may be required with persons who, in addition to their obesity, have a personality or affective disorder (7).

Time-Limited, Closed Groups

Treatment sessions are held weekly, usually for 15 to 25 weeks, although treatment as long as 52 weeks has been reported (45). The use of time-limited, as contrasted with open-ended therapy, helps patients to pace themselves. They appear better able to sustain motivation knowing that there is a clear beginning and end to the initial phase of treatment.

The use of closed treatment groups, in which the same patients begin and end treatment together, appears preferable to the use of open groups, in which new members may be added to the group at any point in time (46). The addition of new members after the first few weeks impairs the development of group cohesiveness, and may be a factor contributing to the high attrition rates that characterize programs using open groups (47,48). Moreover, it is difficult to establish a curriculum of behavior change, in which one week's session builds upon another, if patients in the same group are at different stages of treatment (7).

Group Sessions

Weekly group sessions usually last 60 to 90 minutes and follow a structured agenda, which may be provided by the use of a manual (25). Most of the group's time is spent reviewing the previous week's homework assignment and patients' efforts to modify their eating, exercise, and thinking habits. As such, treatment is patient oriented and focuses on the process of behavior change. The group leader also briefly introduces a new weight control skill at each session and explains the homework assignment to be practiced to acquire the behavior. The group leader, however, spends minimal time lecturing to participants. It is assumed that patients know what they should do to control their weight but need assistance in implementing needed behaviors.

Practitioners Skills

Insufficient attention has been paid to the skills and training required to provide behav-

ioral treatment. Several early studies indicated that patients treated by professional therapists lost significantly more weight than those treated by peer counselors, despite the use of the same treatment materials (49–51). In practice, however, the vast majority of care in commercial programs is provided by persons without professional training.

Training in psychopathology and group psychotherapy is likely to help practitioners lead more effective groups through increasing sensitivity to nonbehavioral events (7,24). When behavioral treatment is not effective, clinical experience suggests that it is because of a failure to establish a supportive and cohesive group. Unfavorable group dynamics, which can be introduced by patients with personality disorders or by those experiencing significant life distress, must be addressed with the group in order to establish a secure and trusting atmosphere (52). Maintenance of a sound working group should take precedence over weight control issues, which means that at some meetings, the practitioner may have to set aside the planned agenda.

RESULTS OF BEHAVIORAL TREATMENT

Table 1 provides a summary analysis of the results of behavioral treatment as delivered in university and hospital clinics. The data were taken from reports that appeared in four behaviorally oriented journals: *Addictive Behaviors; Behavior Therapy; Behaviour Research and Therapy;* and *Journal of Consulting and Clinical Psychology.* For each of the years shown, all relevant articles were reviewed and summary statistics calculated.

Short-Term Weight Losses

Data from the years 1985 to 1990 indicate that patients in behavioral programs are treated for approximately 15 to 20 weeks and lose about 8.5 kg in this time. Thus both the

TABLE 1. *Summary analysis of selected studies from 1974 to 1990 providing treatment by behavior therapy and conventional reducing diet*

	1974	1978	1984	1985–87	1988–90
No. of studies included	15	17	15	13	5
Sample size	53.1	54.0	71.3	71.6	21.2
Initial weight (kg)	73.4	87.3	88.7	87.2	91.9
Initial % overweight	49.4	48.6	48.1	56.2	59.8
Length of treatment (weeks)	8.4	10.5	13.2	15.6	21.3
Weight loss (kg)	3.8	4.2	6.9	8.4	8.5
Loss per week (kg)	0.5	0.4	0.5	0.5	0.4
Attrition (%)	11.4	12.9	10.6	13.8	21.8
Length of follow-up (weeks)	15.5	30.3	58.4	48.3	53
Loss at follow-up	4.0	4.1	4.4	5.3	5.6

From ref. 20, with permission.

length of treatment and the size of the weight losses have more than doubled since 1974 when patients were treated for an average of only 8.4 weeks and lost 3.8 kg. This change reflects the fact that many of the early studies consisted of doctoral dissertations, which students may have been motivated to complete as quickly as possible.

It is of note that the weekly rate of weight loss has remained constant at 0.4 to 0.5 kg/week in early and later behavioral studies. Thus the larger weight losses observed in more recent studies appear to be attributable simply to increasing the length of treatment. This finding has led investigators to extend treatment to up to 1 year in the hope that the 0.5 kg/week loss would be maintained throughout this period (45). Perri et al. (53) investigated a 40-week program and observed that patients lost 9.9 kg in the first 20 weeks, but only an additional 3.6 kg in the second 20 weeks. Wadden et al. (45), in a 52-week study, observed a loss of 11.9 kg in the first 26 weeks of treatment, with only an additional 2.5 kg during the second 26 weeks. Thus there appear to be limits to the size of the weight losses that can be produced by traditional behavioral interventions, a finding that has led investigators to explore the use of very-low-calorie diets, surgery, and other options. It is not clear whether these limits are based primarily on metabolism or motivation.

Long-Term Weight Losses

Researchers have paid increasing attention to the long-term results of treatment during the past decade. Table 1 shows that the mean length of follow-up increased from 15.5 weeks in the 1974 studies to 53 weeks in the most recent studies (1988 to 1990). Several papers have reported follow-up data for periods of 5 years or more (40,54,55).

Data from studies published between 1984 and 1990 indicate that patients, on average, regain about one-third of their weight loss in the year following treatment. For example, patients treated between 1988 and 1990 lost 8.5 kg during treatment but 1 year later maintained a loss of only 5.6 kg. In none of the five studies published during this period did patients, on average, continue to lose weight during follow-up.

Patients in the 1974 and 1978 studies maintained, on average, their full end-of-treatment weight losses at the time of follow-up, suggesting that current behavioral treatment is less effective than its predecessor (20). This impression is not warranted, however. Follow-up in the earlier studies was limited to 30 weeks or less, which allowed less time for the observation of weight gain. In addition, earlier studies were associated with significantly smaller weight losses, which may elicit fewer compensatory mechanisms associated with weight regain (28).

Alternative Therapies

Patients regain greater amounts of weight with increasing time after therapy. Several studies have shown that a majority will regain all of their weight loss within 5 years (54,55). These long-term data leave little doubt that maintenance of weight loss, as contrasted to the induction of weight loss, is the critical problem in obesity therapy (and one that will be discussed later).

These poor long-term data have led some investigators to conclude that behavioral treatment is of limited efficacy (56) and that better results might be obtained with interventions modeled upon Overeaters Anonymous or comparable approaches, which view obesity as an addictive disorder (57). The author is sympathetic to such suggestions but believes that alternative approaches must be empirically evaluated in the same manner as has behavioral treatment. Although several authors, including Roth (58), have provided eloquent testimony of their recovery from overeating, no controlled investigations have been published, and there are only perhaps a handful of case studies. Further clarification is also required of the conceptualization of obesity as an addictive disorder because it clearly does not meet the classic criteria of addiction (59).

TREATMENT OF MODERATE OBESITY: VERY-LOW-CALORIE DIETS

Very-low-calorie diets (VLCDs), providing 400 to 800 kcal/day, have been a popular treatment option in recent years for persons 30% or more overweight who have failed to reduce using conventional approaches (60). In contrast to the liquid protein diets of 1976 to 1977, current VLCDs providing protein of high biological quality appear to be safe when used under medical supervision for 16 or fewer weeks by appropriate persons (61). The development and clinical use of these diets have been described in detail by a number of investigators (62–66), as have the criteria for patient selection and the schedule of medical monitoring required for safe use (67).

Types of Diets

Very-low-calorie diets produce weight losses almost as great as those associated with fasting, but they preserve lean body tissue through the provision of approximately 50 to 100 g of protein daily (61). The greater the individual's ideal body weight, the greater the amount of protein that should be provided. Protein may be obtained from lean meat, fish, and fowl served in food form (64) or from milk- or egg-based protein formulas served as a liquid diet (65,66).

Patients who consume either diet are instructed to drink at least 2 liters of noncaloric fluid daily and to avoid the consumption of all other foods (62–66). The two approaches are associated with comparable weight losses (68). The liquid diets are more widely used because of their provision by commercial manufacturers, but one study found that the diet of conventional foods (lean meat, fish, and fowl) was associated with greater reductions in hunger and with less disruption of social eating than was a liquid diet (68).

Clinical Course and Complications

Most investigators believe that successful treatment by VLCD requires multidisciplinary care provided by a physician, behavioral psychologist, dietitian, and, preferably, an exercise specialist (60). The physician is responsible primarily for the medical evaluation and monitoring of the patient. The remainder of the team works in the short term to facilitate the patient's adherence to the modified fast and in the long term to improve eating and exercise habits using the behavioral methods described in the previous section.

Treatment is frequently provided in groups and covers four principal stages:

1. During an introductory period of 1 to 4 weeks, patients consume a 1,000 to 1,500 kcal/day diet of conventional foods and prepare themselves and family members for the VLCD (69,70).
2. The VLCD is usually consumed for 8 to 16 weeks, during which time patients are instructed in methods to facilitate adherence to the diet (including self-monitoring of food and fluid intake) and to increase their physical activity (49,69,70).
3. Conventional foods are slowly reintroduced over a 4 to 8 week period commonly referred to as "refeeding," during which patients are instructed in consuming a well-balanced, low-fat diet and in practicing the stimulus control procedures previously described (46,69,70).
4. Intensive instruction in behavioral methods of weight control is provided during the last phase of treatment, with particular emphasis on relapse prevention (46,69,70).

Complications

When consumed under appropriate medical supervision, VLCDs are generally associated with only mild complications, which may include fatigue, dizziness, muscle cramping, headache, gastrointestinal distress, and cold intolerance (61). These and two other symptoms occasionally reported, dry skin and hair loss, remit fully with termination of the diet (71).

An exception to this generally favorable picture is the report of increased risk of symptomatic gallstones in persons who consume these diets. Two controlled trials reported that approximately 26% of persons treated by a VLCD developed gallstones, as detected by ultrasound (72,73). Supersaturation of the biliary cholesterol and gallbladder stasis are two mechanisms believed responsible for this occurrence (72,73). Further research is required to determine the incidence of clinically significant gallstones associated with consumption of a VLCD, as compared with a conventional

reducing diet. In the meantime, Kanders and Blackburn (12) have suggested that the risk of gallstones can be reduced by the use of diets that provide sufficient protein (i.e., 14 g) and fat (i.e., 10 g) at one meal to ensure gallbladder contraction and that limit weight loss to 2% or less of body weight/week.

Short-Term Weight Losses

Very-low-calorie diets produce average losses of 15 to 20 kg in 12 weeks—losses that are more than double the size of those produced by a conventional 1,000 to 1,500 kcal/day diet (61). Although longer treatment is associated with greater weight losses, there appears to be a point of diminishing return. Thus women treated by Donnelly et al. (74) for 13 weeks lost 20.5 kg, whereas those treated by Hovell et al. (75) for 16 to 26 weeks lost only 4 kg more (mean loss of 24.5 kg). Our research team observed a loss of 17.3 kg in women during the first 3 months of treatment by a 420 kcal/day diet. This average monthly loss of 5.8 kg slowed to 3.1 kg, however, when the diet was extended to a fourth month, despite the fact that patients remained more than 50% overweight on average (76). We believe that it is hard to justify the increased cost of VLCDs when the monthly rate of weight loss falls below 4 kg.

Attrition

The large weight losses reported for VLCDs could reflect selective reporting in which the results for persons who discontinue treatment are not included in group means (75,77). Approximately 25% of patients treated by Kirschner et al. (77), for example, dropped out of treatment in the first 3 weeks, a fact not reflected in their report of a mean weight loss of 23.4 kg. In a recent multicenter study of a proprietary program, we found that 44% of patients did not complete the full 26 weeks of treatment (46). Nevertheless, individuals who dropped out still achieved large weight losses; women lost 14 kg and men 22 kg, respectively, as compared with losses of 22 kg and 32 kg for women and men, respectively, who completed treatment. Thus VLCDs appear to be associated with large weight losses even when the effects of attrition are taken into account.

Long-Term Weight Losses

Research on the long-term efficacy of VLCDs lags far behind that for traditional behavioral treatment (78). This is an alarming and regrettable state of affairs, given that during the past 5 years several hundreds of thousands of persons were treated by VLCDs in hospital-based programs. There have been only six controlled evaluations of this approach that included a follow-up evaluation of 1 year or longer (39,70,79–82). Results of the four studies that provide the most

easily interpretable data are summarized in Table 2.

Three of the four studies agree in showing that weight gain is a significant problem following treatment by VLCD. Patients in the Wadden and Stunkard (70) study who were treated by VLCD alone (without training in behavior modification) regained approximately 64% of their weight loss in the year following treatment. Those who received the same diet combined with behavior therapy fared significantly better but still regained 38% of their weight loss. Patients in the study by Wing et al. (82), who received a similar program of VLCD and behavior modification, regained a full 53% of their weight loss 1 year after treatment, whereas patients treated by Sikand et al. (81) regained almost their entire weight loss within 2 years. These findings are consistent with those of several uncontrolled studies (75,77,83) and with the re-

TABLE 2. *Summary analysis of randomized clinical trials of a very-low-calorie diet that include follow-up data*

Reference	Subjects[a]	Mean pretreatment weight (kg)	Mean age (years)	Treatment regimen[b]	Mean treatment duration (weeks)	Mean weight loss (kg)[c]	Mean weight loss at follow-up (kg)
Miura et al., 1989 (80)	46 F, 24 M	148% of ideal weight	35.4	1. VLCD for 4–8 weeks followed by conventional diet	16	8.6	1 year: 5.0; 2 years: 4.1
				2. BT + conventional diet	16	4.5	1 year: 5.5 2 years: 5.8
				3. BT + VLCD for 4–8 weeks followed by conventional diet	16	10.7	1 year: 11.5 2 years: 12.0
Sikand et al., 1988 (81)	30 F (21; 15)	102.7	38.8	1. BT + VLCD for 16 weeks	16	17.5	2 years: 0.8
				2. BT + exercise + VLCD for 16 weeks	16	21.8	2 years: 9.1
Wadden et al., 1989 (55)	89 F (76; 68; 55)	106.0	42.1	1. PSMF for 8 weeks; 1,000–1,200 kcal/ day for 8 weeks	16	13.1*	1 year: 4.7* 5 years: +1.0
				2. BT + 1,200 kcal/day	26	13.0*	1 year: 6.6*† 5 years: +2.7
				3. BT + PSMF for 8 weeks; 1,000–1,200 kcal/day for 18 weeks	26	16.8†	1 year: 10.6† 5 years: +2.9
Wing et al., 1991 (82)	26 F, 10 M (33; 33)	103.8	51.0	1. BT + 1,000–1,500 kcal/day	20	10.1*	1 year: 6.8
				2. BT + PSMF/VLCD for 8 weeks; 1,000–1,500 kcal/day for 12 weeks	20	18.6†	1 year: 8.6

[a] Numbers in parentheses indicate the number of persons remaining at the end of treatment and at successive follow-up evaluations.
[b] VLCD, very low-calorie diet; BT, behavior therapy; PSMF, protein-sparing modified fast.
[c] Dissimilar superscripts—* and †—indicate significant differences.
From ref. 20, with permission.

sults of our multicenter evaluation, in which patients regained approximately 40% of their weight loss in the year following treatment (46).

Results of the three American studies summarized in Table 2 stand in sharp contrast to those reported from Japan by Miura et al. (80). These investigators found, as did Wadden et al. (70), that patients treated by VLCD alone regained weight rapidly. In sharp contrast, those who received VLCD combined with behavior modification continued to lose weight in the 2 years following therapy. Reasons for Miura et al.'s superior results are not clear but may include cultural differences between Japanese and American dieters and the fact that the Japanese patients were significantly less overweight than their American counterparts, and lost one-third to one-half less weight. Briefer treatment and smaller weight losses may not be associated with as severe biological pressures to regain weight (28).

Controlled Treatment Comparisons

The studies by Wadden et al. (70) and Wing et al. (82) provided randomized comparison of behavior therapy combined with either a 1,000 to 1,500 kcal/day diet or a VLCD. In both studies, the VLCD was associated with significantly greater end-of-treatment weight losses than was the conventional reducing diet. At 1-year follow-up, however, significant differences in weight losses were not observed between treatment conditions in either study. Patients in both conditions (in both studies) regained weight, but those who had received the VLCD regained substantially more.

These findings raise questions about the value of VLCDs as compared with conventional reducing diets, which are both safer and less expensive to administer (78). Careful studies are required to assess the short- and long-term benefits of both approaches in relationship to their costs. It will be important to assess not only long-term changes in

weight but also changes in health status. Wing et al. (82), for example, found that type II diabetics treated by VLCD showed significantly better glycemic control 1 year after treatment than did patients treated by a conventional reducing diet, despite patients in the two conditions showing comparable weight losses at this time. Thus VLCDs may be particularly useful in managing certain disorders.

Understanding Very-Low-Calorie Diets

A separate line of research has also raised questions about the necessity of severely restricting caloric intake. Two uncontrolled studies found that patients who consumed a 800 kcal/day diet achieved weight losses comparable to those treated by a 420 kcal/day diet for the same period of time (84,85). We recently confirmed these findings in a controlled trial in which outpatients were randomly assigned to diets providing either 420, 660, or 800 kcal daily (71). Figure 2 shows that there were only marginal differences in the weight losses of patients in the three conditions despite their treatment according to otherwise identical protocols. We were unable in this study to identify reasons why the patients in the 420 kcal/day diet did not lose significantly more weight than those who consumed the 800 kcal/day diet. The clinical implications of the study, however, are clear: there appears to be little benefit to severely restricting caloric intake.

Form of the Diet

These findings suggest that researchers may have misconstrued reasons for the efficacy of VLCDs (78). Investigators have focused almost exclusively on the caloric content of VLCDs and overlooked the form and manner in which the diets are consumed. Very-low-calorie diets—particularly those served in liquid form—provide patients a fixed energy intake and allow them to avoid contact with conventional foods. Thus the

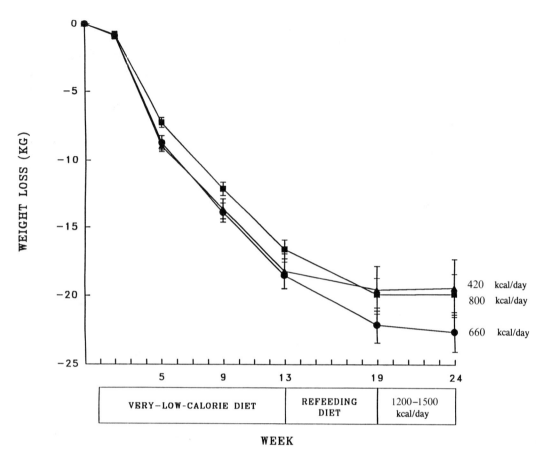

FIG. 2. Mean weight losses of patients randomly assigned to receive a 420, 660, or 800 kcal/day diet. All patients were prescribed a 1,200 to 1,500 kcal diet the first week. One of the three very-low-calorie diets described above was prescribed for weeks 2 to 13, after which patients were refed during weeks 14 to 19. Patients were prescribed a 1,200 to 1,500 kcal/day diet (of their own choosing) for the last 7 weeks of treatment. (From ref. 71, with permission.)

diets appear to facilitate excellent adherence, particularly if patients are warned that they may become ill if they "go off the diet."

The results of our randomized trial lead us to believe that patients who consume a liquid diet providing 1,000 kcal/day would lose approximately the same amount of weight as those who consume a VLCD providing 600 or 750 kcal/day diet. We further believe that persons who consume a 1,000 kcal/day liquid diet will lose significantly more weight than those requested to consume a self-selected diet of 1,000 kcal/day composed of conventional foods, the method followed with behavioral treatment. Recent research using doubly labeled water has shown that when asked to keep a food diary obese indi-

viduals typically underestimate their energy intake by 30 to 40% (86,87). Thus a self-selected diet of 1,000 kcal/day is likely to provide 1,400 kcal/day. Liquid diets take the guesswork out of measuring foods and counting calories.

Further research is required to determine if current liquid diets can be increased to 900 or more kcal/day without significantly reducing weight losses or other benefits of treatment. Increasing the caloric content of the diets should reduce the intensity of the medical supervision required and thus the cost of treatment.

It is of interest that Wing (88) has recently explored methods to increase the size of weight losses associated with traditional behavioral treatment by providing patients with foods that they are to consume or requesting that they eat prepackaged, calorie-controlled meals (i.e., frozen dinners). Preliminary findings have shown that the use of portion-controlled meals is associated with significantly greater short- and long-term weight losses than is the use of a conventional, self-selected diet. Thus there may well be a convergence in the type of dietary intervention used in VLCD and traditional behavioral programs. Both may eventually use prepackaged, portion-controlled diets providing approximately 1,000 kcal/day. It will be of interest to compare the short- and long-term effectiveness of a liquid diet with that of a portion-controlled diet composed of conventional foods.

TO LOSE OR NOT TO LOSE: THE PROBLEM OF WEIGHT LOSS MAINTENANCE

This review has shown that behavioral treatment combined with a 1,000 to 1,500 kcal/day reducing diet produces average losses of approximately 8.5 kg and VLCDs average losses of 15 to 25 kg. These are impressive findings when one considers the results of treatment described by Stunkard and McLaren-Hume (89) some 30 years ago. Clearly, investigators have made important advances in the induction of weight loss.

This review has also shown, however, that weight regain following treatment is a significant problem. Patients treated by behavior therapy and a 1,000 to 1,500 kcal/day diet regain about one-third of their weight loss in 1 year, while those treated by behavior therapy combined with a VLCD regain this amount or more. Several studies have suggested that a majority of patients are likely to regain all of their weight loss within 5 years (41,55,56).

As noted earlier, findings of significant weight regain have led some investigators to question the utility and ethics of current treatment (57,90,91) and to suggest that foregoing treatment may prove less damaging to

physical and psychological health than repeated cycles of weight loss and regain (56,90). The option of no treatment deserves serious consideration, particularly in the case of older individuals with lower body obesity who are free of health complications. It is an option, however, that cannot be universally endorsed until there are definitive research data. Although results of some epidemiological studies have suggested that weight cycling may increase the risk of illness and premature death (5,92), better controlled investigations are needed, as discussed by Wing (93).

Effects of Treatment versus No Treatment

A definitive evaluation of the long-term results of treatment produced by behavior therapy, VLCDs, and other approaches ultimately requires comparison of treated subjects with a group of untreated controls who are observed for the same period of time, preferably 5 years or more (40). Such an evaluation might reveal that treated individuals lose 10 to 20 kg but regain to their baseline weight over a 5-year period. Epidemiological data, however, suggest that untreated individuals will also gain weight during this time and thus may be 5 kg or more above baseline weight at the 5-year follow-up (94,95). In addition, persons who did not reduce are unlikely to experience any of the improvements in health enjoyed, at least temporarily, by those who lose weight. From this perspective, treatment—even with full weight regain—may still confer important advantages over no treatment.

Maintenance of Weight Loss

Rather than abandoning current methods of inducing weight loss because they do not provide good long-term results, it would seem more prudent to tackle the problems associated with maintaining weight loss. Research on this topic has been under way for less than a decade but has already yielded significant findings, as described in Perri's chapter in this volume.

Two important shifts must incur in our conceptualization of obesity in order to improve the long-term management (24,31). First, patients and their practitioners must realize that obesity, particularly in persons 40% or more overweight, is likely to be a chronic condition requiring life-long care. Practitioners would not expect 15 to 25 weeks of treatment for essential hypertension or diabetes to show effects 5 years after treatment. These disorders cannot be cured by brief therapy, only managed to varying degrees with ongoing care. Obesity and its treatment should be viewed similarly.

The second issue is that there are critical differences in the behaviors required for losing weight versus maintaining a weight loss, as illustrated in Table 3 (24). Most weight-loss programs, commercial or otherwise, provide little instruction in the maintenance of

TABLE 3. *Comparison of behaviors and reinforcement associated with losing weight versus maintaining a weight loss*

Weight loss	Maintenance of weight loss
The goal of treatment is to lose a large amount of weight, after a prolonged period of weight gain	The goal of treatment is to lose small amounts of weight, as small increases in weight occur
The dieter's principal strategy is to *avoid* eating all of the foods that have caused the weight problem	The dieter's principal task is to learn to eat troublesome foods in a controlled fashion (mastery) and to eat new foods, low in fat and calories
Treatment is time-limited, usually 15 to 25 weeks	Treatment is on-going and life-long
The dieter receives support from the diet program and from family and friends	The dieter receives little or no support from professionals or family members
Weight loss is highly reinforcing; it is very noticeable and pleasing to dieters and their families	Maintenance of weight loss is not reinforcing; dieters forget about their accomplishments, as do their family members
Dieters do not have to exercise to lose weight	Exercise appears to be critical to maintenance of weight loss

From ref. 24, with permission.

weight loss. If included, such information is usually presented while patients are still losing weight and do not have the opportunity to practice relevant skills. Such opportunity usually occurs only after patients have left treatment and have experienced their first crisis with weight regain. Thus it is imperative that programs provide instruction in the maintenance of weight loss that is distinct in both its timing and content from the initial treatment used to induce weight loss.

Factors Associated with Maintenance of Weight Loss

Research has revealed several factors associated with long-term weight control. These include: (a) continued contact with a health-care provider; (b) increased physical activity; and (c) adherence during the weight-loss program.

Continued Contact

Perri has conducted an outstanding series of studies on treatment variables associated with the maintenance of weight loss (31,96,97). He and his colleagues have shown that following weight loss, patients who continue to have regular contact with their provider maintain their weight losses significantly better than individuals not receiving such care. Posttreatment contact may consist of regularly scheduled telephone calls (96) or patients' participation in biweekly treatment sessions (31). Perri's chapter in this volume provides a detailed summary of his findings.

Physical Activity

Results of correlational studies have suggested that individuals who exercise regularly maintain their weight losses better than sedentary persons (39,98). Similar findings have been obtained in randomized clinical trials (81,99), including that of Pavlou and colleagues (39), in which patients assigned to an exercise condition maintained the great majority of their weight loss 3 years after treatment. Mechanisms responsible for the favorable effects of exercise on body weight have not been clearly identified, as discussed by Grillo, Brownell, and Stunkard in this volume. The message is clear, however; increased physical activity is critical to long-term weight control.

Adherence during Weight Loss

Although not as impressive a predictor as the two preceding variables, adherence to behavioral treatment during weight reduction correlates with maintenance of weight loss 1 year or more later (29,31,100). Thus persons who during the initial period of treatment show the best attendance and keep diet diaries most faithfully achieve larger weight losses in both the short and long term.

FUTURE DIRECTIONS

This last section briefly considers recommendations for practice and research. Recommendations for research are limited to treatment, although the most significant advances in treatment undoubtedly will depend upon advances in our understanding of the etiology of obesity.

Individualizing Treatment

Obese individuals frequently have different treatment needs and preferences. Greater attention must be paid to the initial evaluation of patients, as described by Stunkard, in order to assess these needs and then select the most appropriate intervention (Fig. 1). Some patients, for example, may require adjunct dietary counseling, psychotherapy, or marital therapy. As a general rule, such interventions should be provided in addition to group treatment for obesity, rather than replacing it as the primary therapeutic modality.

Treatment of Binge Eating

Binge eating represents an excellent example of the need to individualize care. Approximately 25 to 40% of obese individuals who seek treatment at university and hospital clinics indicate that they engage in binge eating, in which they consume a large amount of food in a short period of time and feel unable to control this behavior (101–103). Unlike persons with bulimia nervosa, obese binge eaters do not compensate (by vomiting or other means) for their binge episodes, which may contribute to their weight problem. Obese binge eaters as compared with obese nonbingers are more likely to display significant psychopathology (104,105), and, with some types of therapy, to discontinue treatment prematurely and to regain weight more rapidly (105).

Investigators have recently begun to explore the use of cognitive–behavioral interventions designed to reduce the frequency of binge episodes (106). From this perspective, control of the binge eating is thought to be more important than is weight reduction per se and with its control may lead to weight loss. Research is needed on this and other approaches including that advocated by Overeaters Anonymous.

Weight Maintenance Therapy

Continuing patient–therapist contact, as described by Perri, clearly facilitates long-term weight control. Anecdotal reports, however, have suggested that it is difficult in many cases to keep patients in therapy, even when treatment is offered free of charge or at a greatly reduced rate. Patients frequently complain of boredom in attending treatment sessions in the same room with the same individuals for a period of a year or more. In addition, some participants indicate that they are demoralized by other members' reports of overeating and weight gain—reports that are inevitable in a weight loss maintenance program.

Research is needed to answer a host of questions concerning maintenance therapy including:

1. Which is preferable, group or individual therapy? Group therapy clearly has advantages for weight loss but may have some disadvantages in the maintenance of weight loss, as suggested above.
2. If group treatment is used, should patients remain with the same participants with whom they lost weight or should they be placed in a group with a large percentage of new members? Should the therapist who provided instruction in weight loss also provide instruction in the maintenance of weight loss, or would the introduction of a new therapist have advantages? Continuity of care would suggest that patients should remain with the same group members and therapists. The need, however, to renew expectations of success and provide new learning might favor the introduction of a new group and therapist.
3. Are there new interventions that can be introduced in a maintenance program to increase patient learning, in addition to increasing their interest in therapy? A maintenance curriculum, for example, might be created in which patients meet at a health club for several months to obtain supervised instruction in physical activity rather than simply talking about exercise in group meetings. Similarly, classes that provide hands-on experience with low-fat cooking would seem preferable to verbal descriptions of such cuisine.

Clearly, there are many questions about the optimal structure and content of programs designed to facilitate the maintenance of weight loss. Bold innovation is required in this area.

PRESERVING PATIENTS' SELF-ESTEEM

This chapter began with a discussion of the difficulties that obese individuals face today in deciding whether they should attempt to lose weight. It concludes with a reminder of the daily despair many obese individuals experience as a consequence of living in a society that abhors fat. In all too many cases overweight individuals have been ridiculed, scorned, and rejected, not only by passing strangers but by family, friends, and, sadly, even their health-care providers. Practitioners must realize that the frustration and occasional anger they experience in working with unsuccessful patients is only a small fraction of the frustration and self-loathing that many obese individuals feel because of their failure to control their weight. No good comes when practitioners express their negative feelings (understandable as they may be) to patients. On the contrary, patients are deeply harmed by such criticism, which is likely to increase their burden of shame and their desire to avoid treatment.

Patience and constancy are two of the most important tools in the treatment of obesity—patience to accept the inevitable difficulties that an obese individual will encounter with his or her weight and constancy to remain available and supportive at such times. The patient will not always achieve successful weight control with such therapy but will experience the provider's respect and concern, both of which are remarkable healers of injured self-esteem.

ACKNOWLEDGMENTS

This chapter was completed with the support of a Research Scientist Development Award from the National Institute of Mental Health and a grant from the Sandoz Nutrition Company. The author thanks Ms. Kathy Letizia for her superb editorial assistance.

REFERENCES

1. Manson JE, Colditz GA, Stampfer MJ, et al. A prospective study of obesity and risk of coronary heart disease in women. *N Engl J Med* 1990;322:882–9.
2. VanItallie TB. The perils of obesity in middle-aged women. *N Engl J Med* 1990;320:928–9.

3. US House of Representatives, Committee on Small Business, Subcommittee on Regulation, Business Opportunities, and Energy. Deception and fraud in the diet industry: Part I. Washington: US Government Printing Office; 1990; 101-50.

4. O'Neill M. Dieters, craving balance, are battling fears of food. *New York Times* 1990;139(48,192):1.

5. Lissner L, Odell PM, D'Agostino RB, et al. Variability of body weight and health outcomes in the Framingham population. *N Engl J Med* 1991;324:1839–44.

6. Stunkard AJ. The current status of treatment for obesity in adults. In: Stunkard AJ, Stellar E, eds. *Eating and its disorders.* New York: Raven Press;1984;157–74.

7. Wadden TA, Foster GD. Behavioral assessment and treatment of markedly obese patients. In: Wadden TA, VanItallie TB, eds. *Treatment of the seriously obese patient.* New York: Guilford Press; 1992;290–330.

8. Bjorntorp P. Regional patterns of fat distribution: health implications. *Ann Intern Med* 1985; 103:994–5.

9. Sjöström L. Mortality of severely obese subjects. *Am J Clin Nutr* 1992;55:516S–21S.

10. Brownell KD, Wadden TA. The heterogeneity of obesity: fitting treatments to individuals. *Behav Ther* 1991;22:153–77.

11. Brownell KD, Wadden TA. Etiology and treatment of obesity: understanding a serious, prevalent, and refractory disorder. *J Consult Clin Psychol [in press]*.

12. Kanders BS, Blackburn GL. Reducing primary risk factors by therapeutic weight loss. In: Wadden TA, VanItallie TB, eds. *Treatment of the seriously obese patient.* New York: Guilford Press, 1992; 213–30.

13. Garrow JS. *Treat obesity seriously.* New York: Churchill Livingstone, 1981.

14. Guy-Grand B. Long-term pharmacological treatment of obesity. In: Wadden TA, VanItallie TB, eds. *Treatment of the seriously obese patient.* New York: Guilford, 1992;478–95.

15. Marcus MD, Wing RR, Ewing L, Kern E, McDermott M, Gooding W. A double-blind, placebo-controlled trial of fluoxetine plus behavior modification in the treatment of obese binge eaters. *Am J Psychiatry* 1990;147:876–81.

16. Miller PM, Sims KL. Evaluation and component analysis of a comprehensive weight control program. *Int J Obes* 1981;5:57–65.

17. Stuart RB. Behavioral control of overeating. *Behav Res Ther* 1967;5:357–65.

18. Stunkard AJ. The management of obesity. *NY State J Med* 1958;58:79–87.

19. Stunkard AJ. Obesity. In: Bellack AS, Hersen M, Kazdin AE, eds. *International handbook of behavior modification and therapy.* New York: Plenum Press, 1982;535–73.

20. Brownell KD, Wadden TA. Behavior therapy for obesity: modern approaches and better results. In: Brownell KD, Foreyt JP, eds. *Handbook of eating disorders: physiology, psychology, and treatment of obesity, anorexia, and bulimia.* New York: Basic Books, 1986;180–97.

21. Ravussin E, Lillioja S, Knowler WC, et al. Reduced rate of energy expenditure as a risk factor for body-weight gain. *N Engl J Med* 1988;318:462–72.

22. Sjöström L. Fat cells and body weight. In: Stunkard AJ, ed. *Obesity.* Philadelphia: WB Saunders, 1980;72–100.

23. Stunkard AJ, Harris JR, Pedersen NL, McClearn GE. A separated twin study of the body mass index. *N Engl J Med* 1990;322:1483–7.

24. Wadden TA, Bell ST. Obesity. In: Bellack AS, Hersen M, Kazdin AE, eds. *International handbook of behavior modification and therapy, vol II.* New York: Plenum Press, 1990;449–73.

25. Brownell KD. *The LEARN Program for weight control.* Dallas: American Health Pub Co, 1990.

26. Beck AT. *Cognitive therapy and the emotional disorders.* New York: International Universities Press, 1976.

27. Stunkard AJ. Some perspectives on human obesity: its causes. *Bull NY Acad Med* 1988;64:902–23.

28. Brownell KD. Obesity: understanding and treating a serious, prevalent, and refractory disorder. *J Consult Clin Psychol* 1982;50:820–40.

29. Wadden TA, Letizia KA. Predictors of attrition and weight loss in patients treated by moderate and severe caloric restriction. In: Wadden TA, VanItallie TB, eds. *Treatment of the seriously obese patient.* New York: Guilford, 1992;383–410.

30. Black DR. A minimal intervention program and a problem-solving program for weight control. *Cognitive Ther Res* 1987;11:107–20.

31. Perri MG, McAllister DA, Gange JJ, Jordan RC, McAdoo WG, Nezu AM. Effects of four maintenance programs on the long-term management of obesity. *J Consult Clin Psychol* 1988;56:529–34.

32. Donato K. Efficiency and utilization of various energy sources for growth. *Am J Clin Nutr* 1987;45:164–7.

33. Sclafani A. Dietary obesity. In: Stunkard AJ, ed. *Obesity.* Philadelphia: WB Saunders, 1980; 161–81.

34. Lissner L, Levitsky DA, Strupp BJ, Kalkwarf HJ, Roe DA. Dietary fat and the regulation of energy intake in human subjects. *Am J Clin Nutr* 1987;46:886–92.

35. Spiegel TA, Wadden TA, Foster GD. Objective measurement of eating rate during behavioral treatment of obesity. *Behav Ther* 1991;22:61–7.

36. Mahoney MJ, Mahoney K. *Permanent weight control: a total solution to a dieter's dilemma.* New York: WW Norton, 1976.

37. Collins RL, Rothblum ED, Wilson GT. The comparative efficacy of cognitive and behavioral approaches in the treatment of obesity. *Cognitive Ther Res* 1986;10:299–317.

38. Kayman S, Bruvold W, Stern J. Maintenance and relapse after weight loss in women: behavioral aspects. *Am J Clin Nutr* 1990;52:800–7.

39. Pavlou KN, Krey S, Steffee WP. Exercise as an adjunct to weight loss and maintenance in moderately obese subjects. *Am J Clin Nutr* 1989; 49:1115–23.

40. Brownell KD, Jeffery RW. Improving long-term weight loss: pushing the limits of treatment. *Behav Ther* 1987;18:353–74.

41. Epstein LH, Wing RR, Koeske R, Ossip D, Beck S. A comparison of lifestyle change and programmed aerobic exercise on weight and fitness changes in obese children. *Behav Ther* 1982;13:651–65.
42. Blair SN, Kohl HW, Paffenbarger RS, Clark DG, Cooper KH, Gibbons LW. Physical fitness and all-cause mortality: a prospective study of healthy men and women. *JAMA* 1989;262:2395–401.
43. Renjilian DA, Perri MG, Nezu AM, McKelvey WF, Schein RL. Individual versus group therapy for obesity: matching clients with treatments. Paper presented at the American Psychological Association Convention, New Orleans, LA, August, 1990.
44. Stunkard AJ, Cohen RY, Felix MRJ. Weight loss competitions at the worksite: how they work and how well. *Prev Med* 1989;18:460–74.
45. Wadden TA, Foster GD, Letizia KA. Long-term treatment of obesity with and without very-low-calorie diet. Unpublished manuscript, 1990.
46. Wadden TA, Foster GD, Letizia KA, Stunkard AJ. A multi-center evaluation of a proprietary weight reduction program for the treatment of marked obesity. *Arch Intern Med* 1992;152:961–6.
47. Volkmar FR, Stunkard AJ, Woolston J, Bailey RA. High attrition rates in commercial weight reduction programs. *Arch Intern Med* 1981;141:426–8.
48. Feuerstein M, Papciak A, Shapiro S, Tannenbaum S. The weight loss profile: a biopsychosocial approach. *Int J Psychiatr Med* 1989;19:181–92.
49. Jeffery RW, Wing RR, Stunkard AJ. Behavioral treatment of obesity: the state of the art in 1976. *Behav Ther* 1978;9:189–99.
50. Levitz L, Stunkard AJ. A therapeutic coalition for obesity: behavior modification and patient self-help. *Am J Psychiatry* 1974;131:423–27.
51. Wilson GT. Behavior modification and the treatment of obesity. In: Stunkard AJ, ed. *Obesity.* Philadelphia: WB Saunders, 1980;325–44.
52. Yalom I. *The theory and practice of group psychotherapy,* 2nd ed. New York: Basic Books, 1975.
53. Perri MG, Nezu AM, Patti ET, McCann KL. Effect of length of treatment on weight loss. *J Consult Clin Psychol* 1989;57:450–4.
54. Kramer FM, Jeffery RW, Forster JL, Snell MK. Long-term follow-up of behavioral treatment for obesity: patterns of weight regain in men and women. *Int J Obes* 1989;13:123–36.
55. Wadden TA, Sternberg JA, Letizia KA, Stunkard AJ, Foster GD. Treatment of obesity by very low calorie diet, behavior therapy, and their combination: a five-year perspective. *Int J Obes* 1989;13[Suppl 2]:39–46.
56. Garner DM, Wooley SC. Confronting the failure of behavioral and dietary treatments for obesity. *Clin Psychol Rev* 1991;11:1–52.
57. Goodrick GK, Foreyt JP. Why treatments for obesity don't last. *J Am Diet Assoc* 1991;91:1243–7.
58. Roth G. *Breaking free from compulsive eating.* New York: Bobbs-Merrill 1984.
59. Wilson GT. The addiction model of eating disorders: a critical analysis. *Adv Behav Res Ther* 1991;13:27–72.
60. Wadden TA, Van Itallie TB, Blackburn GL. Responsible and irresponsible use of very-low-calorie diets in the treatment of obesity. *JAMA* 1990;263:83–5.
61. Wadden TA, Stunkard AJ, Brownell KD. Very low calorie diets: their efficacy, safety, and future. *Ann Intern Med* 1983;99:675–84.
62. Apfelbaum M. Traitement de l'obésité par la diète protodique. *Entriens e Bichat* 1967;1:62.
63. Bistrian BR. Clinical use of a protein sparing modified fast. *JAMA* 1978;240:2299–302.
64. Blackburn GL, Lynch ME, Wong SL. The very-low-calorie diet: a weight-reduction technique. In: Brownell KD, Foreyt JP, eds. *Handbook of eating disorders: physiology, psychology, and treatment of obesity, anorexia, and bulimia.* New York: Basic Books, 1986;198–212.
65. Genuth S. Supplemented fasting in the treatment of obesity and diabetes. *Am J Clin Nutr* 1979;32:2579–86.
66. Vertes V, Genuth SM, Hazelton IM. Supplemented fasting as a large scale outpatient program. *JAMA* 1977;238:1251–3.
67. Atkinson RL. Medical evaluation and monitoring of patients treated by severe caloric restriction. In: Wadden TA, VanItallie TB, eds. *Treatment of the seriously obese patient.* New York: Guilford Press, 1992;273–89.
68. Wadden TA, Stunkard AJ, Brownell KD, Day SC. A comparison of two very-low-calorie diets: protein-sparing-modified fast versus protein liquid formula diet. *Am J Clin Nutr* 1985;41:533–9.
69. Palgi A, Read JL, Greenberg I, Hoffer MA, Bistrian BR, Blackburn GL. Multidisciplinary treatment of obesity with a protein-sparing modified fast: results in 688 outpatients. *Am J Public Health* 1985;75:1190–4.
70. Wadden TA, Stunkard AJ. Controlled trial of very low calorie diet, behavior therapy, and their combination in the treatment of obesity. *J Consult Clin Psychol* 1986;54:482–8.
71. Foster GD, Wadden TA, Peterson FJ, Letizia KA, Bartlett SJ, Conill AM. A controlled comparison of three very-low-calorie diets: effects on weight, body composition, and symptoms. *Am J Clin Nutr* 1992;55:811–7.
72. Broomfield PH, Chopra R, Sheinbaum RC, et al. Effects of ursodeoxycholic acid and aspirin on the formation of lithogenic bile and gallstones during loss of weight. *N Engl J Med* 1988;319:1567–72.
73. Liddle RA, Goldstein RB, Saxton J. Gallstone formation during weight-reduction dieting. *Arch Intern Med* 1989;149:1750–3.
74. Donnelly JE, Pronk NP, Jacobsen DJ, Pronk SJ, Jakicic JM. Effects of a very-low-calorie diet and physical training regimens on body composition and resting metabolic rate in obese females. *Am J Clin Nutr* 1991;54:56–61.
75. Hovell MF, Loch A, Hofstetter CR, et al. Long-term weight loss maintenance: assessment of a behavioral and supplemental fasting regimen. *Am J Public Health* 1988;78:663–6.
76. Wadden TA, Foster GD, Letizia KA, Mullen JL. Long-term effects of dieting on resting metabolic rate in obese outpatients. *JAMA* 1990;264:707–11.
77. Kirschner MA, Schneider G, Ertel NH, Gorman J. An eight-year experience with a very-low-calorie

formula diet for control of major obesity. *Int J Obes* 1988;12:69–80.

78. Wadden TA, Bartlett SJ. Very low calorie diets: an overview and appraisal. In: Wadden TA, VanItallie TB, eds. *Treatment of the seriously obese patient.* New York: Guilford Press, 1992;44–79.

79. Andersen T, Backer OG, Stokholm KH, Quaade F. Randomized trial of diet and gastroplasty compared with diet alone in morbid obesity. *N Engl J Med* 1984;310:352–6.

80. Miura J, Arai K, Tsukahara S, Ohno M, Kideda Y. The long term effectiveness of combined therapy by behavior modification and very low calorie diet: 2 year follow up. *Int J Obes* 1989;13[Suppl 2]:73–7.

81. Sikand G, Kondo A, Foreyt JP, Jones PH, Gotto AM. Two year follow-up of patients treated with very low calorie dieting and exercise testing. *J Dietet Assoc* 1988;88:487–8.

82. Wing RR, Marcus MD, Salata R, Epstein LH, Miaskiewicz S, Blair EH. Effects of a very-low-calorie diet on long-term glycemic control in obese type II diabetics. *Arch Intern Med* 1991;151:1334–40.

83. Genuth SM, Vertes V, Hazelton J. Supplemented fasting in the treatment of obesity. In: Bray G, ed. *Recent advances in obesity research.* London: Newman, 1978;370–8.

84. Kanders BS, Blackburn GL, Lavin PT, Norton D. Weight-loss outcome and health benefits associated with the Optifast Program in the treatment of obesity. *Int J Obes* 1989;13[Suppl 2]:131–4.

85. Vertes V. Clinical experience with a very low calorie diet. In: Blackburn GL, Bray GA, eds. *Management of obesity by severe caloric restriction.* Littleton: PSG Publishing Company, 1985;349–58.

86. Bandini LG, Schoeller DA, Cyr HN, Dietz WH. Validity of reported energy intake in obese and nonobese adolescents. *Am J Clin Nutr* 1990;52:421–5.

87. Schoeller DA. Measurement of energy expenditure in free-living humans by using doubly labeled water. *J Nutr* 1988;118:1278–89.

88. Wing RR. Advances in the treatment of obesity. Presented at the annual meeting of the Association for the Advancement of Behavior Therapy, New York, NY, November 21, 1991.

89. Stunkard AJ, McLaren-Hume M. The results of treatment for obesity. *AMA Arch Intern Med* 1959;103:79–85.

90. Wooley SC, Garner DM. Obesity treatment: the high cost of false hope. *J Am Diet Assoc* 1991;91:1248–51.

91. Lustig A. Weight loss programs: failing to meet ethical standards. *J Am Diet Assoc* 1991;91:1252–4.

92. Hamm P, Shekelle RB, Stamler J. Large fluctuations in body weight during young adulthood and twenty-five year risk of coronary heart disease in men. *Am J Epidemiol* 1989;129:312–8.

93. Wing RR. Weight cycling in humans: a review of the literature. *Ann Behav Med* [in press].

94. Shah M, Hannan PJ, Jeffery RW. Secular trend in body mass index in the adult population of three communities in the upper midwestern part of the USA: the Minnesota Heart Health Program. *Int J Obes* 1991;15:499–503.

95. Williamson DF, Kahn HS, Remington PL, Anda RF. The 10-year incidence of overweight and major weight gain in US adults. *Arch Intern Med* 1990;150:665–72.

96. Perri MG, Shapiro RM, Ludwig WW, Twentyman C, McAdoo WG. Maintenance strategies for the treatment of obesity: an evaluation of relapse prevention training and posttreatment contact by mail and telephone. *J Consult Clin Psychol* 1984;52:404–13.

97. Perri MG, McAdoo WG, Spevak PA, Newlin DB. Effect of a multicompartment maintenance program on long-term weight loss. *J Consult Clin Psychol* 1984;52:480–1.

98. Gormally J, Rardin D, Black S. Correlates of successful response to a behavioral weight control clinic. *J Consult Clin Psychol* 1980;27:179–91.

99. Dahlkoetter J, Callahan EJ, Linton J. Obesity and the unbalanced energy equation: exercise versus eating habit change. *J Consult Clin Psychol* 1979;47:898–905.

100. Jeffery RW, Björnson-Benson WM, Rosenthal BS, Lindquist RA, Kurth CL, Johnson SL. Correlates of weight loss and its maintenance over two years of follow-up among middle-aged men. *Prev Med* 1984;13:155–68.

101. Gormally J, Black S, Daston S, Rardin D. The assessment of binge eating severity among obese persons. *Addict Behav* 1982;7:47–55.

102. Marcus MD, Wing RR, Lamparski DM. Binge eating and dietary restraint in obese patients. *Addict Behav* 1985;10:163–8.

103. Spitzer RL, Devlin M, Walsh BT, et al. Binge eating disorder: a multisite field trial of the diagnostic criteria. *Int J Eating Disord* 1992;11:191–202.

104. Marcus MD, Wing RR, Hopkins J. Obese binge eaters: affect, cognitions, and response to behavioral weight control. *J Consult Clin Psychol* 1988;56:433–9.

105. Telch CF, Agras WS, Rossiter E, Wilfley D, Kenardy J. Group cognitive-behavioral treatment for the non-purging bulimic: an initial evaluation. *J Consult Clin Psychol* 1990;58:629–35.

106. Malenbaum R, Herzog D, Eisenthal S, Wyshak G. Overeaters anonymous: impact on bulimia. *Int J Eating Disord* 1988;7:139–43.

Obesity: Theory and Therapy, Second Edition, edited by A. J. Stunkard and T. A. Wadden. Raven Press, Ltd., New York © 1993.

13

Estimation of the Effect of Obesity on Health and Longevity

A Perspective for the Physician

Theodore B. VanItallie and Edward A. Lew

Department of Medicine, Columbia University College of Physicians and Surgeons, St. Luke's-Roosevelt Hospital Center, New York, New York 10025

"Depend on it, Sir (said Dr. Samuel Johnson in 1777), when a man knows he is to be hanged in a fortnight, it concentrates his mind wonderfully" (1). In the same psychological vein, albeit under less extreme and more hopeful circumstances, the awareness of being at relatively high risk of developing a severe illness or dying prematurely can concentrate the minds of patients and impel them to begin to correct potentially reversible risk factors (like overweight) and to adopt a generally healthier life style. In such situations, the challenge facing the physician is to provide the patient with an estimate of degree of health and/or mortality risk that is reasonably accurate and yet not excessively frightening. At the same time the physician should not be so reassuring that the patient will feel too comfortable to take any corrective action.

Another dimension of the same problem is to help the patient find ways to sustain the motivation necessary to continue to adhere to whatever program will be most effective in staving off the illness that portends. To this end, the physician may have to keep reminding uncooperative patients that some avoidable health risk still threatens, and to provide positive reinforcement (praise and enthusi-

asm) to patients who are successful in bringing their risk attributes under better control.

A good part of the effectiveness of physicians in helping patients adhere to a treatment and/or prevention regime arises from their ability to elicit a patient's trust, respect, and cooperation. Apart from the clear value of applying such interpersonal skills in patient management, it has become increasingly important for physicians to gain a sufficient working knowledge of morbidity and mortality risk to be able to give their patients a reasonable understanding of the hazards they face and the long-term consequences to health and survival of continuing certain self-damaging behaviors.

THE CONCEPT OF RISK

Perceptions of health risks stem from estimates of the probabilities of contracting specific diseases, the probability of dying early, or the probability of surviving for an extended period of time. Estimates of the probabilities of surviving many years lead to the concept of life expectancy.

Risks can be expressed either as absolute numbers or in relative terms (Table 1). Mor-

TABLE 1. *Terminology of morbidity and mortality risk: some commonly used expressions*

Mortality rate (m)	Usually calculated as the quotient of the number of deaths over a period of time (customarily 1 year) divided by the average number of subjects exposed to risk of death over that period
Mortality ratio (MR)	The quotient of the probability of death (q) in the population under examination (e.g., an overweight population) divided by the corresponding probability of death calculated from the experience in a defined population regarded as an appropriate standard for judging normal mortality levels
Morbidity rate	
Incidence rate	Calculated as the quotient of new morbid events (e.g., myocardial infarctions) reported over a period of time (customarily 1 year) divided by the average number of subjects exposed to the risk of morbidity over that period, not including those who had already succumbed to such morbid events
Prevalence rate	Calculated as the quotient of existing subjects with a morbid condition (e.g., diabetes) divided by the total number of subjects in the population
Relative risk ratio (i.e., mortality ratio or relative prevalence)	Ratio of the risk of dying or of developing a morbid condition (e.g., diabetes) over a period of time in a population under study (e.g., overweight individuals) to the risk of dying or of developing the same morbid condition in a comparable population not possessing the risk attribute in question; *relative prevalence* is the prevalence of a health problem in a population possessing a certain risk attribute (e.g., overweight) divided by the prevalence of the same problem among an otherwise comparable nonoverweight population; the resulting quotient is a *relative risk ratio*
Attributable risk	The maximum proportion of a particular disease (or group of diseases) that may be attributed to a particular cause, such as overweight
Proportional hazards model	Mathematical model used to assess the independent effect of a risk attribute (e.g., overweight) on risk of a morbid condition (e.g., coronary heart disease) in the presence of other risk factors such as cigarette smoking or hypercholesterolemia

Adapted from ref. 32, with permission.

bidity rates, mortality rates, and life expectancies exemplify absolute risks. More light is shed on such risks by comparing them with corresponding risks in more broadly representative or simply other populations. Thus it is illuminating to compare mortality rates among grossly obese persons in whom we may be particularly interested with corresponding mortality rates among persons of average weight. The ratio of the absolute risk to the risk selected for comparison provides a relative measure of the risk. When mortality rates are so compared the result is called a mortality ratio (MR). It is usually calculated as the quotient of the probability of death in the population under study (q) divided by the corresponding probability as determined from a defined population (q′).

The magnitude of the MR (or other measure of the relative risk) is strongly affected by the value of the denominator, that is, by the

choice of the comparison population. If the MR for a group in which we are interested is derived by dividing the mortality rates in that group by the corresponding mortality rates in an ostensibly "normal" population, much clearly depends on how this population is selected. If we are concerned with a group of persons with a body mass index (BMI) equal to or greater than 28 kg/m^2, we can compare their mortality either with that of persons of average weight or with that of persons 80 to 90% of average; since the mortality of the latter is lower, the MR will be correspondingly higher, as shown in Table 2.

Relative risk of developing a particular illness is calculated from morbidity rates, which can be expressed as either incidence rates or prevalence rates (Table 1). As an example, if the prevalence rate of diabetes among overweight individuals 20 to 45 years of age is 38 per 1,000, but 10 per 1,000

TABLE 2. *Mortality ratios (MRs) from coronary heart disease in men aged 50 to 59 years*

| Weight index (% of average weight) | MRs (%)[a] | |
	In relation to death rates of those 90–109% of average weight	In relation to death rates of those <80% of average weight
<80	77	100
80–89	86	112
90–109	100	130
110–119	128	166
120–129	141	183
130–139	176	229
>139	216	281

[a] In men aged 50 to 59 years, the most favorable mortality experience occurred among those whose weight index (percent of average weight) was <80. Data from ref. 22 and ref. 23.

among nonoverweight, but otherwise comparable individuals in the same population, then the *relative* prevalence of this particular health problem among the overweight is 3.8. In this context, relative prevalence is the same as the relative risk ratio. Another way of expressing the relative risk ratio is as a percentage; thus a ratio of 3.8 is the same as 380%.

From the relative risk ratio, the physician can estimate the extent to which a particular risk attribute such as overweight increases the probability of developing any of a number of obesity-associated health problems. Examples include hypertension, diabetes, coronary heart disease, gout, and cholelithiasis.

HELPING PATIENTS CONCEPTUALIZE RISK

If one is attempting to help patients conceptualize relative risk, they should be made aware that, within the population of which they are members, people can be grouped according to numerous characteristics such as age, sex, race, ethnicity, socioeconomic status, etc. Such a defined group or "cohort" can be determined to have a particular mortality rate. If the patient is a member of such a cohort, this rate represents the patient's abso-

lute risk of dying over some given period of time—usually a year. If the same cohort is then subdivided into subgroups (for example, into quintiles) according to cholesterol concentration in plasma, BMI, or the presence of some other trait thought to affect health or life expectancy, one can compare the adverse outcomes subgroup by subgroup.

An example of such a comparison can be found in a recent report of a prospective study of obesity and risk of coronary heart disease (2). As reported by the authors, for increasing levels of BMI, the age- and cigarette smoking-adjusted relative risk (computed as the incidence rate in a specific BMI category) of combined nonfatal myocardial infarction and fatal coronary heart disease among middle-aged women increased more than threefold when subjects in the highest BMI quintile (>29 kg/m^2) were compared with those in the lowest quintile (<21 kg/m^2).

What overweight patients may need to be told is that, within the population of which they are members, there are otherwise comparable non-overweight individuals whose risk of dying (mortality rate) or of developing certain obesity-related illnesses (morbidity rate) is very much lower than theirs.

Some longitudinal cohort studies can be used to demonstrate that individuals who manifest such attributes as severe overweight (e.g., a BMI > 32 kg/m^2) or a sedentary life style have an enhanced risk of developing certain illnesses and/or of dying prematurely (3–6). It does not necessarily follow, however, that weight reduction or adoption of a physically more active life style will enable people to reduce such risks to normal. Large-scale prospective cohort studies suitably designed to quantify changes in morbidity and mortality risk in association with sustained body fat reduction, with or without increased exercise, have yet to be reported. The results of one small study on morbidly obese patients (7) are encouraging; however, until the results of more definitive investigations become available, health professionals will have to continue to extrapolate from a host of data showing that sustained weight reduction can help bring a variety of risk attributes such as an elevated blood pressure or a high plasma low-density lipoprotein (LDL) concentration to safer levels. Unfortunately, physicians cannot truthfully tell their patients that, if their weight returns to and remains at the recommended level, all excess risk will have been eliminated. There is evidence, however, that men who have reduced their weights to not more than 20% above average at first experienced distinctly lower mortality lasting for some years; it then tended to increase with the passage of time (5,6,8,9).

THE NATURE OF THE ASSOCIATION BETWEEN OVERWEIGHT AND ENHANCED RISK OF ILLNESS

It has been known since Greco-Roman times that manifest obesity can be hazardous to health; however, the strength of the association between overweight and increased morbidity and mortality has been found to vary from one epidemiologic investigation to another (10). Factors believed to explain such variability include differences in the duration of the period of observation and in the size and nature of the subject population, whether adjustment was made for cigarette smoking, etc. (11). As pointed out by Sjöström in this volume, and by others (10,11), cohort studies that have been unable to demonstrate a relationship between body weight and mortality have (a) involved a relatively small population (usually fewer than 7,000 subjects); (b) had follow-up periods of insufficient duration (generally less than 10 years); (c) failed to control for the fact that cigarette smoking is more frequent among the nonobese than the obese; (d) failed to adjust for early mortality among subjects in whom clinical or subclinical illness was present at the outset of the study; (e) selected unsuitable subjects [as in the Seven Countries Study (12), which focused on working populations, which tend to be much fitter by virtue of the "healthy worker effect"]; and (f) improperly controlled for "intermediate" risk attributes like hypertension and hyperlipidemia that are at least in part caused by obesity.

In contrast, studies of sufficient size and heterogeneity (with 20,000 or more participants) and longer duration (10 to 30 years) have all shown a positive relationship between overweight and increased relative mortality. Unfortunately, in many of these positive population studies, the adverse effects of obesity have been materially underestimated owing to defects such as lack of control for cigarette smoking, failure to start out with a population consisting only of ostensibly healthy individuals, and reliance on a period of observation too short to permit the adverse effects of obesity to be fully observed.

Yet, even in studies that take into account all the above-described confounding factors, the hazards associated with being obese may continue to be underestimated if the anatomical measurement being used as the surrogate for obesity is insufficiently sensitive or specific.

In 1985, Björntorp (13) proposed two theories to explain the relatively weak association between obesity and coronary (ischemic) heart disease:

> First, a primary factor both causes obesity and precipitates ischemic heart disease (or some other illness) as a secondary phenomenon. Second, the association with cardiovascular disease (or other illness) is found only in a subgroup of persons with obesity. This effect would then be diluted in large populations after a long period of observation.

Björntorp expressed the belief that the second theory is more likely to be the correct one and cited evidence to indicate that the waist-hip circumference ratio (WHR), an index of upper-body or abdominal obesity, is more sensitive and specific than the BMI as a predictor of morbidity and mortality risk in obese individuals.

Since 1984, when two longitudinal studies were reported demonstrating the value of the WHR as a relatively sensitive index of increased morbidity and mortality risk in Swedish men and women (14,15), many investigations have shown that upper body or abdominal obesity (as disclosed by a high WHR) is associated with an increased incidence of metabolic disorders and cardiovascular disease (16). Abdominal obesity reflects excessive accumulation of visceral fat and, apparently, it is the enlargement of the visceral fat depot ("visceral obesity") that gives rise to a sequence of metabolic events that, in their turn, result in a variety of metabolic changes including impaired glucose tolerance, hyperlipidemia, and possibly hypertension (17). Some of these postulated relationships are shown in Fig. 1.

The principal problem in testing the hypothesis that visceral fat content is a more sensitive and specific indicator of obesity-related risk than the WHR, skinfold thicknesses at various sites, or the BMI resides in the nature of the technology required to estimate visceral fat mass. Until recently, an expensive and radiologically somewhat hazardous procedure, computed tomography (CT), has been the only method available for determining the intraabdominal fat area [visceral adipose tissue (AT)] (18,19). By means of this procedure, a positive relationship of increased visceral fat content to a variety of metabolic disorders has been demonstrated (20).

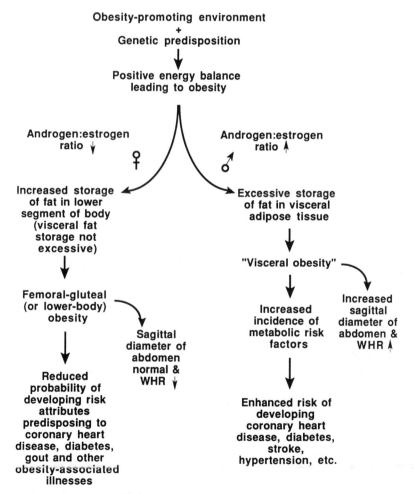

FIG. 1. A simplified representation of sequences of events postulated to give rise to either visceral (android) obesity or femoral-gluteal (gynoid) obesity. WHR, waist-hip circumference ratio.

However, as Sjöström clearly explains in this volume, the use of area determinations (which are two-dimensional) are less than satisfactory, considering that the body has three dimensions. For this reason, according to Sjöström, results obtained by conventional CT imaging cannot be used to express regional areas of AT as percentages of the total AT volume. To overcome this problem, Sjöström et al. (21) developed a multiscan CT procedure that permits determination of the volume of 20 different compartments from 28 scans and the distance between them. Obviously, the use of such a multiscan procedure in clinical practice is not feasible; however, as Sjöström and his colleagues have discovered, it is possible to identify CT-calibrated anthropometric predictors of the visceral AT volume that are reasonably satisfactory for use in surveys or for estimating morbidity and mortality risk in individual patients. Indeed, after testing several hundred possible indicators of visceral AT volume, Sjöström et al. (21) found that, by using weight, height, and the sagittal diameter of the supine patient measured at the level of the iliac crest, one can estimate the composition of the human body in terms of the weights of three clinically important important compartments, namely, fat-free mass (FFM), subcutaneous fat (SF), and visceral fat (VF). In this context, the expression "sagittal diameter" refers to the anterior–posterior (A-P) diameter of the median plane of the body at the level of the iliac crest. (The median plane divides the trunk into right and left halves.) This particular sagittal diameter can be determined on a supine subject by placing a carpenter's level at right angles to the median plane so that, while horizontal, its inferior surface touches the highest point of the abdomen at the level of the iliac crests. After a normal expiration by the subject, the perpendicular distance from the inferior surface of the carpenter's level to the surface of the examining table is measured. This distance corresponds to the sagittal diameter of interest.

In the studies of Sjöström et al. (21), when the results of predictive equations based on height, weight, and sagittal diameter (herein abbreviated to the *HWSD method*) are compared with those obtained by multiscan CT volumetric analysis, the errors of estimation of VF by the HWSD method are approximately 20% in both primary and cross-validation studies of men and women. In contrast to the ability of the HWSD method to predict VF with at least fair accuracy, it appears that the WHR is poorly related to VF (21).

Use of the HWSD method is based on the notion that, in the supine position, intraabdominal fat increases the A-P diameter of the abdomen, while subcutaneous fat tends to increase its lateral diameter. According to Sjöström (*this volume*), "This is probably the reason why sagittal diameter is able to discriminate between visceral and subcutaneous adipose tissue in individuals with similar waist circumferences."

In preliminary studies, Sjöström et al. (*this volume*) have found that the visceral fat mass estimated by HWSD is a more sensitive indicator than the WHR in predicting the metabolic abnormalities and other health problems (Table 3) believed to be associated with excess visceral fat accumulation. If these find-

TABLE 3. *Some metabolic abnormalities and diseases linked to "visceral obesity"*

Metabolic abnormalities
    Atherogenic lipid profile
    High fibrinogen levels
    Insulin resistance
    Hyperinsulinemia
    Glucose intolerance
    Hyperuricemia
Diseases
    Non-insulin-dependent diabetes
    Coronary heart disease
    Hypertension
    Stroke
    Sudden death
    Angina pectoris
    Cholecystitis and cholelithiasis
    Gout
    Obstructive sleep apnea
    Uric acid nephrolithiasis
    Breast cancer (in postmenopausal women)

ings are confirmed by other investigators, it would seem that the HWSD estimation of visceral fat content (or some refinement thereof) should be added to the diagnostic armamentarium of physicians who are attempting to assess the effect of overweight on health and mortality risk in their patients.

USE OF THE BMI AS THE POINT OF DEPARTURE IN RISK ASSESSMENT

Despite growing evidence implicating VF as an important determinant of risk, it is as yet unclear just how physicians should make use of information about VF (presumably obtained by means of the HWSD method) in their efforts to formulate the best possible assessment of risk in their overweight patients. Unfortunately, there is no generally agreed upon algorithm for making such an assessment. Indeed, the mere knowledge that it may be important to include consideration of visceral fat content in the risk calculation provides little guidance as to how such information can be applied in any systematic attempt to arrive at a quantitative estimation of risk. Accordingly, until more definitive studies have been carried out, it makes sense to undertake the risk assessment process by using the body mass index (kg/m^2) as the point of departure. This is because a great deal of reliable quantitative information has been acquired over many years concerning the relationship between BMI and risk of ill health and a shortened life span (11).

Sjöström (*this volume*) and others (9–11) have already reviewed in considerable detail the extensive published literature on the hazards of overweight; thus, we have confined the scope of the present discussion largely to the findings of the American Cancer Society (ACS) study (22,23), a prospective investigation that was sufficiently large (750,000 subjects), of substantial duration (14 years), involved subjects who were ostensibly healthy (but not examined by a physician) at the out-

set of the investigation, and distinguished between smokers and nonsmokers. Although our focus is on the results of the ACS study, we believe it worthy of emphasis that the results of several US investigations, particularly the Framingham Heart Study (24,25) and the Seventh Day Adventist study (26), in which there were data on the mortality experience of nonsmokers, have been sufficiently consonant to provide a reasonable basis for defining mortality-optimal BMI ranges for men and women. "Mortality-optimal," of course, can also refer to deaths from specified causes such as coronary heart disease, diabetes, and hypertension as well as to all-cause (AC) mortality. As it turns out, the BMI ranges associated with the lowest relative mortality (22,23,26) and the lowest relative morbidity from coronary heart disease and diabetes (2,24,25) are fairly similar and, for the purposes of this particular analysis, can be merged. The proposed mortality/morbidity optimal BMI ranges are shown in Table 4.

As a part of the risk assessment procedure, one also has to determine how a rising BMI affects AC mortality risk as well as mortality and morbidity risk from specified causes. As regards AC mortality risk, we have chosen (as mentioned earlier) to rely on the findings of the ACS study (23). In Fig. 2, the mortality ratio (percent) for nonsmoking men and nonsmoking women is plotted against BMI. In the figure, the curve denoting the regression of BMI on MR is made sufficiently broad to encompass values for adults of both sexes. (It

TABLE 4. *Body mass indices (BMIs) associated with lowest all-cause mortality in nonsmoking men and women of all ages participating in the American Cancer Society Study*

	Mortality-optimal BMIs[a]
Men	19.9–22.6
Women	18.6–23.0

[a] These BMI ranges were also associated with the lowest (or nearly lowest) mortality rates from coronary heart disease and diabetes.
Adapted from ref. 23.

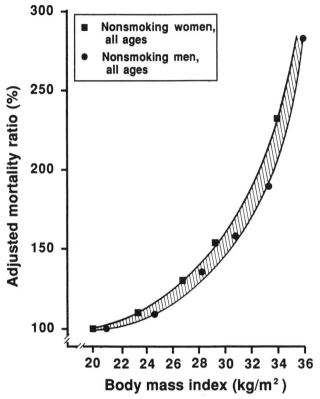

FIG. 2. Mortality ratios by body mass index (kg/m²) for nonsmoking men and women of all ages. From refs. 22 and 23.

should be pointed out that overall BMI values are generally lower for women than for men, at least at ages under 50. Hence, for any fixed value of BMI the mortality ratios tend to be higher for women.)

The ACS study (22,23) has also disclosed the striking rise in diabetes mortality that occurs among the overweight. An example of the dramatic effect of increasing overweight on relative risk of dying from diabetes is given in Table 5, in which mortality ratios from diabetes, coronary heart disease, and cancer are shown for middle-aged women exhibiting various degrees of overweight. The data show clearly that, while coronary heart disease risk is substantial among overweight women aged 50 to 59 years, the relative mortality from diabetes is far higher. The results of the ACS study indicate that, between the ages of 50 and 60, the lowest mortality ratios from diabetes (assigned a value of 64%) occur

TABLE 5. *Mortality ratios from diabetes, coronary heart disease (CHD), and cancer by body mass index (BMI) in women aged 50 to 59 years*

	Mortality ratios (%)[b]		
BMI (kg/m²)[a]	Diabetes	CHD	Cancer
20.0–22.5	64	82	92
22.5–27.5	100	100	100
27.5–30.0	228	145	114
30.0–32.5	435	164	116
32.5–35.0	712	216	112
>35	1,232	311	182

[a] Based on weights in indoor clothing without shoes.
[b] In relation to death rates among those 90 to 109% of average weight. Death rates among women of average weight exceeded those among women with below-average ("optimal") weights.
Adapted from ref. 22.

in men and women who remain 10 to 20% below average weight for their age. These findings provide little encouragement for the proposition that some degree of overweight is safe and may even be desirable in older-age individuals (27).

SOME MODIFIERS OF THE RISKS ASSOCIATED WITH OVERWEIGHT

It is becoming increasingly clear that the morbidity and mortality risks associated with overweight do not simply depend on the severity of the condition, although this is the impression that might be gained from Fig. 2 and Table 5. As mentioned earlier, there is evidence suggesting that the risk of developing diabetes (for example) may be more closely related to the accumulation of visceral fat than to the generalized accumulation of excess fat (20). If this is the case, then the risk of becoming diabetic would be greater in a severely overweight middle-aged man (BMI = 38 kg/m^2) with a visceral fat content of 11 kg [24% of the body fat mass (BFM)] than in an equally overweight man with a visceral fat content of 6 kg (13% of the BFM).

Despite the growing evidence that visceral fat content may be a major determinant of risk in patients with various degrees of overweight, it has to be remembered that almost all of the information currently available about the relation of overweight to morbidity and mortality risk has been generated by investigations that used weight for height as the index of overweight. Although future studies may demonstrate that the principal adverse

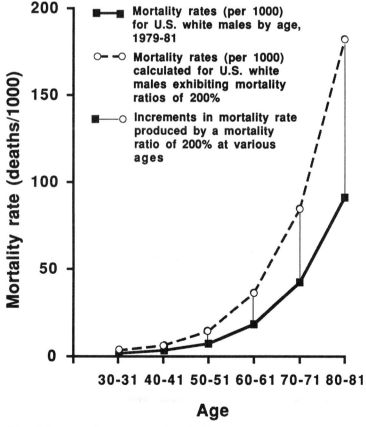

FIG. 3. Effect of the rising mortality rate associated with aging on the magnitude of the increments in mortality rate produced at various ages by a mortality ratio of 200%.

effects of overweight occur only or principally in individuals with "visceral obesity," we believe that it would be premature to discard the BMI as the primary marker for risk estimation in overweight patients. It makes more sense, at this juncture, to use the BMI to reach a first approximation of relative risk. Once that approximation has been obtained, it is then appropriate to consider the effect of various modifying factors on the level of risk.

Some of the potential risk-modifying factors that deserve consideration are listed in Table 6. Unfortunately, not enough is known about the magnitude of their effect—either separately or in combination—on health and longevity to permit one to make a quantitative estimate of the degree to which one or more such "modifiers" will augment risk.

However, it can be said with considerable confidence that, if one were to compare two equally overweight patients of the same age and sex, morbidity and mortality risk would be substantially greater in the individual who possessed one or more exacerbating attributes such as (a) upper-body fat distribution (or other evidence of visceral obesity); (b) hypertension, hyperglycemia, and/or hyperlipidemia; (c) a family history of obesity-relevant illness (diabetes, premature coro-

nary heart disease); and (d) obesity of prolonged duration. [As regards risk in individuals with a family history of cardiovascular disease (those with two or more natural parents or siblings who had degenerative cardiovascular disease diagnosed before age 60), among men with such a history issued standard life insurance policies, the mortality ratio was almost double the expected (28)].

No precise statistical weight can be assigned to the foregoing risk modifiers; however, it is appropriate that the physician call the patient's attention to their presence or absence and explain that the urgency of treatment for obesity becomes greater and greater, depending: first, on the severity of the overweight (see Fig. 2); second, on the presence or absence of risk augmenters; and third, on the gravity of any risk enhancers that happen to be present. In arriving at a judgment about the magnitude of risk exhibited by a given patient and the level of "treatment urgency," physicians will have to form their own judgment based on considerations such as those listed in Table 6.

PUTTING RELATIVE RISK INTO PERSPECTIVE

To gain a better perspective on the concept of relative mortality (and relative morbidity), it may be useful for the physician to consider the effect of age on the death rate. In Fig. 3 the lower curve represents the ever accelerating death rate exhibited by aging US white males after the age of 30 (29). Indeed, in this group, mortality rates rise from 0.1% at age 30 to 9% at age 80, a 90-fold increase. If a 30-year-old male is found to have a mortality ratio of 200%, then his risk of dying will have increased from 0.1% to 0.2%. On the other hand, an 80-year-old male with an MR of 2.0 (200%) will increase his risk of dying from 9 to 18%. Thus, if 1,000 men aged 30 were to exhibit an MR of 200%, the excess death rate (EDR) would be 1 per 1,000. If 1,000 men aged 80 were to exhibit an MR of 200%, the EDR would be 90 per 1,000.

TABLE 6. *Some attributes that may enhance morbidity and mortality risk in overweight patients*

Excess fat in visceral adipose tissue ("visceral obesity") inferred from:
  Measurement of sagittal diameter of the abdomen at iliac crest (see text for details)
  A high waist-to-hip circumference ratio (>0.9 for men; >0.8 for women)
  Upper body fat distribution pattern
Presence of obesity-associated risk factors such as hypertension, hyperglycemia, hyperlipidemia, hyperuricemia, left ventricular hypertrophy
Family history of premature coronary heart disease, diabetes, gout, cholelithiasis, hypertension
Obesity of prolonged duration
Impaired health not attributable to overweight (e.g., valvular heart disease)
Below normal stature
Membership in a race known to be vulnerable to obesity-associated health problems (e.g., diabetes in some Native Americans)

As shown in Fig. 3, the mortality rate (m) of an average man 60 years of age is higher than that of a 50-year-old man with an MR of 200%. Indeed, the death rate in US white men more than doubles every decade between the ages of 40 and 100. What this means is that, as people get older, the significance of having an increased relative risk of dying can change dramatically depending on the normal mortality level for the age under consideration. Thus, if MR doubles for a 30-year-old man, his risk of dying increases from 1.66 per 1,000 to 3.32 per 1,000. For a 60-year-old man to increase his risk by 1.66 per 1,000 would mean an increment from 17.7 per 1,000 to 19.28 per 1,000 a 9% increase. Thus, at age 60, an MR of 109% has the same meaning, expressed in terms of increase in probability of dying, as an MR of 200% at age 30.

These simple calculations are given in some detail in order to remind physicians of the importance of the word "relative" when relative morbidity and mortality are being discussed. Obviously, the significance of an elevated relative risk becomes increasingly ominous if the normal mortality rate is already high, as is the case with advancing age. In contrast, a high MR in a young adult has to be considered in the light of the low mortality rate that normally obtains at that age level.

VARIATION IN VULNERABILITY TO THE ADVERSE EFFECTS OF OVERWEIGHT

It is well known that susceptibility to the adverse effects of overweight is subject to considerable individual variation. Sjöström (*this volume*) and others (30) have suggested that much of this variability may be eliminated if the adverse consequences of obesity are correlated with visceral fat content rather than with BMI (or even WHR). On the other hand, Grundy and Barnett (31) have proposed a somewhat different explanation for the fact that many individuals appear to be

resistant to the potentially harmful effects of overnutrition. In their view, "overnutrition produces clinical disease only in individuals who already possess a metabolic weakness or 'defect' in a given system. In the absence of such underlying defects, overnutrition, or obesity, is well tolerated." Thus, Grundy and Barnett have suggested that "a person may possess an underlying metabolic abnormality that does not manifest as clinical disease unless or until adverse stimuli (such as overnutrition) are superimposed." As these authors point out, such underlying abnormalities or "latent" metabolic defects (presumably of genetic origin) may be present in a number of different metabolic pathways. Examples include pathways involving cholesterol, glucose, insulin, uric acid, and electrolytes.

If susceptibility to certain obesity-related health hazards (i.e., diabetes, hypertension, gout, cholelithiasis) is determined by the presence in a subset of the population of latent metabolic weaknesses that succumb under the stress of overnutrition, then any approach to identifying individuals at risk must take such genetic vulnerability to the adverse effects of obesity into account. In other words, it would seem urgently necessary to attempt to find ways of disclosing metabolic weaknesses in patients while such weaknesses remain subclinical. However, at the present time, the relatively few tolerance tests that might uncover various latent metabolic disorders are expensive and difficult to carry out. It seems possible, however, that a careful family history may provide useful clues pointing to a given patient's vulnerability to obesity-related illness.

Whatever the case, the notion that the development of obesity can give rise to clinically manifest illness (diabetes, hyperlipidemia, etc.) in a metabolically vulnerable individual also carries with it the hopeful connotation that some degree of fat loss can partly or fully alleviate the problem. Another corollary of the metabolic weakness hypothesis is that the degree of overweight needed to bring into being one or more illnesses can be quite variable, depending in part (perhaps) on the pattern of regional fat distribution and in part on the ability of a "faulty" metabolic pathway to tolerate the strain imposed by excess fat in the body or, perhaps more specifically, in the visceral adipose tissue depot.

REFERENCES

1. Boswell J. *Life of Johnson,* vol II, 1776–1784. London: Oxford, 1924:127.
2. Manson JE, Colditz GA, Stampfer MJ, et al. A prospective study of obesity and risk of coronary heart disease in women. *N Engl J Med* 1990;322:882–8.
3. VanItallie TB. Health implications of overweight and obesity in the United States. *Ann Intern Med* 1985;103:983–8.
4. Blair S, Kohl HWTH, Paffenbarger BS Jr, Clark DG, Cooper SH, Gibbons LW. Physical fitness and all-cause mortality: a prospective study of healthy men and women. *JAMA* 1989;262:2395–401.
5. *Build and blood pressure study 1959,* vol 1 Chicago: Society of Actuaries, 1959:117–20.
6. *Build study 1979* Boston: Society of Actuaries and Association of Life Insurance Medical Directors of America, 1980:117.
7. Mason E. The impact of obesity surgery on morbidity, mortality and survival. *Int J Obes* 1989; 13:596(abst).
8. Marks HH. Influence of obesity on morbidity and mortality. *Bull NY Acad Sci* 1960;36:296–312.
9. Simopoulos A, VanItallie TB. Body weight, health, and longevity. *Ann Intern Med* 1984;100:285–95.
10. Manson JE, Stampfer MJ, Hennekens CH, Willett WC. Body weight and longevity. A reassessment. *JAMA* 1987;257:353–8.
11. VanItallie TB, Lew EA. Overweight and underweight. In Lew EA, Gajewski J, eds. *Medical risks 1987: mortality trends by age and time elapsed.* New York: Praeger, 1990;13.1–13.22.
12. Keys A. *Seven Countries. A multivariate analysis of death and coronary heart disease.* Cambridge, MA: Harvard University Press, 1980.
13. Björntorp P. Regional patterns of fat distribution. *Ann Intern Med* 1985;103:994–5.
14. Larsson B, Svardsudd K, Welin L, Wilhelmsson L, Björntorp P, Tibblin G. Abdominal adipose tissue distribution, obesity, and risk of cardiovascular disease and death: 13-year follow-up of participants in the study of 792 men born in 1913. *Br Med J* 1984;288:1401–4.
15. Lapidus L, Bengtsson C, Larsson B, Pennert K, Rybo E, Sjöström L. Distribution of adipose tissue and risk of cardiovascular disease and death: a 12-year follow-up of participants in the population study of 1462 women in Gothenburg, Sweden. *Br Med J* 1984;289:1257–61.
16. Vague J. *Obesities.* London: John Libbey, 1991.
17. Kaplan NM. The deadly quartet. Upper-body obesity, glucose intolerance, hypertriglyceridemia, and hypertension. *Arch Intern Med* 1989;149:1514–20.
18. Borkan GA, Gerzof SG, Robbins AH, Hults DE, Silbert CK, Silbert JE. Assessment of abdominal fat content by computed tomography. *Am J Clin Nutr* 1982;36:172–7.
19. Ashwell M, Cole TJ, Dixon AK. Obesity: new insight into the anthropometric classification shown by computed tomography. *Br Med J* 1985; 290:1692–4.
20. Fujioka S, Matsuzawa Y, Tokunaga K, Tarui S. Contribution of intra-abdominal fat accumulation to the impairment of glucose and lipid metabolism in human obesity. *Metabolism* 1987;36:54–9.
21. Kvist H, Chowdhury B, Grangard V, Tylen U, Sjöström L. Total and visceral adipose-tissue volumes derived from measurements with computed tomography in adult men and women: predictive equations. *Am J Clin Nutr* 1988;48:1351–61.
22. Lew EA, Garfinkel L. Variations in mortality by weight among 750,000 men and women. *J Chron Dis* 1979;32:563–76.
23. Lew EA. Mortality and weight: insured lives and the American Cancer Society studies. *Ann Intern Med* 1985;103:1024–9.
24. Hubert HB, Feinleib M, McNamara PM, Castelli WP. Obesity as an independent risk factor for cardiovascular disease: a 26-year follow-up of participants in the Framingham Heart Study. *Circulation* 1983;67:968–77.
25. Garrison RJ, Feinleib M, Castelli WP, McNamara PM. Cigarette smoking as a confounder of the relationship between relative weight and long-term mortality. The Framingham Heart Study. *JAMA* 1983;249:2199–203.
26. Lindsted K, Tonstad S, Kuzma JW. Body mass index and patterns of mortality among Seventh-day Adventist men. *Int J Obes* 1991;15:397–406.
27. Andres R, Elahi D, Tobin JD, Muller DC, Brant L. Impact of age on weight goals. *Ann Intern Med* 1985;103:1030–3.
28. *Medical impairment study 1983.* Boston: Society of Actuaries and Association of Life Insurance Medicine Directors of America, 1986;73.
29. U.S. Decennial Life Tables for 1979–81, vol 1, no 1. National Center for Health Statistics DHHS Publication no (PHS) 85-1150-1. Washington, DC: US Govt. Printing Office, 1985.
30. Fugimoto WY, Newell-Morris LL, Shuman WP. Intra-abdominal fat and risk variables for non-insulin-dependent diabetes (NIDDM) and coronary heart disease in Japanese American women with android or gynoid fat patterning. In: Oomura Y, Tasui S, Inoue S, Shimazu T, eds. *Progress in obesity research.* London: John Libbey, 1990.
31. Grundy SM, Barnett JP. Metabolic and health complications of obesity. In Bone RC, ed. *Disease-a-month,* vol 36, no 12. St. Louis: CV Mosby-Year Book, 1990:643–731.
32. VanItallie TB, Lew EA. Assessment of morbidity and mortality risk in the overweight patient. In: Wadden TA, VanItallie TB, eds. *Treatment of the seriously obese patient.* New York: Guilford Press, 1992:3–32.

Obesity: Theory and Therapy, Second Edition,
edited by A. J. Stunkard and T. A. Wadden.
Raven Press, Ltd., New York © 1993.

14

Popular Diets for Weight Loss

From Nutritionally Hazardous to Healthful

*†Johanna T. Dwyer and †Diana Lu

*Tufts University Medical School; and †Frances Stern Nutrition Center, New England
Medical Center Hospitals, Boston, Massachusetts 02111*

Health professionals recognize that success in long-term weight management is most likely to occur when a program includes long-term changes in life style such as eating in moderation, a physically active daily life that involves exercise, and behavior modification. However, the public remains convinced that there must be quicker and easier ways to lose weight without addressing all of these issues. Thus, sporadic dieting attempts designed to cut calories and lose weight, are common. Data on the long-term efficacy of various reducing diets, diet foods, and commercial and nonprofit weight-loss programs are unavailable to most consumers. Lay people are vulnerable to advertisements and ill-conceived programs in books, magazines, and elsewhere in spite of scientific evidence that many of the claims of effectiveness are exaggerated or outright false. When overweight patients turn to health professionals for help, they frequently ask questions about these heavily advertised and promoted diets and weight-loss schemes. Therefore, it is important for health professionals to know how weight loss is best achieved and to have the information to answer patients' questions.

This chapter briefly reviews the physiological and psychological means by which diets work. We classify some of the various popular reducing diets that are currently in vogue using widely accepted criteria (1,2). Other diets are analyzed elsewhere (3–7). Some of the sounder schemes that can be recommended for those who wish to lose weight on their own are described. Pitfalls and problems that may arise when the unwary turn to unproven or dangerous diets that are currently popular are highlighted.

HOW DIETS WORK

The means by which body fatness can be reduced are straightforward (8,9). Either energy intake is decreased, energy output is increased, or both are altered simultaneously to produce a net energy deficit. If the energy deficit persists for long enough and other nutrients are provided in adequate amounts, body fat and weight are lost in a linear manner. The slope of the decline is determined by the size of the energy deficit. Furthermore, the loss of fat is directly proportional to the size and duration of the energy deficit. Rate of weight loss depends also on the extent to which the individual adheres to the regime.

Over the short term, such as a few weeks, deviations from this linear relationship between caloric deficit and weight loss often occur. Weight loss also reflects shifts in water balance, especially in the first few weeks. Such alterations are most pronounced early in weight loss, but may occur at other points as well, depending on adherence. Also, the size of the caloric deficit and diet composition can alter the mix of metabolic fuels that are burned for energy, the type of tissue lost, body water balance, and weight loss.

Ultimate success in keeping a leaner physique depends on sustaining somewhat lower levels of energy intake and higher levels of energy output, as compared with those prior to weight reduction.

CRITERIA FOR EVALUATING DIETARY COMPONENTS OF WEIGHT-LOSS PLANS

During the hypocaloric, weight-loss phase of dieting, the eating plan must meet seven essential criteria, easily remembered as the "seven Cs". These are listed in Table 1 and include calories; composition; costs; consumer friendliness; coping with coexisting health problems; all components of a sound weight management program; and continuation provisions for long-term weight maintenance. Weight management plans that meet the seven Cs are generally safe and effective. Those that fail to meet one or more should not be recommended to patients. With some alterations, these same criteria apply to the maintenance phase after weight loss has been achieved (10). Specific considerations with respect to each component are discussed more fully below.

TABLE 1. *Seven essential criteria of healthy weight control plans: the seven Cs*

Calories
Composition
Costs
Consumer friendliness
Coping with existing health problems
Components of sound weight management
    Healthful hypocaloric diet
    Physical activity and exercise
    Behavioral modification
Continuation provisions for long-term maintenance
    Plan for maintaining weight at reduced levels after
      healthier weights achieved by slightly decreased
      foods intakes and increased energy outputs
      compared with before dieting

CALORIES

If fat is to be lost, a caloric deficit from the intake required for energy balance must be created so that the individual achieves a state of negative energy balance. This is best achieved by a combination of a hypocaloric diet and increased physical activity. The size of the caloric deficit depends on the difference between the individual's usual food intake and the calorie level of the diet selected. In addition, changes in physical activity including, but not limited to, increased exercise must also be taken into account.

Average energy intakes of American men are about 2,800 kcal/day, and for women about 1,800 kcal/day. Best estimates vary with size and activity level. The energy needs of a person whose weight is stable can be obtained for clinical purposes by using recently devised formulas for estimating resting metabolism (11,12). First an estimate of resting metabolic rate (RMR) is calculated using the formula:

Male RMR = 900 + 10 (weight in kg)

Female RMR = 700 + 7 (weight in kg)

The result, which is a rough approximation of energy needs at rest, is then adjusted for physical activity by multiplying it by 1.2 for very sedentary, 1.4 for moderately active, or 1.8 for very active individuals. This is an estimate of the individual's total caloric needs in a state of energy balance. It is a good starting point from which to design a weight-loss regime.

To achieve negative energy balance and to lose weight, a caloric deficit must be imposed that is sufficient to permit a reasonable rate of weight loss. One pound of body fat contains about 3,500 kcal. Thus 500 kcal less per day causes a loss of about 1 lb a week (500 × 7), and 1,000 kcal less per day results in a loss of about 2 lb a week (1000 × 7). Weight losses greater than $\frac{1}{2}$ to 1 lb a week are not suggested for self-initiated efforts. Even under medical supervision, however, a loss of no more than 2 lb a week is usually recommended. In actuality, weight losses of 2 lb or more are rarely possible to sustain in outpatient obesity treatment programs. When weight losses are more rapid than this, risks of excessive loss of lean body mass increase, as do risks of nutrient deficiencies, fatigue, and other side effects.

The caloric deficit can be easily calculated. First, make an estimate of the individual's current energy intake using one of the formulas above. Then subtract from it the calories provided by the reducing regime. Weight loss can be predicted from this difference. For example, if a moderately active 176-lb man has energy needs at rest of 1,700 kcal a day, and his total daily needs in energy balance are about 2,380 kcal, the energy deficit would be 640 kcal/day on a diet of about 1,740 kcal, and he would lose a little over 1 lb a week. On a 1,500-kcal/day reducing diet, his energy deficit would be 880 kcal, and he would lose about $1\frac{1}{2}$ lb a week. The calculation would be 2,380 kcal − 1,500 kcal = 880 kcal × 7 days/week = 6,160 kcal/week. 6160 kcal per week divided by 3,500 kcal per pound of fat would yield 1.76 pounds lost per week. On the same 1,500 kcal/day diet, his wife, a 154-lb moderately active woman, with energy needs of about 1,666 kcal/day, would only have an energy deficit of 166 kcal, and she would lose a little less than a pound a week. The important point illustrated in the examples above is that even with perfect adherence, whenever reducing diets at fixed caloric levels are used, people with different energy needs may lose different amounts of weight. Many dieters fail to realize that when it comes to dieting, comparisons are odious.

The caloric level of a reducing diet that is most appropriate for an individual depends on health characteristics, severity of obesity, adequacy of medical supervision, and patient preferences. The metabolic effects of different reducing regimes vary directly with their energy levels and the energy deficits that they create for the individual. The effects are greater when caloric levels are lower and energy deficits are more drastic.

Some adjustments in these rough calculations must be made as weight is lost. Unfortunately for the dieter, homeostatic adaptations occur on low-calorie diets, so that RMR declines. This decrease occurs to the same extent in all individuals when the same degree of caloric deficit is achieved, regardless of how fat or lean the person is. Just as RMR decreases when weight is lost, it rises when weight is gained. However, the fall in RMR never alters energy needs more than about 15% or so. Additional decreases in energy output are possible due to the lesser cost of moving a lighter body around, or because of less movement altogether.

Common reducing regimens today include total fasting, the very-low-calorie diets (VLCD) under 600 to 800 kcal/day, low-calorie diets providing from 800 to 1,200 kcal/day, and more moderate hypocaloric reducing plans of 1,200 kcal/day or above. Because caloric level is so critical in determining the short-term effectiveness of weight reduction, it is discussed in much greater detail below.

Total Fasting

Fasting, or total starvation, is not recommended as an obesity therapy because of the excessive losses of lean body mass that accompany it. However, some people use total fasts of their own volition for dieting. Both fasting and VLCDs are drastic weight reduction methods that have profound metabolic effects. They are diuretic, kaliuretic, and saliuretic, and are insufficient in nutrients unless supplemented. Fasting is self-defeating, since the large losses in lean body mass are accompanied by declines in RMR. Energy outputs at rest, which are reflected in the RMR, result from catabolism in actively metabolizing cells in the vital organs and muscles that constitute the lean body mass. As lean body mass falls, so too does RMR. Lethargy is common, voluntary physical activity tends to fall off dramatically, and exercise tolerance is greatly diminished. Thus energy outputs from physical activity also tend to fall. Some of the more serious possible adverse effects stemming from the use of fasting are described in Table 2. The metabolic changes associated with starvation (13,14), on very hypocaloric diets (15), and during refeeding (16) are well described in the literature.

Very-Low-Calorie Diets
(Less than 600 kcal/day)

Very-low-calorie diets usually provide fewer than 600 kcal daily, but officially they are defined as any regimen under 800 kcal/day (17). They are also below RMRs of virtually all adults and thus it is not surprising that they have potent metabolic effects.

The health risks associated with VLCDs are greatly lessened and become acceptable when they are administered to appropriate types of patients who receive ongoing expert medical supervision, for reasonable lengths of time. VLCDs must also be well formulated from the nutritional standpoint to be safe, meeting the RDA for vitamins, minerals, protein, electrolytes, and water.

Choosing the Right Patients

Patient selection is particularly vital on VLCDs, since the risks of side effects and compromised growth or rehabilitation preclude their use with certain individuals. They are not appropriate therapies for most obese children, growing adolescents under 18 years of age (especially those who are pubertal),

pregnant women, lactating women, the elderly, those who are very fragile emotionally, and those who are ill. Metabolic perturbations and potential losses of lean body mass are particularly dangerous for these individuals.

Table 2 lists some of the serious potential adverse effects. Table 3 lists some of the other disruptive side effects and bothersome problems that may develop. Individuals who are not severely overweight should not use a VLCD. On VLCDs, slightly or moderately overweight people are more at risk of developing side effects such as hypovolemia because they are more likely to be ketosis-prone than are massively obese individuals. For this reason they are not good candidates for such a regimen. Well-supervised VLCD programs, such as some of those discussed later in this chapter, have strict entry criteria so that inappropriate patients are screened out.

Medically supervised VLCDs are an important addition to the therapeutic armamentarium for very obese people who do not fall in the categories mentioned above, especially when weight must be lost quickly because of immediate and urgent health problems that might be lessened with obesity treatment (9). Among very obese people with coexisting medical conditions that are worsened by their obesity, moderately low calorie diets (e.g., those over 1,200 kcal/day) take so long to produce adequate weight loss that the medical risks of delay may be intolerable.

VLCDs are helpful when the person is very

TABLE 2. *Serious potential adverse effects due to misuse of very-low-calorie diets (VLCD)*[a]

Effect	Starvation	VLCD	Periodic fasting
Lean body mass decrease	xxx	xx if unsupervised, x if supervised	x
Linear growth decrease	xxx	xx if unsupervised, x if supervised	x
Cardiac changes	xx	xx if unsupervised	x
Disorder in water balance: diuresis, dehydration	xx	xx	x
Ketosis	xx	xx	x
Electrolyte imbalances	x	x	x
Nutrient deficiencies if not supplemented	xxx	xx	x

[a] xxx, most pronounced; x, least pronounced.

TABLE 3. *Side effects of fasting and very-low-calorie diets (VLCD)*

Effect	Starvation: total fast	VLCD	Periodic fasts
Lowered resting metabolism	xxx	xx	x
Lethargy, decreased voluntary physical activity and exercise tolerance	xxx	xx	x
Lightheaded feeling, with dizziness, weakness, feeling faint on standing	xxx	xx	xx
Anemia	xxx	xx	x
Constipation	xxx	xx	x
Menstrual irregularity, ketosis, hair loss	xxx	xx	?

xxx, most pronounced; x, least pronounced.

obese [body mass index (BMI) over 32 or over 140% of desirable weight] and when very large amounts of weight [e.g., over 50 lb (22.7 kg)] must be lost quickly. They demonstrate that weight loss is possible, accelerate the rate of weight loss, give visible cosmetic and symptom relief, and decrease health risks. They may also increase the determination required of the very obese to make a long-term commitment to achieve healthier weights. Many such patients have repeatedly tried low-calorie diets and failed. Adherence is difficult when the weight-loss phase must continue for many months or years, and so the dieter needs all the assistance possible to facilitate the process. For the very obese who must lose very large amounts of weight the process can be eased by alternating an occasional 4-month VLCD with more moderate weight control methods the rest of the time. Excessive depletion of lean body mass is avoided and the weight loss is speeded up.

VLCDs are also useful therapy for those very obese people who are being evaluated for gastric restriction surgery. Using a VLCD before surgery reduces weight slightly and thus may decrease some surgical risks. It also gives both the physician and patient an opportunity to assess ability and determination to adhere to a rigorous dietary regimen. Discipline in diet will be required following gastric restriction surgery since the patient will have a smaller stomach capacity (see Mason and Doherty, *this volume*). Consequently only very small solid meals can be tolerated without gastric distress or vomiting. Even with a smaller stomach, caloric solids and liquids must be restricted to promote weight loss. A large number of calories can still be ingested from liquids even after surgery. While it is true that a smaller stomach and gastric distress inhibit eating temporarily, eventually the stomach stretches, and larger amounts of food can be consumed. Therefore moderation in food intake is still mandatory. Candidates for gastric restriction who are unable to adhere to a VLCD would probably not be able to limit their intake after surgery and thus can be expected to have poor weight loss.

Medical and Health Surveillance

VLCDs are not panaceas; they are simply a rapid way to lose weight. The VLCD should be medically supervised and administered in the context of an overall long-term weight management program provided by a multidisciplinary team. The team should include a physician who is skilled in the use of VLCDs and knowledgeable of clinical nutrition, a registered dietitian, a nurse, and a psychologist, all specially trained in the treatment of high-risk obesity. An exercise physiologist is also helpful, particularly when patients have health problems that make the usual types of exercise difficult.

Achieving the benefits of VLCD therapy without incurring unnecessary risks requires medical judgment. Starvation and VLCDs lower basal metabolism, and often also give rise to lethargy, which may lead to unconscious decreases in voluntary physical activity. The combination of the two results in less overall energy output and decreased energy needs, making it more difficult to lose weight. Central nervous system disturbances may result from the very low intake of dietary carbohydrate, which is usually limited to 100 g daily and frequently 50 g or less. The side effects that may accompany such low levels include dizziness, feelings of weakness, and light-headedness, especially when the individual suddenly rises from reclining or sitting positions (see Table 3). Other less serious side effects include constipation, menstrual irregularities, anemia, headaches, irritability, anxiety, and apathy.

Without medical supervision, VLCDs pose considerable health risks. Self-prescribed VLCDs remain a dangerous dieting choice, especially if the person is already at risk by virtue of the degree of massive obesity, has other health problems, or is taking medications. Medication schedules often need adjustment to avoid inadvertent overdoses due to altered drug metabolism, volume of distribution, or other characteristics.

Duration of Use

In order to minimize the risk of cardiac problems associated with loss of lean body mass, which may include both arrhythmias and wasting of the heart muscle itself, the duration of the VLCD should be limited to no more than 12 to 16 weeks. If adequate weight loss has not been achieved by then, diets with more modest energy deficits can then be employed to complete the weight loss and to reintroduce the dieter to regular foods. Because other types of diets and health advice must also be provided, it is important that the VLCD be integrated into an overall treatment program.

Nutritional Adequacy

The earliest versions of VLCDs were formulas that provided 300 to 400 kcal/day from protein sources of variable and sometimes very poor biological value. Some preparations also lacked sufficient amounts of essential micronutrients. These protein and mineral deficits (including possibly both potassium and magnesium deficiency) were as-

sociated with disturbances in cardiac function, including arrhythmias, prolonged QT intervals, ventricular fibrillation, and premature ventricular contractions (18,19). In the mid-1970s deaths were reported from the use of some liquid protein supplements bought in drugstores or sold door to door (20). A few, such as the Last Chance Diet, were also popularized in books. Consequently, the Food and Drug Administration took a more proactive role in developing and enforcing regulations to govern the use of VLCDs, and health professionals became more aware of the possible dangers involved in the use of such products.

Two types of more satisfactory, medically supervised VLCDs are in use today. Both provide most of their calories from protein, and for this reason they are sometimes referred to as protein-supplemented modified fasts, or protein-sparing modified fasts (PSMFs). The two approaches, described more fully later, produce similar weight losses (21,22). To prevent nutrient deficits, PSMFs need to be supplemented with vitamins and minerals. With appropriate supplementation, these PSMFs are relatively safe and are associated with less depletion of lean body mass than is total starvation (23) since energy deficits are not as great.

The first type of PSMF relies on animal protein foods (such as meat, fish, or fowl), and is accompanied by mineral, electrolyte, and vitamin supplements. These are sometimes prescribed by physicians in outpatient practice and are used in a few commercial programs. Their main advantage is that the individual can obtain most of the foods at the local supermarket, and food costs are relatively low. The disadvantage is that vitamin, mineral, and electrolyte supplements must be taken separately, and other aspects of long-term weight management (such as nutrition education, physical activity, and behavior modification) may be neglected.

The second type of PSMF consists of a milk- or egg-based liquid formula diet. Many such products are commercially available today through medically supervised programs. These include hospital- or clinic-based commercial programs such as Health Management Resources (HMR), Medifast, Optifast, and Medibase. Some of these options are described in Table 4. Details on others are available in recent publications on diet and weight loss programs (24,25). The advantage of these diets is that the formulas, foods, and supplements provided are nutritionally complete. In addition, they are provided under a physician's direction. Some, such as Optifast and HMR, are provided as part of larger programs that include appropriate exercise and physical activity (of a low intensity), a refeeding period after the VLCD period is over, nutrition education, and some attention to problems of long-term maintenance. As noted, these VLCDs are usually found in health-care settings so that adequate medical and behavioral supervision are usually included. The potential for abuse, such as using less formula than recommended, or development of unrecognized complications, is decreased.

These VLCDs do, however, have several disadvantages. Some of the side effects described in Table 3 occur even with well-managed programs. One risk is that the coexisting medical difficulties of some patients may be unrecognized or not dealt with adequately in treatment, especially if very-high-risk patients are treated. These risks can be overcome by the dedication and expertise of the health professionals who are involved in the weight control program. Both initial differences in mood and hunger (26,27) and effectiveness of the various VLCD and PSMF programs 1 year after therapy on weight loss (28,29) seem to be slight, nor is there evidence that long-term effectiveness measured by ability to sustain weight losses 5 years after treatment is any better with a VLCD than with less expensive programs. The programs are very expensive, ranging from at least a thousand to several thousand dollars. In many cases these costs are not covered by health insurance and must be paid out of pocket by patients. Thus this treatment option may not be available to some patients who may need it.

The VLCD programs often involve joint ventures with marketing-oriented private entrepreneurs or special revenue enhancement for medical staff or departments that participate. Profit margins for these programs are large and are less highly regulated than they are for most other medical services. Perhaps partly as a consequence of these financial arrangements, many of the medically based VLCD programs have very aggressive marketing, sales and follow-up components, urging patients to enroll in and stay in treatment (see Taylor and Stunkard, *this volume*). Similar diligence in marketing and follow-up is often not exhibited by health providers in pursuing patients with even more serious conditions such as high serum cholesterol levels, for which long-term effectiveness is better if dietary adherence is maintained. The marketing, sales, and follow-up techniques are often very much more aggressive than the low-key approaches that are usual for other medical and nutritional services of greater long-term effectiveness, such as serum cholesterol and cardiovascular risk reduction lowering strategies. Unfortunately, the advertising of most medical facilities that sponsor these programs is just as uninformative to consumers as that of commercial, free-standing facilities. In addition, many programs lack adequate provision for free or reduced price care for those patients who otherwise could not afford treatment.

The adverse publicity about the dangers of VLCD, the weight rebound experienced by Oprah Winfrey (the television star who lost and then regained 67 pounds in a highly publicized bout of dieting using a PSMF), and the widespread availability of medically supervised VLCD programs in the past few years may have lessened the tendency of consumers to undertake these diets on their own. Some people, however, including obese adolescent girls, still often self-prescribe fasts to lose weight. These and all other misuses of VLCDs should be discouraged.

Diet books suggesting that VLCDs need not be accompanied by medical supervision are also still available, although fortunately

TABLE 4. *Analyses of some popular weight-loss programs*

Diet	Entry criteria	Cost	Medical supervision?	Nutrition education, behavior modification, exercise included?	Description, comments
<600–800 kcal/day **Reasonable:** Health Management Resources (HMR)	20% above ideal body weight or 40 lb overweight for VLCD diet	$115/week for medically supervised program, $90/week for moderate program	Yes	Yes	Medically supervised VLCD (520 to 800 kcal) program and moderate program with less intensive supervision (800 to 1,000 kcal) available. 3 phases: Weight loss Refeeding Maintenance Use of liquid formula diet and/or HMR frozen entrees (150 to 230 kcal)
Medifast	20% above ideal body weight	$62.50 to $75/week	Yes	Prescribed but not necessarily provided by a multidisciplinary team of professionals	4-phase program: Medical evaluation Weight reduction (450 kcal liquid diet for women; 480 kcal for men) Realimentation Maintenance
Optifast	30% above ideal body weight; 20% if medically at risk or 50 lb overweight	$100/week	Yes	Yes	4-phase program: Modified fast (420 to 800 kcal liquid diet) Refeeding Stabilization Maintenance (optional)
Unreasonable: Total fasting	Not appropriate for anyone	—	No	No	Not advised due to high loss of lean body mass, vitamin and mineral deficiencies and other complications
800–1,200 kcal/day **Reasonable:** Diet Center	Physician approval needed for individuals more than 40% or 50 lb overweight or who have preexisting health problems	$50/week for reducing phase; less for other phases	? (Nurse travels to different sites)	Prescribed, but not necessarily provided by a multidisciplinary team of professionals	4-phase program Conditioning (unlimited kcal) Reducing (minimum of 1,000 kcal) Stabilizing Maintenance Individual differences in caloric needs are taken into consideration for all phases. Vitamin/mineral supplement taken daily. 1,000 mg of vitamin C is recommended daily, which seems excessive

Program	Candidates	Cost		Professional involvement	Description
Diet Workshop	Physician approval needed for individuals with preexisting health problems	Registration fee of $14, $9/week	No	Prescribed but not provided by a multidisciplinary team of professionals	Based on system of food "units" Reducing phase (900 to 1,000 kcal increased gradually to 1,200 kcal until goal weight is achieved) Maintenance (kcal according to individual needs) Vitamin/mineral supplement recommended
Jenny Craig Weight Loss Centers	Physician approval needed for individuals with preexisting medical conditions	$185 for membership; $60 to $70/week for food	No	Prescribed but not provided by a multidisciplinary team of professionals	2 phases: Reducing (about 1,000 kcal for women; 1,200 to 1,400 kcal for men) Maintenance (kcal according to individual needs) Complete reliance on packaged foods initially
Nutri/System	Physician approval needed for individuals more than 100 lb overweight or who have preexisting medical problems	Variable according to location and goal weight; $60 to $69/week for food	No	Prescribed but not provided by a multidisciplinary team of professionals	2 phases: Weight loss (minimum of 1,000 kcal for women; 1,200 kcal for men) Maintenance (kcal according to individual needs) Complete reliance on packaged foods until maintenance phase; low-fat (14%), high-carbohydrate (61%) diet; special diet modifications for medical conditions
Weight Watchers	More than 10 lb overweight	$12 to $20 registration fee, $7 to $9/week	No	Prescribed but not provided by a multidisciplinary team of professionals	Based on system of food exchanges Weight loss (1,040 to 1,450 kcal for women; 1,440 to 1,910 kcal for men) Maintenance (kcal according to individual needs)
Not recommended Slim Fast/Ultra Slim Fast	Physician approval recommended for individuals who are pregnant, nursing, under 18 years old, have health problems, or who want to lose more than 30 lb or more than 15% of their body weight	$8 to $12/week	No	Limited	Over the counter meal replacement is mixed with low-fat milk (Slim Fast) or water (Ultra Slim Fast). Slim Fast is 190 kcal/serving, Ultra Slim Fast is 220 kcal/serving. 2 phases: Weight loss (2 to 3 formulas, 1 fruit, 1 meal of 410 kcal; 1,100 to 1,200 kcal/day) Maintenance (1 to 2 formulas, 2 meals; 3 fruits; 6 oz milk; 1,450 to 1,520 kcal/day) Frozen entrees (230 to 400 kcal) also available. This diet can be dangerous if instructions are not followed properly

they are few in number. These include such titles as *The Rice Diet Report,* which is about 700 kcal/day, and older books, now fortunately off most bookshelves, such as *Fasting As a Way of Life, Nutraerobics,* and the *Last Chance Diet.* People who rely on such books to devise and use VLCDs on their own run substantial and unnecessary health risks (24).

In addition to the major metabolic hazards that have already been mentioned in Table 2, Table 3 shows that fasting and weight reduction methods that provide fewer than 600 to 800 kcal/day pose other undesirable side effects. Although these are not life threatening, they may discourage or frighten the patient. Therefore medical supervision is mandatory, and self-devised VLCDs are not to be recommended.

Self-prescribed VLCDs are sometimes concocted in an idiosyncratic manner from commercial over the counter (OTC) diet products. Powdered diet formulae and meal replacement products such as Slim Fast or Ultra Slim Fast, which are available OTC in drugstores and supermarkets, are particularly amenable to such abuses. These products range in energy levels from about 190 to 220 kcal per serving. If the meal replacements were used three times a day as directed, along with one or two fruit and snacks and a low-calorie dinner, daily calorie intakes would fall somewhere between 1,100 and 1,200 kcal. If directions are followed, intakes of nutrients other than calories and electrolytes should be satisfactory. Meal replacements, however, have a high potential for abuse since instructions may not be followed and medical supervision is absent. When the menu replacement shakes are alternated with the use of periodic fasting, the result could be hazardous. Because of the potential for abuse and the lack of medical supervision, Ultra Slim Fast and Slim Fast are not recommended.

Other Aspects of Safe VLCD Use

For safe use, a careful medical evaluation prior to embarking on VLCD, an exercise prescription limited to activities of low intensity (most OTC products simply exhort the person to exercise without providing specifics), review of the nutritional adequacy of the diet, adjustment of any medications, ongoing medical monitoring during use, and a duration on VLCD of not more than 3 to 4 months are mandatory. Plans for refeeding by gradually increasing energy and carbohydrate intakes are mandatory. Additional nutrition information and guidance are needed for long-term maintenance of weight loss while consuming a diet of conventional foods.

Low-Calorie Diets (800 to 1,200 kcal/day)

There is no sharp line of demarcation, in terms of their biological effects, between VLCD and more moderate low-calorie diets (LCD) providing 800 to 1,200 kcal/day. A rule of thumb is that the less severe the caloric restriction, the less likely are the risks of metabolic complications and other side effects. Diets of 800 to 1,200 kcal/day are still below RMR for most adults, so they too have noticeable effects on metabolism as well as on loss of adipose tissue.

Diets that are this hypocaloric should not be embarked upon without physician approval. They are most suited for individuals who have significant medical reasons for losing weight, such as non-insulin-dependent diabetes mellitus, hyperlipidemia, and hypertension. In addition to a diet plan, the patient also needs help in developing a physical activity and exercise plan, and in learning some behavior modification techniques that will facilitate adoption of life-style changes.

When 800 to 1,200 kcal/day LCDs are based on regular foods rather than on specially formulated or fortified products, they usually require vitamin and mineral supplementation to be nutritionally adequate. Therefore, multivitamin–multimineral supplements are usually recommended. For women, iron and calcium supplementation needs special attention.

Frequent health supervision and follow-up

are essential since the patient may become dehydrated, particularly if the diet is very low in carbohydrate (and thus ketogenic). Tables 2 and 3 summarize some of the potential side effects that may arise if care is not taken to prevent them.

Table 4 lists several of the more reasonable LCD commercial weight loss programs. These programs include Weight Watchers, Diet Workshop, Diet Center, Jenny Craig, Weight Loss Centers, and Nutri/System. The Physicians' Weight Loss Clinics, New Directions, and other programs also use reasonable LCD. Many of these regimens start off with a low-carbohydrate, hypocaloric diet of 900 to 1,000 kcal/day to stimulate diuresis and a more rapid weight loss in the first few weeks of dieting than would be achieved from fat loss alone. If carbohydrate levels are very low, a state of relative dehydration may be present, but as either carbohydrate or calorie levels rise, weight may suddenly increase due to rehydration and antidiuresis. Most of the regimes gradually increase energy levels after a few weeks to over 1,200 kcal/day.

Many books advocate LCDs. A few recent offerings are reviewed in Table 5. Recent favorites that are relatively reasonable include the New Pritikin Program (30). This is a very-low-fat high-carbohydrate diet, which must be supplemented with vitamins and minerals to achieve the RDA. The Hilton Head diet is questionable since it does not meet standards for minimum numbers of servings from the Basic Four Food Groups, nor does it include a well-developed behavior modification component (31). Among the unreasonable books are the Rotation Diet (32), which is based on unproven and unlikely theories, and Dr. Berger's immune power diet (33), which makes many inappropriate claims and which is unsound nutritionally.

Years ago, most of the diet meal replacements were milk-based formula products such as Metrecal, which were sold over the counter in drugstores. Today, frozen microwavable meals, dried products, and canned meals are also available. Some are sold as part of commercial weight-loss programs, such as those foods provided by the Nutri/System program and Jenny Craig Weight Loss Centers.

Some people use drugstore OTC items to help with dieting. These include Slim Fast and Ultra Slim Fast (described above), the Cambridge/Food For Life Program, and Diet Ayds. Herbalife and the many Shaklee products may also be obtained from door to door salesmen. Dieters sometimes use these products to devise diets that restrict calories more severely than label directions specify. These products are specially formulated powders or foods that are designed as meal replacements. Label directions or package inserts usually suggest consulting a physician if the individual falls in a high-risk group, but there is no guarantee that any dieter will do so. Even though directions recommend a regimen that would be in the 1,100 to 1,200 kcal/day range, and thus well above 800 kcal if followed precisely, there is no assurance that dieters will do this.

An interesting new development in products for self-initiated weight-loss regimes is the advent of frozen low-calorie main dishes, which are widely available in grocery stores and supermarkets. Such products include Healthy Choice, Ultra Slim Fast Frozen Entrees, Weight Watchers, Stouffers' Lean Cuisine, and Budget Gourmet Light, among others. These frozen low-calorie products usually provide about 200 to 300 kcal/serving (Ultra Slim Fast Entrees ranging from 230 to 400 calories) from a variety of recipes. Most of the dishes are low in fat and cholesterol and relatively high in carbohydrate. They vary in their vitamin and mineral contributions. They can be convenient, quickly prepared entrees that are useful as adjuncts to a total weight management program. However, the potential for abuse is present, as noted below.

One of the frozen entrees, Ultra Slim Fast, specifies on the label that it can be used as part of a total weight-loss program. The back panel of the package shows a daily meal plan consisting of two Ultra Slimfast formula shakes, which are about 220 kcal each, and

TABLE 5. *Analyses of some popular diet books*

Diet	Meets Basic 4 Food Groups?	Nutrition education, behavior modification, exercise included?	Description, comments
800–1,200 kcal/day			
Questionable:			
Hilton Head Over-35 Diet by Peter Miller. New York: Warner Books, 1989	No—low in milk and fruit/ vegetable groups during low-calorie phase	Yes—but limited behavior modification	3 phases: Low calorie (rotates between 900 kcal/day on weekdays and 1,200 kcal/day on weekends) Reentry (about halfway between low-calorie and maintenance phases) Maintenance (kcal equal to resting metabolic rate plus activity factor) Varying energy intakes in weight loss has not been proved to prevent drops in RMR
The New Pritikin Program by Robert Pritikin. New York: Simon and Schuster, 1990	Yes—heavy emphasis on fruit/ vegetable and bread/ cereal groups	Yes	Energy intakes of 1,000 kcal/day for women, 1,200 kcal/day for men on "maximum weight loss" plan. Does not take individual needs for weight loss into account. Low-fat (10%), high-carbohydrate (75% to 80%) diet that is also low in sodium and high in fiber. May be difficult to follow such a low-fat diet
Unreasonable:			
Dr. Berger's Immune Power Diet by Stewart Berger. New York: New American Library, 1985	No—low in milk and bread/ cereal groups	Limited	Diet to improve immune system but includes weight loss as an added benefit; based on unsupported claims that certain foods affect immune system and levels of energy, creativity, mood, and emotion 3 phases: Elimination (about 1,050 kcal/day) Reintroduction (about 1,400 kcal/day) Maintenance (about 1,650 kcal/day) Individual differences in caloric needs for weight loss are not considered; recommends megadoses of supplements, which can be dangerous
Rotation Diet by Martin Katahn. New York: Bantam Books, 1987	No—low in milk and bread/ cereal groups for most phases	Yes	Energy intakes of 600 to 1,500 kcal/day rotated over 4 weeks; maintenance level is 1,800 kcal/day. Individual differences in caloric needs for weight loss are not considered. Varying energy intakes in weight loss has not been proved to prevent drops in RMR
>1,200 kcal/day			
Reasonable:			
Fat Attack Plan by Annete Natow and Jo-Ann Heslin. New York: Pocket Books, 1990	May be low in meat or bread/ cereal groups depending on what dieter chooses	Yes	Teaches dieter to count grams of fat in foods 3 phases: "Super start" (about 1,350 kcal/day) "Getting ahead"—15 g fat (about 1,400 kcal/day) "In control"—45 g of fat for women (about 1,700 kcal/day), 60 g of fat for men (about 1,900 kcal/day) May be difficult to follow such a low-fat diet
Fit or Fat Target Diet by Covert Bailey. Boston: Houghton and Mifflin, 1984	Yes	Limited—more guidance may be needed for weight loss; focus is on long-term weight management	Emphasis on healthy balanced diet rather than weight loss. Recommended minimum calorie level to promote weight loss is 1,000 to 1,400 kcal/day for women; 1,400 to 1,800 kcal/day for men. Diet is based on Basic Four Food Groups with emphasis on low-fat, low-sugar, and high-fiber foods (about 1,500 kcal/day)

TABLE 5. *Continued.*

Diet	Meets Basic 4 Food Groups?	Nutrition education, behavior modification, exercise included?	Description, comments
Set Point Diet by Gilbert Leveille. New York: Ballantine Books, 1985	Yes	Yes	1,200 to 2,400 kcal/day food plans. Maintenance adds 300 kcal/day. More research is needed regarding the set-point theory of body weight being confined to narrow range, and whether or not diet can lower one's set-point weight

T-Factor Diet by Martin Katahn. New York: WW Norton, 1989	Yes	Yes	Two diets provided:
			  T-factor diet is relatively low in calories and involves counting fat grams (20 to 40 g fat for women or about 1,200 kcal/day, 30 to 60 g fat or about 1,800 kcal/day for men).
			  "Quick Melt Diet" restricts women to 1,000 to 1,300 kcal/day and men to 1,500 to 1,800 kcal/day. Does not take individual caloric differences for weight control into account
			May be difficult to follow such low-fat diet. Based on thermogenesis studies suggesting that dietary fat is more efficiently converted into body fat than carbohydrates

Callaway Diet by Wayne Callaway. New York: Bantam Books 1990	No—low in milk group	Yes—but limited advice on maintenance	1,400 to 2,000 kcal/day menus. Geared toward dieters who are "starvers" (periodically fast or near fast with VLCD), "stuffers" (compulsive eaters), or "skippers" (skip meals)
Unreasonable: *Fit For Life* by Harvey and Marilyn Diamond. New York: Warner Books, 1985	No—low in milk, meat, and bread/cereal groups; *very* high in fruit/vegetable groups	Yes—but little emphasis on behavior modification and weight maintenance	Based on unsupported claims that fat deposits are caused by improper food combinations. Diet is high in fat (41%) and lacks variety. Individual differences in caloric needs for weight control are not considered, and high bulk may make it difficult to consume adequate calories

are recommended as meal replacements at breakfast and lunch, a fruit for a snack, and a frozen entree which is to be eaten with a vegetable salad, a slice of bread, and a low-fat dessert. If used as directed, such an eating plan would provide well over 800 kcal/day, although levels would vary depending on how the items were used. When the entrees, however, are used as the only meal of the day, or when they are combined with periodic fasting on several other days during the week, they may lead to the kind of acute problems outlined in Tables 2 and 3 that frequently accompany unsupervised VLCDs. For example, if one entree were used per day, with no additional calories aside from a breakfast consisting of a glass of skim milk, a half-cup of orange juice, and a cup of high-fiber bran cereal (and only noncaloric fluids throughout the day) the intake would be lower than 600 kcal/day and would fail to meet the RDA for several vitamins and minerals. Some individuals who habitually use these meals are also compulsive exercisers who embark on very ambitious aerobic exercise programs at the same time, further increasing the caloric deficit.

Weight Watchers frozen entrees also specify use as part of an overall weight-loss plan.

If these entrees are used along with attendance at one of the Weight Watchers formal commercial weight-loss groups, which are available in most localities, ongoing surveillance and group support would be provided. The other major disadvantage is that the frozen entrees are relatively costly.

When 800 to 1,200 kcal/day diets are based on regular foods and do not consist of specially developed recipes or synthesized and fortified products developed specifically for weight control purposes, they also require vitamin and mineral supplementation.

Balanced Deficit Diets (1,200 or more kcal/day)

Diets that provide 1,200 or more kcal/day are often referred to as balanced deficit diets (BDD), since deficits in calories and the distribution of energy providing nutrients are better balanced than they are in the high-protein, low-fat, low-carbohydrate VLCDs. With wise menu choices from ordinary foods, moderately low calorie BDDs provide most individuals with adequate nutrient intakes. Their higher calorie level makes adherence easier, and minimizes undesirable physiological effects (34). Some diets permit the dieter to choose from a variety of regular foods, from a variety of frozen entrees, or from foods sold through the weight-loss program. Others restrict choice to a set menu or exchange plan.

A 1,200 kcal/day diet is usually low enough to induce weight loss in most people. Indeed, in very large people, even a 1,200 kcal/day diet may be too low. For example, a 209-lb (95-kg) man who is moderately active and whose energy needs are about 2,590 kcal/day would experience weight losses well in excess of 2 pounds a week on a diet product such as Slim Fast, which recommends energy intakes of about 1,100 to 1,200 kcal/day. Such very rapid losses are inadvisable without medical supervision, since they are likely to be accompanied by troublesome and some-

times frightening side effects. Thus all reducing diets must be tailored to the user. There is no level that is safe for everyone. Consultation with a physician will ensure that there are no medical contraindications to dieting or vigorous exercise. If the diet is nutritionally adequate and well balanced, diets at this caloric level can usually be undertaken without close medical supervision. Metabolic disturbances are extremely unlikely on moderately low-calorie diets, although they do occur occasionally in massively obese individuals whose energy needs are extremely high. Higher calorie diets may be called for with such individuals.

At the same time the dieting begins, a program of aerobic exercise and increased daily physical activity should also be prescribed. Exercise, in addition to expending calories to move the body, may counteract the diet-induced decrease in RMR, so that even greater energy deficits can be achieved without further dietary deprivation (35). A behavior modification component is also an essential part of all sound weight-loss programs. It is important to stress to the dieter that just as the eating plan must be followed, so too must the exercise plan be scheduled and built into daily life.

For those who want an individualized moderately low-calorie diet plan, one option is to consult a registered dietitian. Often they work in conjunction with a physician, exercise physiologist, and psychologist, who can supply additional inputs in other areas needed for sound weight management.

Formal LCD programs operated by health centers or hospitals (and in some instances commercial group weight-loss programs) offer patients the group support, nutritional advice and instruction in physical activity and behavior modification that they need. There are many commercial weight-loss programs that are generally sound. Some of these are described in Table 4. Those that use conventional or low-calorie foods available in supermarkets include the Diet Center, Physicians' Weight Loss Centers, and Weight

Watchers. Others, including Nutri/System and Jenny Craig Weight Loss Centers, provide packaged foods to the dieter at weekly classes. Each program has strengths and weaknesses and should be evaluated carefully before patients are referred to them, since they change over time (36). The programs usually include some attention to weight maintenance, but drop-out rates are very high, even during the weight-loss phase (see Taylor and Stunkard, *this volume*).

Other approaches that cost little or no money may also be helpful, including Take Off Pounds Sensibly (TOPS) and Overeaters Anonymous (OA). These programs provide psychological support and social contacts through self-help groups. OA also suggests a "Grey Svelte Diet," which is high in fruits and vegetables, high in protein and carbohydrate, but not necessarily highly restricted in calories. Years ago OA participants often used a high-protein, very-low-carbohydrate diet that was very dangerous, so this safer diet represents an improvement.

There are many examples of reasonable, moderately low-calorie diet books. Table 5 reviews several, using the seven Cs discussed earlier as the criteria for evaluation. Three-day sample menus were also analyzed and nutrient levels evaluated. These were judged adequate if they met the minimum number of servings specified in the Basic Four Food Guide of the US Department of Agriculture. Reasonable books at this calorie level include the *Set Point Diet* (37), the *Fat Attack Plan* (38), the *Fit or Fat Target Diet* (39), and the *T Factor Diet* (40). *The Callaway Diet* for Starvers, Stuffers and Skippers (41) is slightly low in calcium, but may be useful for those who binge eat and skip meals to help get them back on track. However, it places less emphasis on the principle of long-term maintenance than might be desirable. Other books, including *Fit for Life* (42) by Harvey and Marilyn Diamond, in all of its editions, and all books written to date by Stewart Berger, author of *Dr. Berger's Immune Power Diet,* cannot be recommended because of the large number of unjustified scientific claims they make.

COMPOSITION

Composition of the diet, the second of the seven Cs, is important in many respects, not the least of which is its influence on the loss of fat and weight. Fasting causes excessive breakdown of lean tissue with consequent water losses. Conscious limitations of fluid intake, or excessive sweating in steam baths and saunas may also lead to relative dehydration and rapid, although transient, weight losses (43).

Some other weight-loss regimes also stimulate endocrine responses, which give rise to ketosis with a secondary diuresis. Diuresis is common during fasting, on VLCDs providing less than 600 to 800 kcal/day, such as Medifast or Optifast, and on other higher calorie but still very-low-carbohydrate diets, such as Dr. Atkins' Diet Revolution, which was popular a decade ago (44).

Protein

In hypocaloric states the hormonal milieu favors the sparing of nitrogen and preferential use of adipose tissue for energy, but inevitably some lean body mass and nitrogen are also lost. Losses of water, calcium, phosphorus, potassium, and vitamins follow. Depletion of more than 40% of initial normal lean body mass is life threatening (45). It is vital to preserve lean body mass as much as possible during weight loss, since these are the actively metabolizing cells of the body. Lesser losses of lean body mass can also be hazardous, affecting cardiovascular function, exercise tolerance, and possibly resistance to infection, so they, too, should be avoided.

Protein is of major concern on total fasts and VLCDs because extremely hypocaloric states increase protein needs above recommended levels (46,47). When energy intakes are insufficient, some amino acids are used to maintain blood sugar levels and others are used for energy, so the overall protein requirement increases.

As a rule of thumb, a minimum of 65 to 70 g of protein are needed daily. On a VLCD, nitrogen balance depends on maintaining intakes of nitrogen, ideally with at least 1.5 g of high-quality protein per kilogram of ideal body weight per day, with intakes no less than about 65 to 70 g daily (48,49). Recommendations may be even higher if the dieter suffers from certain diseases or is physically stressed, since nitrogen losses are further accelerated in these states (50).

When the patient consumes 600 to 1,200 kcal/day, protein intake should equal at least 1 g per/kg of ideal body weight. Some diet books, such as the recently popular *Fit for Life* diet book (43), and the previously popular *Fasting As A Way of Life* diet, recommend eating patterns that tend to be low in protein and are unsound in numerous other ways. Hence they should be avoided. Reducing diets over 1,200 kcal/day should provide at least 0.8 g of protein per kg of ideal body weight.

Carbohydrate

Carbohydrate levels are particularly important on low-calorie diets since adequate carbohydrate is necessary to maintain blood sugar levels and fluid balance. The daily carbohydrate requirement for those eating less than 600 kcal/day is at least 50 g. The brain requires about 100 g/day of glucose for fuel, and other tissues use about 50 g, so that even at 50 g/day, ketosis is likely. Over time some adaptations can be made, but even as insulin–glucagon ratios induce adipose tissue breakdown causing the body to burn more and more fatty acids, there are some tissues that cannot do this and that must rely on glucose supplied either exogenously or from proteolysis of muscle. Fifty grams of carbohydrate is the amount supplied in about 2 potatoes, 4 slices of bread, or 4 tablespoons of sugar. One hundred grams or more of carbohydrate a day, preferably mostly complex carbohydrate, is recommended both to spare protein and to avoid large shifts in weight due to changes in water balance. When carbohydrate levels are below about 100 g, insulin levels fall and protein is catabolized to provide the glucogenic amino acids. These can be converted to glucose, the preferred fuel of the brain, and other glucose-requiring cells. Most diets providing under 100 g/day of carbohydrate or under approximately 800 kcal/day are ketogenic. Examples include the previously popular Scarsdale diet, the Magic Mayo (or Grapefruit) Diet, Dr. Atkin's Diet, and the Drinking Man's Diet. They induce a relative insulin deficit, and secondary to the ketosis that then arises, a diuresis and loss of fluid weight follow quickly in the first few days on the diet (51). When protein is burned to preserve blood sugar levels, additional water is liberated by the protein catabolic process. In general, for every gram of protein or glycogen that is broken down, 3 g of water are released. The rapid weight loss in the first few days on VLCDs is often welcomed by dieters. However, individuals on such regimens are also relatively dehydrated (52). Dieters may have negative side effects including fatigue, postural hypotension, a fetid taste in their mouths, and elevated serum uric acid levels, and may be more subject to negative nitrogen balance.

With diets providing 800 to 1,200 kcal/day, the carbohydrate goal should be as close to 55% of calories as possible. Over 1,200 kcal/day, 55% or more of total calories should be from carbohydrate, mostly complex carbohydrate.

Dietary fiber, which is usually but not always chemically similar to carbohydrate but is virtually noncaloric, also needs to be considered. On a VLCD, intakes usually recommended for best health and laxation may not be feasible. On 800 kcal/day diets and above, however, 20 to 30 g/day from various food sources is recommended. Inclusion of five fruits and vegetables a day and whole grain breads and cereals help meet this goal.

Electrolytes

Electrolytes are extremely important on VLCDs; occasionally cardiac arrhythmias resulting from hypokalemia have been reported (53,54). Hypokalemia can be fatal, and therefore patients, especially those who are at high risk of electrolyte problems, should be very carefully monitored.

Fluids

Hydration is also important. Much of the initial, very rapid weight loss that occurs in the first few days of dieting is due to diuresis and dehydration. This is especially likely when the diet is very low in carbohydrate and/or very low in calories. Quite aside from symptoms of thirst, dehydration poses considerable health risks.

Vitamins and Minerals

The lower the diet is in calories, the more likely it is that other essential nutrients and electrolytes such as potassium, magnesium, and other minerals and vitamins will be lacking. Some of the VLCDs in the 1970s may have been limited in a number of these respects, as well as in protein quality. These features may have contributed to the illness and sudden death that were reported. Fortunately, these particular formulas are no longer on the market (21). As a general rule of thumb, diets below 1,200 kcal/day are likely to require vitamin and mineral supplements. Above 1,200 kcal/day, food sources of nutrients are preferred, and needs can usually be met by inclusion of the Basic Four Food Groups. In any event, all reducing diets must meet the RDA for age and sex. These nutritional underpinnings of a sound reducing diet include electrolytes, trace elements, and water, as well as the better recognized vitamins and minerals.

Adjustments for Special Needs

Special adjustments may be necessary for women, especially for calcium and iron needs. If physical activity is extremely vigorous, electrolytes and water may need special attention. Other health considerations may also necessitate special adjustments in other nutrients.

COST

The costs of various diets and other obesity therapies range from modest to exorbitant. Obesity is big business; billions of dollars are spent each year on its treatment. The good news for dieters is that there is no association between cost and effectiveness. The bad news is that standardized disclosures of the effectiveness of various treatments for obesity are simply unavailable. Therefore the buyer must beware.

Table 4 describes various reducing diets and provides a rough idea of relative prices. In general, medically supervised programs, particularly those that supply food or extensive interventions such as special exercise programs, are among the more costly programs. To date, few medically supervised programs provide monitored exercise components. Some programs demand that the dieter pay all costs, regardless of the services actually used or the weight loss that is achieved. Other programs, such as Nutri/System, provide rebates to those who are able to keep their weight off over the long term.

CONSUMER FRIENDLINESS

Ethical marketing and business practices are mandatory in obesity treatment programs, whether they be for profit or nonprofit. There is a need for greater documentation of the various effects, both positive and negative, of existing weight control services. For example, 1- and 5-year cure rates should be included in descriptions of the programs.

Although many high-quality programs and regimens exist, professional and operational standards for consumer safety and protection in the weight-loss industry are insufficient and need to be improved. No ready and specific means of redress is available for consumers who are affected by abusive practices. Weight loss involves a health-related human service and the ethical standards that apply to it should incorporate those involved in any sort of health care. A new Canadian government task force report on weight control and recent Congressional Hearings held in this country have been devoted to exploring ways to improve consumer-related aspects of weight control programs (55,56). Other problems also need to be addressed in the weight-loss field. Access to treatment, especially for the poor, and for those who lack adequate health insurance, must be improved. Another problem is to develop voluntary, industry-wide codes for marketing. Advertising should provide enough information so that consumers can judge if they truly need weight reduction, and, if so, which programs will be safe and effective for them. These problems apply to medically supervised as well as to other endeavors involving weight loss.

COPING WITH COEXISTING HEALTH PROBLEMS

For any program, adequate provisions should be made for the diagnosis, treatment, and surveillance of coexisting medical and psychological conditions and risks. At the very minimum, this includes medical assessment and determination of individual readiness from the psychological and behavioral standpoint prior to embarking on the diet. The hypocaloric diets that are prescribed should also incorporate other therapeutic considerations including medical monitoring for coexisting health problems and ongoing surveillance of health, exercise, mental health, and behavioral as well as dietary status. Client safety issues, particularly for those with significant health risks who may embark

on programs with little or no medical supervision, must not be ignored. Individuals who are at high risk of health complications from dieting, particularly when self-imposed regimes are used, include children, adolescents, pregnant and nursing women, persons with eating disorders, those who would become underweight with weight loss, underweight persons, the massively obese (e.g., those with a BMI of 37 or greater, which is at least 200% of desirable weights), and those who are currently or who have previously experienced emotional difficulties associated with weight loss.

CONTAINS ALL ESSENTIAL COMPONENTS FOR SOUND WEIGHT MANAGEMENT

It is relatively easy to take weight off. It is much more difficult to maintain weight loss. Chances of success are improved when information and tools are provided for making life-long changes.

A hypocaloric diet that is adequate in nutrients is only one of several essential components of a sound weight management program. There is also a need for nutrition education, practice in low-calorie eating under a variety of social situations, and making wise food choices that are nutritionally adequate. Nutrition information and practice are especially important in preparing the dieter for sustaining and maintaining lower weights once they have been achieved. The adoption of a healthy eating plan as part of the maintenance phase of long-term weight management is also critical. If the dieter simply returns to his or her previous calorie levels, weight will be regained quickly.

The individual dieter also needs to be aware of other issues concerning his or her specific weight-loss regimen. For example, when the individual has been on a VLCD, after sufficient fat is lost to accomplish goals, a gradual refeeding period is likely to be necessary before the patient is able to readjust to a higher calorie diet suitable for maintenance.

If intakes are suddenly increased, abdominal distress and edema may occur. Also, if the individual binges or greatly increases carbohydrate intake while consuming a VLCD, weight gains of 5 to 10 lb of edema fluid may suddenly occur. This edema is due to the rapid reversal of the glycogen depletion and dehydration that are common on VLCD. Carbohydrate intakes are very low on VLCDs, thereby depleting body glycogen stores and inducing a state of low-grade ketosis, which in itself helps to perpetuate the relative dehydration further. During refeeding or binging, carbohydrate intakes greatly increase, and glycogen with its water of hydration suddenly accumulates, with consequent weight gains. Although these are not fat gains, many dieters are disappointed and surprised by their rapid weight gain. During the refeeding phase, if refeeding occurs too quickly, sharp upward spikes in weight may also occur. This can be prevented by increasing carbohydrate and energy intakes gradually.

On LCD and diets providing 1,200 or more kcal/day, gradual transitions to maintenance levels give the dieter a chance to introduce additional food choices slowly while continuing to maintain lowered weights.

In addition to dietary guidance, an exercise prescription with additional attention devoted to increased daily physical activity of less demanding sorts is mandatory for long-term weight management. During the weight-loss phase, the exercise prescription will vary, depending on the calorie level of the diet. As the transition to weight maintenance is made, even those on a VLCD need to increase their exercise levels gradually.

Limitations secondary to medical problems must also be considered in planning physical activity and exercise programs. For individuals with disabilities, exercise physiologists and physical therapists may be helpful in formulating both more active ways of daily living and more structured aerobic exercise that can be well tolerated.

Finally, psychological support that includes motivation and remotivation, lapse and relapse prevention, and the practice of behavior modification strategies must be included in both the weight-loss and weight-maintenance phases. Excellent materials are now available to help dieters. These include the *Lean Program for Weight Control* (57), the *Weight Maintenance Survival Guide* (58), and the *Weight Control Digest,* which is available in both lay and professional editions (59). Other reasonable approaches include the *I Don't Eat A Lot* program (60).

CONTINUATION PROVISIONS FOR LONG-TERM MAINTENANCE

At minimum, a reasonable diet, physical activity, and behavior modification plans for both weight reduction and long-term maintenance of healthy weights need to be specified. Although the prescriptions for weight loss and maintenance share some common elements, they are dissimilar. During maintenance, energy intakes must be somewhat lower, and physical activity levels must be higher, than they were prior to embarking on the reducing diet in order to maintain lowered weights. Long-term eating plans that conform to the recent recommendations of the National Academy of Sciences (published in the *Diet and Health Report*), the *Dietary Guidelines for Americans,* and other authoritative groups are appropriate (61,62). For those who want additional practical guidance in healthy life styles to control weight over the long term, several books on overall diet, including the *Optimal Diet Book* (63), *Tufts University Guide to Total Nutrition* (64), and *Dr. Jean Mayer's Diet and Nutrition Guide* are available (65).

Unfortunately, weight cycling, with losses and rapid regains, are the rule rather than the exception for many dieters (66). When people succeed in keeping the weight off, they appear to share common factors. These factors include an emphasis on exercise, gradual changes in diet, and, in some cases, therapy that treats obesity as a food-dependency disorder best dealt with through external social control groups rather than through self-control alone (67). Such strategies are particularly helpful for the mildly obese and, if combined with low-calorie diets to produce greater weight loss, they may also help those whose obesity is more serious (68).

LONG-TERM MAINTENANCE

The ultimate test of any diet is that weight remains lower over the long term. In this respect, the results of all weight-loss therapies have been disappointing. In one study, 90% of one group of patients who lost over 25 lb on a variety of diets gained much of the weight back within 2 years (69). Most of the weight is regained after 5 years, regardless of what therapies are employed, and ultimate maintenance of lower weights is poor. The challenge to those who design weight reduction programs in the 1990s is to improve long-term weight loss. This will involve greater understanding of the factors that regulate energy intake and expenditure.

ANALYSES OF TODAY'S COMMON WEIGHT LOSS SCHEMES

Table 4 presents our evaluation, using the seven Cs, of some of the more popular weight loss programs in use today. Table 5 provides similar information on some diet books on the best-seller list.

As new diets join this list in the future, health professionals and lay people should assess their merits using the criteria listed in the seven Cs discussed above. Those that generally conform to all of these criteria are rated as reasonable. Those that fall short and are weak on only a few criteria are rated as questionable. Finally, those that are deemed unsafe for general or nutritional health, or are fraudulent, are considered unreasonable. Clearly a diversity of diets will always be available, ranging from the scientifically and nutritionally unsound to the sublime. Consumers and health professionals need to keep

up with them and to eschew unreasonable or questionable offerings (70).

CONCLUSIONS

The notion that diets alone are the answer to weight loss is no longer subscribed to by health experts. Over the past decade, awareness has grown that if obesity risks are to be decreased, comprehensive, long-term weight management efforts are essential. Diet plans that do not emphasize increasing physical activity are not likely to be helpful. In spite of this, a variety of weight-loss programs, ranging from unsound to excellent, continue to be available in the American and Canadian markets. Therefore there is every reason for both dieters and their counselors to analyze these products and programs before they use them.

ACKNOWLEDGMENTS

Partial support for preparing this manuscript was provided by grant MCJ 91210 to Dr. Dwyer from the Maternal and Child Health Services, US Department of Health and Human Services, and training grant MCH 8421. Partial support was also provided for salary support with Federal funds from the US Department of Agriculture, Agricultural Research Service under contract number 53-3K06-5-10. The contents of this publication do not necessarily reflect the views or policies of the US Department of Agriculture, nor does mention of trade names, commercial products, or organizations imply endorsement by the US government.

REFERENCES

1. Weinsier RL, Wadden TA, Ritenbaugh C, Harrison GG, Johnson FS, Wilmore JH. Recommended therapeutic guidelines for professional weight control programs. *Am J Clin Nutr* 1984;40:865–72.
2. Bierman EL (ed). *Contemporary management of the overweight patient: opinion leaders' symposium pro-*

ceedings. Little Falls, NJ: Health Learning Systems, 1991.

3. Berland, T. *Rating the diets.* New York: Signet Books, 1986.

4. Bennion LJ, Bierman EL, Ferguson JM, Editors of Consumer Reports Books. *Straight talk about weight control: taking pounds off and keeping them off.* New York: Consumers Union, 1991.

5. Nicholas P, Dwyer J. Diets for weight reduction: nutritional considerations. In: Brownell K, Foreyt J, eds. *Physiology, psychology, and treatment of the eating disorders.* New York: Academic Press, 1986;122–44.

6. Dwyer JT. Analyses of popular diets. In: Paige D, ed. *Clinical nutrition,* 2nd ed. St. Louis: CV Mosby, 1988;838–48.

7. Dwyer JT. Treatment of obesity: conventional programs and fad diets. In: Bjorntorp BM, Bradoff I, eds. *Obesity.* Philadelphia: JB Lippincott, 1992;662–76.

8. Dwyer JT. Sixteen popular diets: brief nutritional analyses. In: Stunkard AJ, ed. *Obesity.* Philadelphia: WB Saunders, 1980;276–91.

9. VanItallie TB. Dietary approaches to the treatment of obesity. In: Stunkard AJ, ed. *Obesity.* Philadelphia: WB Saunders, 1980;249–61.

10. Federal Trade Commission. *Facts for consumers: diet programs.* Washington, DC: Federal Trade Commission, 1990.

11. Owen OE, Kavle E, Owen RS, et al. A reappraisal of caloric requirements in healthy women. *Am J Clin Nutr* 1986;44:1–19.

12. Owen OE, Holup JL, D'Allessio DA, et al. A reappraisal of the caloric requirements of men. *Am J Clin Nutr* 1987;46:875–85.

13. Cahill GF. Starvation in man. *Clin Endocrinol Metab* 1976;5:397–415.

14. Aoki TT, Finley RJ. The metabolic response to fasting. In: Rombeau J, Caldwell M, eds. *Parenteral Nutrition.* Philadelphia: WB Saunders, 1986;9–28.

15. Aoki TT, Finlley RJ. The effect of insulin on renal handling of sodium, potassium, calcium, and phosphate in man. *J Clin Invest* 1975;55:845–55.

16. Dulloo AG, Girardier L. Adaptive changes in energy expenditure during refeeding following low calorie intake: evidence for a specific metabolic component favoring fat storage. *Am J Clin Nutr* 1990;52: 415–20.

17. Life Sciences Research Office. *Research needs in management of obesity by severe caloric restriction.* Washington, DC: Federation of American Societies for Experimental Biology. FDA contract 223-75-2090, 1979.

18. Wadden TA, Van Itallie TB, Blackburn GL. Responsible and irresponsible use of very low calorie diets in the treatment of obesity. *JAMA* 1990;263:83–5.

19. Paulsen BK. Position of the American Dietetic Association: very low calorie weight loss diets. *J Am Diet Assoc* 1990;90:722–6.

20. Sours HE, Frattali VP, Brand CD, et al. Sudden death associated with very low calorie weight reduction regimens. *Am J Clin Nutr* 1981;34:453–61.

21. Wadden TA, Stunkard AJ, Brownell KD. Very low calorie diets: their efficacy, safety, and future. *Ann Intern Med* 1983;99:675–84.

22. Wadden TA, Stunkard AJ, Brownell KD, Day SC. A comparison of two very low calorie diets: protein sparing modified fast versus protein formula liquid diet. *Am J Clin Nutr* 1985;41:533–9.

23. Fisler JS, Drenick EJ. Starvation and semistarvation diets in the management of obesity. *Ann Rev Nutr* 1987;7:465–84.

24. Quincy M. *Diet right! The consumer's guide to diet and weight loss programs.* Berkeley, CA: Canari Press, 1991.

25. Yetiv JZ. *Popular nutritional practices: a scientific appraisal.* Toledo, OH: Popular Medicine Press, 1986.

26. Wadden TA, Stunkard AJ, Day SC, Gould RA, Rubin CJ. Less food less hunger: reports of appetite and symptoms in a controlled study of PSMF. *Int J Obes* 1987;11:239–49.

27. Wing RR, Marcus MD, Blair EH, Bustin LR. Psychological responses of obese type II diabetics to very low calorie diets. *Diabetes Care* 1991; 14:576–99.

28. Wing RR, Marcus MD, Salata R, Epstein LH, Miaskiewicz S, Blair EH. Effects of VLCD on long term glycemic control in obese type II diabetic subjects. *Arch Intern Med* 1991;151:1334–40.

29. Wadden TA, Stunkard AJ. Controlled trial of VLCD, behavior therapy, and their combination in the treatment of obesity. *J Consult Clin Psychol* 1986;54:482–8.

30. Pritikin R. *The new Pritikin program.* New York: Simon and Schuster, 1990.

31. Miller P. *Hilton Head—Over 35.* New York: Warner Books, 1989.

32. Katahn M. *Rotation Diet.* New York: Bantam Books, 1987.

33. Berger S. *Dr. Berger's immune power diet.* New York: New American Library, 1985.

34. Wing RR. Behavioral strategies for weight reduction in obese type II diabetics. *Diabetes Care* 1989;12:139–44.

35. Health Services and Promotion Branch. *Report of the task force on the treatment of obesity.* Ottawa: Minister of Supply and Services, Canada Health and Welfare, 1991.

36. Byerly L, Day M, Hack S, et al. *Popular diets: how they rate,* 2nd ed. Santa Monica, CA: California Dietetic Association, 1987.

37. Leveille G. *Set point diet.* New York: Ballantine Books, 1985.

38. Natow A, Heslin JA. *Fat attack plan.* New York: Pocket Books, 1990.

39. Bailey C. *Fit or fat target diet.* Boston: Houghton and Mifflin, 1984.

40. Katahn M. *T factor diet.* New York: WW Norton, 1989.

41. Callaway W. *Callaway diet.* New York: Bantam Books, 1990.

42. Diamond H, Diamond M. *Fit for life.* New York: Warner Books, 1985.

43. Forbes GB. *Human body composition: growth, aging, nutrition and activity.* New York: Springer-Verlag, 1987.

44. Atkins RC. *Dr. Atkins' nutrition breakthrough.* New York: Bantam Books, 1981.

45. Roubenoff R, Kehayias JJ. The meaning and measurement of lean body mass. *Nutr Rev* 1991; 49:163–75.

46. Committee on Dietary Allowances. *Food and Nutrition Board: recommended dietary allowances.* Washington, DC: National Academy Press, 1989.

47. Calloway DH. Nitrogen balance of men with marginal intakes of protein and energy. *J Nutr* 1975;105:914–23.

48. Gelfand RA, Hendler R. Effect of nutrient composition on the metabolic response to very low calorie diets: learning more and more about less and less. *Diabetes Metab Rev* 1989;5:17–30.

49. Weck M, Fischer S, Hanefeld M, et al. Loss of fat, water, and protein during very low calorie diets and complete starvation. *Klin Wochenschr* 1987;65: 1142–50.

50. Moore FC. Energy and the maintenance of the body cell mass. *J Parenter Enter Nutr* 1980;4:228–30.

51. Van Itallie TB, Yang MU. Current concepts in nutrition: diet and weight loss. *N Engl J Med* 1977;297:1158–60.

52. Van Itallie TB. Diets for weight reduction: mechanisms of action and physiological effects. In: Bray G, ed. *Obesity: comparative methods of weight control.* London: John Libbey, 1980;15–24.

53. Atkinson RL. Low and very low calorie diets. *Med Clin North Am* 1989;73:203–15.

54. Amatruda JM, Biddle TL, Patton ML, et al. Vigorous supplementation of a hypocaloric diet prevents cardiac arrhythmias and mineral depletion. *Am J Med* 1982;74:1016–22.

55. US House of Representatives, Committee on Small Business, Subcommittee on Regulation, Business Opportunities, and Energy. Deception and fraud in the diet industry, Parts I and II. Washington, DC: Government Printing Office, 1990; Serial no 101-50.

56. US House of Representatives, Committee on Small Business, Subcommittee on Regulation, Business Opportunities, and Energy. Juvenile dieting, unsafe over the counter diet products, and recent enforcement efforts by the Federal Trade Commission.

Washington, DC: US Government Printing Office, 1990; Serial no. 101-80.

57. Brownell KD. *The LEARN program for weight control.* Dallas: Brownell and Hager, 1990.

58. Brownell KD, Rodin J. *The weight maintenance survival guide.* Dallas: Brownell and Hager, 1991.

59. Learn Education Center. *Weight control digest.* Dallas: Learn Education Center, 1991.

60. Aronson V, and Jonas S. *The I don't eat a lot (but I can't lose weight) weight loss program.* New York: Rawson Press, 1989.

61. Committee on Diet and Health, Food and Nutrition Board, National Academy of Sciences. *Diet and health: recommendations to reduce chronic disease risk.* Washington, DC: National Academy Press, 1989.

62. US Department of Agriculture and US Department of Health and Human Services. *Dietary guidelines for americans,* 3rd ed. Washington, DC: US Government Printing Office, 1990.

63. Dwyer JT, St. Jeor SK. *The Optimal Diet.* New York: Brownell and Hager, 1992.

64. Gershoff S, Whitney C, Editorial Advisory Board of the Tufts University Diet and Nutrition Letter. *The Tufts University Guide to Total Nutrition.* New York: Harper and Row, 1991.

65. Mayer J, Goldberg JP. *Dr. Jean Mayer's diet and nutrition guide.* New York: Pharos Books, 1990.

66. Blackburn GL, Wilson GT, Kanders BS, et al. Weight cycling: the experience of human dieters. *Am J Clin Nutr* 1989;49:1105–9.

67. Foreyt JP, Goodrick GK. Factors common to successful therapy for the obese patient. *Med Sci Sports Exerc* 1991;23:292–7.

68. Foreyt JP. Issues in the assessment and treatment of obesity. *J Consult Clin Psychol* 1987;55:677–84.

69. Beck M, Springen K, Beachy L, Hager M, Buckley L. The losing formula. *Newsweek* 1990 Apr 30.

70. Bierman EL, Brownell KD, Dwyer JT, Horton ES, Pi-Sunyer FX, Sherger JE, eds. *Contemporary management of the overweight patient.* Little Falls, NJ: Health Learning Systems, 1991.

Obesity: Theory and Therapy, Second Edition,
edited by A. J. Stunkard and T. A. Wadden.
Raven Press, Ltd., New York © 1993.

15

The Metabolic and Psychological Importance of Exercise in Weight Control

*Carlos M. Grilo, *Kelly D. Brownell, and †Albert J. Stunkard

*Department of Psychology, Yale University, New Haven, Connecticut 06520; and
†Department of Psychiatry, University of Pennsylvania, Philadelphia, Pennsylvania
19104-2648

Obesity, the surplus of adipose tissue, results from excess energy intake relative to energy expenditure. Physical activity is a critical aspect of energy expenditure. It is not possible to understand many aspects of obesity without understanding the role played by physical activity. For example, despite stable caloric intake (1), the prevalence of obesity has increased during this century (2–4). Daily energy expenditure has decreased as society has progressed from agricultural to industrial to service to information-based economies, in part because fewer persons have jobs requiring strenuous physical exertion. Daily energy expenditure dropped an estimated 200 kcal/day from 1965 to 1977 (5). The Centers for Disease Control estimate that fewer than 20% of U.S. adults engage in vigorous and frequent physical activity, whereas roughly half of the adult population leads sedentary lives (6,7). Our current reliance on computers and widespread "convenience devices" (home shopping, garage door openers, etc.) appears to parallel the continued rise of obesity (2,4,8).

During this century, more has changed than physical activity. Despite lower caloric intake, the percentage of calories from fat has increased dramatically, and meal patterns have changed (fewer regular meals are consumed) (2). These factors undoubtedly contribute to the increased prevalence of obesity, but must be considered in concert with the significant decline in physical activity. Given the effects of exercise on metabolism, body composition, and psychological factors related to eating, it is not difficult to posit a causal relationship between inactivity and obesity.

ASSOCIATIONS BETWEEN PHYSICAL ACTIVITY AND OBESITY

The role of energy expenditure in the development of human obesity has been studied primarily by comparing the activity of obese and normal weight persons. Measurement of physical activity under daily living conditions is difficult. Researchers have employed a variety of methods including self-report (9), activity monitors (pedometer and actometer) (10), and time-lapse photography (11). Each of these methods is subject to problems (12,13).

Physical activity, in general, appears inversely related to body weight, body composition (14,15), and waist-to-hip ratio (16), although its relation to different degrees of obesity is less clear (17,18). The findings regarding the level of physical activity of obese persons are in serious conflict. Six studies on childhood obesity concluded that obese children are less active than nonobese children (11,19–23), while four others found no differences (24–27). Among adult males, nine studies found lower levels of activity among obese than among nonobese (9,10,28–34), while four found similar activity levels (18,35–37). Obese women were found to be less active than nonobese women in five studies (10,30,32,38,39) and equally active in five other studies (18,25,34,35,40). One study (41) found no differences between obese and nonobese persons in spontaneous physical activity (e.g., fidgeting) measured in a room by radar; such activity may account for as much as 9% of total energy expenditure (42).

Thus the findings regarding physical activity and obesity are equivocal. Roughly equal numbers of studies with both children and adults have reported significant and nonsignificant differences in activity levels between obese and nonobese persons. Even studies that have employed similar methods (e.g., activity monitors) have produced conflicting results (25,38).

Degree of obesity may account, in part, for these conflicting findings (13,18). Two studies that failed to observe differences in physical activity sampled "obese" subjects who were, on average, only 20% overweight (18,25) whereas two studies that observed lower activity levels among obese persons sampled clinically obese subjects (on average over 54% overweight) (10,38). Thus an inverse relationship between physical activity and obesity may be more salient among the highly obese, whereas the activity levels of mildly obese persons may be indistinguishable from that of the nonobese (13,18). Presently, it remains uncertain whether this decrement in physical activity may be gradual and linear as weight increases, or whether a substantial drop in activity occurs when a particular degree of obesity is reached (18).

Studies showing less activity in obese persons must be interpreted with caution not only because of methodological limitations (e.g., problems with definition and reliability of assessment of activity, different forms of activity) (12,14,17), but for conceptual reasons as well. First, it is possible that physical inactivity represents a consequence rather than a cause of obesity. Cross-sectional designs and comparisons of obese and nonobese persons preclude causal interpretation. A recent longitudinal study represents the first attempt to address this question of causality. Klesges and colleagues (17) found that lower levels of leisure and work activity predicted increases in body weight over time for women. Levels of leisure and work activity, however, were not consistent predictors of weight change over time for men. Interestingly, for both men and women, higher levels of sports activity were related to *higher* levels of weight gain over time. Further longitudinal research is needed to examine this issue, particularly with attention paid to resting energy expenditure, measurement of energy expenditure in different physical activities, and classification by degree of overweight. The flip side of this issue was partially addressed in a recent study that found no differences in physical activity between post-obese and naturally lean subjects as determined by diary recordings (37).

Lower levels of activity may not represent lower levels of energy expenditure, because of the greater caloric cost of activities for the obese person. No study of adults and only two studies of children (23,43) have converted measures of physical activity into measures of caloric expenditure. Waxman and Stunkard (23) did this in children by measuring oxygen consumption, and found that despite being less active than their nonobese male siblings, obese boys actually expended more calories through activity. This finding [replicated for girls (43)], coupled with other reports that many light activities have higher energy costs in obese compared with nonobese persons, questions whether the failure of most studies to adjust for body mass produces an overestimation of the association between physical activity level and obesity (13). However, because obese persons require more energy for a given activity as weight increases, and at a certain weight may actually burn more calories than a lean person who exercises far more, it is still possible, and even likely, that low levels of exercise contribute to the onset of obesity.

EXERCISE AND WEIGHT CONTROL

In the complex and often uncertain world of obesity research, one fact can be stated with authority: exercise is associated with weight loss. This association has been examined extensively with a variety of correlational (e.g., comparing maintainers with regainers) and experimental designs (e.g., group studies evaluating only exercise, single group studies with multiple intervention components including exercise, and controlled group studies comparing exercise with other interventions) (44,45).

Correlational studies consistently find that exercise is associated with successful weight loss and maintenance (46–50). Kayman and colleagues (49) compared obese women who regained lost weight to formerly obese women who were successful maintainers. Ninety percent of the successful maintainers exercised regularly (minimum of three times a week for more than 30 minutes) whereas only 34% of the weight regainers reported regular exercise.

Experimental studies with random assignment and control groups comparing exercise to no exercise provide the strongest evidence for the role of exercise in weight control. Many experimental studies (51–58) but not all (59–61) have found that exercise plus diet produces greater weight loss than just diet.

Although the magnitude of the effect of exercise on weight loss in such studies is generally modest, its prediction of weight loss maintenance is impressive. Exercise is one of the best predictors of maintenance (51,55,62, 63). Exercise enhances maintenance with both balanced diets (55,64) and very-low-calorie diets (55,56). Modest increases in lifestyle (e.g., using stairs instead of elevators and increased walking) to increase energy expenditure by as little as 200 to 400 calories/day results in improved maintenance in children (65–67).

An experimental study by Pavlou and colleagues (55) provides strong evidence for the importance of exercise regardless of diet intervention. Overweight subjects were assigned to one of four diets [balanced caloric-deficit diet of 1,000 kcal (BCDD), a protein-sparing modified fast (PSMF), and two liquid forms of these balanced and ketogenic diets (DPC-70 and DPC-800)] and to exercise and nonexercise groups for 12 weeks. Posttreatment and follow-up weight data obtained for 8 and 18 months are summarized in Fig. 1. The exercise group maintained weight loss at an 18-month follow-up regardless of diet, whereas those who did not exercise showed no difference in weight between pretreatment and the 18-month follow-up. Pavlou and colleagues also extended existing knowledge by showing that the addition or cessation of exercise after treatment predicts weight loss at follow-up. As shown in Fig. 2, subjects who ceased exercise at the end of treatment regained weight, whereas those who began exercise at the end of treatment maintained weight loss at the 18-month follow-up.

MECHANISMS LINKING EXERCISE AND WEIGHT CONTROL

Exercise produces a complex series of metabolic and psychological consequences. Exercise can alter body weight, body composition, appetite, and basal metabolism, and can effect health, independent of weight loss. Perhaps most important, exercise can enhance psychological well-being, improve self-esteem, and maintain motivation. Therefore, there are multiple pathways by which exercise may aid in weight control (Table 1).

Exercise, Body Weight, and Body Composition

Exercise Expends Energy

Exercise expends energy [see McArdle and colleagues (68) for caloric expenditure of physical activities]. Many persons are surprised, if not discouraged, however, when learning that even the most rigorous physical activities produce relatively small energy defi-

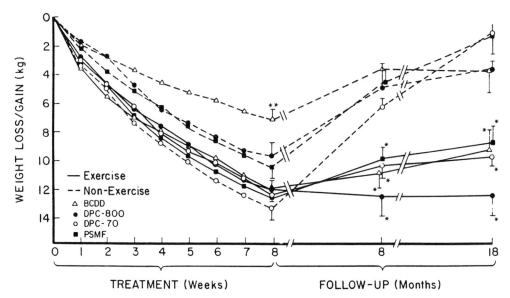

FIG. 1. Eighteen-month follow-up data of the main study confirms the long-term effectiveness of exercise intervention for as short a period as 8 weeks. There is no difference between initial and 18-month follow-up weight for those who did not exercise, regardless of diet used for weight loss. In contrast, the exercise group maintained weight lost. *, $p < 0.001$ vs. nonexercise; **, $p < 0.01$ vs. all exercise and ○ group. BCDD, balanced calorie-deficit diet; PSMF, protein-sparing modified fast. (From ref. 55, with permission.)

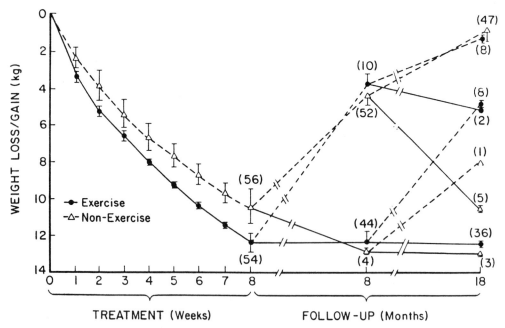

FIG. 2. The addition or removal of learned exercise would appear to be a major contributing factor relative to weight maintenance. Subjects who ceased exercise regained or demonstrated a strong tendency to return to prestudy weights. Poststudy introduction of exercise (learned but nonsupervised) creates a positive effect. $\bar{x} \pm$ SEM; number of subjects given in parentheses. (From ref. 55, with permission.)

TABLE 1. *Likely mechanisms linking exercise with success at weight control*

1. Energy expenditure
2. Minimization of lean body mass loss
3. Appetite suppression
4. Increased metabolic rate
5. Diminished dietary fat preferences
6. Improvement of risk factors associated with obesity
7. Positive psychological effects

cits. Björntorp (69) has reported that the Vasaloppet, a grueling 49-mile cross-country ski race in Sweden that lasts approximately 10 hours, requires the energy equivalent of only 2 lb of adipose tissue. Nevertheless, even though the immediate effects are limited, the cumulative effect of small changes in physical activity may have beneficial consequences over the long term. For example, walking up and down two flights of stairs a day, in lieu of using an elevator, would account for approximately 6 lb of weight loss per year for an average weight (176-lb) man (29).

Weight loss through exercise is generally greater than would be expected through the direct expenditure of energy (70). This suggests that physical activity influences physiological and psychological processes that in turn influence body weight. Body composition, appetite, and basal metabolism are three likely processes.

Exercise May Minimize the Loss of Lean Body Mass

Weight loss due to dieting results in loss of both lean and fat body mass. Exercise has variable effects on body weight and body composition (the ratio of lean to fat tissue) (71–73). Physical training usually increases the lean to fat ratio, but since lean tissue is more dense than the fat it replaces, body weight may not change (68). The often observed slowing of the rate of weight loss over time (68) is dependent on the amount of weight loss, in general, and on the amount of lean tissue loss, in particular (72). Recent studies have found that regular aerobic exercise, even in the absence of dietary restriction, can produce significant body fat loss and slow the loss of lean tissue (74–76).

Resistance forms of weight training added to caloric restriction result in greater maintenance of lean tissue compared with diet without exercise (77). The use of resistance training to improve lean to fat tissue ratio may have the added benefit of increasing energy expenditure through increased resting metabolic rate (see below) (78). These findings, however, are not unequivocal; several studies have failed to observe this protective role of exercise (79–81). One study found that resistance training exercise plus a 1,200 kcal diet did not result in greater changes in body mass, fat mass, or fat-free mass than did low-intensity exercise plus a 1,200 kcal diet (82). Thus the apparent benefits of exercise in limiting the loss of lean tissue may be in comparison to lack of exercise.

Exercise May Maintain or Suppress Appetite

A common misconception is that exercise has limited value for weight reduction because increased energy expenditure is offset by a corresponding increase in appetite. This is generally incorrect, although the effects of activity on intake are complex and depend on a number of factors including the type of exercise, sex and age effects, and level and type of obesity.

Mayer and colleagues (83,84) first studied the relationship between activity and appetite in animals. Although food intake of normal weight rats increased with increasing energy expenditure over a wide range of energy demands, intake did not decrease proportionally when physical activity fell below a minimum level. These initial results have been replicated many times (85–95).

The intensity of the physical activity influences the regulatory effect on appetite and food intake (96). Increasing activity in the sedentary range decreases food intake and body weight, whereas increasing activity in the more active range leads to increased food intake and stable body weight (68). Although fewer studies of the regulatory effect of food intake have been done on humans, available findings are consistent with those of the animal literature. Studies have found decreased food intake and body weight following increased activity in the low to moderate range and increased food intake and stable body weight in the vigorous range (45,97–100).

The relationships between physical activity, weight, and food intake are also affected by sex. A number of animal studies have shown that activity decreases food intake in males (86,89,92,94,101–103) but not in females (89,101,103,104) although one study found a decrease in female rats (83). Human studies have found no compensatory increase in energy intake among males (97) but significant increases among females (97,100,105) following increased physical activity. However, three studies found increased food intake in male rats after the termination of exercise (106–108).

These apparent sex differences in the food-intake response to exercise appear more troublesome to normal-weight women than obese women. A series of studies found that whereas lean women maintain their weight and body composition by adjusting food intake commensurate with exercise level, obese women do not appear to adjust food intake (109). Thus exercise in obese women may create a negative energy balance, since no compensatory food increase occurs.

In summary, exercise is unlikely to increase appetite beyond the level needed to keep body weight stable, and in many cases may lead to decreased intake, although this is less clear for women than for men. The danger lies in people *believing* that they will be hungrier after they exercise. Scheduling exercise when people are prone to eat may be particularly helpful.

Exercise May Counter the Metabolic Decline Produced by Dieting

Decreased caloric intake produces a decline in resting metabolic rate (RMR) (68,70,110–115). This decline begins within 24 to 48 hours after caloric restriction begins and can exceed 20% in as little as 2 weeks (70). The decline in RMR associated with caloric restriction is generally 20 to 30% in both obese and lean persons (70). Since RMR is responsible for 60 to 70% of total energy expenditure (70,116–118), this decline may exert a strong influence on body weight (2). Decreased caloric intake also produces alterations in body mass and composition (119) that may also contribute to increased food efficiency (120).

Thus dietary restriction and weight reduction create adaptive changes in energy expenditure that can be a barrier to further weight reduction. Decreased metabolic rate and increased energy efficiency are the important effects. Exercise may help counteract the decrease in metabolic rate (68,121,122). Moderate exercise is associated with elevated RMR across different training levels and weight categories (123,124). RMR is significantly higher among exercise-trained individuals than nontrained individuals (122). Significant increases in RMR can be achieved in obese persons through regular exercise. An 11-week training program involving 5 hours of aerobic exercise a week performed at 50% VO_2 max resulted in a significant increase in RMR (8% of pretraining value) despite significant reductions in body weight and body fat mass (see Fig. 3) (122).

Exercise May Alter Increased Dietary Fat Preference Produced by Weight Cycling

A single bout of caloric restriction and refeeding increases food efficiency in animals (125,126). It is also possible that with successive episodes of caloric restriction, metabolic rate falls more rapidly with each episode, and that the return to baseline levels takes longer each time the restriction ends. Recent research has begun to address the metabolic (127) and health (128,129) consequences of repeated episodes of weight loss followed by weight regain (i.e., weight cycling), which is commonplace among dieters (130) and almost universal for certain populations such as wrestlers (131). While findings regarding the negative effects of weight cycling on

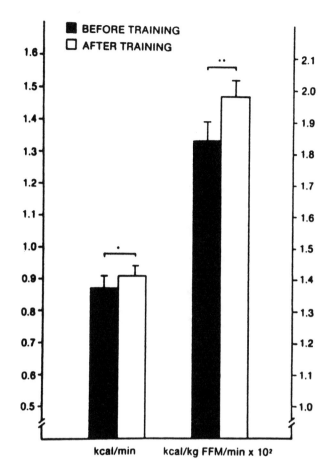

FIG. 3. The influence of exercise training. Resting metabolic rate in moderately obese women before and after an 11-week training program. Mean ± SEM. *, p = 0.05; **, p = 0.01. FFM, fat-free mass. (From ref. 122, with permission.)

health appear robust (128,129,132), the effects on efficiency of energy utilization remain uncertain. Several studies with rats (127,133–137) and humans (138–140) have found increased food efficiency following weight cycles, but other studies in rats (134,135,141–146) and humans (58,147, 148) have not. Accumulating evidence, however, does point to higher consumption of dietary fat in rats following weight cycles (137,149). Reed and colleagues (137) found that female rats with three cycles of restriction and refeeding consumed a significantly greater percentage of calories as fat than did non-weight-cycled controls. This increased fat consumption was also accompanied by larger adipose tissue depots in the weight-cycled rats.

Thus weight cycling may decrease metabolic rate and increase energy efficiency and dietary fat selection. Exercise may help coun-

teract these metabolic effects (58,113,120, 149). The addition of exercise to diet results in a significantly smaller decline in RMR among weight-cycled women (58). The addition of exercise to diet significantly increases weight loss and body fat loss in both weight-cycled and non-weight-cycled obese females (58). Gerardo-Gettens and colleagues (149) found that exercise prevents increased dietary fat selection in weight-cycled female rats and reduces the amount of body fat regained during refeeding periods.

Exercise May Improve Health

Exercise may benefit obese persons by producing positive effects on blood pressure, blood lipid levels, plasma insulin levels, and cardiorespiratory function (150–155). Exercise can provide these benefits independently of weight loss (151,155–157). Moreover, improvements in health and disease prevention can be accomplished with modest levels of activity (152,158–162).

In a prospective study of physical fitness and mortality with over 13,000 individuals, Blair and colleagues (158) found significantly lower mortality rates in more physically fit individuals. Individuals were given medical examinations and maximal treadmill exercise tests to determine physical fitness and then categorized into five fitness levels ranging from very unfit (level I) to very fit (level I to V). Subjects were then followed for 5 years. Results showed a strong inverse relationship between physical fitness and mortality for men and women even after statistical adjustment for age and other risk factors such as smoking, cholesterol level, systolic blood pressure, fasting blood glucose level, and parental level of heart disease (158). Equally important was the finding that modest levels of fitness are associated with substantially reduced mortality risk. Figure 4 represents a graphic summary of these findings provided by Brownell (163). This figure shows health risk ratio by fitness level separately for males and females. Risk ratio was determined by giving the most fit group (level 5) a value of 1 and determining mortality risk for the four other fitness categories in reference to that number. The greatest decline in mortality risk occurs for both men and women by moving from the lowest level of fitness (level 1) to the second level of fitness (level 2) (158,163). For instance, men in the lowest level of fitness have a risk ratio of 3.44 compared with 1.37 for men in level 2. A shift from level 1 to level 2 results in a substantial reduction in mortality risk among men. Thus a modest increase in fitness has great health benefits. Figure 4 shows that further increases in fitness are associated with continued but less impressive reductions in mortality risk.

Exercise May Have Positive Psychological Effects

Physical activity is associated with a number of positive psychological changes (164).

We have a strong clinical impression that collectively these psychological effects serve to enhance self-esteem, self-efficacy (165), and a general sense of well-being. These in turn appear to lead to better dietary adherence. Although this topic has received less attention than the possible physiological mechanisms linking exercise to weight control, we believe that the psychological effects may be *the* most important mechanism. Hence we will review the literature on this topic in some detail.

Exercise and Psychological Functioning

Reviews conclude consistently that physical fitness and mental health are positively associated—higher levels of physical fitness predict more positive mental health (166–170; see refs. 171,172 for problems of overuse and abuse of exercise). Reviews have also concluded that exercise improves mood and psychological well-being and enhances self-concept and self-esteem (164,173). Exercise is associated with reduced stress, anxiety (164,168), and depression (164,168,174) and improved self-esteem and self-concept (164,167,170). Similar conclusions were offered by an NIMH Consensus Panel in 1987 (175). Although the question of causality remains uncertain and merits careful experimental attention, these findings suggest that exercise is associated with positive improvements in psychological functioning.

Level of Intensity

Studies have reported that low-level and moderate-level physical activity can have both short-term and sustained effects on psychological well-being and mood (151,164, 173,176). A recent review of methodologically strong studies since 1980 (excluding treatment studies) concluded that four of the six experimental studies that employed random assignment to exercise found that moderate exercise improved psychological well-being and mood (164). High-intensity exercise, however, can increase tension, anxiety, and fatigue in some individuals (177).

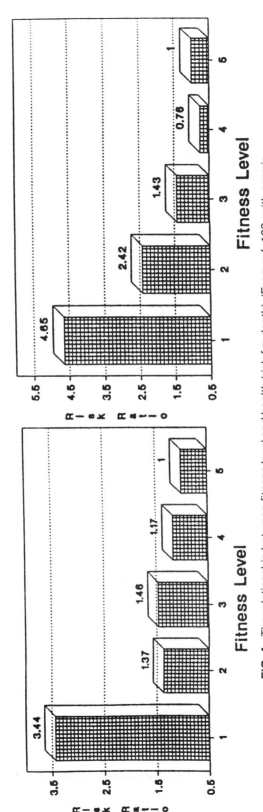

FIG. 4. The relationship between fitness level and health (risk for death). (From ref. 163, with permission, based on findings from ref. 158.)

EXERCISE ADHERENCE

Adherence to exercise is a major challenge (151,178,179). Regardless of potential benefits, an exercise program is useful only to the extent it is followed. Dishman (180) reports that the typical dropout rate from supervised exercise programs worldwide has remained at roughly 50% during the past 20 years. Not surprisingly, exercise adherence among the obese is poor. Gwinup (181) found that 68% of obese women dropped out of a 1-year program requiring walking. On a more positive note, exercise adherence may be enhanced in several ways. Brief discussions of adherence, issues specific to working with overweight persons, and program development follow.

Exercise Adherence

Most research on exercise adherence focuses on individual strategies based on social-learning and behavioral approaches (179). Useful information on adherence is now available not only from clinical studies, but from community interventions with large populations (182). Most of the work has not focused on obese persons, but the results provide a general framework from which a program for the overweight individual can be formed.

Behavioral Approaches

A variety of behavioral approaches have been found to increase adherence both individually as well as when part of a larger intervention. These include behavior contracts (183–185), contingency reinforcement (186), incentives (185), and cognitive-behavioral interventions such as self-monitoring, goal-setting, and detailed feedback (187). Dishman (179) concludes that cognitive-behavioral interventions are associated with 10 to 25% increases in the frequency of physical activity when compared with control approaches. The impact of these interventions on duration and intensity of physical activity, however, is less clear (179).

Unfortunately, increased physical activity associated with behavioral interventions may not endure after the intervention ends (151,178,179). A promising avenue to maintain exercise adherence is the incorporation of relapse prevention strategies (188,189). Cognitive behavioral programs for exercise adherence that have incorporated components of Marlatt and Gordon's (189) relapse prevention model result in superior physical activity rates at follow-up (187,190–193). Flexible exercise goals are associated with less drop-out and greater adherence than are rigid exercise goals (187). Training individuals in specific techniques to cope with missed exercise sessions predicts superior exercise adherence posttreatment (192). Studies have found that minimal intervention strategies such as monthly mailings and telephone contacts can also enhance long-term exercise adherence and predict maintenance of weight loss (194,195). Minimal intervention strategies may be more effective in maintaining exercise than diet following treatment (194). A recent study, however, found that therapist-supported relapse prevention is superior to minimal posttreatment interventions (190). Careful supervision of exercise during treatment is needed for continued success following treatment (55,196).

Large-Scale Community Interventions

One study found that the placement of a sign encouraging stair use at the base of escalators was associated with a dramatic increase in the use of stairs in both obese and nonobese persons (29). A recent research development is the use of large-scale community interventions to increase health behavior compliance (182,197). Public health approaches, which focus on larger segments of the population, in contrast to clinical and high-risk interventions, represent promising avenues for increasing exercise and other health-related behaviors (182).

King, in a review of comprehensive, integrated, community-based interventions for promoting physical activity, concluded that these are feasible, acceptable to communities, and potentially effective (182). Positive and sustained changes in physical activity have been observed in several ongoing multi-community risk reduction studies in the United States (182). The findings of one community project are particularly relevant for our discussion. The Community Health Assessment and Promotion Project (198) attempted to modify health behaviors relevant to obesity in roughly 400 individuals (predominately black women). The program emphasized the cultural and practical needs of this population (safety, privacy, free transportation, child-care) and focused on nutrition and exercise information and the importance of moderate-intensity activity (e.g., walking, low-impact aerobics). Significant weight losses and improvements in health such as reductions in blood pressure were observed. Client participation at 4 months remained over 60%. This program demonstrated the promise of large-scale community interventions that consider the needs and characteristics of the target population and remove barriers in a sensitive manner.

Community worksite interventions have also produced positive social influences on exercise (185,199,200), and weight loss (201). Worksite competitions can produce significant weight losses, particularly among men (202). A study by King and colleagues (203) further underscores the importance of considering the characteristics of the target population. This study targeted blue-collar employees, who are less likely to participate in worksite physical activity programs than white-collar employees (182). The project began with an assessment of the physical activity history, needs, and preferences of the blue-collar employees, provided a nearby exercise area, and integrated motivational and competition elements. Exercise participation increased substantially, fitness levels improved, and weight losses occurred (203).

Social Support

Social support from family, friends, and others plays an important role in the health of the individual (204). Adherence to exercise programs, like other health-related behaviors, is influenced by social context. These factors are potentially powerful and have been the focus of increased attention.

Exercise adherence similarly appears responsive to social influence, although this has received less attention than dietary adherence (205,206). Reviews report that spouse support is associated with increased exercise compliance (207,208). King and Frederiksen (192) found that subjects assigned to exercise with comembers exercised more than subjects instructed to exercise alone at posttreatment but not at follow-up. Males' adherence to exercise may be related to their spouses' attitudes. One study found that 80% of men whose wives were positive toward their exercise had good adherence versus 20% of men whose wives had either neutral or negative attitudes (209). Positive spouse participation is associated with increased compliance to exercise programs in cardiac rehabilitation (210).

Further research is needed to examine the factors that mediate success or failure with spouse, family, or peer interventions. In addition, examining these issues applied to exercise in obese persons will be important. Specific guidelines for structuring the social interactions of significant others to aid in the attainment of physical activity goals are available from several sources (163,211). This may be important, given findings regarding potential negative effects of social relationships such as undermining. Determination of who is likely to benefit from specific social support techniques relevant to exercise initiation and adherence is important (211).

Sensitivity to the Needs of Overweight Persons

Careful attention to potential physical and psychological barriers to exercise among overweight persons appears critical (212). Table 2 summarizes barriers to exercise. Failure to attend to these barriers may exacerbate the adherence problem. Careful assessment and creative problem-solving may enhance adherence.

TABLE 2. *Psychological and physical barriers to exercise in obese persons*

Psychological barriers
  Previous negative experiences
    Teased by peers
    Poor performance
    Picked last for teams
    Feeling inadequate
  Lack of confidence
  Lack of knowledge or experience
  Shame of being observed
Physical barriers
  Burden of excess weight
  Low level of fitness

Physical Burden

Excess weight itself represents a hurdle that must be overcome. Increased activity for an obese person may be difficult, tiring, and painful. Care should be taken to set reasonable goals and develop healthy expectations. It must be understood that high levels of activity may not be attainable immediately, nor should this be the goal. Because high-intensity exercise can increase tension, anxiety, and fatigue, excessive activity is likely to deter subsequent efforts. Both men and women are more likely to adopt a moderate-intensity program than they are to adopt a high-intensity one (213,214). Changes in life style activity predict better long-term weight losses than more strenuous activity among obese children (65,67). Moreover, the dropout rate for vigorous programs can be as much as twice that for moderate-intensity programs (213). It is important therefore, for the overweight person to select the type and amount of exercise that is both feasible and enjoyable.

Previous Learning

Negative associations that plague obese persons, particularly those who have been overweight since childhood, represent another hurdle. The social cost of obesity is well documented (215–217). Early negative experiences with peers and others (e.g., being teased, being picked last for teams) leave many obese persons self-conscious and embarrassed about their bodies (218,219). These negative experiences create an atmosphere in which thoughts of exercise evoke unpleasant memories, feelings of incompetence, and shame at the prospect of being observed. Indeed, overweight persons are less likely to adopt exercise programs than are nonobese persons (213). Support is important so that people undertake exercise in a way that enhances self-efficacy (165) before the psychological and physical barriers become insurmountable.

Developmental Issues

Exercise initiation and adherence may also be enhanced by addressing developmental issues (182). Our discussion has emphasized the importance of tailoring interventions to the characteristics of the target population. Consideration of life periods, transitions, and developmental milestones that present specific needs and barriers to physical activity may lead to more effective interventions. A young single male executive will have different developmental and practical issues than a single working mother with three children. Table 3 presents features and examples of physical activity programs for several important periods proposed by King (182).

Program Recommendations

The three basic issues confronting the clinician are the type of exercise to prescribe, ways to maximize adherence, and relapse prevention. Table 4 outlines a program for the obese patient. Important components are discussed below.

Avoid an Exercise Threshold

The three-part cardiorespiratory equation involving frequency, intensity, and duration (68) is a common answer to the frequently asked question, "How much exercise?" A typ-

TABLE 3. *Features and examples of physical activity programs for several major developmental milestones*

Milestone (critical period)	Specific features	Goals/strategies
Adolescence	Rapid physical and emotional changes	Exercise as part of a program of healthy weight regulation (both sexes)
	Increased concern with appearance and weight	Noncompetitive activities that are fun, varied
	Need for independence	Emphasis on independence, choice
	Short-term perspective	Focus on proximal outcomes (e.g., body image, stress management)
	Increased peer influence	Peer involvement, support
Initial work entry	Increased time and scheduling constraints	Choice of activities that are convenient, enjoyable
	Short-term perspective	Focus on proximal outcomes
	Employer demands	Involvement of worksite (environmental prompts, incentives)
		Realistic goal-setting/injury prevention
		Coeducational noncompetitive activities
Parenting	Increased family demands and time constraints	Emphasis on benefits to self and family (e.g., stress management, weight control, well-being)
	Family-directed focus	Activities appropriate with children (e.g., walking)
	Postpartum effects on weight, mood	Flexible, convenient, personalized regimen
		Inclusion of activities of daily living
		Neighborhood involvement, focus
		Family-based public monitoring, goal-setting
		Availability of child-related services (child care)
Retirement age	Increased time availability and flexibility	Identification of current and previous enjoyable activities
	Longer term perspective on health; increased health concerns, "readiness"	Matching of activities to current health status
		Emphasis on mild- and moderate-intensity activities, including activities of daily living
		Use of "life path point" information and prompts
	Caregiving duties, responsibilities (parents, spouse, children or grandchildren)	Emphasis on activities engendering independence
		Garnering support of family members, peers
		Availability of necessary services (e.g., caretaking services for significant other)

(From ref. 182, with permission.)

ical exercise prescription is that exercise must be performed 3 times a week at 70% maximum heart rate for a minimum of 15 minutes. This equation follows extensive exercise physiology research (168) showing that such exercise is required to improve cardiorespiratory conditioning. We suggest that this is *not* the primary goal for obese persons.

The exercise equation implies an "exercise threshold," i.e., for exercise to be beneficial, it must be performed at specific levels for specific lengths of time. This equation may produce an "all-or-none" effect (e.g., "I've exercised enough to do me some good" or "That effort fell short so why exercise at all?"). The threshold may motivate physically fit persons, but may deter others.

We recommend that professionals avoid the use of the traditional exercise equation and any prescription that implies a threshold.

This recommendation is based on three assumptions: (a) even modest exercise can produce impressive health benefits (158–160,162); (b) psychological benefits can occur even at low levels of activity (164); and (c) a regimen of moderate exercise will enhance self-efficacy and in turn, improve adherence (173,183).

We would like to draw special attention to the psychological benefits of moderate activity. Each attempt at increased physical activity, no matter how trivial from a physiological perspective, represents a positive achievement. For example, parking an extra distance from the entrance to a mall is a symbolic gesture showing accomplishment, positive change, and commitment. Each bout of activity represents a positive experience that can buffer the dieter against the stresses of dietary change. This psychological benefit

TABLE 4. *Recommendations for maximizing exercise adherence in obese persons*

General principles
Be sensitive to psychological barriers
Be sensitive to physical barriers
Decrease focus on exercise threshold
Increase focus on enhanced self-efficacy
Emphasize consistency and enjoyment, not amount and type
Begin at person's level of fitness
Encourage person to define routine activities as "exercise"
Focus on compliance and avoid emphasis of minor metabolic issues (e.g., whether to exercise before or after a meal)
Consider life-span developmental context
Consider sociocultural issues
Evaluate social support network

Specific interventions
Prescription
Provide clear information about importance of activity, including the psychological benefits
Maximize routine activity; daily activities are exercise
Maximize walking (e.g., park a greater distance from work)
Increase use of stairs in lieu of escalators
Incorporate a programmed activity that is enjoyable, fits with lifestyle, and is feasible as client's fitness improves
Behavioral
Introduce self-monitoring, feedback, and goal-setting techniques
Identify important targets other than weight loss, including physical changes, increased endurance, lowered resting heart rate
Use physical activity when tempted to overeat or when distressed
Stimulus control: increase exercise cues (e.g., reminders for increasing activity) and decrease competing cues (e.g., do not schedule exercise when it might conflict with work or social obligations)
Maintenance and relapse prevention
Use flexible guidelines and goal-setting, but avoid rigid rules
Identify potential high-risk situations for skipping exercise (e.g., stressful times, busy schedule)
Develop plans to cope with high-risk situations
Use exercise following dietary lapses to counteract caloric effects physically and, more importantly, to regain psychologically a sense of control, mastery, and commitment
Convey philosophy that one day lapsed does not a failure make
Use of minimal intervention strategies including phone contacts may foster exercise maintenance

can ultimately be more important that the physical effects of exercise.

Other psychological benefits are also likely. Modest activity can be gradually increased, which can sustain motivation and increase self-esteem. Self-monitoring of activity is helpful in providing reinforcement, because it is a tangible record of accomplishments. This type of feedback may be especially valuable for the obese person. Records of exercise and improvements in physiological measures (e.g., resting heart rate, blood pressure, endurance) that are responsive to exercise can be useful nonweight indicators of progress.

Exercise may also decrease stress and anxiety, which represent common overeating situations for dieters (220). Exercise can also be employed as a coping strategy to overcome difficult or tempting dietary situations (221). For instance, walking when tempted to overeat or when emotionally distressed may be a powerful strategy. In addition to coping with a specific challenge, action may enhance self-efficacy (165). This may generalize to continued success in overcoming such difficult situations.

Consistency May Be More Important than the Type or Amount of Exercise

Using traditional approaches to exercise, much attention is given to prescribing specific types and amounts of exercise. It is our belief that the fundamental question is not "What is the best type of exercise," but "What will the individual be doing a year from now?" Therefore, developing a *consistent* form of activity, or a consistent group of activities, is the primary focus. It is preferable for a person to regularly play golf twice a week and walk for 1 additional day, than to run 5 miles a day for a week and then stop entirely.

Provide Thorough Education

It is important to emphasize the importance of exercise for weight control. The professional can describe the physical and psychological benefits of exercise and dispel erroneous notions such as "no pain, no gain." Poor health behaviors can reflect lack of knowledge as well as nonadherence.

SUMMARY

Obesity is a significant health problem in our society. Exercise is an important predictor of weight loss maintenance, so increased physical activity represents a key intervention for the treatment of obesity. Activity may facilitate weight reduction through direct energy expenditure, but changes in body weight cannot be explained solely by increased caloric expenditure due to exercise. Exercise may promote weight loss through several possible physiological and psychological mechanisms, including decreased appetite, basal metabolic changes, increased lean body mass, and enhanced medical and psychological well-being. Exercise may promote long-term weight maintenance, which remains the dieter's greatest challenge (222). Exercise adherence, which represents a major challenge, is threatened by the special physical and psychological burdens of obesity. Based on this review and our clinical experience with obese persons, we offer a number of recommendations for the development, prescription, and maintenance of exercise programs for the obese client. Focus on life style change and consistency may represent the best treatment philosophy.

REFERENCES

1. Marston R, Raper N. Nutrient content of the U.S. food supply. *Natl Food Rev* 1987;36:1392–8.
2. Brownell KD, Wadden TA. The heterogeneity of obesity: fitting treatments to individuals. *Behav Ther* 1991;22:153–77.
3. Brownell KD, Wadden TA. Etiology and treatment of obesity: towards understanding a serious, prevalent, and refractory disorder. *J Consult Clin Psychol* [*in press*].
4. VanItallie TB. Health implications of overweight and obesity in the United States. *Ann Intern Med* 1985;103:983–8.
5. US Department of Agriculture, Consumer Nutrition Division, Human Nutrition Information Service. Nationwide food consumption survey. Nutrient intakes, individuals in 48 years, year 1977–1978. Hyattsville, MD: US Department of Agriculture, 1984; Report no I-2.
6. Centers For Disease Control. Sex-, age-, and region-specific prevalence for sedentary lifestyle in selected states in 1985—the behavioral risk factor surveillance system. *MMWR* 1987;36:195–204.
7. Centers for Disease Control. CDC surveillance summaries. *MMWR* 1990;39[SS-2]:8.
8. Stephens T. Secular trends in adult physical activity: exercise boom or bust? *Res Q Exerc Sport* 1987;58:94–105.
9. Mayer J, Roy P, Mitra KP. Relation between caloric intake, body weight, and physical work: studies in an industrial male population in West Bengal. *Am J Clin Nutr* 1956;4:169–75.
10. Chirico A, Stunkard AJ. Physical activity and human obesity. *N Engl J Med* 1960;263:935–40.
11. Bullen BA, Reed RB, Mayer J. Physical activity of obese and non-obese adolescent girls appraised by motion picture sampling. *Am J Clin Nutr* 1974;14:211–33.
12. LaPorte RE, Montoye HJ, Caspersen CJ. Assessment of physical activity in epidemiologic research: problems and prospects. *Public Health Rep* 1985;100:131–46.
13. Shah M, Jeffery RW. Is obesity due to overeating and inactivity, or to a defective metabolic rate? A review. *Ann Behav Med* 1991;13:73–81.
14. Klesges RC, Eck LH, Isbell TR, Fulliton W, Hanson CL. Physical activity, body composition, and blood pressure: a multimethod approach. *Med Sci Sports Exerc* 1991;23:759–65.
15. Strazzulo P, Cappuccio FP, Trevisan M, et al. Leisure time physical activity and blood pressure in schoolchildren. *Am J Epidemiol* 1988;127:726–33.
16. Laws A, Terry RB, Barrett-Connor E. Behavioral covariates of waist-to-hip ratio in Rancho Bernardo. *Am J Public Health* 1990;80:1358–62.
17. Klesges RC, Klesges LM, Haddock CK, Eck LH. A longitudinal analysis of the impact of dietary intake and physical activity on weight change in adults. *Am J Clin Nutr* 1992;55:818–22.
18. Tyron WW. Activity as a function of body weight. *Am J Clin Nutr* 1987;46:451–5.
19. Dietz WH, Gortmaker SL. Do we fatten our children at the television set? Obesity and television viewing in children and adolescents. *Pediatrics* 1985;75:807–12.
20. Johnson ML, Burke MS, Mayer J. Relative importance of inactivity and overeating in the energy balance of obese high school girls. *Am J Clin Nutr* 1956;4:37–44.
21. Rose HE, Mayer J. Activity, caloric intake, and the energy balance of infants. *Pediatrics* 1968; 41:18–29.
22. Stefanick AS, Heald FP, Mayer J. Caloric intake in relation to energy output of obese and non obese adolescent schoolboys. *Am J Clin Nutr* 1959; 7:55–62.
23. Waxman M, Stunkard AJ. Caloric intake and expenditure of obese boys. *J Pediatr* 1980;96:187–93.
24. Bradfield RB, Paulos J, Grossman L. Energy expenditure and heart rate of obese high school girls. *Am J Clin Nutr* 1971;24:1482–8.
25. Maxfield E, Konishi F. Patterns of food intake and physical activity in obesity. *J Am Diet Assoc* 1966;49:406–8.
26. Stunkard AJ, Pestka J. The physical activity of obese girls. *Am J Dis Child* 1962;103:812–7.
27. Wilkinson PW, Parkin JM, Pearlson G, Strong H, Sykes P. Energy intake and physical activity in obese children. *Br Med J* 1977;1:756(abst).

28. Bloom WL, Eidex MF. Inactivity as a major factor in adult obesity. *Metabolism* 1967;16:679–84.

29. Brownell KD, Stunkard AJ, Albaum JM. Evaluation and modification of exercise patterns in the natural environment. *Am J Psychiatry* 1980; 137:1540–5.

30. Forman MR, Trowbridge FL, Gentry EM, Mark JS, Hogelin GC. Overweight adults in the United States: the behavior risk factor surveys. *Am J Clin Nutr* 1986;44:410–6.

31. Hickey N, Mulcahy R, Bourke GJ, Graham I, Wilson-Davies K. Study of coronary risk factors related to physical activity in 15,171 men. *Br Med J* 1975;3:507–9.

32. Hutson EM, Cohen NL, Kunkel ND, Steinkamp RC, Rouke MH, Walsh HE. Measures of body fat and related factors in normal adults. *J Am Diet Assoc* 1965;47:179–86.

33. Meyers AW, Stunkard AJ, Coll M, Cooke CJ. Stairs, escalators, and obesity. *Behav Modif* 1980;4:355–9.

34. Shah M, Jeffery RW, Hannan PJ, Onstad L. The relationship between sociodemographic and behavior variables and body mass index in a population with high-normal blood pressure: hypertension prevention trial. *Eur J Clin Nutr* 1989;43:583–96.

35. Baecke JAH, van Staveren WA, Burema J. Food consumption, habitual physical activity, and body fatness in young Dutch adults. *Am J Clin Nutr* 1983;37:278–86.

36. Lincoln JE. Calorie intake, obesity, and physical activity. *Am J Clin Nutr* 1972;25:350–4.

37. Tremblay A, Sauve L, Despres J-P, et al. Metabolic characteristics of post-obese individuals. *Int J Obes* 1989;13:357–66.

38. Doris RJ, Stunkard AJ. Physical activity: performance and attitudes of a group of obese women. *Am J Med Sci* 1957;223:622–8.

39. Romieu I, Willet WC, Stampfer MJ, et al. Energy intake and other determinants of relative weight. *Am J Clin Nutr* 1988;47:406–12.

40. McCarthy MC. Dietary and activity patterns of obese women in Trinidad. *J Am Diet Assoc* 1966;48:33–7.

41. Schutz Y, Ravussin E, Diethelm R, Jequier E. Spontaneous physical activity measured by radar in obese and control subjects studied in a respiration chamber. *Int J Obes* 1982;6:23–8.

42. Ravussin E, Lillioja S, Anderson TE, Christin L, Bogardus C. Determinants of a 24-hour energy expenditure in man. Methods and results using a respirometry chamber. *J Clin Invest* 1986;78: 1568–78.

43. Waxman M. *Fat families and thick descriptions: a naturalistic study of obese girls and their nonobese sisters* [Dissertation]. University of Pennsylvania, 1988 (reference no L0011988B655).

44. Epstein LH, Wing RR. Aerobic exercise and weight. *Addict Behav* 1980;5:371–88.

45. Thompson JK, Jarvie GJ, Lahey BB, Cureton KJ. Exercise and obesity: etiology, physiology, and intervention. *Psychol Bull* 1982;91:55–79.

46. Colvin RH, Olson SB. A descriptive analysis of men and women who have lost significant weight and are highly successful at maintaining the loss. *Addict Behav* 1983;8:287–95.

47. Gormally J, Rardin D. Weight loss and maintenance changes in diet and exercise for behavioral counseling and nutrition education. *J Consult Clin Psychol* 1981;28:295–304.

48. Gormally J, Rardin D, Black S. Correlates of successful response to a behavioral weight control clinic. *J Counseling Psychol* 1980;27:179–91.

49. Kayman S, Bruvold W, Stern JS. Maintenance and relapse after weight loss in women: behavioral aspects. *Am J Clin Nutr* 1990;52:800–7.

50. Marston AR, Criss J. Maintenance of successful weight loss: incidence and prediction. *Int J Obes* 1984;8:435–9.

51. Dahlkoetter J, Callahan EJ, Linton J. Obesity and the unbalanced energy equation: exercise vs. eating habit change. *J Consult Clin Psychol* 1979; 47:898–905.

52. Duddleston AK, Bennion M. Effect of diet and/or exercise on obese college women. Weight loss and serum lipids. *J Am Diet Assoc* 1970;56:126–9.

53. Harris MB, Hallbauer ES. Self-directed weight control through eating and exercise. *Behav Res Ther* 1973;11:523–9.

54. Hill JO, Schundlt DG, Sbrocco T, et al. Evaluation of an alternating-calorie diet with and without exercise in the treatment of obesity. *Am J Clin Nutr* 1989;50:248–54.

55. Pavlou KN, Krey S, Steffee WP. Exercise as an adjunct to weight loss and maintenance in moderately obese subjects. *Am J Clin Nutr* 1989; 49:1115–23.

56. Sikand G, Kondo A, Foreyt JP, Jones PH, Gotto AM. Two-year followup of patients treated with a very-low-calorie-diet and exercise training. *J Am Diet Assoc* 1988;88:487–8.

57. Stalonas PM, Johnson WG, Christ M. Behavior modification for obesity: the evaluation of exercise, contingency management, and program adherence. *J Consult Clin Psychol* 1978;46:463–9.

58. van Dale D, Saris WHM. Repetitive weight loss and weight regain: effects on weight reduction, resting metabolic rate, and lipolytic activity before and after exercise and/or diet treatment. *Am J Clin Nutr* 1989;49:409–16.

59. Phinney SD, LaGrange BM, O'Connell M, Danforth E. Effects of aerobic exercise on energy expenditure and nitrogen balance during very low calorie dieting. *Metabolism* 1988;37:758–65.

60. Lennon D, Nagle F, Stratman F, Shrago E, Dennis S. Diet and exercise training effects on resting metabolic rate. *Int J Obes* 1985;9:39–47.

61. Belko AZ, Van Loan M, Barbieri TF, Mayclin P. Diet, exercise, weight loss, and energy expenditure in moderately overweight men. *Int J Obes* 1987;11:93–104.

62. King AC, Frey-Hewitt D, Dreon D, et al. Diet versus exercise in weight maintenance: the effects of minimal intervention strategies on long-term outcomes in men. *Arch Intern Med* 1989;149:2741–6.

63. Perri MG, McAdoo WG, McAllister DA, Lauer JB, Yancey DZ. Enhancing the efficacy of behavior therapy for obesity: effects of aerobic exercise and a multicomponent maintenance program. *J Consult Clin Psychol* 1986;54:670–5.

64. Hill JO, Sparling PB, Shields TW, Heller PA. Effects of exercise and food restriction on body com-

position and metabolic rate in obese women. *Am J Clin Nutr* 1987;46:622–30.

65. Epstein LH, Wing RR, Koeske R, Ossip DJ, Beck S. A comparison of lifestyle change and programmed aerobic exercise on weight and fitness changes in obese children. *Behav Ther* 1982; 13:651–65.

66. Epstein LH, Wing RR, Koeske R, Valoski A. The effects of diet plus exercise on weight change in parents and children. *J Consult Clin Psychol* 1984;52:429–37.

67. Epstein LH, Wing RR, Koeske R, Valoski A. A comparison of lifestyle exercise, aerobic exercise, and calisthenics on weight loss in obese children. *Behav Ther* 1985;16:345–56.

68. McArdle WD, Katch FI, Katch VL. *Exercise physiology: Energy, nutrition, and human performance.* Philadelphia: Lea & Febiger, 1991.

69. Bjorntorp P. Exercise and obesity. *Psychiatr Clin North Am* 1978;1:691–6.

70. Bray G. *The obese patient.* Philadelphia: WB Saunders, 1976.

71. Forbes GB. *Human body composition: growth, aging, nutrition, and activity.* New York: Springer-Verlag, 1987.

72. Forbes GB. Exercise and body composition. *J Appl Physiol* 1991;70:994–7.

73. Forbes GB. The companionship of lean and fat: some lessons from body composition studies. In: *New techniques in nutritional research.* New York: Academic Press, 1991;317–29.

74. Bouchard C, Tremblay A, Nadeau A, et al. Long-term exercise training with constant energy intake. 1: Effect on body composition and selected metabolic variables. *Int J Obes* 1990;14:57–73.

75. Despres JP, Bouchard C, Tremblay A, Savard R, Marcotte M. Effects of aerobic training on fat distribution in male subjects. *Med Sci Sports Exerc* 1985;17:113–8.

76. Segal KR, Pi-Sunyer FX. Exercise, resting metabolic rate, and thermogenesis. *Diabetes Metab Rev* 1986;2:19–34.

77. Ballor DL, Katch VI, Becque MD, Marks CR. Resistance weight training during caloric restriction enhances lean body weight maintenance. *Am J Clin Nutr* 1988;47:19–25.

78. Donnelly JE, Pronk NP, Jacobsen DJ, Pronk SJ, Jakicic JM. Effects of a very-low-calorie diet and physical-training regimens on body composition and resting metabolic rate in obese females. *Am J Clin Nutr* 1991;54:56–61.

79. Hagan RD, Upton SJ, Wong L, Whittman J. The effects of aerobic conditioning and/or caloric restriction in overweight men and women. *Med Sci Sports Exerc* 1986;18:87–94.

80. Nieman DC, Haig JL, Fairchild KS, DeGuia ED, Dizon GP, Register UD. Reducing-diet and exercise-training effects on serium lipids and lipoproteins in mildly obese women. *Am J Clin Nutr* 1990;52:640–5.

81. van Dale D, Saris WHM, Schoeffelen PFM, Ten Hoor F. Does exercise give an additional effect in weight reduction regimes? *Int J Obes* 1987; 11:367–75.

82. Ballor DL, McCarthy JP, Wilterdink EJ. Exercise intensity does not affect the composition of diet-

and exercise-induced body mass loss. *Am J Clin Nutr* 1990;51:142–6.

83. Mayer J, Marshall NB, Vitale JJ, et al. Exercise, food intake, and body weight in normal rats and genetically obese adult mice. *Am J Physiol* 1954;177:544–8.

84. Mayer J, Thomas D. Regulation of food choice and obesity. *Science* 1967;156:328–37.

85. Ahrens RA, Bishop CL, Berdanier CD. Effect of age and dietary carbohydrate source on the responses of rats to forced exercise. *J Nutr* 1972;102:241–8.

86. Crews EL, Fuge KW, Oscai LB, Holloszy JO, Shank RE. Weight, food intake, and body composition: effects of exercise and of protein deficiency. *Am J Physiol* 1969;216:275–87.

87. Holloszy JO, Skinner JS, Toro G, Cureton TK. Effects of a six month program of endurance exercise on the serum lipids of middle-aged men. *Am J Cardiol* 1964;14:753–60.

88. Katch VL, Martin R, Martin J. Effects of exercise intensity on food consumption in the male rat. *Am J Clin Nutr* 1979;32:1401–7.

89. Nance DM, Bromley B, Barnard RJ, Gorski RA. Sexually dimorphic effects of forced exercise on food intake and body weight in the rat. *Physiol Behav* 1977;19:155–8.

90. Oscai LB, Holloszy JO. Effects of weight changes produced by exercise, food restriction, or overeating on body consumption. *J Clin Invest* 1969;48:2124–8.

91. Oscai LB, Spirakis CN, Wolff CA. Effects of exercise and of food restriction on adipose tissue cellularity. *J Lipid Res* 1972;13:588–92.

92. Oscai LB, Mole PA, Brei B, Holloszy JO. Cardiac growth and respiratory enzyme levels in male rats subjected to a running program. *Am J Physiol* 1971;220:1238–41.

93. Stern JS, Johnson PR. Spontaneous activity and adipose cellularity in the genetically obese Zucker rat (fafa). *Metabolism* 1977;26:371–80.

94. Stevenson JAF, Box BM, Feleki V, Beaton JR. Bouts of exercise and food intake in the rat. *J Appl Physiol* 1966;21:118–22.

95. Sclafani A, Springer D. Dietary obesity in adult rats: similarities to hypothalamic and human obesity syndromes. *Physiol Behav* 1976;17:461–71.

96. Wilmore JH. Body composition in sport and exercise: directions for future research. *Med Sci Sports Exerc* 1983;15:21–31.

97. Andersson B, Xu X, Rebuffe-Scrive M, Terning K, Krotkiewski M, Bjorntorp P. The effects of exercise training on body composition and metabolism in men and women. *Int J Obes* 1991;15:75–81.

98. Epstein LH, Wing RR, Thompson JK. The relationship between exercise intensity, caloric intake, and weight. *Addict Behav* 1978;3:185–90.

99. Holm G, Bjorntorp P, Jagenberg R. Carbohydrate, lipid, and amino acid metabolism following physical exercise in man. *J Appl Physiol* 1978; 45:128–32.

100. Woo R, Garrow JS, Sunyer FXP. Effect of exercise on spontaneous calorie intake in obesity. *Am J Clin Nutr* 1982;36:470–7.

101. Applegate EA, Upton DE, Stern JS. Food intake, body composition, and blood lipids following

treadmill exercise in male and female rats. *Physiol Behav* 1982;28:917–20.

102. Katch FI, Martin R, Martin J. Effects of exercise intensity on food consumption in the male rat. *Am J Clin Nutr* 1979;32:1401–7.

103. Oscai LB, Mole PA, Holloszy JO. Effects of exercise on cardiac weight and mitochondria in male and female rats. *Am J Physiol* 1971;220:1944–8.

104. Oscai LB, Mole PA, Krusack LM, Holloszy JO. Detailed body composition analysis on female rats subjected to a program of swimming. *J Nutr* 1973;103:412–8.

105. Woo R, Pi-Sunyer FX. Effect of increased physical activity on voluntary intake in lean women. *Metabolism* 1985;34:836–41.

106. Applegate EA. Exercise and detraining: effect on food intake, adiposity, and lipogenesis in Osborne-Mendel rats made obese on a high fat diet. *J Nutr* 1984;114:447–59.

107. Thomas BM, Miller AT, Jr. Adaptation to forced exercise in the rat. *Am J Physiol* 1958;193:350–4.

108. Walhberg M, Mole PA, Stern JS. Effect of swim training on development of obesity in the genetically obese rat. *Am J Physiol* 1982;242:R204–R211.

109. Pi-Sunyer FX. Effect of exercise on food intake. In: Bjorntorp P, Brodoff BN, eds. *Obesity.* Philadelphia: JB Lippincott, 1992;454–62.

110. Apfelbaum M, Bostsarron J, Lacatis D. Effect of caloric restriction and excessive caloric intake on energy expenditure. *Am J Clin Nutr* 1971;24:1405–9.

111. Barrows K, Snook JT. Effect of a high-protein, very-low-calorie diet on resting metabolism, thyroid hormones, and energy expenditure of obese middle-aged women. *Am J Clin Nutr* 1987;45:391–8.

112. Elliot DL, Goldberg L, Kuehl KS, Bennett WM. Sustained depression of resting metabolic rate after massive weight loss. *Am J Clin Nutr* 1989;49:93–6.

113. Mole PA, Stern JS, Schultz CL, Bernauer EM, Holcomb BJ. Exercise reverses depressed metabolic rate produced by severe caloric restriction. *Med Sci Sports Exerc* 1989;21:29–33.

114. Ravussin E, Burnand B, Schutz Y, Jequier E. Energy expenditure before and during energy restriction in obese patients. *Am J Clin Nutr* 1985;41:753–9.

115. Welle SL, Amatruda JM, Forbes GB, Lockwood DH. Resting metabolic rates of obese women after rapid weight loss. *J Clin Endocrinol Metab* 1984;59:41–4.

116. Danforth E, Landsberg L. Energy expenditure and its regulation. In: Greenwood, MRC, ed. *Obesity.* New York: Churchill Livingstone, 1983;103–21.

117. Garrow JS. *Energy balance and obesity in man.* New York: Elsevier, 1974.

118. Ravussin E, Lillioja S, Anderson TE, Christen L, Bogardus C. Determinants of 24-hour energy expenditure in man. Methods and results using a respirometry chamber. *J Clin Invest* 1986;78:1568–78.

119. Harris RBS, Kasser TR, Martin RJ. Dynamics of recovery of body composition after overfeeding, food restriction, or starvation of mature female rats. *J Nutr* 1986;116:2536–46.

120. Wainwright PE, Simpson JR, Cameron R, Hoffman-Goetz L, Winfield D, McCutcheon D, MacDonald M. Effects of treadmill exercise on weight cycling in female mice. *Physiol Behav* 1991;49:639–42.

121. Tremblay A, Despres J-P, Bouchard C. The effects of exercise-training on energy balance and adipose tissue morphology and metabolism. *Sports Med* 1985;2:223–33.

122. Tremblay A, Fontaine E, Poehlman ET, Mitchell D, Perron L, Bouchard C. The effect of exercise-training on resting metabolic rate in lean and moderately obese individuals. *Int J Obes* 1986;10:511–7.

123. Brehm BA. Elevation of metabolic rate following exercise: implications for weight loss. *Sports Med* 1988;6:72–8.

124. Ekblom B. Energy expenditure during exercise. In: Bjorntorp P, Brodoff BN, eds. *Obesity.* Philadelphia: JB Lippincott, 1992;454–62.

125. Bjorntorp P, Yang M. Refeeding after fasting in the rat: effects on body composition and food efficiency. *Am J Clin Nutr* 1982;36:444–9.

126. Boyle PC, Storlien H, Keesey RE. Increased efficiency of food utilization following weight loss. *Physiol Behav* 1978;21:261–4.

127. Brownell KD, Greenwood MRC, Stellar E, Shrager EE. The effects of repeated cycles of weight loss and regain in rats. *Physiol Behav* 1986;38:459–64.

128. Hamm P, Shekelle RB, Stamler J. Large fluctuations in body weight during young adulthood and twenty-five year risk of coronary heart disease in men. *Am J Epidemiol* 1989;129:312–8.

129. Lissner L, Odell PM, D'Agostino, et al. Variability of body weight and health outcomes in the Framingham population. *N Engl J Med* 1991;324:1839–44.

130. Rossner S. Weight cycling—a new risk factor. *J Intern Med* 1989;226:209–11.

131. Steen SN, Brownell KD. Patterns of weight loss and regain in wrestlers: has the tradition changed? *Med Sci Sports Med* 1990;22:762–8.

132. Lissner L, Brownell KD. Weight cycling, mortality, and cardiovascular disease: a review of epidemiologic findings. In: Bjorntorp P, Brodoff BN, eds. *Obesity.* Philadelphia: JB Lippincott, 1992;653–61.

133. Archambault CM, Czyewski D, Cruz GD, Foreyt JP, Mariotto MJ. Effects of weight cycling in female rats. *Physiol Behav* 1989;46:417–21.

134. Cleary MP. Consequences of restricted feeding/refeeding cycles in lean and obese female Zucker rats. *J Nutr* 1986;116:290–303.

135. Cleary MP. Response of adult lean and obese female Zucker rats to intermittent food restriction/refeeding. *J Nutr* 1986;116:1489–99.

136. Hill JO, Fried SK, DiGirolamo M. Effects of fasting and restricted refeeding on utilization of ingested energy in rats. *Am J Physiol* 1984;247:R318–R327.

137. Reed DR, Contreras RJ, Maggio C, Greenwood MRC, Rodin J. Weight cycling in female rats increases dietary fat selection and adiposity. *Physiol Behav* 1988;42:389–95.

138. Blackburn G, Kanders B, Brownell KD, et al. The

effect of weight cycling on the rate of weight loss in man. *Int J Obes* 1987;11:448A(abst).

139. Blackburn GL, Wilson GT, Kanders BS, et al. Weight cycling: the experience of human dieters. *Am J Clin Nutr* 1989;49:1105–9.

140. Steen SN, Oppliger RA, Brownell KD. Metabolic effects of repeated weight loss and regain in adolescent wrestlers. *JAMA* 1988;260:47–50.

141. Bell RR, McGill TJ. Body composition in mice maintained with cyclic periods of food restriction and refeeding. *Nutr Res* 1987;7:173–82.

142. Desautels M, Dulos RA. Effects of repeated cycles of fasting-refeeding on brown adipose tissue composition in mice. *Am J Physiol* 1988;255:E120–E128.

143. Gray DS, Fisler JS, Bray GA. Effects of repeated weight loss and regain on body composition in obese rats. *Am J Clin Nutr* 1988;47:393–9.

144. Hill JO, Newby FD, Thacker SV, Sykes MN, DiGirolamo M. Influence of food restriction coupled with weight cycling on carcass energy restoration during ad libitum refeeding. *Int J Obes* 1988;12:547–55.

145. Hill JO, Thacker S, Newby D, Nickel M, DiGirolamo M. A comparison of constant feeding with bouts of fasting-refeeding at three levels of nutrition in the rat. *Int J Obes* 1987;11:201–12.

146. Wheeler J, Martin R, Yakubu F, Lin D, Hill JO. Weight cycling in female rats subjected to varying meal patterns. *Am J Physiol* 1990;258:R124–R129.

147. Melby CL, Schmidt WD, Corrigan D. Resting metabolic rate in weight-cycling collegiate wrestlers compared with physically active, noncycling control subjects. *Am J Clin Nutr* 1990;52:409–14.

148. Wadden TA, Bartlett SJ, Letizia TA, Foster GD, Stunkard AJ, Conill A. Relationship of dieting history to resting metabolic rate, body composition, eating behavior, and subsequent weight loss. *Am J Clin Nutr* 1992;56:203S–8S.

149. Gerardo-Gettens T, Miller GD, Horwitz BA, et al. Exercise decreases fat selection in female rats during weight cycling. *Am J Physiol* 1991;260:R518–R524.

150. Blair SN, Goodyear NN, Gibbons LW, Cooper KH. Physical fitness and incidence of hypertension in healthy normotensive men and women. *JAMA* 1984;252:487–90.

151. Dubbert PM. Exercise in behavioral medicine. *J Consult Clin Psychol* [in press].

152. Leon AS, Connett J, Jacobs DR, Rauramaa R. Leisure-time physical activity levels and risk of coronary heart disease and death. *JAMA* 1987;258:2388–95.

153. Martin JE, Dubbert PM, Cushman WC. Controlled trial of aerobic exercise in hypertension. *Circulation* 1990;81:1560–7.

154. Paffenbarger RS, Hyde RT, Wing AL, Hsieh CC. Physical activity, all-cause mortality, and longevity of college alumni. *N Engl J Med* 1986;314:605–13.

155. Powell KE, Caspersen CJ, Koplan JP, Ford ES. Physical activity and chronic disease. *Am J Clin Nutr* 1989;49:999–1006.

156. Bjorntorp P. Physical exercise in the treatment of obesity. In: Bjorntorp P, Brodoff BN, eds. *Obesity.* Philadelphia: JB Lippincott, 1992;708–11.

157. Wood PD, Stefanick ML, Dreon DM, et al. Changes in plasma lipids and lipoproteins in overweight men during weight loss through dieting as compared with exercise. *N Engl J Med* 1988;319:1173–9.

158. Blair SN, Kohl HW III, Paffenbarger RS, Clark DG, Cooper KH, Gibbons LW. Physical fitness and all-cause mortality. *JAMA* 1989;262:2395–401.

159. DeBusk RF, Stenestrand U, Sheehan M, Haskell WL. Training effects of long versus short bouts of exercise in healthy subjects. *Am J Cardiol* 1990;65:1010–3.

160. Duncan JJ, Gordon NF, Scott CB. Women walking for health and fitness: how much is enough? *JAMA* 1991;266:3295–9.

161. Helmrich SP, Ragland DR, Leung RW, Paffenbarger RS. Physical activity and reduced occurrence of non-insulin-dependent diabetes mellitus. *N Engl J Med* 1991;325:147–52.

162. Tremblay A, Despres J-P, Maheux J, et al. Normalization of the metabolic profile in obese women by exercise and a low fat diet. *Med Sci Sports Exer* 1991;23:1326–31.

163. Brownell KD. *The LEARN program for weight control.* Dallas: American Health Publishing Company, 1991.

164. Plante TG, Rodin J. Physical fitness and enhanced psychological health. *Curr Psychol: Res Rev* 1990;9:3–24.

165. Bandura A. *Social learning theory.* Englewood Cliffs, NJ: Prentice-Hall, 1977.

166. Folkins CH, Sime WE. Physical fitness training and mental health. *Am Psychol* 1981;36:373–89.

167. Gruber JJ. Physical activity and self-esteem development in children: a meta-analysis. In: Stull GA, Eckert HM, eds. *Effects of physical activity on children.* Champaign, IL: Human Kinetics, 1986;30–48.

168. Mihevic PM. Anxiety, depression, and exercise. *Quest* 1981;33:140–53.

169. Morgan WP. Affective beneficence of vigorous exercise. *Med Sci Sports Exer* 1985;17:94–100.

170. Sonstroem RL. Exercise and self-esteem. In: Terjung RL, ed. *Exercise and sports sciences reviews.* Lexington, MA: Collamore, 1984;123–55.

171. Brownell KD, Rodin J, Willmore JH. *Eating, body weight, and performance in athletes: disorders of modern society.* Philadelphia: Lea & Febiger, 1992.

172. Thompson JK, Pasman L. The obligatory exercise questionnaire. *Behav Ther* 1991(May);137.

173. Rodin J, Plante TG. The psychological effects of exercise. In: Williams RS, Wallace A, eds. *Biological effects of physical activity.* Champaign, IL: Human Kinetics, 1989.

174. Raglin JS, Morgan WP. Influence of vigorous exercise on mood states. *Behav Ther* 1985;8:179–83.

175. Morgan WP, Goldston SE, eds. *Exercise and mental health.* New York: Hemisphere, 1987.

176. Goldwater BC, Collins ML. Psychologic effects of cardiovascular conditioning: a controlled experiment. *Psychosom Med* 1985;47:174–81.

177. Steptoe A, Cox S. Acute effects of aerobic exercise on mood. *Health Psychol* 1988;7:329–40.

178. Dishman RK. *Exercise adherence: its impact on public health.* Champaign, IL: Human Kinetics, 1988.

179. Dishman RK. Increasing and maintaining exercise and physical activity. *Behav Ther* 1991;22:345–78.
180. Dishman RK. Determinants of participation in physical activity. In: Bouchard C, Shephard RJ, Stephens T, Sutton JR, McPherson BD, eds. *Exercise, fitness and health.* Champaign, IL: Human Kinetics, 1990;75–102.
181. Gwinup G. Effect of exercise alone on the weight of obese women. *Arch Intern Med* 1975;135:676–80.
182. King A. Community intervention for promotion of physical activity and fitness. In: Pandolf KB, Holloszy JO, ed. *Exercise and sport sciences reviews.* Baltimore: Williams & Wilkins, 1991; 19:211–59.
183. Epstein LH, Woodall K, Goreczny AJ, Wing RR, Roberston RJ. The modification of activity patterns and energy expenditure in obese young girls. *Behav Ther* 1984;15:101–8.
184. Neale AV, Singleton SP, Dupuis MH, Hess JW. The use of behavioral contracting to increase exercise activity. *Am J Health Promotion* 1990; 4:441–4.
185. Robison JI, Rogers MA, Carlson, et al. Effects of a 6-month incentive-based exercise program on adherence and work capacity. *Med Sci Sport Exerc* 1992;24:85–93.
186. Perkins KA, Rapp SR, Carlson CR, Wallace CE. A behavioral intervention to increase exercise among nursing home residents. *Gerontologist* 1986;26: 479–81.
187. Martin JE, Dubbert PM, Katell AD, et al. Behavioral control of exercise in sedentary adults: studies 1 through 6. *J Consult Clin Psychol* 1984; 52:795–811.
188. Brownell KD, Marlatt GA, Lichtenstein E, Wilson GT. Understanding and preventing relapse. *Am Psychol* 1986;41:765–82.
189. Marlatt GA, Gordon J, eds. *Relapse prevention: maintenance statiegies in the treatment of addictive behaviors.* New York: Guilford, 1985.
190. Baum JG, Clark HB, Sandler J. Preventing relapse in obesity through posttreatment maintenance systems: comparing the relative efficacy of two levels of therapist support. *J Behav Med* 1991;14: 287–302.
191. Belisle M, Roskies E, Levesque MM. Improving adherence to physical activity. *Health Psychol* 1987;6:159–72.
192. King AC, Frederiksen LW. Low-cost strategies for increasing exercise behavior: relapse preparation training and social support. *Behav Modif* 1984;8:3–21.
193. King AC, Taylor CB, Haskell WL, DeBusk RF. Strategies for increasing early adherence to and long-term maintenance of home-based exercise training in healthy middle-aged men and women. *Am J Cardiol* 1988;61:628–32.
194. King AC, Frey-Hewitt B, Dreon D, et al. Diet versus exercise in weight maintenance: the effects of minimal intervention strategies on long-term outcomes in men. *Arch Intern Med* 1989;149:2741–6.
195. Perri MG, McAllister DA, Gange JJ, Jordan RC, McAdoo WG, Nezu AM. Effects of four maintenance programs on the long-term management of obesity. *J Consult Clin Psychol* 1988;56:529–34.
196. Craighead LW, Blum MD. Supervised exercise in behavioral treatment for moderate obesity. *Behav Ther* 1989;20:49–59.
197. Owen N, Dwyer T. Approaches to promoting more widespread participation in physical activity. *Community Health Stud* 1988;12:339–47.
198. Lasco RA, Curry RH, Dickson VJ, Powers J, Menes S, Merritt RK. Participation rates, weight loss, and blood pressure changes among obese women in a nutrition-exercise program. *Public Health Rep* 1989;104:640–6.
199. Blair SN, Piserchia PV, Wilbur CS, et al. A public health intervention model for worksite health promotion: impact on exercise and physical fitness in a health promotion plan after 24 months. *JAMA* 1986;255:921–6.
200. Gebhardt DL, Crump CE. Employee fitness and wellness programs in the workplace. *Am Psychol* 1990;45:262–72.
201. Stunkard AJ. The control of obesity: social and community perspectives. In: Brownell KD, Foreyt JP, eds. *Handbook of eating disorders: physiology, psychology, and treatment of obesity, anorexia, and bulimia.* New York: Basic Books, 1986;213–28.
202. Brownell KD, Felix MRJ. Competitions to facilitate health promotion: review and conceptual analysis. *Am J Health Promotion* 1987;2:28–36.
203. King AC, Carl F, Burkel L, et al. Increasing exercise among blue-collar employees: the tailoring of worksite competitions to meet specific needs. *Pre Med* 1988;17:357–65.
204. Cohen S, Syme SL. *Social support and health.* New York: Academic Press, 1985.
205. Black DR, Gleser LJ, Kooyers KJ. A meta-analytic evaluation of couples weight-loss programs. *Health Psychol* 1990;9:330–47.
206. Lassner JB. Does social support aid in weight loss and smoking interventions? Reply from a family systems perspective. *Ann Behav Med* 1991;13: 66–72.
207. Knapp DN. Behavioral management techniques and exercise promotion. In: Dishman RK, ed. *Exercise adherence: its impact on public health.* Champaign, IL: Human Kinetics, 1988;203–35.
208. Wankel LM. Exercise adherence and leisure activity: patterns of involvement and interventions to facilitate regular activity. In: Dishman RK, ed. *Exercise adherence: its impact on public health.* Champaign, IL: Human Kinetics, 1988;369–96.
209. Heinzelmann F, Bagley RW. Response to physical activity programs and their effects on health behavior. *Public Health Rep* 1970;85:905–11.
210. Erling J, Oldridge NB. Effect of a spousal-support program on compliance with cardiac rehabilitation. *Med Sci Sport Exerc* 1985;17:284A.
211. Brownell KD, Rodin J. *The weight maintenance survival guide.* Dallas: American Health Publishing Company, 1990.
212. Brownell KD, Grilo CM. Weight maintenance. In: Blair SN, et al, eds. *ACSM resource manual for guidelines for exercise testing and prescription.* Philadelphia: Lea & Febiger [in press].
213. Sallis JF, Haskell WL, Fortmann SP, et al. Predictors of adoption and maintenance of physical activity in a community sample. *Prev Med* 1986; 15:331–41.
214. Sallis JF, Hovell MF. Determinants of exercise be-

havior. In: Pandolf KB, Holloszy JO, eds. *Exercise and sport sciences reviews,* vol 18. Baltimore: Williams & Wilkins, 1990.

215. Allon N. The stigma of overweight in everyday life. In: Wolman B, ed. *Psychological aspects of obesity: a handbook.* New York: Van Nostrand Reinhold, 1982;130–74.

216. Bray GA. Effects of obesity on health and happiness. In: Brownell KD, Foreyt JP, eds. *Handbook of eating disorders: Physiology, psychology, and treatment of obesity, anorexia, and bulimia.* New York: Basic Books, 1986;3–44.

217. Wadden TA, Stunkard AJ. Social and psychological consequences of obesity. *Ann Intern Med* 1985;103:1062–7.

218. Thompson JK. *Body image disturbance: assessment and treatment.* Elmsford, NY: Pergamon, 1990.

219. Thompson JK, Fabian LJ, Moulton DO, Dunn ME, Altabe MN. Development and validation of the physical appearance related testing scale. *J Pers Assess* 1991;56:513–21.

220. Grilo CM, Shiffman S, Wing RR. Relapse crises and coping among dieters. *J Consult Clin Psychol* 1989;57:488–95.

221. Grilo CM, Shiffman S, Wing RR. Coping with dietary relapse crises and their aftermath [*submitted for publication*].

222. Brownell KD. Relapse and the treatment of obesity. In: Wadden TA, VanItallie TB, eds. *Treatment of the seriously obese patient.* New York: Guilford, 1992;437–55.

Obesity: Theory and Therapy, Second Edition,
edited by A. J. Stunkard and T. A. Wadden.
Raven Press, Ltd., New York © 1993.

16

The Place of Appetite-Suppressant Drugs in the Treatment of Obesity

Trevor Silverstone

Department of Psychological Medicine, Medical College of St. Bartholomew's Hospital, University of London, London EC1 7BE, United Kingdom

Over 50 years ago the first appetite-suppressant drug, amphetamine (Benzedrine), was introduced into clinical practice for the treatment of obesity. Shortly afterwards, the dextro rotatory isomer d-amphetamine (Dexedrine) was found to be the active anorectic constituent of the racemic mixture and came to supplant it. Unfortunately, not only was d-amphetamine an appetite suppressant, it was also discovered to be a drug with marked central stimulant and euphoriant properties, which led to widespread abuse (along with a similar drug, phenmetrazine, Preludin). They can thus no longer be recommended for use in the treatment of obesity, and in many countries, including the United States and United Kingdom, their prescription is narrowly restricted by legislation.

Since then a number of other centrally acting appetite drugs have been developed with less of an abuse potential than d-amphetamine. The centrally acting appetite-suppressant compounds that are currently licensed and recommended for the treatment of obesity fall into two broad pharmacological categories, those that act on central catecholamine neurotransmitter systems within the brain, and those that act on serotoninergic systems.

Appetite-suppressant drugs, through reducing hunger drives, can help overweight patients resist the many physiological and psychological pressures to eat; such drugs thus assist patients in keeping to a reduced calorie diet. This will in turn lead to weight loss with a consequent improvement in health.

Despite clear differences in pharmacology and abuse potential, there is still an unfortunate tendency to refer to all centrally acting appetite suppressants as "amphetamine-like," (whatever their pharmacology) and to view them all with equal suspicion. This has led to what I consider ill-informed and misguided warnings against using such drugs *at all* in the management of obesity. Such negative attitudes to appetite-suppressant drugs are not only wrong in substance, they are unhelpful in clinical practice. In this chapter I shall show why I believe this to be the case.

CLINICAL APPLICATION

There is no consensus on the use of anorectic drugs in clinical practice. On the contrary, views range widely, from total rejection, to grudging acceptance, to a clear recommendation in appropriate patients. The British National Formulary (1) dismisses them out of hand as being, "of no real value in the treatment of obesity since they do not improve the long-term outlook." The American Medical Association (2), while less extreme in its condemnation, remains clearly unenthusiastic: "Occasionally, *adjunctive* use of anorexiants will help patients who respond unsatisfactorily." The Royal College of Physicians

(3) adopts a more measured tone: "Anorectic drugs may be a useful adjunct to dietary and behaviour therapy . . . but should not be used on their own."

In order to place anorectic drugs in perspective, it should be recognized that most obese patients do not eat more than their contemporaries; therefore what they need is help in reducing their dietary intake *below the norms of their society.* Unfortunately, despite evidence to the contrary, obese patients are frequently viewed as self-indulgent gluttons totally lacking in will-power for whom moral exhortation rather than pharmacological assistance is required.

When given as part of an integrated dietary program to patients thought to be medically at risk, anorectic drugs can be of real benefit in helping them lose weight. The major charges levelled against anorectic drugs, and the reasons they are not more widely accepted include: (a) the rate of weight loss slows with time (this is usually attributed to tolerance developing); (b) when the patient stops taking the drug, he or she regains the lost weight; (c) anorectic drugs do not reeducate patients to adopt "good" eating habits; and (d) they lead to drug dependence and abuse and are therefore dangerous (as well as useless).

Let us examine each of these charges in turn:

1. While it is true that the rate of weight loss plateaus after some 5 to 6 months of continuous treatment, this happens with all effective weight loss regimes (even surgical). It occurs largely because the body adapts to a lowered calorie intake by reducing the resting metabolic rate and because of the decreased amount of metabolically active tissues. Thus there comes a time when the lowered energy intake is matched by the reduced energy output, and weight loss ceases. Hardly the fault of the drug. In fact, true drug tolerance rarely develops. In a study designed to investigate this point, we allocated a series of obese patients into three groups: one group received

diethylpropion 75 mg daily continuously for 4 months, another group received active diethylpropion in the first and third months and placebo in the intervening months, and the third group received active diethylpropion during the second and fourth months with placebo in months 1 and 3 (4). If tolerance were the cause of the falling rate of weight loss seen over time, then the patients in the third group who received diethylpropion for the first time in the second month should have shown a greater drug effect than those in the first group who had been receiving it continuously. They did not; the weight lost was almost identical.

2. What about weight regain after stopping anorectic drug treatment? I believe that this reflects the release from the continuing anorectic effect these drugs exert for as long as they are taken, despite no further weight loss occurring. The fact that the drugs cease to work when they are no longer being taken is hardly surprising; this is a totally unrealistic expectation of any drug (5).

3. Finally, what about the problem of dependence and abuse? The only evidence for physical dependence, with consequent withdrawal symptoms, relates to the nonstimulant anorectic fenfluramine. Suddenly stopping fenfluramine can occasionally lead to a depressive syndrome. The risk of this happening is minimized by gradual dose reduction. Psychological dependence is similarly uncommon; most patients prescribed the anorectic drugs recommended for use in obesity have little or no difficulty in stopping. The term *drug abuse* refers to the self-administration of a substance taken for *nontherapeutic purposes,* usually in greater than therapeutic doses, by *nonpatients.* Such abuse has really only occurred with amphetamine, dexamphetamine, and phenmetrazine, drugs that are no longer recommended for the treatment of obesity and that are the subject of rigid restriction and control in most countries. For the anorectic compounds considered in this chapter, examples of abuse are rare.

Anorectic drugs can play a useful role in the overall management of obesity provided it is recognized that the rationale of such treatment is to help the patient keep to a restricted calorie diet. Therefore they should be given only in conjunction with appropriate dietary information and advice, which itself should be reinforced at frequent intervals and accompanied by instruction in the range of strategies that have been found to assist patients avoid overeating (behavior modification).

It is my view that these drugs should be given only to those who are medically at risk either because of the degree of their obesity (that is, when the body mass index is 30 or more) or if they suffer from a serious complication of overweight such as non-insulin-dependent diabetes or hypertension. Their place in promoting weight loss purely for cosmetic purposes is questionable, and they should not be used at all in childhood.

When to start treatment with anorectic drugs depends more on individual preferences by the doctor and by the patient. A good case can be made for starting on active anorectic drug treatment (combined with dietary instruction and behavioral advice) when the patient presents, provided such treatment is appropriate on clinical grounds. It is likely that he or she has tried to lose weight before, either unaided or using some other dietary aid such as attending a diet group. The greater immediate weight loss together with the reduced discomfort of dieting associated with anorectic drug treatment is likely to provide a much needed boost to morale and increase motivation. On the other hand, there are those who think that anorectic drugs should be held in reserve to be used only when resolution is flagging and weight loss waning. It is a matter that in my view should largely be left to the patient to decide after full discussion of the advantages and disadvantages of anorectic drug treatment and the relative merits of starting earlier or later in the comprehensive treatment program (which should include graded exercise).

Patients by and large find anorectic drugs helpful (6).

CHOICE OF DRUG

Before a drug can be considered, it has to be shown to possess true anorectic properties, that is, reduce both hunger and food intake, lead to significant loss of body weight, and be well tolerated and safe.

The choice of which anorectic drug to use lies first of all between one of the catecholaminergic or one of the serotoninergic compounds. For patients with a history of significant depression, one of the catecholamine-mediated drugs (diethylpropion, phentermine or mazindol) are to be preferred. They appear to be equally effective, with a similar side-effect profile. Intermittent treatment with these drugs appears to be as good as continuous treatment. For the more anxious patient, a serotoninergic drug (fenfluramine, d-fenfluramine, or fluoxetine) is preferable.

Combining a catecholaminergic and serotonin anorectic may be more effective than giving either alone (7), but this approach is relatively untried and requires further study.

Catecholamine Anorectics

Diethylpropion (Tenuate, Apisate)—Dose: 75 mg daily

Diethylpropion is a phenylethylamine with minor sympathomimetic properties and much less stimulant activity than amphetamine (8). It has clear appetite-suppressant activity. In both normal weight and obese subjects, it has been found to lower subjective hunger ratings and to reduce food intake (9,10). It is well absorbed from the gastrointestinal tract with peak plasma levels occurring some 2 hours after administration. Metabolism within the liver gives rise to active metabolites that have an elimination half-life of 8 hours.

Several placebo-controlled double-blind clinical trials attest to its efficacy in helping obese patients lose weight, at least in the short term (8–11). Combining the results of four such studies, each lasting 12 weeks and involving a total of over 200 patients, the mean weight loss among patients taking diethylpropion was 7.2 kg (0.60 kg/week) compared with 3.8 kg (0.32 kg/week) in those taking placebo.

McKay (12) conducted a double-blind placebo-controlled trial, lasting 23 weeks, of diethylpropion [given as a 75-mg sustained-release tablet daily (Tenuate dospan)] in 20 obese patients (10 on diethylpropion, 10 on placebo). All the patients taking diethylpropion completed the trial, whereas six of the ten on placebo failed to complete (three because of inefficacy). Among the completers, diethylpropion had a clear advantage: by 23 weeks there was a mean weight loss of 11.7 kg in the diethylpropion group compared with 2.4 kg in the placebo group. Intermittent treatment, with alternate months on diethylpropion, is as effective as continuous medication in uncomplicated obesity (4,13,14) and in obese diabetic patients (15). Direct comparison with dl-fenfluramine (16) and with mazindol (17) revealed no significant differences in efficacy among these compounds over the short term.

Unwanted side effects are relatively uncommon (11). Some patients experience insomnia, particularly if they take diethylpropion in the afternoon. Although cases of abuse have been reported, the risk appears to be small (18) and is largely confined to those who had previously abused amphetamine or phenmetrazine (8).

Phentermine (Duromine, Ionamin)—Dose: 15 to 30 mg daily

Phentermine significantly reduces both hunger ratings and food intake in normal and overweight subjects (10,19). It is well absorbed from the small intestine and has a half-life of 20 to 24 hours. Given as a sustained release resin complex, peak plasma levels occur within 8 hours of oral administration, and therapeutic levels persist for at least 20 hours. Phentermine is more effective than placebo in promoting weight loss in patients with uncomplicated obesity (20,21) and in obese diabetics (22). Intermittent treatment with alternative months on phentermine resinate, 30 mg daily, with the intervening months on placebo, is as effective as continuous treatment (20,23).

In a longer term crossover study in which obese diabetic patients received either phentermine resinate 30 mg daily for 6 months ($n = 34$) or placebo ($n = 32$), the mean weight loss among the patients when receiving phentermine was 5.3 kg, compared with 1.5 kg on placebo ($p < 0.001$) (22). Phentermine is equal in efficacy to dl-fenfluramine (21,23).

Adverse effects, which are generally minor and rarely require treatment, reflect the mild sympathomimetic and stimulant properties of the drug. They include insomnia, nervousness, irritability, and headache (24). Phentermine has been given successfully to patients with moderate hypertension and to diabetics. Abuse is very uncommon (18).

Mazindol (Teronac, Sanorex)—Dose: 2 mg daily

Mazindol is a potent appetite suppressant, with 1 mg significantly reducing food intake in normal subjects over an 8-hour period (10). It is well absorbed from the gastrointestinal tract; the peak plasma level is reached 2 hours after administration. The elimination half-life of mazindol (and its metabolites) ranges from 33 to 55 hours; despite this relatively long half-life, no evidence of accumulation was found in patients receiving 6 mg daily for up to 6 months.

Mazindol is significantly more effective than placebo in helping obese patients lose weight over the short term. In a trial involving 90 patients (80 of whom were women), treatment with mazindol 1 mg t.i.d. led to a mean weight loss of 2.8 kg over 6 weeks compared to 1.4 kg on placebo (25). In a rather complex study comparing mazindol to placebo, with the treatment being administered by one of 12 therapists, mazindol similarly appeared to be more useful than placebo (26). In a 12-week trial involving 228 obese patients conducted in Japan, the mean weight loss on mazindol was 4.2 kg compared with 1.2 kg on placebo, a highly significant difference (27). A crossover trial of mazindol 2 to 3 mg/day given for 20 weeks, followed by (or preceded by) 20 weeks on placebo, also showed a clear-cut superiority for mazindol (especially when mazindol was given first) (28).

The moderate stimulant properties of mazindol can cause nervousness, irritability, and insomnia. In addition, dry mouth, sweating, nausea, and constipation have been reported (13). When given to patients with preexisting heart disease, dysrhythmias and a worsening of angina may occur (29). Because mazindol may potentiate the pressor effects of catecholamines, it should not be given in conjunction with sympatheticomimetic drugs, or with antihypertensive agents of the adrenergic neuron blocking type such as guanethidine and debrisoquine. Mazindol has been used rarely as a drug of abuse, and only by subjects with a previous history of addiction to other drugs.

Phenylpropanolamine

Phenylpropanolamine is a phenylethylamine derivative, being the racemic mixture of the isomers of norephedrine. It is a constituent of a number of nonprescription remedies for coughs and colds, and is also marketed as an antiobesity agent. There are few direct quantitative data concerning the effect of phenylpropanolamine on hunger and food intake in human subjects, although some 45% of obese patients prescribed phenylpropanolamine for weight reduction report appetite reduction. It is well absorbed from the gastrointestinal tract [see Lasagna (30) for review of the pharmacology]. Its elimination half-life is 3.9 to 4.6 hours, with most of the drug being excreted unchanged. Thus far,

only relatively short-term clinical trials of phenylpropanolamine have been carried out in obesity. It has proved more effective than placebo; in one study the mean overall weight loss was 6.1 kg on phenylpropanolamine and 4.3 kg on placebo (31). It is equivalent to diethylpropion: the mean weight loss was 3.10 kg on phenylpropanolamine (plus caffeine), and 3.61 kg on diethylpropion (32).

Although phenylpropanolamine has mild stimulant properties, its abuse potential seems low (30) and in normal volunteers no euphoriant effect was detected using the Addictive Research Centre Inventory (33,34). The risk of other adverse effects is also low (30). Even though it is a sympathomimetic compound, it has little effect on blood pressure in healthy normal volunteer subjects when given at the recommended dose (33,35,36). Overweight patients who were also hypertensive were treated with phenylpropanolamine 25 mg t.i.d. for 6 weeks and experienced no adverse effects on blood pressure compared with placebo, although there was a greater weight loss on phenylpropanolamine (37).

Drugs Acting on Central Serotoninergic Pathways

Fenfluramine (Ponderax, Pondamin)—Dose: 60 mg daily

Fenfluramine is the racemic mixture of the two enantioners d- and l-fenfluramine. While chemically a phenylethylamine like most of the centrally acting drugs considered in the preceding section, it has a markedly different spectrum of pharmacological activity. In particular, its anorectic action appears to be mediated through activating serotoninergic rather than catecholaminergic pathways in the brain (38). As a consequence, it has no stimulant activity; if anything, it has slight depressant effects (39). Fenfluramine has a marked anorectic action. In normal volunteer subjects, hunger ratings are reduced in a dose-related manner following administration of single doses of 20, 40, and 80 mg, with the degree of anorexia closely paralleling the plasma level (40). Food intake is also significantly suppressed by single doses of 40, 60, and 80 mg fenfluramine given to healthy subjects, following an overnight fast (10). It is rapidly absorbed from the gastrointestinal tract, with peak plasma level being reached in 4 hours, and is rapidly metabolized into norfenfluramine. Fenfluramine and norfenfluramine have a plasma half-life of some 20 hours, and after multiple dosage, steady-state plasma levels are reached within 4 to 5 days (41).

A considerable number of placebo-controlled trials attest to the efficacy of fenfluramine in helping obese patients lose weight (14,42). Given as a sustained release formulation at a daily dose of 60 mg, it leads to greater weight loss than placebo, even when patients receive regular dietary advice and supervision and enter a behavioral modification program (7). In a direct comparison of (a) fenfluramine (up to 120 mg daily) plus group counseling, (b) behavior modification, and (c) a combination of the two, fenfluramine with or without behavior modification proved superior over a 6-month treatment period (43). However, after treatment was stopped, the drug-treated patients regained more weight than patients who had been given behaviour modification alone. Fenfluramine is as effective as diethylpropion (16), d-amphetamine (44), and phentermine (23).

Fenfluramine can cause gastrointestinal disturbances (nausea or diarrhea), possibly as a direct consequence of its serotoninergic enhancing action. Drowsiness and lethargy are often experienced during the initial stages of treatment. While it is devoid of stimulant properties, abrupt withdrawal of fenfluramine can lead to severe depression; the dose should therefore always be reduced gradually. The incidence of side effects can be minimized by increasing the dose gradually over several weeks to the maximum tolerated dose. As it is devoid of stimulant properties, fenfluramine has not been used as a drug of abuse.

Dexfenfluramine (Adifax Isomerase)— Dose: 30 mg daily

Dexfenfluramine possesses twice the anorectic potency of the racemic mixture dl-fenfluramine; 30 mg d-fenfluramine suppresses food intake to the same degree as 60 mg dl-fenfluramine, suggesting that the greater part of the anorectic activity of the racemic mixture lies in the d-isomer (45). In a direct comparison, the overall anorectic effect of the dextrorotatory isomer of fenfluramine, dexfenfluramine, was found to be greater than that of the levo-isomer fenfluramine (46). In keeping with the view that d-fenfluramine is acting via central serotoninergic pathways, its anorectic activity in humans is markedly attenuated by the serotonin receptor blocking drug metergoline (47).

Dexfenfluramine tends to reduce the intake of foods high in carbohydrate content more than that of foods containing a greater proportion of protein (46). This finding accords with the observation that dexfenfluramine reduces the frequency of snacking in obese patients prone to consume a lot of carbohydrate-containing snacks (sometimes referred to as "carbohydrate cravers") (48). However, this observation is not in keeping with the findings of an even greater differential effect between sweet and nonsweet food and in the opposite direction. Thus the intake of sweet foods is more resistant to the anorectic effect of dexfenfluramine (46). Obese subjects are as responsive to the anorectic action of d-fenfluramine as normal weight volunteers (49).

Dexfenfluramine 30 mg daily is superior to placebo over the shorter term (12 weeks) in uncomplicated obesity, in obesity associated with hypertension, and in neuroleptic-induced obesity, with the weight loss on active dexfenfluramine being uniformly at least twice as much as that on placebo. Weight loss is clearly attributable to an appetite-suppressant effect: Finer et al. (50) noted that 28 (80%) of the 35 patients on dexfenfluramine "reported a decrease in hunger and/or food intake," compared with 14 (34%) of the 41 on placebo; Sriwatanakul et al. (51) similarly remarked: "patients receiving d-fenfluramine reported a significant decrease in hunger," as assessed by a visual analog scale. Finer et al. (52) extended their observations for a further 3 months on an open-label basis in 31 patients. Weight loss continued throughout the whole 6-month observation period, although the rate of loss appeared to slow during the last 2 or 3 months.

In a formal 6-month placebo-controlled study involving 39 obese women, only those whose obesity was of the android type ("apples") appeared to benefit from d-fenfluramine; those whose obesity was gluteofemoral ("pears") did not (53). Overall, there was gratifying weight loss on both treatments, probably due to more strict adherence to the dieting regime than is usually the case, allowing less room for a drug effect to be seen.

In the most comprehensive longer term (1 year) study of any anorectic drug, Guy-Grand et al. (54) enlisted 782 obese patients, (160 men, 622 women) in 24 centers in nine European countries. The patients, who were all at least 20% above their ideal body weight, were randomly allocated to receive either dexfenfluramine (15 mg b.d.) or placebo; all were prescribed a calorie-restricted diet. They were seen monthly for the first 2 months, and every 2 months thereafter. By the end of 12 months, 189 (45%) of the patients on placebo had withdrawn, 84 (44%) because they were dissatisfied with their weight loss; this compares with 49 (33%) of the 150 patients on d-fenfluramine who failed to complete. By the end of the trial, weight loss was significantly greater on active treatment, with more than twice as many patients on d-fenfluramine losing at least 10% of their initial body weight. However, the time course of mean weight loss in the 256 patients on d-fenfluramine and the 227 on placebo who completed the trial was similar. Both groups showed plateauing, with no further weight being lost after the first 6 months; there was,

however, a tendency to weight regain in the placebo group.

It appears that after 6 months, the action of d-fenfluramine was more one of preventing weight regain than of promoting further weight loss; when the trial ended, the patients who had been receiving d-fenfluramine gained rather more weight (2 kg) than those on placebo (1 kg) in the following 2 months (54). In a subgroup of obese diabetics, the patients receiving d-fenfluramine not only achieved a greater weight loss but also better diabetic control (55). It may be that d-fenfluramine has a direct effect on glucose utilization and insulin sensitivity: after 1 week it has been shown to reduce insulin resistance independently of weight reduction (56). d-fenfluramine is also effective in neuroleptic-induced obesity (57).

Side effects are relatively minor and short-lived (58). In the 12-month placebo-controlled trial involving 782 patients (54), rather more complaints of tiredness occurred on d-fenfluramine than placebo (28% versus 20% of patients), of diarrhea (15% versus 9%), of dry mouth (12% versus 4%), of increased urinary frequency (7% versus 3%), and of drowsiness (5% versus 2%). There appears to be no risk of drug dependence with this compound. It should be noted that d-fenfluramine is not currently available in the United States.

Fluoxetine (Prozac)—Dose: 60 mg daily

Fluoxetine is an antidepressant drug that acts by enhancing central serotoninergic neurotransmission through inhibiting the reuptake of serotonin into the presynaptic neuron (59). In normal weight healthy human volunteers, 60 mg fluoxetine taken daily for 2 weeks caused a statistically significant decrease in food intake and body weight in a placebo-controlled double-blind crossover trial (60). A subsequent 1-month placebo comparison in obese subjects has revealed an even greater appetite-suppressant effect (61). Its effect on nutrient selection is uncertain; while some (61,62) find that fluoxetine curtails the intake of carbohydrate more than protein, others do not (63). Fluoxetine is well absorbed orally. It has a long plasma half-life of some 5 days, while that of its active metabolite (norfluoxetine) is even longer, 7 to 13 days. Giving fluoxetine in fixed daily doses of 10, 20, 40, and 60 mg and placebo for 8 weeks to 131 obese patients revealed that the greatest mean weight loss (3.9 kg) was seen in the group that received 60 mg daily (64).

In a much longer trial lasting 52 weeks and involving obese patients who were binge eaters ($n = 45$), as well as those who were not ($n = 23$), both types of patients responded to behavior therapy plus fluoxetine (mean weight change -13.9 kg) than to behavior therapy alone (mean weight change $+ 0.6$ kg) (65). Weight loss on fluoxetine plateaued after 20 weeks, particularly in the binge eaters but not in the nonbingers. Obese diabetics with non-insulin-dependent diabetes show an improvement in glucose tolerance as well as weight loss after relatively short-term treatment (8 to 12 weeks) with fluoxetine but not placebo (66–68).

In obese patients the adverse events profile is different from that seen when the drug is given to patients suffering from depressive illness, perhaps reflecting the higher (60 mg) daily dose for obesity than for depression (20 mg) (69). In the dose-ranging study previously referred to (64), the side effects most commonly reported by the patients were insomnia, drowsiness, and diarrhea; in depressed patients the most frequent side effect is nausea. Serious adverse effects other than drug-related allergic rashes are uncommon (69) and there appears to be little risk of drug dependence. It has no detectable effect on psychomotor performance.

HOW LONG TO TREAT?

Obesity is a life-long condition; the great majority who lose weight regain it. Thus it follows that treatment should similarly be long-term. Even modest weight loss, *provided it is maintained,* brings real advantages in terms of health. Longer term treatment with anorectic drugs maintains greater weight loss than placebo; this is reversed when the anorectic drugs are stopped (28,70). A good case could therefore be made out for continuing such treatment for several years, if not for life. Others take a similar view on this point (5,71). Such a perspective flies in the face of the usual recommendations that if anorectic drugs are to be used at all, they should only be given for a short time, say 3 to 4 months.

Short-term use (up to 6 months) is indicated in patients with significant obesity in whom there is a well-defined short-term objective such as an impending operation. Longer term use can be justified on theoretical and practical grounds to prevent weight regain (often referred to as weight maintenance), but we need more data on efficacy and safety before we can be categorical about recommending continuous treatment for over a year.

As obesity is a life-long problem, a much longer term view of management than is usually taken needs to be adopted at the outset. It is unlikely that any single tactic will work over the long term. What is required is a range of therapeutic interventions that can be combined and/or alternated over years. Such a policy of "ringing the changes" is likely to be more effective in maintaining motivation and prolonging success. Alternating treatments can also help: giving d-fenfluramine, following successful weight loss on a very-low-calorie diet, was much more successful than placebo in preventing weight regain. Thus for the management of severe obesity, a short (1 to 2 months) period on a very-low-calorie diet followed by a more lenient diet accompanied by anorectic drug treatment for, say 3 to 6 months, followed by an active exercise program together with regular behavioral modification instructions, followed by attendance at a weight-loss group for a while, may be more effective than relying on any one of these approaches alone. Imaginative choreography of all these various treatments is what is required. Anorectic drugs can play a key role in such a program.

CONCLUSIONS

Anorectic drugs have the property their name implies: they suppress appetite. This results in a reduction in food intake, which over time leads to a loss of weight. All the compounds licensed for use in obesity are more effective than placebo in helping obese patients lose weight when taken in conjunction with a calorie-restricted diet. Although the rate of weight loss falls with time, they continue to exert some effect on food intake, as weight regain occurs when they are stopped. They thus have a potential role in weight maintenance. There is little to choose between them in terms of efficacy. All the drugs listed are relatively safe and unlikely to give rise to dependence; they are very rarely used as drugs of abuse.

Anorectic drugs can play a valuable role in an overall weight-reduction program, but should only be prescribed as part of such a program. In many cases short-term use is sufficient, but longer term administration, either intermittently or in combination, is likely to be of benefit. The indications and disadvantages of long-term administration warrant further study.

Obesity poses a serious health hazard. Obese patients need all the help they can get in the difficult task of losing weight and keeping it down; anorectic drugs should certainly not be withheld on the basis of prejudice and misconceptions.

REFERENCES

1. British National Formulary. *Appetite suppressants.* London: British Medical Association and the Royal Pharmaceutical Society of Great Britain, 1992;160.
2. American Medical Association. Drugs used in obesity. *Drug Evaluations Subscriptions,* vol 3. 1990;6:1–616.
3. Royal College of Physicians. Obesity. *J R Coll Physicians* Lond 1983;17:3–58.
4. Silverstone JT. Intermittent treatment with anorectic drugs. *Practitioner* 1974;212:245–52.
5. Bray GA. Barriers to the treatment of obesity. *Ann Intern Med* 1991;115:152–3.
6. Ashwell M. A survey of patients' views on doctors' treatment of obesity. *Practitioner* 1973;211:653–61.
7. Weintraub M, Sriwatanakul K, Sundaresan PR, Weis OF, Dorn M. Extended release fenfluramine: patient acceptance and efficacy of evening dose. *Clin Pharmacol Ther* 1983;33:621–7.
8. Hoekenga MT, O'Dillon RH, Leyland HM. A comprehensive review of diethylpropion hydrochloride. In: Garattini S, Samanin R, eds. *Central mechanisms of anorectic drugs* New York: Raven Press, 1978.
9. Silverstone JT, Turner P, Humpherson PL. Direct measurement of the anorectic activity of diethylpropion (Tenuate Dospan). *J Clin Pharmacol* 1968;8[Suppl 3]:172–9.
10. Silverstone T, Kyriakides M. Clinical pharmacology of appetite. In: Silverstone T, eds. *Drugs and appetite.* London: Academic Press, 1982;93–123.
11. Sullivan AC, Comai K. Pharmacological treatment of obesity. *Int J Obes* 1978;2:167–89.
12. McKay RHG. Long-term use of diethylpropion in obesity. *Curr Med Res* 1973;1:489–93.
13. Munro JF. The clinical use of anti-obesity agents. In: Munro JF, eds. *The treatment of obesity.* Lancaster: MTP, 1979;85–121.
14. Munro JF, Ford FM. Drug treatment of obesity. In: Silverstone T, eds. *Drugs and appetite.* London: Academic Press, 1982;125–57.
15. Silverstone JT, Buckle RM. Obesity in diabetes: some considerations on treatment. *Am J Clin Nutr* 1966;19:158–67.
16. Silverstone JT, Cooper RM, Begg RR. A comparative trial of fenfluramine and diethylpropion in obesity. *Br J Clin Practitioners* 1970;24[Suppl 10]:423–5.
17. Allen GS. A double-blind trial of diethylpropion hydrochloride, mazindol and placebo in the treatment of exogenous obesity. *Curr Ther Res* 1977;22: 678–83.
18. Carabillo EA. USA drug abuse warning network. In: Garattini S, Samanin S, eds. *Central mechanisms of anorectic drugs.* New York: Raven Press, 1978.
19. Silverstone T. The anorectic effect of a long-acting preparation of phentermine (Duromine). *Psychopharmacoligia* 1972;25:315–20.
20. Truant AP, Olon LP, Cobb S. Phentermine resin as an adjunct in medical weight reduction: a controlled randomised double-blind prospective study. *Curr Ther Res* 1972;14:726–38.
21. Tuominen S, Hietula M, Kuusankoski M. Double-blind trial comparing fenfluramine, phentermine and dietary advice on treatment of obesity. *Int J Obes* 1990;14[Suppl 2]:138.
22. Campbell C, Bhalla IP, Steel JM, Duncan LJP. A controlled trial of phentermine in obese diabetic patients. *Practitioner* 1977;218:851–5.
23. Steel JM, Munro JF, Duncan LJP. A comparative trial of different regimes of fenfluramine and phentermine in obesity. *Practitioner* 1973;211:232–6.
24. Douglas A, Douglas JG, Robertson CE, Munro JF. Plasma phentermine levels, weight loss and side-effects. *Int J Obes* 1983;7[Suppl 6]:591–5.
25. Grapin B, Cohen A. Drug therapy in simple obesity: controlled trial of mazindol. *Intern Med Dig* 1974;9:15–21.
26. Atkinson RL, Greenway FL, Bray GA, Dahms WT, Molitch ME. Treatment of obesity: comparison of physician and non-physician therapists using pla-

cebo and anorectic drugs in a double-blind trial. *Int J Obes* 1977;1:113–20.

27. Onishi T. Clinical evaluation of mazindol, an anorexiant, on obesity. *Int J Obes* 1990;14[Suppl 2]:34.

28. Miach P, Thomson W, Doyle A, Louis W. Double-blind cross-over evaluation of mazindol in the treatment of obese hypertensive patients. *Med J Aust* 1976;2:378.

29. Bradley MJ, Blum NJ, Scheib RK. Mazindol in obesity with known cardiac disease. *J Int Med Res* 1974;2:347–54.

30. Lasagna L. Anorectic activity. In: *Phenylpropanolamine—a review*. New York: Wiley-Interscience, 1988;132–46.

31. Weintraub M, Ginsberg G, Stein E, Sundaresan P, Schuster B. Phenylpropanolamine OROS (Acutrim) vs placebo in combination with calorie restriction and physician managed behaviour modification. *Clin Pharmacol Ther* 1986;39:501–9.

32. Altschuler S, Conte A, Sebok M, Marlin R, Winick C. Three controlled trials of weight loss with phenylpropanolamine. *Int J Obes* 1982;6:549–56.

33. Liebson I, Bigelow G, Griffiths R, Funderburk F. Phenylpropanolamine: effects on subjective and cardiovascular variables at recommended over the counter dose levels. *J Clin Pharmacol* 1987;27:685–93.

34. Morgan JP, Funderburk F, Blackburn GL, Noble R. Subjective profile of phenylpropanolamine: absence of stimulant or euphorigenic effects at recommended dose levels. *J Clin Psychopharmacol* 1989;9:33–8.

35. Goodman R, Wright J, Barlascini C, McKenney J, Lambert C. The effect of phenylpropanolamine on ambulatory blood pressure. *Clin Pharmacol Ther* 1986;40:144–7.

36. Blackburn G, Morgan J, Lavin P, Noble R, Funderburk F. Determinants of the pressor effect of phenylpropanolamine in healthy subjects. *JAMA* 1989;261:3267–72.

37. Bradley MH, Raines J. The effects of phenylpropanolamine hydrochloride in overweight patients with controlled stable hypertension. *Curr Ther Res* 1989;46:74–84.

38. Silverstone T, ed. *Drugs and appetite*. London: Academic Press, 1982;23–39.

39. Fink M, Shapiro DM, Itil TM. EEG profiles of fenfluramine, amobarbital and dextroamphetamine in normal volunteers. *Psychopharmacologia* 1971;22:369–83.

40. Silverstone JT, Fincham J, Campbell DB. The anorectic activity of fenfluramine. *Postgrad Med J* 1975;51[Suppl 1]:171–4.

41. Campbell DB. Plasma concentration of fenfluramine and its metabolite, norfenfluramine, following single and repeated oral administration. *Br J Pharmacol* 1971;43:465–9.

42. Pinder RM, Brogden RN, Sawyer PR, Speight TM, Avery GS. Fenfluramine: a review of its pharmacological properties and therapeutic efficacy in obesity and diabetes mellitus. *Drugs* 1975;10:241–323.

43. Craighead LW, Stunkard A, O'Brien RM. Behavior therapy and pharmacotherapy for obesity. *Arch Gen Psychiatry* 1981;38:763–8.

44. Stunkard A, Rickels K, Hesbacher P. Fenfluramine in the treatment of obesity. *Lancet* 1973;1:503–5.

45. Silverstone T, Smith G, Richards R. A comparative evaluation of dextrofenfluramine and dl-fenfluramine on hunger, food intake, psychomotor function and side effects in normal human subjects. In: Bender A, Brookes L, eds. *Body weight control*. Edinburgh: Churchill Livingstone, 1987;240–6.

46. Goodall E, Feeney S, McGuirk J, Silverstone T. A comparison of the effects of d- and l-fenfluramine and d-amphetamine on energy and macronutrient intake in human subjects. *Psychopharmacology* 1992;106:221–7.

47. Goodall E, Silverstone T. Differential effect of d-fenfluramine and metergoline on food intake in human subjects. *Appetite* 1988;11:215–28.

48. Wurtman J, Wurtman R, Reynolds S, Tsay R, Chew B. Fenfluramine suppresses snack intake among carbohydrate cravers but not among non-carbohydrate cravers. *Int J Eating Disord* 1987;6:687–99.

49. Hill AJ, Blundell JE. Sensitivity of the appetite control system in obese subjects to nutritional and serotoninergic challenges. *Int J Obes* 1990;14:219–33.

50. Finer N, Craddock D, Lavielle R, Keen H. Dextrofenfluramine in the treatment of refractory obesity. *Curr Ther Res* 1985;38:847–54.

51. Sriwatanakul K, Yuthavong K, Kominor S. Double-blind study to determine the efficacy and safety of dexfenfluramine in the treatment of obesity. *Eur J Clin Pharmacol* [Suppl] 1989;36:A322.

52. Finer N, Craddock D, Lavielle R, Keen H. Prolonged weight loss with dexfenfluramine treatment in obese patients. *Diabetes Metab* 1987;13:598–602.

53. Van Gaal L, Vansant G, Vandevoorde K, Biasi B, De Leevw, I. Long-term evaluation of dexfenfluramine treatment in obese women. *Int J Obes* 1989;13[Suppl 1]:abst 141.

54. Guy-Grand B, Apfelbaum M, Crepaldi G, Gries A, Lefebvre P. International trial of long-term dexfenfluramine in obesity. *Lancet* 1989;2:1142–5.

55. Tauber-Lassen E, Damsbo P, Enrikson JE, Palmvig B, Beck-Nielsen H. Improvement of glycaemic control and weight loss in type 2 (non-insulin-dependent diabetics) after one year of dexfenfluramine treatment. *Diabetologica* 1990;33:abst A230.

56. Scheen AJ, Paolisso G, Salvatore T, Lefebvre PJ. Dexfenfluramine reduces insulin resistance independently of weight reduction in obese type 2 (non-insulin-dependent) diabetic patients. *Diabetologica* 1988;31:640A.

57. Goodall E, Oxtoby C, Richards R, Watkinson G, Brown D, Silverstone T. A clinical trial of the efficacy and acceptability of d-fenfluramine in the treatment of neuroleptic-induced obesity. *Br J Psychiatry* 1988;153:208–13.

58. Turner P. Dexfenfluramine: its place in weight control. *Drugs* 1990;39[Suppl 3]:53–62.

59. Fuller RW, Wong DT. Fluoxetine and serotoninergic appetite suppressant drugs. *Drug Dev Res* 1989;17:1–15.

60. McGuirk J, Silverstone T. The effect of the 5-HT reuptake inhibitor fluoxetine on food intake and body weight in healthy male subjects. *Int J Obes* 1990a;14:361–72.

61. McGuirk J, Silverstone T. Effects of fluoxetine on

appetite, food intake and body weight in obese subjects. *Int J Obes* 1990b;14[Suppl 2]:141.

62. Pijl H, Koppeschaar H, Meinders A, Willekens F, Op De Kamp I. Fluoxetine and dietary intake and composition. *Int J Obes* 1989;13[Suppl 2]:131–145 (abst).

63. Breum L, Moller S, Bjerre U, Jacobsen S. Effect of fluoxetine on amino acids and macro-nutrient selection in obese patients. *Int J Obes* 1990;14[Suppl 2]:141.

64. Levine L, Enas G, Thompson W, Byyny R, Daver A. Use of fluoxetine, a selective serotonin-uptake inhibitor in the treatment of obesity: a dose-response study (with a commentary by Michael Weintraub). *Int J Obes* 1989;13:635–45.

65. Marcus MD, Wing RR, Ewing L, Kern E, McDermott M. A double-blind, placebo controlled trial of fluoxetine plus behaviour modification in the treatment of obese binge-eaters and non-binge eaters. *Am J Psychiatry* 1990;147:876–81.

66. Rosenstock J, Cercone S, Koffler M, Ramirez L, Raskin P. The effects of the serotonin reuptake inhibitor fluoxetine on weight loss, glycaemic control and lipid levels in non-insulin dependent diabetes mellitus. *Diabetes* 1987;36[Suppl 1]:66A.

67. Wise S. Fluoxetine, efficacy and safety in treatment of obese type 2 (non-insulin-dependent) diabetes. *Diabetologica* 1989;32:557A.

68. Kutnowski M, Daubresse J, Friedman H, Kolanowski J, Krzentowski G. Eight weeks fluoxetine therapy in obese patients with impaired glucose tolerance. *Int J Obes* 1990;14[Suppl 2]:48.

69. Zerbe RL. Safety of fluoxetine in the treatment of obesity. *Int J Obes* 1987;11[Suppl 3]:191–9.

70. Guy-Grand B, Apfelbaum M, Crepaldi G, Gries A, Lefebvre P, Turner P. Effect of withdrawal of dexfenfluramine on body weight and food intake after a one year's administration. *Int J Obes* 1990;14[Suppl 2]:48.

71. Stunkard AJ. Anorectic agents lower a body weight set point. *Life Sci* 1982;30:2043–55.

Obesity: Theory and Therapy, Second Edition,
edited by A. J. Stunkard and T. A. Wadden.
Raven Press, Ltd., New York © 1993.

17

Preventing Relapse Following Treatment for Obesity

*Michael G. Perri and †Arthur M. Nezu

*Department of Clinical and Health Psychology, University of Florida, Gainesville, Florida
32610-0165; and †Department of Mental Health Sciences, Hahnemann University,
Philadelphia, Pennsylvania 19102-1192

Clinicians who treat obese individuals are well aware that helping patients to lose weight is but a preliminary skirmish in what for most patients is a life-long battle with obesity. Numerous studies have documented the problem of poor maintenance of weight loss following treatment for obesity. Indeed, long-term follow-ups often reveal that the *majority* of patients regain virtually the entire amount of weight loss in treatment, regardless of the specific therapy used (1–3). Such findings suggest that preventing relapse may be the most pressing challenge in the treatment of obesity. In this chapter, we view the problem of poor maintenance of weight loss from a biobehavioral perspective, and we summarize a series of research studies on interventions specifically designed to prevent weight-loss relapse. We also describe a continuous care/problem solving model that can be used as a guide to clinical decision making in the long-term management of obesity.

A BIOBEHAVIORAL PERSPECTIVE ON RELAPSE

Why do the majority of patients experience relapse following treatment of obesity? Poor maintenance of treatment-induced weight loss appears to stem from the interplay of biological and behavioral factors.

Treatments for obesity often fail because they do not adequately equip the patient to cope with the relentless physiological processes that compensate for weight loss and the negative psychological reactions that result from the inability to sustain weight loss.

Losing weight seems to trigger a variety of physiological mechanisms, such as increased energetic efficiency (4,5) and increased production of adipose tissue lipoprotein lipase (6), which prime the obese person for regaining weight. Moreover, continuous exposure to an environment rich in fattening foods, combined with a dieting-induced heightened sensitivity to palatable foods, further disposes the patient to lapses in dietary control (7). Thus, when "on their own" following weight-loss treatment, many patients become discouraged by the significant problems that they encounter in trying to maintain weight loss. Often, they attribute their lack of success to personal failings (8). Such attributions frequently lead to feelings of frustration and guilt, and sometimes to anxiety, depression, and anger. Many patients utilize ineffective means of coping with these distressful emotions. For example, some resort to rationalizations and avoidance, saying to themselves, "I'm too stressed out to deal with a diet right now, but on Monday, I'll get back on the wagon." Such an approach provides "permission" to deviate even further from behaviors required to sustain their weight loss, and an accumulation of broken resolutions to resume "appropriate" eating behaviors often precipitates an abandonment of the entire weight-loss effort. As a consequence, many obese patients ultimately regain much or all of the weight that they had lost in treatment.

RESEARCH ON THE PREVENTION OF RELAPSE

Given that a complex interaction of physiological and psychological factors makes long-term weight loss difficult to achieve, what interventions are available to help patients sustain the behavioral changes (i.e., decreased energy intake and increased energy expenditure) required for the maintenance of weight loss? In a series of prospective investigations, we have examined the effectiveness of several maintenance strategies, including: (a) continued patient–therapist contact following initial weight-loss treatment; (b) skills training to equip patients to cope more effectively with the challenges of the posttreatment period; (c) social influence programs to provide patients with enhanced social support after treatment; (d) increased physical activity to provide patients with positive physical and psychological effects that may enhance long-term success; and (e) multicomponent interventions that marshal several combinations of strategies to help patients sustain behavior change and maintain weight loss.

In each of our studies, the patients were mildly and moderately obese (i.e., 20 to 100% over ideal weight) volunteers who responded to announcements of a weight-loss research program. Our typical subject was a 45-year-old, middle-class, married, white woman who at the start of treatment weighed approximately 200 lb and was about 50% over ideal body weight. In each study, patients were treated initially with a conservative program consisting of behavior therapy and low-calorie diet (e.g., 1,200 kcal/day for women) and were then assigned randomly either to an experimental maintenance program or to a control condition with no additional therapeutic contact. Subjects in the control conditions in each study had no contact with their therapists following initial treatment except for periodic follow-up evaluations.

Continued Professional Contact and Skills Training

After undergoing weight-loss treatment, patients are faced with the challenge of maintaining behavioral changes accomplished in treatment or returning to prior patterns of eating and inactivity. Addressing this challenge requires ongoing vigilance and an active awareness of critical aspects of their eating and exercise. Posttreatment professional contacts may be a useful means of helping patients to be continuously mindful of their weight-loss progress. Such contacts may enhance motivation, and may also enable patients to reframe weight-loss difficulties in a positive and constructive fashion. The contacts can also provide an opportunity for trouble-shooting when difficulties in weight-loss maintenance arise.

Posttreatment therapist–patient contacts by *telephone* and *mail* can be used to provide professional support and advice during the period following initial treatment. Having patients mail to their therapists self-monitoring data, including information about eating, exercise, and weight, may enhance both their awareness and their maintenance of behaviors critical to weight control. Moreover, the use of frequent, posttreatment telephone contacts between therapists and patients has shown promise as an effective maintenance strategy across a variety of problem areas (9).

A number of researchers have noted that an effective maintenance program may also need to equip patients with a *new* set of abilities to succeed in the posttreatment period (10). Specifically, patients may need to learn the skills to anticipate, avoid, and cope with those circumstances that increase the risk of their experiencing a relapse (11,12). Following initial weight-loss treatment, patients inevitably face a wide variety of circumstances in which they are tempted to exceed a prescribed calorie goal or deviate from the weight-management procedures that they learned in treatment. If the patient does not have the ability to handle the "high-risk situation" effectively, he or she may experience a slip or lapse in self-control. Furthermore, if the person interprets the lapse as evidence of failure at self-control, he or she is likely to experience a sense of hopelessness and a decrease in self-efficacy. Thus a seemingly minor slip may initiate the start of a full-blown relapse.

Marlatt and Gordon (11) have recommended several specific strategies to prevent or minimize relapse following treatment. First, it is necessary to teach patients to recognize and identify those situations that pose a high risk for relapse. Second, training in problem solving can be used to help patients generate coping strategies for high-risk situations. Third, patients require practice in coping with actual high-risk situations. Finally, it is important to teach patients cognitive strategies to overcome guilt feelings and the sense of failure often associated with slips.

In the first study in our series (13), we evaluated whether providing patients with relapse prevention training (B + R), or posttreatment therapist contacts by mail and telephone (B + C), or the combination of both strategies (B + R + C) would enhance the long-term maintenance of weight loss, compared to behavioral treatment alone (B). The results showed that neither strategy by itself

improved the maintenance of weight loss, but when the two approaches were combined, significantly better maintenance of weight loss was observed ($p < 0.05$). The findings indicated that the combination of relapse prevention training plus posttreatment contact was the only condition in which patients did *not* suffer significant relapse over a 12-month follow-up period (Table 1). Self-report data suggested that the superior performance of participants in this condition may have resulted from their greater use during follow-up of key strategies including self-monitoring, stimulus control, and exercise.

The superior performance of the group that received the posttreatment contact strategy *and* relapse prevention training suggests that the *content* of patient–therapist interactions may be a crucial factor in posttreatment success. Therapists' advice about specific coping techniques may have helped patients to negotiate and avoid relapses. Thus, when combined with training targeted at the specific problems of the posttreatment period, therapist contact by mail and telephone appears to have potential as an effective maintenance strategy.

Social Support and a Multicomponent Maintenance Program

Effective maintenance of weight loss may require a *multifaceted* set of posttreatment strategies. Stuart (14) suggested that effective maintenance programs require a combination of strategies, including continued self-

TABLE 1. *Mean weight losses (kg) for B + R + C, B + R, B + C, and B alone*

Time of assessment	Condition[a]			
	B + R + C (n = 17)	B + R (n = 15)	B + C (n = 15)	B (n = 21)
Posttreatment	9.63	8.55	8.72	7.51
Follow-up (months)				
3	11.76	7.25	10.55	8.49
6	10.78	4.90	8.69	7.65
12	10.34	2.96	5.77	6.28

[a] B, behavior therapy; R, relapse prevention training; C, posttreatment therapist contact. (Adapted from ref. 34, with permission.)

monitoring of positive behaviors, frequent posttreatment patient–therapist contacts, and active patient participation in self-help groups.

In our second study (15), we incorporated social support into a maintenance package by instructing patients how to form "buddy groups" based on the structure and procedures of a problem-solving approach (16). Following initial treatment, patients received instructions to meet regularly, to monitor each other's weight, to use praise to encourage weight loss progress, and to problem solve as a group when an individual was experiencing difficulties with weight-loss efforts. In addition, patients in the multicomponent maintenance program were asked to mail weekly postcards to their therapists specifying details of their weight-loss progress. The therapists, in turn, made brief weekly phone calls to these patients to provide additional support and guidance during the year following treatment.

The effects of the multicomponent maintenance program (B + M) were compared with a standard program of behavioral treatment (B) over the course of a 21-month follow-up period. The results showed that the multicomponent program of posttreatment social support combined with continued self-monitoring and patient–therapist contacts significantly enhanced the maintenance of weight loss ($p < 0.05$; Table 2). This positive finding was tempered, however, by the modest amount of weight loss maintained and the substantial cost of therapist time to provide telephone contacts with patients for an entire year following treatment.

Exercise and a Multicomponent Maintenance Program

Exercise is often associated with long-term success in weight management (17–19). Exercise can enhance the treatment of obesity by increasing the rate at which fat is lost while decreasing the loss of lean body mass. Exercise may also facilitate weight loss by increasing metabolic rate. The psychological bene-

TABLE 2. *Mean weight losses (kg) for behavior therapy plus multicomponent treatment and for behavior therapy alone*

	Condition	
Time of assessment	Behavior therapy plus multicomponent program (n = 26)	Behavior therapy (n = 17)
Posttreatment	6.13	5.64
Follow-up (months)		
3	8.15	6.95
6	8.02	5.69
9	7.75	3.10
15	5.82	2.09
21	4.56	0.36

(Adapted from ref. 34, with permission.)

fits of regular exercise include improvements in mood and self-concept and an increased sense of well-being (20). In the third study in our series (21), we examined whether the additions of an aerobic exercise regimen during treatment and a multicomponent maintenance program following treatment would improve the efficacy of behavior therapy for obesity. The goals of this study were first, to increase the magnitude of initial weight loss in behavioral treatment and second, to improve the maintenance of weight loss by replicating the effects of the multicomponent program developed in our previous study. The effects of an aerobic program consisting of two specific types of activity (i.e., brisk walking and stationary cycling) with fixed levels of intensity, duration, and frequency were tested, and the impact of a multicomponent maintenance program was also examined. Thus patients were randomly assigned to one of four conditions: behavior therapy (B), behavior therapy plus aerobic exercise (B + A), behavior therapy plus a multicomponent maintenance program (B + M), or behavior therapy plus aerobic exercise and a multicomponent maintenance program (B + A + M).

The results showed that the groups that received the aerobic exercise program lost significantly more weight than those that did not. The net effect of the aerobic exercise program was a 29% improvement in weight loss beyond that accomplished in the behavior therapy only condition ($p < 0.001$; Table 3). At each follow-up assessment, patients who received the multicomponent maintenance program demonstrated significantly better weight loss progress than subjects in the behavior therapy only condition (Table 3). The maintenance program appeared to be effective because of its participants' greater adherence to behavioral self-management procedures (22). The combination of continued monitoring of key behaviors, frequent phone contacts with therapists, and peer group support appears to increase adherence and foster maintenance of weight loss.

Posttreatment Therapist Contact and Peer Support

In our next study (23), we tested the specific effectiveness of peer support versus therapist contact as maintenance strategies for weight loss. The major question that we addressed was whether maintenance programs of peer support (B + P) or therapist contact (B + T) would foster better weight-loss progress compared with a control condition (B) in which patients received no additional contacts during the period following treatment.

The peer-support group maintenance program consisted of a series of 15 biweekly (i.e., every other week) meetings that implemented the structure and procedures of a problem-solving treatment within the context of a self-help group. In the therapist-contact maintenance program, patients also attended 15 biweekly sessions. In these sessions, therapists directed the patients' use of problem-solving strategies to cope with difficulties in weight-loss maintenance.

At the conclusion of the maintenance program (i.e., 7 months posttreatment), the therapist-contact group showed significantly better weight-loss progress than the peer support and control conditions (Table 4). Both the peer support and control groups regained weight during this period, with the amounts regained not differing significantly from each other. Although subjects in all groups tended to regain weight from the 7-month to 18-month follow-up, both the therapist-contact and peer-support programs showed better weight loss maintenance than the control group ($p < 0.05$; Table 4). These results suggest that posttreatment programs consisting of either peer group or therapist contacts can foster better long-term weight loss progress than therapy that does not include a posttreatment maintenance program.

Posttreatment Therapist Contact and Relapse Prevention Training

In our next study (24), we tested the effectiveness of relapse prevention training versus frequent therapist contacts as maintenance strategies for weight loss. The major question we addressed was whether *year-long* posttreatment maintenance programs consisting of either comprehensive training to prevent and overcome relapse (B + R) or a high frequency of therapist contacts (B + T) would

TABLE 3. *Mean weight losses (kg) for B + A + M, B + M, B + A, and B alone*

Time of assessment	Condition[a]			
	B + A + M (*n* = 17)	B + M (*n* = 15)	B + A (*n* = 15)	B (*n* = 21)
Posttreatment	10.96	8.60	10.25	7.85
Follow-up (months)				
3	12.30	9.90	9.67	6.28
6	11.45	9.57	8.40	3.98
12	9.67	6.78	5.15	0.66
18	7.59	5.07	3.07	0.95

[a] B, behavior therapy; A, aerobic exercise program; M, multicomponent maintenance program. (Adapted from ref. 34, with permission.)

TABLE 4. *Mean weight losses (kg) for B + T,*
B + P, and B alone

Time of assessment	Condition[a]		
	B + T ($n = 27$)	B + P ($n = 32$)	B ($n = 16$)
Posttreatment	10.70	10.90	10.26
Follow-up (months)			
7	11.54	9.31	7.82
18	6.39	6.47	3.07

[a] B, behavior therapy; T, therapist-contact program;
P, peer-support program. (Adapted from ref. 34, with
permission.)

yield better weight loss progress compared
with behavioral treatment without posttreatment contact (B). Both the relapse prevention and therapist-contact maintenance programs were conducted in 26 biweekly
meetings scheduled during the year after initial treatment. The relapse prevention program included the following procedures:
identification of high-risk situations; training
in problem-solving; practice in coping with
high-risk situations; and the development of
cognitive coping strategies for overcoming
setbacks. The therapist-contact maintenance
program consisted of therapist-led problem-
solving sessions aimed at helping patients
maintain the behavioral changes accomplished during the initial treatment period.

At the 6- and 12-month follow-up evaluations, both maintenance conditions showed
significantly better weight-loss progress than
the no-posttreatment-contact condition ($p <
0.05$), but the differences in weight loss be-
tween the relapse prevention and therapist-
contact maintenance programs were not statistically significant (Table 5). Collectively,

TABLE 5. *Mean weight losses (kg) for B + R,*
B + T, and B alone

Time of assessment	Condition[a]		
	B + R ($n = 29$)	B + T ($n = 33$)	B ($n = 26$)
Posttreatment	8.89	7.98	9.32
Follow-up (months)			
6	9.65	10.13	7.00
12	7.33	9.42	4.52

[a] B, behavior therapy; T, therapist-contact program;
R, relapse prevention program. (Adapted from ref. 35,
with permission.)

these findings suggest that structured posttreatment programs can facilitate the maintenance of weight loss and that a high frequency of therapist contacts may be as
effective as relapse prevention training in
helping patients to maintain weight losses accomplished in treatment.

Posttreatment Therapist Contact, Social Influence, and Exercise

In the sixth study in our series (25), the
effectiveness of four year-long maintenance
programs for the management of obesity was
compared with a control condition that received initial behavioral treatment only (B).
The four maintenance conditions were: posttreatment therapist contact (B + C); posttreatment therapist contact plus an aerobic
exercise maintenance program (B + C + A);
posttreatment therapist contact plus a social
influence maintenance program (B + C + S);
and posttreatment therapist contact plus a
combination of both the aerobic exercise and
social influence maintenance programs (B +
C + A + S).

All four maintenance programs were conducted in 26 biweekly sessions scheduled
during the 12 months following initial treatment. Patients in the B + C condition received the initial treatment plus the year-long
program of therapist contacts. These subjects
were asked to maintain their aerobic exercise
levels at 80 minutes per week, i.e., 20 minutes
a day, 4 days a week.

Patients in the B + C + A condition received the initial behavioral treatment and
the posttreatment therapist contact programs
and also received an aerobic exercise maintenance program consisting of a new set of exercise goals for the posttreatment period and
therapist-led exercise bouts during the biweekly posttreatment sessions. During the
maintenance program, the prescribed frequency and duration of aerobic exercise were
increased gradually from 80 to 180 minutes a
week (i.e., from 20 minutes a day, 4 days a
week, to 30 minutes a day, 6 days a week).

Patients in the B + C + S condition received the initial behavioral treatment and the posttreatment therapist-contact program, and they received a multifaceted program of social influence strategies designed to enhance motivation and to provide incentives for continued weight-loss progress. The social influence program included monetary group contingencies for program adherence and continued weight loss, active patient participation in preparing and delivering lectures on maintaining weight loss, and instructions on how to provide peer support for weight loss through ongoing telephone contacts and peer group meetings during the posttreatment period.

Patients in the fourth experimental condition (B + C + A + S) received the initial behavioral treatment and the posttreatment therapist contact programs. In addition, these participants also received both the aerobic exercise and social influence maintenance programs previously described.

At the 12-month follow-up, all four experimental conditions demonstrated significantly better maintenance of weight loss than the behavior therapy only condition ($p < 0.01$). The superiority of the four maintenance conditions was still evident at the 18-month follow-up assessment (Table 6). Moreover, on average, participants in the four experimental conditions maintained 82.7% of their mean posttreatment losses, whereas patients in the behavior therapy alone condition maintained only 33.3% of their original weight loss. No significant differences between the four experimental conditions were

evident at the follow-up evaluations. However, the B + C + A + S condition was the only group that showed a significant *additional* weight loss during the follow-up period ($p < 0.05$). From posttreatment to the 6-month follow-up evaluation, subjects in the B + C + A + S condition demonstrated an additional mean weight loss of 4.1 kg. Furthermore, at the 18-month follow-up, this group maintained 99% of its mean posttreatment weight loss.

These results suggest that year-long maintenance programs can help sustain behavior change and weight-loss progress begun during the initial treatment period. Moreover, the magnitude of long-term weight losses sustained by maintenance program participants at the 18-month follow-up (i.e., $M = 10.7$ kg) compares favorably with results reported in the obesity literature. These findings indicate that an intensive therapist-led program directed toward teaching patients how to overcome specific problems of the posttreatment period can indeed enhance the long-term maintenance of weight loss. The results also suggest that the combination of high-frequency exercise coupled with intensive support from peers and therapists holds potential as a multifaceted approach to improving the long-term management of obesity.

Research on helping patients to sustain the behavioral changes required to maintain weight loss is in the early stages of development. Our work represents an initial foray that has suggested directions for future investigations. In many cases, successful long-term management of obesity may require mainte-

TABLE 6. *Mean weight losses (kg) for B + C + A + S, B + C + A, B + C + S, B + C, and B alone*

Time of assessment	Condition[a]				
	B + C + A + S (*n* = 17)	B + C + A (*n* = 15)	B + C + S (*n* = 15)	B + C (*n* = 21)	B (*n* = 16)
Posttreatment	13.67	13.05	11.34	13.17	10.80
Follow-up (months)					
6	17.75	15.19	13.54	15.79	8.94
12	15.70	12.97	13.35	12.88	5.67
18	13.54	9.14	8.43	11.41	3.60

[a] B, behavior therapy; C, posttreatment therapist contact; A, aerobic exercise maintenance program; S, social influence maintenance program. (Adapted from ref. 34, with permission.)

nance programs and periods of follow-up care numbering *years* rather than months. There is little research available on the effectiveness of maintenance programs that extend beyond 1 year. One notable exception is an investigation by Björvell and Rössner (26,27) that examined the impact of a comprehensive 4-year-long, continuous care approach to the management of obesity.

Björvell and Rössner (26) posited that successful management of obesity would require long-term care and a multifaceted approach to treatment. Thus they constructed an intensive, comprehensive, and long-lasting treatment regimen, including behavior therapy, nutritional training, and supervised exercise. Participants in the comprehensive treatment program included 53 women who at the start of treatment averaged 245 lb and were 69% over ideal body weight. Initial treatment was conducted during a 6-week period of inpatient hospitalization. Treatment was conducted in small groups of five patients. Participants had two behavioral treatment sessions per week that included standard behavior therapy techniques plus training in relapse prevention strategies, and they had three supervised exercise sessions per week plus a program of additional activities that included walking and swimming. The subjects also received extensive training from a dietitian in techniques of low-calorie cooking. In addition, during the 6-week course of their hospitalization, the patients were placed on a very-low-calorie diet consisting of approximately 600 calories per day (including 60 g of protein, 16 g of fat, and 54 g of carbohydrate).

Following this initial phase of treatment, participants received a 4-year-long maintenance program. All patients were expected to attend one of two group sessions that were offered each week. Therapists made vigorous efforts to contact any patient who missed a scheduled appointment. Posttreatment contacts by both telephone and mail were used to keep patients actively involved in participating in the maintenance sessions. Finally, whenever it appeared that a patient was in jeopardy of a relapse, the investigators had

the individual return to the hospital for short-term (i.e., 2-week) "refresher" courses of treatment. Over the 4 years of the investigation, virtually all the participants returned for at least one course of rehospitalization.

Table 7 presents the results for the women who underwent the four years of comprehensive treatment in the Björvell and Rössner (26,27) study. It is not surprising that the women lost a significant amount of weight after 6 weeks of inpatient treatment; the long-term results, however, are both surprising and heartening. At 1 year, the subjects improved their initial weight losses on average by 50%, and at the 4-year assessment, the participants had maintained 77% of their peak losses. Even more impressive are the 10-year results, showing that the subjects succeeded in maintaining an average weight loss of almost 10 kg 6 years after the end of active treatment. These findings strongly suggest that providing obese patients with an intensive program of continuous care can result in successful long-term management of obesity.

Thus the results from research on weight-loss maintenance strategies present a "good news/bad news" picture regarding the long-term treatment of obesity. The bad news is that *without* a maintenance program, patients generally abandon the self-management strategies taught in treatment and gradually regain weight. The good news is that when initial therapy is supplemented with posttreatment care, patients exhibit greater adherence to weight-loss techniques and better maintenance of weight loss. Indeed, the most consistent finding in our studies was that structured programs of posttreatment

TABLE 7. *Mean weight losses (kg) over 10 years for women who participated in 4-year comprehensive treatment program for obesity*

Assessment	N	M
6 weeks	53	10.0
1 year	50	14.5
2 years	49	12.3
3 years	46	10.5
4 years	47	11.5
10 years	42	9.5

Adapted from refs. 26 and 27.

therapist contact helped patients to maintain weight-loss progress. Posttreatment contact appears to be effective because the longer patients remain in contact with health-care professionals, the longer they adhere to the eating and exercise habits needed to sustain weight loss (28).

Effective maintenance programs appear to require a multifaceted set of strategies. Continued self-monitoring of eating and exercise behaviors seems to be a prerequisite for continued weight-loss progress, and a high frequency of patient–therapist contacts following treatment also appears essential to maintenance. Although skills training and social support strategies by themselves may not be sufficient to help patients sustain maintenance on their own, these strategies may be helpful to particular patients and may be useful components of multifaceted maintenance programs. Exercise can play a key role in the management of obesity. A program of regular physical activity can facilitate both initial and long-term weight loss. Moreover, the results from our sixth study (25) demonstrated that a maintenance program that included therapist contact combined with high-frequency exercise and social support produced significant *additional* weight loss during the posttreatment period.

After initial treatment, most patients require the help of a health-care professional to cope with the array of problems they face in maintaining their weight-loss progress. Posttreatment contacts that utilize a problem-solving approach can provide a basic structure for therapists to assist patients in coping with the challenges of the posttreatment period. In the next section, we describe a problem-solving model that can serve as a useful guide to clinical decision making in the long-term management of obesity.

TOWARD A CONTINUOUS CARE/ PROBLEM SOLVING MODEL OF OBESITY MANAGEMENT

A common question raised by clinicians who treat obese patients is "What techniques can I use to help my patients maintain weight loss?" At the present time, attempts to match individuals to specific maintenance strategies are bound to rely more heavily on the clinician's judgment than on a "cookbook" derived from the empirical literature (29,30). Under such circumstances, a problem-solving approach can be utilized to guide the clinician's decision making (31), and a formal model of decision making may help the clinician determine the most appropriate treatment strategy for a given patient under a specific set of circumstances (32). Let us consider how a problem-solving model of decision making might be applied to the long-term management of obesity (33). Within this framework, clinical decision making can be viewed as comprised of five component processes: (a) problem orientation; (b) problem definition and formulation; (c) generation of alternatives; (d) decision making; and (e) solution implementation and verification.

Problem Orientation

This initial process represents the response set that the clinician uses in relation to understanding and reacting to problems. In working with obese patients, it is helpful for clinicians to adopt an orientation that recognizes several key features of the etiology and treatment of obesity. Specifically, clinicians must recognize that obesity is a *multidetermined* condition and that the particular biological, psychological, and social factors that contribute to poor maintenance of weight loss may vary from patient to patient, and may also differ from time to time within the same patient. Consequently, clinical interventions are more likely to be effective when conceptualized as strategies based on an *idiographic* assessment of a particular individual rather than as techniques uniformly applied across all patients. In addition, since obesity constitutes a *chronic* rather than an acute problem, clinicians must orient obese patients to understand the need for long-term management of their obesity. Similar to the diabetic or hypertensive patient, obese individuals may never be cured of their "disease." Rather they must be resigned to keeping their condition under control through *active efforts* at self-management for the *rest of their lives.* Accordingly, clinicians must be prepared to structure treatments that will provide patients with long-term, perhaps life-long, assistance in managing their obesity. Long-term success is unlikely unless the obese patient develops a life style that sustains the decreased energy intake and increased energy expenditure necessary to maintain a lower weight.

Problem Definition and Formulation

Whereas the problem orientation component may be viewed as a general set or approach to the problem of obesity, the next four problem-solving processes may be viewed as specific skills or tasks for the clinician to accomplish in the care of the obese patient. The major objectives of the problem definition and formulation task are to identify the particular aspects of the situation that make it a problem for a given patient, and to specify a realistic set of goals or objectives. Given individual differences among patients, it is essential that problems be idiographically defined. To increase the probability of accurately defining the problem, the clinician and patient need to work together to: (a) seek all relevant facts about the problem; (b) describe these facts in clear and unambiguous terms; (c) separate objective information from unverified inferences; (d) identify those factors that actually make the situation a problem; and (e) set a series of realistic and attainable goals.

"I'm depressed because I stopped losing weight" is a common "problem" reported by patients during the period following initial weight-loss treatment. In deciding what to do in this situation, the clinician needs to define the problem accurately by assessing a variety of variables, including: the patient's *affect,* to determine whether a significant change in mood has occurred; the patient's *behavior,* to evaluate whether the individual's level of calo-

ric intake and expenditure would be expected to produce a weight change; the patient's *cognitions,* to determine whether expectations for a weight loss are realistic in the given situation; and the patient's *social circumstances,* to determine the impact of significant others on the patient's thoughts, feelings, and actions. A full and accurate formulation of the patient's problem will enhance the clinician's chances of successfully helping the patient to resolve the problem.

Generation of Alternatives

The next task for the clinician is to make available as many potential solutions as possible and to maximize the likelihood that the most effective alternatives will be among them. Accordingly, it is helpful for clinicians to initially *defer judgment* while "brainstorming" to develop a number of potential solutions. The more alternatives that are produced, the greater the likelihood that effective solutions will be generated. Moreover, higher quality ideas will be generated if the clinician defers critical evaluation until after an exhaustive list of possible solutions has been compiled.

Patients often expect that there is *one* "right answer" for a weight problem or that a solution that has worked in the past will work in the present. Thus, an individual who is distressed over not losing weight during the period following initial treatment may become convinced that further weight loss is only possible through indefinite use of a very-low-calorie diet (e.g., 400 kcal/day). If the clinician and patient conduct a thorough assessment and define the problem in terms of the patient's *affective* response to not losing weight, then an appropriate goal for generation of alternatives would be potential solutions that can help the patient "feel better" about him- or herself while coping with the weight problem. In generating potential solutions to achieve this goal, it is often helpful for the clinician and patient to develop a variety of *strategies* (i.e., general courses of action to resolve the identified problem) and *tactics* (i.e., specific steps to implement the strategy in a particular situation). Thus, in uncritically brainstorming for a large number of potential solutions, the clinician and patient can generate a wide range of possible strategies and tactics, as in the brief example described below:

Strategy 1: improve physical appearance

Tactics: get a new hair style; color your hair; go to an expensive beauty parlor; get a facial; get a make-up consultation; learn to use make-up to make your face look thinner; get a manicure; get a pedicure; go to a tanning salon; get a color analysis

Strategy 2: use exercise for self-improvement

Tactics: take up jogging; sign up for a tennis class; join a bowling league; buy a Jane Fonda videotape; buy an exercise bike; buy a 10-speed bike; join a bicycle club; walk 2 miles a day; run 2 miles a day; learn how to use free weights; join a health spa; learn how to use a universal exercise machine

Strategy 3: work on self-acceptance

Tactics: say to yourself, "It doesn't matter how I look"; refuse to look in the mirror; refuse to buy new clothes; look in the mirror and say to yourself, "You're all right just the way you are"; make up a list of ten good things about yourself; say to yourself "It's not awful to be overweight"; say to yourself, "There are a lot of neat things that I like about me."

Decision Making

The clinician's objectives in the decision-making process are to evaluate the potential solutions, select the most effective alternatives for implementation, and develop an overall solution plan. It is important that the clinician assess the *likelihood* that the patient will actually implement a particular alternative. Then, in judging the *value* of various

alternatives, the clinician and patient should consider the short- and long-term consequences of each alternative for both the patient and for significant others in the patient's life. By conducting a cost-benefit analysis of various alternatives, the clinician and patient can decide upon a course of action that has a high probability of being implemented and producing positive consequences.

In weighing the relative costs and benefits associated with a potential course of action, the clinician can consider the impact of potential solutions across a number of categories, including: (a) *time/effort*—the amount of personal time and effort involved in implementing an alternative and the extent to which it might impinge upon time committed for other important personal concerns; (b) *emotional cost/gain*—the emotional ramifications that the individual might incur by implementing a particular alternative; (c) *consistency with patient's values*—the extent to which potential courses of action will be consistent with the patient's moral and ethical value system; (d) *effects on personal growth*—the impact of potential solutions on the patient's sense of achievement, self-esteem, and self-efficacy; (e) *physical well-being*—the effect a potential course of action might have on the patient's health; (f) *effects on family and friends*—the impact that potential solutions will have on those people involved in significant relationships with the patient; and (g) *effects on others in the social environment*—the effects of possible courses of action on coworkers, neighbors, or others in the patient's social network.

Solution Implementation and Verification

The objectives of this task are threefold: (a) to implement the proposed solution; (b) to observe the actual consequences that occur after carrying out the solution; and (c) to evaluate the effectiveness of the solution. Once the clinician and patient decide upon a course of action, it is essential that they agree upon a means of monitoring the implementation of the plan to determine its effectiveness. Although weight change would appear to be the most likely measure of outcome, it is generally more helpful to include additional measures to evaluate whether changes in certain hypothesized moderating factors (e.g., caloric intake, minutes of exercise, attendance at sessions, etc.) lead to the expected change or maintenance of weight.

In the evaluation process, the clinician compares the observed outcome with the desired outcome initially specified in the problem definition and formulation step. If this match is satisfactory, then the problem can be considered resolved. If the match is *not* satisfactory, the clinician then needs to discover the source of the discrepancy. The actual difficulties may involve suboptimal performance of the solution response by the patient, misapplication of certain aspects of the problem-solving process itself, or both. For example, the discrepancy may be due to deficient performance by the patient, and the clinician and patient may need to improve upon the means of solution implementation. It may be, however, that the problem was not adequately defined and formulated, or that various mediating factors that contribute negatively to treatment outcome were not previously identified. Additionally, it is possible that insufficient ideas were initially generated or that the consequences of the solution were not evaluated accurately. These types of discrepancies between expected outcome and actual outcome highlight the need for the clinician to return to earlier stages in the problem-solving process. The therapist may want to redefine and reformulate the problem or identify an alternative strategy to the one already implemented. Thus continuous monitoring and evaluation of the effectiveness of maintenance strategies is critical to achieving long-term success in weight control.

CONCLUSIONS

In this chapter, we examined the problem of poor maintenance of weight loss from a biobehavioral perspective. We argued that a complex interplay of biological and behavioral factors contributes to the poor maintenance of weight loss that occurs following treatment for obesity. We suggested that treatments for obesity often fail because they do not adequately prepare patients to deal with (a) the relentless physiological processes that compensate for weight loss, and (b) the negative psychological reactions that result from the patient's failure to maintain weight loss.

In this chapter, we also summarized a series of research studies on interventions specifically designed to prevent weight-loss relapse. Our review showed that when initial therapy for obesity is supplemented with posttreatment care, patients exhibit greater adherence to weight-loss techniques and better maintenance of weight loss. Indeed, the accumulated research evidence reveals that the longer patients remain in contact with health-care professionals, the longer they adhere to the eating and exercise habits needed to sustain weight loss.

In the final section of this chapter, we presented a continuous care/problem-solving model of obesity management. We argued that the clinician must view his or her role as that of an *active problem solver,* who is prepared to aid the patient systematically and continuously in identifying effective strategies to sustain the behavioral changes needed for maintenance of weight loss. Accordingly, we described a problem-solving approach to clinical decision making that health-care professionals can use to help their patients achieve success in the long-term management of obesity.

REFERENCES

1. Bennett, W. Dietary treatments of obesity. In: Wurtman RJ, Wurtman JJ, eds. *Human obesity.* New York: New York Academy of Sciences, 1987;55–65.
2. Kramer FM, Jeffery RW, Forster JL, Snell MK. Long-term follow-up of behavioral treatment for obesity: patterns of weight gain among men and women. *Int J Obes* 1989;13:123–36.
3. Wadden TA, Sternberg JA, Letizia KA, Stunkard AJ, Foster GA. Treatment of obesity by very low

calorie diet, behavior therapy, and their combination: A five-year perspective. *Int J Obes* 1989; 13:39–46.

4. Bray GA. Effect of caloric restriction on energy expenditure in obese patients. *Lancet* 1969;2:397–8.

5. Geissler CA, Miller DS, Shah M. The daily metabolic rate of the post-obese and the lean. *Am J Clin Nutr* 1987;45:914–20.

6. Kern PA, Ong JM, Saffari B, Carty J. The effects of weight loss on the activity and expression of adipose tissue lipoprotein lipase in very obese humans. *N Engl J Med* 1969;322:1053–9.

7. Rodin J, Schank D, Striegel-Moore R. Psychological features of obesity. *Med Clin North Am* 1989; 73:47–66.

8. Marlatt GA. Relapse prevention: theoretical rationale and overview of the model. In: Marlatt GA, Gordon JR, eds. *Relapse prevention: maintenance strategies in the treatment of addictive behaviors.* New York: Guilford, 1985;3–70.

9. Spevak PA. Maintenance of therapy gains: strategies, problems, and progress. *JSAS Cat Select Doc Psychol* 1981;11,35 (no. 2255).

10. Wadden TA, Bell ST. Obesity. In: Bellack AS, Hersen M, Kazdin AE, eds. *International handbook of behavior modification and therapy,* vol II. New York: Plenum, 1990;449–73.

11. Brownell KD, Marlatt GA, Lichtenstein E, Wilson GT. Understanding and preventing relapse. *Am Psychol* 1986;41:765–82.

12. Marlatt GA, Gordon JR, eds. *Relapse prevention: maintenance strategies in the treatment of addictive behaviors.* New York: Guilford Press, 1985.

13. Perri MG, Shapiro RM, Ludwig WW, Twentyman CT, McAdoo WG. Maintenance strategies for the treatment of obesity: an evaluation of relapse prevention training and posttreatment contact by mail and telephone. *J Consult Clin Psychol* 1984; 52:404–13.

14. Stuart RB. Weight loss and beyond: are they taking it off and keeping it off? In: Davidson PO, Davidson SM, eds. *Behavioral medicine: changing health lifestyles.* New York: Brunner/Mazel, 1980;151–94.

15. Perri MG, McAdoo WG, Spevak PA, Newlin DB. Effect of a multicomponent maintenance program on long-term weight loss. *J Consult Clin Psychol* 1984;52:480–1.

16. D'Zurilla TJ, Nezu AM. Social problem solving in adults. In: Kendall PC, ed. *Advances in cognitive-behavioral research and therapy,* vol 1. New York: Academic Press, 1982;202–74.

17. Colvin RH, Olson SB. A descriptive analysis of men and women who have lost weight and are highly successful at maintaining the loss. *Addict Behav* 1983;8:287–96.

18. Katahn M, Pleas J, Thackrey M, Wallston KA. Relationship of eating and activity reports to follow-up weight maintenance in the massively obese. *Behav Ther* 1982;13:521–8.

19. Kayman S, Bruvold W, Stern JS. Maintenance and relapse after weight loss in women: behavioral aspects. *Am J Clin Nutr* 1990;52:800–7.

20. Folkins CH, Sime WE. Physical fitness training and mental health. *Am Psychol* 1981;36:373–89.

21. Perri MG, McAdoo WG, McAllister DA, Lauer JB, Yancey DZ. Enhancing the efficacy of behavior therapy for obesity: effects of aerobic exercise and a multicomponent maintenance program. *J Consult Clin Psychol* 1986;54:670–5.

22. Stalonas PM, Kirschenbaum DS. Behavioral treatments for obesity: eating habits revisited. *Behav Ther* 1985;16:1–14.

23. Perri MG, McAdoo WG, McAllister DA, Lauer JB, Jordan RC, Yancey DZ. Effects of peer support and therapist contact on long-term weight loss. *J Consult Clin Psychol* 1987;55:615–7.

24. Perri MG, McKelvey WF, Schein RL, Renjilian DA, Viegener BJ, Nezu AM. Relapse prevention training versus frequent therapist contacts as weight-loss maintenance strategies. Paper presented at the annual meeting of the Association for Advancement of Behavior Therapy, San Francisco, CA, 1990.

25. Perri MG, McAllister DA, Gange JJ, Jordan RC, McAdoo WG, Nezu AM. Effects of four maintenance programs on the long-term management of obesity. *J Consult Clin Psychol* 1988;56:529–34.

26. Björvell H, Rössner S. Long-term treatment of severe obesity: four year follow-up of results of combined behavioural modification programme. *Br Med J* 1985;291:379–82.

27. Björvell H, Rössner S. A ten year follow-up of weight change in severely obese subjects treated in a behavioural modification program. *Int J Obes* 1990;14[Suppl 2]:88.

28. Perri MG, Nezu AM, Patti ET, McCann KL. Effect of length of treatment on weight loss. *J Consult Clin Psychol* 1989;57:450–2.

29. Brownell KD, Wadden TA. The heterogeneity of obesity: fitting treatments to individuals. *Behav Ther* 1991;22:153–77.

30. Foreyt JP, Goodrick GK. Factors common to successful therapy for the obese patient. *Med Sci Sports Exer* 1991;23:292–7.

31. Perri MG, Nezu AM, Viegener BJ. *Improving the long-term management of obesity: theory, research, and clinical guidelines.* New York: John Wiley & Sons, 1992.

32. Nezu AM, Nezu CM, eds. *Clinical decision making in behavior therapy: A problem-solving perspective.* Champaign, IL: Research Press, 1989.

33. Perri MG. Obesity. In: Nezu AM, Nezu CM, eds. *Clinical decision making in behavior therapy: a problem-solving perspective.* Champaign, IL: Research Press, 1989;193–226.

34. Perri MG. Maintenance strategies for the management of obesity. In: Johnson WG, ed. *Advances in eating disorders,* vol. 1. Greenwich, CT: JAI Press, 1987;177–94.

35. Perri MG. Improving maintenance of weight loss following treatment by diet and lifestyle modification. In: Wadden TA, VanItallie TB, eds. *Treatment of the seriously obese patient.* New York: Guilford Press, 1992;456–77.

Obesity: Theory and Therapy, Second Edition,
edited by A. J. Stunkard and T. A. Wadden.
Raven Press, Ltd., New York © 1993.

18

New Developments in Childhood Obesity

Leonard H. Epstein

*Department of Psychiatry, University of Pittsburgh School of Medicine,
Pittsburgh, Pennsylvania 15213*

Obesity is a major pediatric health problem. The prevalence of obesity in children is rising, and estimates suggest that 27.1% of 6- to 11-year-old children and 21.9% of 12- to 18-year-old children are obese (1). This represents a problem in part because of the immediate consequences of obesity in youth, which can include changes in health risk or health status, such as lowered fitness (2), increased blood pressure, increased total cholesterol, and decreased high-density lipoprotein concentrations (3). In addition, obesity in childhood is predictive of adult obesity (4–9). Given the poor success rate of treating obesity in adulthood (10), a better understanding of factors that promote obesity in children, and effective treatments for obesity in childhood to prevent adult obesity are needed.

The goal of this chapter is to provide an overview of recent research on obesity in children. Several areas will be covered, including research on epidemiology, risk and etiological factors, and treatment. By necessity, this overview will be selective, and will cover topical or newer research that may be relevant for setting future directions for obesity research rather than covering material presented in previous reviews. The interested reader should consult other reviews (11) to put flesh on the skeleton presented here.

TRACKING CHILDHOOD OBESITY

Epidemiological research tracking obesity in children has shown that overweight children are more likely than nonobese children to become obese adults. The most common approach to tracking is to correlate estimates of obesity over time (12,13). Studies with repeated correlations show that estimates of obesity in later childhood are more predictive of adult obesity than estimates taken in early childhood (12,13). For example, for men relative weight at age 7 correlates moderately with relative weight at age 11 ($r = 0.62$), but this correlation decreases ($r = 0.28$) by age 36. The correlation of relative weight at two points in adulthood (ages 26 and 36) is high, $r = 0.75$ (12).

The most relevant studies of tracking are those that assess whether overweight children are more likely than their lean peers to become obese adults. Several studies use this design, which provides the opportunity to establish relative risks of obese children becoming obese adults.

Charney and colleagues (6) assessed the development of adult obesity in 6-month-old infants who were above or below the 75th percentile for weight. Fourteen percent of obese children became obese adults, while only 8% of nonobese children did, a relative risk of 1.75, suggesting that obese infants are at almost twice the risk of becoming obese adults than are thin infants. However, these data also suggest that weight at 6 months of age is not very predictive of adult status, and the majority of overweight children will outgrow their infant obesity.

Rolland-Cachera and colleagues (7) also

tracked infants 1 year of age to adulthood. Based on body mass index (BMI) values, they divided 1-year-old children and adults into lean, medium, and obese categories. They found that 9 of 44 lean children became obese adults (20%), while 19 of 46 (41%) obese children became obese adults. The relative risk of 2 for obese infants becoming obese adults was very close to the relative risk observed by Charney et al. (6).

Garn and colleagues (8) assessed adult obesity status for children 6 months to 3 years of age. They found that 26.6% of obese children became obese adults, compared with an estimated 15% of all children, a relative risk of 1.77. Data were not provided for the percentage of lean children who became obese adults. Relative risk was greater for the 7-year-old children studied by Stark (9), who showed that the percentage of obese and non-obese children who became overweight adults was approximately 40% and 10%, respectively, a relative risk of 4.

The relative risk of obesity was further increased for preadolescent 10- to 13-year-old children (4,5), who are between 8 and 18 times more likely than nonobese children to become obese adults, dependent on child sex and characteristics of the study sample. Not only is it important to consider that the relative risk increases with age, but also that almost 70% of obese preadolescent children became obese adults. Few of these children outgrew their obesity.

These five long-term epidemiological studies show that the relative risk of an obese child becoming an overweight adult increases with the child's age, and the prospective risk of an obese child becoming an obese adult is greater than for a thin child. However, childhood obesity is only one risk factor for adult obesity, since most obese adults were not obese children. The retrospective risk, which assesses whether obese adults were in fact obese as children, shows a different picture, dependent on child age. For example, Braddon and colleagues (12) studied child relative weight of 36-year-old subjects at five intervals beginning at age 7. They showed that the majority of obese men (71.4%) and women

(63.5%) were underweight or of normal weight at age 7. The pattern began to change at age 11, when 38.5% of obese men and 46.2% of obese women were underweight or normal weight children. Thus, by preadolescence the majority of people who will become obese adults are already overweight, but a sizeable percentage are still nonobese, and on the basis of child weight would not be considered to be at risk for adult obesity.

The major new development in epidemiology of childhood obesity has been the demonstration by Rolland-Cachera and colleagues (14,15) that BMI (kg/m^2) shows reliable developmental patterns, and that differences in these patterns may be predictive of childhood and adult obesity. These investigators showed that BMI increases from birth through about age 1, due to large increases in weight with smaller increases in height. From ages 1 to 6, height increases relatively faster than weight, causing the decrease in BMI, but from age 6 through adulthood weight increases faster than height and thus BMI increases. The investigators have labeled the pattern of change from decreasing BMI to increasing BMI as a rebound.

Rolland-Cachera (7,14) noted that children who show the rebound faster are more likely to become obese children and adults than children who show a more gradual progression of BMI change from decrease to increase. In some sense this is obvious, since obesity in children is caused by increased weight in relationship to height. The new finding provided by Rolland-Cachera is the presentation of developmental curves that provide for the more accurate understanding of a developmental period when children may be at greater risk for developing obesity.

These epidemiological data must be kept in perspective in two ways. First, they examine the role of childhood obesity as a risk for adult obesity, and the verdict is clear that obese children are at a greater risk for developing adult obesity than are lean children. It is also important to acknowledge that most obese adults were not obese children. Obesity is a disorder of energy balance, and it can develop at any time that intake exceeds expenditure. Thus children who were lean throughout development can become obese in late adolescence or adulthood if they remain in positive energy balance for sufficient periods. Second, Rolland-Cachera has provided data that allow us to understand further ages at which the risk of obesity is increased, and perhaps developmental periods that are more sensitive to behavioral and/or biological influences on positive energy balance than other periods.

It remains to be seen whether obesity that develops in childhood is a different disorder from that which develops in adulthood. One obvious consequence is that at the same age, obese adults who were also obese as children will have been obese longer, which may have implications for disease and treatment (15). For example, Abraham and colleagues (4) showed that persons who became obese as adults, but were not obese as children, were at greater risk for cardiovascular disease and diabetes than obese adults who were also obese children. These authors suggest that the weight gain in adulthood is the reason for the excess risk, and that being obese in childhood does not confer the same risk if the obesity is maintained. In contrast, in a 40-year follow-up of obese children, Mossberg (16) found increased rates of cardiovascular (relative risk 1.98) and digestive diseases (relative risk 3.82) in Swedish adults who had been obese as children, as compared with the expected rates of disease for all Swedish adults. Obesity does confer risks, but additional research is needed before it is clear whether the risks of obesity in adulthood are increased or decreased if the adult was also an obese child. Other data have shown that risks associated with obesity, such as elevated blood pressure and elevated serum cholesterol levels, track along with obesity. Obese children are likely to have an elevated risk of cardiovascular disease and this risk persists during development (3).

A second interest for obesity investigators is the influence that obesity in childhood exerts on adult obesity. Given the longer duration of the disorder, it was thought that adults who were obese as children might have a dif-ferent etiology or course of development, and thus might do worse in treatment than adults who became obese in adulthood. Using a prospective design to assess age of attainment of obesity, Garn et al. (17) did not observe differences in the new incidence of obesity as a function of age, and few differences in the familial or sociodemographic factors that contribute to obesity. In addition, age of onset of obesity is not consistently related to treatment outcome in adults (18).

Perhaps the most important conclusion from the epidemiological data is that obesity is a developmental disorder. The relative risk of obesity increases with the age of the child, suggesting that the older an obese child, the more likely he/she will become an obese adult. The probability of outgrowing obesity declines with age. In addition, developmental patterns of weight gain in relation to height suggest that changes at certain ages may increase the risk of childhood obesity.

ETIOLOGICAL FACTORS IN THE DEVELOPMENT OF OBESITY

A variety of etiological factors have been studied that may shed light on why certain types of children are more likely than others to become obese and thus are at greater risk for developing adult obesity. These factors can be broken down into broad categories of biological and sociodemographic risk factors.

Biological Risk Factors: The Role of Energy Balance

Obesity is a disorder of energy balance, and a significant amount of research in obesity has focused on how disorders of intake or expenditure may contribute to the development of obesity. Exciting new measurement advances have increased our understanding of energy balance, and led to the proposal of new hypotheses on the role of intake and expenditure in the development of obesity.

While common sense suggests that people become obese because they eat too much, there has been considerable controversy in regard to the role of overeating in the development of this disorder. Mayer and colleagues (19,20) focused on the role of inactivity in the development of obesity, and they suggested obesity was due to decreased activity, rather than overeating. Other investigators fueled the controversy by also suggesting that obese persons did not eat more than nonobese persons, again suggesting that people become obese as a result of inactivity (21,22).

There is a methodological flaw in concluding that obese children burn fewer calories than nonobese children on the basis of lowered activity levels, and that these lower activity levels contribute to the development of obesity. Activity measures do not measure caloric expenditure, and it must be taken into account that expenditure depends upon both activity and body weight. Thus a person who weighs twice as much as another person may have the same expenditure doing half the amount of the same activity. When this problem was corrected, as by Waxman and Stunkard (23), obese children did not burn fewer calories than nonobese during voluntary activity.

There is a new paradigm that may provide insight into the role of intake and expenditure in regulating body weight, and this is the observation of small and large eaters. Based on the idea that there is considerable variability in intake among persons who weigh the same, George and colleagues (24,25) divided women on the basis of self-reported caloric intake per kg (or kj) of body weight, and identified the upper quartile as large eaters and the lower quartile as small eaters. It was possible to find two people who weighed the same amount but who reported a twofold difference in intake. Small eaters were heavier than large eaters, consistent with the idea that obese persons do not in fact eat more than nonobese. However, there were no differences in activity level or fat-free mass. Macronutrient content of the diets of the small and large eaters was generally similar, though small eaters did eat fewer meals than large eaters, consistent with previous research (26).

These studies of self-reported intake run counter to controlled energy balance studies showing that caloric intake is positively related to body weight—obese individuals require more calories (27–29). While these studies do indicate variability in intake as a function of weight, there generally is not an overlap in the distributions of caloric intake for obese and nonobese samples. On the basis of these studies, it is unlikely that obese and nonobese persons consume the same number of calories.

A recent advance is the use of the doubly labeled water methodology to integrate energy expenditure in the natural environment over repeated days. This methodology has provided new data to resolve this controversy. Bandini et al. (30) compared self-reported caloric intake with integrated energy expenditure over a 2-week period for obese and nonobese adolescents. On the basis of changes in body weight, they could estimate the daily caloric intake. While self-reported intake of these subjects was similar, the doubly labeled water results showed that obese adolescents underreported caloric intake by 40%, while nonobese adolescents underreported caloric intake by only 20%. These results suggest that misconceptions about caloric intake may be the result of overreliance on self-report of caloric intake, and a failure to place adequate emphasis on laboratory studies.

A large body of research has also been completed on the influence of metabolic rate and energy expenditure in childhood obesity. Comparisons of resting metabolic rate and diet-induced thermogenesis in obese and nonobese subjects have shown that obese children have higher metabolic rates than nonobese children, and that even when corrected for lean body mass, the obese do not have a lower metabolic rate (31–33). No differences in diet-induced thermogenesis have been observed between obese and nonobese children (32–34).

Despite the above findings, a low metabolic rate could contribute to the development of obesity. Two investigators have attempted to assess this by studying nonobese children who had lean or obese parents. Roberts and colleagues (35) studied 18 infants at birth, 3 months of age, and 1 year. Six of the infants had non-overweight mothers, and were not overweight themselves, six had overweight mothers but remained non-overweight, and six had overweight mothers and went from non-overweight at 3 months of age to overweight at 1 year. At 3 months of age, resting metabolic rate was measured, total daily energy expenditure was assessed by doubly labeled water methodology, and food records were kept by the mothers for 24 hours. Results showed no differences among the three groups in resting metabolic rate or dietary intake. However, total daily expenditure was less among the children who would become obese relative to the other two groups, suggesting that the activity levels contributed to the differences.

Griffiths and Payne (36) studied normal weight 3- to 5-year-old children with obese and nonobese parents. The investigators used heart rate monitors to estimate caloric expenditure, and on the basis of activity recording attempted to separate activity into resting metabolic rate and additional caloric expenditure. Caloric intake was also measured. Results showed that children of obese parents had lower intake and expenditure than children of nonobese parents, and differences were observed both in caloric expenditure, based on estimated resting metabolic rate, and in estimated additional expenditure. Thus these results suggest that children who have a positive family history maintain normal weight by consuming fewer calories per day than children without a positive family history of obesity. Based on this study, if children of obese parents consumed a caloric intake equivalent to children of nonobese parents, they would become obese.

Griffiths and colleagues (37) followed these children 12 years later, and at that time directly measured their metabolic rate and assessed body composition. The results did not

show the offspring of obese parents to be more likely to be obese than offspring of nonobese parents. Boys with obese parents were taller and heavier than boys with nonobese parents, but these boys were less obese as determined by measures of body fat. No differences in body composition were observed between girls of obese and nonobese parents. The striking finding of this study was that the caloric intake of the girls at age 3–5 was strongly (and negatively) correlated with body mass index and body fat 12 years later.

Both the Griffiths and Payne (36) and Roberts et al. (35) studies suggest that decreased total energy expenditure is a risk factor for the development of adiposity. However, these are only two studies and the results obtained by Roberts et al. (35) are limited by the short follow-up until only 1 year of age. Griffiths and Payne's (37) study indicates that decreased total energy predicts adiposity in adolescence in girls but not, or not yet, in boys. Clearly, further research is needed to validate these suggestive findings.

The potential role of inactivity in the development of obesity has been revitalized by Dietz and colleagues (38). They showed that television watching, a major source of inactivity in children's lives, was positively associated with obesity. The more television a child watched, the more obese he/she was. This analysis assumes that excess television watching or engagement in other sedentary activities precludes time spent being more active, such that excess sedentary behavior becomes a marker for inactivity and a risk factor for obesity. The observation that obese children are more likely to choose sedentary activities than nonobese children has been replicated in our laboratory using behavioral economic analyses of choice (39).

Sociodemographic Risk Factors

The two major sociodemographic risk factors that have been studied are familial obesity and socioeconomic level. A large body of research has shown that obesity runs in families. Obese children are more likely to have obese parents (40) and obese siblings (41) than nonobese children. Parental obesity and child obesity also interact in the prediction of obesity. Obese infants with obese parents are at twice the risk of developing obesity in adulthood than obese infants with nonobese parents (6).

One of the fastest growing areas in obesity research is that of attempting to understand the contribution of genetic and environmental variables that determine the role of familial influence on obesity. This research is reviewed in depth in this volume by Meyer and Stunkard. In an extensive review of behavioral genetic influences on obesity, Grilo and Pogue-Geile (42) hypothesize that the major influences on obesity represent experiences that are not shared by family members. As these investigators note, this conclusion is in contrast to the majority of hypotheses about familial influences, which always stress shared familial influences. Grilo and Pogue-Geile (42) indicate that the nature of the nonshared influences have not been determined, but that they are not simply a result of age or sex differences.

Plomin (43) has reviewed a diverse body of evidence demonstrating that the majority of psychological variables studied using behavioral genetic methods show the greater influence of nonshared than shared environmental influences. This suggests in obesity that family weight similarities are due to genetics and that the environmental influences not shared by each member of the family may have a greater effect on weight than those that are shared. While it is common to assume that shared family influences are important for development, there are many influences in the family that are not shared. Rowe and Plomin (44) present a model for categorizing nonshared environmental influences that are based on four types of variance: sibling interaction, parental treatment, family structure, and extrafamilial networks. Research has shown that many of the important influences on eating and activity are not in fact shared.

For example, Waxman and Stunkard (23) have shown that parents differentially treat obese and nonobese children, feeding the obese children more and suppressing their activity. We have shown that family size (45) can influence short-term weight change, with large families showing less effectiveness of treatment. Parental obesity has also been shown to influence treatment outcome over 5-year observation intervals (46), with children of nonobese parents responding better to treatment than children of obese parents.

Another variable that has received attention recently is socioeconomic status. Sobal and Stunkard (47), in reviewing this literature, showed that weight was inversely related to socioeconomic status (SES) for women but not for men or children in developed countries. In developing countries, SES is positively related to weight for women, men, and children. An interesting new finding in relationship to SES is presented by Rolland-Cachera and colleagues (48,49) on differential susceptibility to environmental challenges for children from low and high SES families. These investigators attempt to explain the apparent contradiction between caloric intake and body weight in terms of socioeconomic level. They (48,49) assessed caloric intake and body mass index in 1- to 3-year-old and 7- to 12-year-old children of families with fathers in unskilled versus skilled occupations. Several interesting findings emerged in both samples. As others have reported, there were no differences in intake across body composition, even when comparing lean versus obese children. Likewise, children of unskilled fathers had higher caloric intake than children of skilled fathers, and there was more obesity in families with unskilled fathers. These results suggest that given the same intake, children with unskilled fathers are more likely to become obese than children with skilled fathers. The individual susceptibility to obesity is either due to or correlated with father's occupation.

This provocative hypothesis could help explain how similar intakes can result in different degrees of fatness. It is important to keep in mind the controversy regarding whether obese persons do or do not consume excess calories, problems with self-report of intake, and the fact that SES has been shown to be inversely related to obesity in developed countries, but SES has not been reliably related to obesity for men or children (47). If the Rolland-Cachera (48,49) results are replicated using more carefully controlled measures of intake, then mechanisms for this effect must be considered. Broadly conceived, it is possible that socioeconomic status could influence obesity in one of two ways. First, there may be something different about the life styles of families of skilled versus unskilled fathers that changes susceptibility, such as eating patterns, dietary and macronutrient composition, or activity patterns.

Second, the relationship between obesity and SES may be an example of what behavioral geneticists call genotype–environment correlation. Children may be differentially exposed to environments on the basis of their predispositions. Families with obese children, (and also obese parents) may select environments for family members that are consistent with these traits, and these children will thus be more likely to be exposed to factors that promote obesity. The mechanisms responsible for the influence of environments associated with unskilled fathers remain to be identified.

Socioeconomic status has received little attention as a factor influencing response to treatment in controlled outcome research. Since treatment for obesity in children involves diet, exercise, and parenting, factors influencing parenting are likely to influence outcome, and many SES-related variables may influence parenting. An interesting new theoretical approach to understanding the relationship between SES and parenting is the theory of insularity and attentional deficits proposed by Wahler and Dumas (50). These investigators suggest that factors associated with low SES shift parental attention away from appropriate behavior to inappropriate behavior, leading to increases in inappropriate behavior and limiting parental social influence in increasing appropriate behavior. The cycle then becomes one of parents always attempting to decrease inappropriate behavior, and selectively attending to inappropriate behavior.

Low SES families may also experience increased stress, which can directly influence child as well as parent behavior (51). Numerous studies have found that parents who are depressed or in conflict show general reductions in parenting skills (52). These parents are unable to cope with daily requirements of parenting, and their attention to their own problems shifts attention from their children's behavior.

Other sociodemographic and familial variables can also influence the response to treatment. Family size (44) and single parent status (53) have been shown to influence treatment of childhood obesity. In addition, there are familial variables that have not been studied but may influence obesity treatment by directly modifying parental parenting skills, such as spacing between children (54). Parental psychopathology has been shown to increase in families with children very close together in age. This may be the result of increased daily parenting demands, with reduced parenting effectiveness.

TREATMENT FOR OBESE CHILDREN

Research on the treatment of childhood obesity has been quite limited in comparison to research on treatments for adult obesity (55). The majority of interventions have focused on treatments of preadolescent children in clinical settings. Fewer studies have been completed on younger children or adolescent children in clinical settings, and only a handful of studies on school-based programs or preventive programs have been completed. Research in this area of childhood obesity is moving very slowly, and only a few studies on treatment have appeared since our last review of behavioral treatments in 1987 (11). Given the limited progress, this section of the review will briefly summarize the findings of the previous review and update findings based on newer and more innovative methods.

Basic components of clinical treatment for obese children involve changing the child's diet, providing an exercise program, and implementing parent training. Since obesity is often a family problem, the success of the program may be in part a function of the degree to which parents can influence changes in their child's behavior. There have been several studies on how to include the family and on parent training. In preadolescent children long-term results are superior when parents and children are targeted for treatment, in comparison with nonspecific targets (56). Families that are provided specific parent training show superior weight loss and weight maintenance than those who do not receive this training (57), and it is better to emphasize positive rather than negative motivational techniques (58). One new and innovative treatment study with preadolescents assessed the role of family problem solving in family-based treatment. Graves and colleagues (59) showed large and sustained reductions in percent overweight for families given a family-based behavioral program that included problem-solving training, in comparison with a similar family-based behavioral program that did not include problem-solving training. Research with adolescents has shown that better outcomes are obtained when both parents and children are treated, but they should be treated separately (60). However, these results did not generalize to treatment of lower SES black adolescent girls (61).

Research on obesity in children has repeatedly demonstrated the importance of exercise. We have shown in two studies that a life-style exercise program was associated with improved weight loss versus a structured aerobic exercise program, in part due to better adherence to the life-style program (62,63). In an innovative uncontrolled program in Japan (64), obese 11-year-old children were provided supervised exercise over a 2-year period. The children reduced their body fat by 40%, while weight remained generally constant, with the fat replaced by lean body mass. Reductions in overweight of 55% in boys and 48% in girls were significant. High-density lipoprotein cholesterol levels increased during the 2 years of observation. While the study lacks controls to assess comparative normal development, or comparison groups to isolate the effective components of treatment, the results suggest the power of exercise.

Reybrouck and colleagues (65) compared diet versus diet plus exercise in a sample of obese adolescent children. After 4 months of therapy both groups showed significant decreases in percent overweight, with the diet plus exercise group showing larger decreases in percent overweight than the diet alone group (-25% versus -15.8%). Not all studies showed changes this large, or favor exercise. Becque and colleagues (66) randomized obese adolescents to a control group and a 20-week diet or diet plus exercise group. While no significant differences were observed in body weight or body fat across groups, results showed approximately equivalent changes in percent body fat in the diet plus exercise and diet group (-3.0% and -3.5%, respectively) while the control group showed a slight increase ($+.7\%$). Both intervention groups showed significant changes in diastolic blood pressure, but the diet plus exercise group showed larger changes in diastolic blood pressure than the diet alone group. Lipid values were not differentially changed across groups.

An important finding is the demonstration that the effects of family-based treatment can persist in preadolescent children for up to 10 years after treatment. In a 10-year follow-up we found obese children who began treatment at approximately 10 years of age were significantly less obese if both parent and child were targeted for treatment in comparison with a nontargeted control (57). The 10-year results were consistent with the 5-year outcome, suggesting that treatment effects were maintained throughout development.

One common concern for treating young

children is the possible negative effects of dieting on growth and height (67). We had previously published 5-year outcomes across multiple studies that suggested diet did not adversely affect growth, and that children resembled their parents in height (68). The 10-year data provided the first opportunity to assess whether young adult height was influenced by dieting (56). Results showed no relationship between weight control success and height. The average child was very close in height to their same sex parent, which provides a good estimate of expected growth.

The demonstration of long-term weight control provides the opportunity of studying the effects of weight control on cardiovascular risk factors associated with obesity. Other investigators have shown the beneficial short-term effects of obesity reduction on cardiovascular risk factors (60,64,66). Recently we demonstrated that reductions in percent overweight and beneficial changes in lipids were maintained over a 5-year interval (69).

In spite of the importance of experimental research on prevention and treatment with young children, no new studies have been identified since the previous review. At that time only one prevention study had been completed, with very encouraging results (70). In addition, we did not identify any new school-based obesity treatment programs, although community-based studies for family health improvement have been reported (71,72). It has become popular to implement general health modification programs in schools or communities for children (73,74). However, it is not clear if the programs are intense enough to produce significant weight change in obese children.

IDEAS FOR NEW RESEARCH

Research is needed in several areas. First, obesity should be considered a developmental problem. The risk of an obese child becoming an obese adult increases with age. Changes in body composition also show developmental characteristics that may be important in delimiting the most effective periods for intervention (13,14). It has been previously noted that child treatment should be linked to developmental differences (75), but no research has attempted to study how treatments may interact with development. Children's cognitive and motor abilities to perform treatment-related skills, their cognitive perceptions of obesity related phenomena (76), and the extent to which they share in the control of eating and exercise-related behaviors vary as function of age. Intervention programs need to take these behavioral and cognitive differences into account.

Second, research programs should be based on or derived from basic research on ingestive behavior and exercise. In children, they should focus on the development and maintenance of child eating (77) and activity regulation. Research on child food choice and ways to modify short-term intake (78–81) can easily be adapted to clinical research studies (82). A better exchange of research methods between developmental research on eating and exercise regulation and clinical research is needed.

Third, clinical research in children needs to take into account treatment innovations that have been identified for adults. For example, one simple but powerful innovation is lengthening treatment, with longer treatment yielding larger weight losses (10). In addition, treatments for childhood obesity have not tested new ways to prevent relapse (83), another important research area for adult treatment. Finally, while a wide variety of pharmacological and dietary programs have been tried with adults, there have only been limited attempts to use with children the newer and innovative very-low-calorie diet interventions developed for obese adults. This is partly because of questions raised about the effects of very-low-calorie diets on growth and development (85,86), and partly because of the failure of these dietary regimens to produce long-term success in adults (86,87). There may be a place for these programs in treatments for grossly obese adolescents, however, and their long-term success may be better with adolescents than with adults.

CONCLUSIONS

Childhood obesity is important both because of its adverse health effects on children, and because of the risks that obesity in childhood convey for adulthood. Research has begun to focus on risk factors that are related to the development of obesity. New hypotheses have been generated to understand better how eating and activity contribute to the development of obesity, and how they may interact with other risk factors, such as social class as determinants. Behavioral genetic research has suggested the role of nonshared family influences on the development of obesity, and further research needs to address these differences both as differential experiences within families and different extrafamilial networks. Finally, treatment research has shown that the effects of behavioral family-based treatments for preadolescent children can be maintained throughout development. Additional research is needed to enhance both treatment and long-term maintenance, and by understanding and incorporating new findings in basic research, it may be possible to push this clinical research to a new level of effectiveness.

ACKNOWLEDGMENTS

This manuscript was supported in part by grants HD20829, HD23713, and HD25997. Appreciation is expressed to Lucene Wisniewski and Alice Valoski for helpful comments on earlier versions of this manuscript.

REFERENCES

1. Gortmaker SL, Dietz WH, Sobol AM, Wehler CA. Increasing pediatric obesity in the United States. *Am J Dis Child* 1987;141:535–40.
2. Cumming GR, Everatt D, Hastman L. Bruce treadmill test in children: normal values in a clinic population. *Am J Cardiol* 1978;41:69–75.
3. Berenson GS. *Cardiovascular risk factors in children: The early natural history of atherosclerosis and essential hypertension.* New York: Oxford University Press, 1980.
4. Abraham S, Collins C, Nordsieck M. Relationship of childhood weight status to morbidity in adults. *Public Health Rep* 1971;86:273–84.
5. Abraham S, Nordsieck M. Relationship of excess weight in children and adults. *Public Health Rep* 1960;75:263–73.
6. Charney E, Goodman HC, McBride M, Lyon B, Pratt R. Childhood antecedents of adult obesity. Do chubby infants become obese adults? *N Engl J Med* 1976;295:6–9.
7. Rolland-Cachera M-F, Deheeger M, Guilloud-Bataille M. Tracking the development of obesity from one month of age to adulthood. *Ann Hum Biol* 1987;14:219–29.
8. Garn SM, Lavelle M. Two-decade follow-up of fatness in early childhood. *Am J Dis Child* 1985;139:181–5.
9. Stark O, Atkins E, Wolff OH, Douglas JWB. Longitudinal study of obesity in the National Survey of Health and Development. *Br Med J* 1981;283:13–7.
10. Brownell KD, Wadden TA. Behavior therapy for obesity: modern approaches and better results. In: Brownell KD, Foreyt JP, eds. *Handbook of eating disorders.* New York: Basic Books, 1986;180–97.
11. Epstein LH, Wing RR. Behavioral treatment of childhood obesity. *Psychol Bull* 1987;101:91–5.
12. Braddon FEM, Rodgers B, Wadsworth MEJ, Davies JMC. Onset of obesity in a 36 year birth cohort study. *Br Med J* 1986;293:299–303.
13. Rolland-Cachera MF, Bellisle F, Sempe M. The prediction in boys and girls of the weight/height² index and various skinfold measurements in adults: a two decade followup study. *Int J Obes* 1989;13:305–11.
14. Rolland-Cachera MF, Deheeger M, Bellisle F, Sempe M, Guilloud-Bataille M, Patois E. Adiposity rebound in children: a simple indicator for predicting obesity. *Am J Clin Nutr* 1984;39:129–35.
15. Wadden TA, Foster GD. Behavioral assessment and treatment of markedly obese patients. In: Wadden TA, VanItallie TB, eds. *Treatment of the seriously obese patient.* New York: Guilford Press, 1992;290–330.
16. Mossberg HO. 40-Year follow-up of overweight children. *Lancet* 1989;II:491–3.
17. Garn SM, Sullivan TV, Hawthorne VM. The juvenile-onset, adolescent-onset and adult-onset obese. *Int J Obes* 1991;15:105–10.
18. Wing RR, Nowalk MP, Epstein LH, Scott N, Ewing L. Methodological issues related to age of onset of obesity. *Addict Behav* 1985;10:69–73.
19. Johnson ML, Burke BS, Mayer J. Relative importance of inactivity and overeating in the energy balance of obese high school girls. *Am J Clin Nutr* 1956;4:37–44.
20. Rose HE, Mayer J. Activity, caloric intake, fat storage, and the energy balance of infants. *Pediatrics* 1968;41:18–29.
21. Corbin CB, Fletcher P. Diet and physical activity patterns of obese and nonobese elementary school children. *Res Q* 1968;39:922–8.
22. Wilkinson PW, Parkin JM, Pearlson G, Strong H, Sykes P. Energy intake and physical activity in obese children. *Br Med J* 1977;284:756.
23. Waxman M, Stunkard AJ. Caloric intake and expenditure of obese boys. *J Pediatr* 1980;96:187–93.
24. George V, Tremblay A, Despres JP, LeBlanc C, Perusse L, Bouchard C. Evidence for the existence of small eaters and large eaters of similar fat-free mass and activity level. *Int J Obes* 1989;13:43–53.

25. George V, Tremblay A, Despres JP, et al. Further evidence for the presence of "small eaters" and "large eaters" among women. *Am J Clin Nutr* 1991;53:425–9.

26. Metzner HL, Lamphiear EE, Wheeler NC, Larkin FA. The relationship between frequency of eating and adiposity in adult men and women in the Tecumseh Community Health Study. *Am J Clin Nutr* 1977;30:712–5.

27. Blair D, Buskirk ER. Habitual daily energy expenditure and activity levels of lean and adult-onset and child-onset obese women. *Am J Clin Nutr* 1987; 45:540–50.

28. DeBoer JO, van Es AJH, van Raaij JMA, Hautvast JGAJ. Energy requirements and energy expenditure of lean and overweight women, measured by indirect calorimetry. *Am J Clin Nutr* 1987;46:13–21.

29. Ravussin E, Burnand B, Schutz Y, Jequier E. Twenty-four-hour energy expenditure and resting metabolic rate in obese, moderately obese, and control subjects. *Am J Clin Nutr* 1982;35:566–73.

30. Bandini LG, Schoeller DA, Cyr HN, Dietz WH. Validity of reported energy intake in obese and nonobese adolescents. *Am J Clin Nutr* 1990;52:421–5.

31. Bandini LG, Schoeller DA, Dietz WH. Energy expenditure in obese and non-obese adolescents. *Pediatr Res* 1990;27:198–203.

32. Epstein LH, Wing RR, Cluss P, et al. Resting metabolic rate in children: relation to child and parent weight and percent overweight change. *Am J Clin Nutr* 1989;49:331–6.

33. Molnar D, Varga P, Rubecz I, Hamar A, Mestyan J. Food-induced thermogenesis in obese children. *Eur J Pediatr* 1985;144:27–31.

34. Bandini LG, Schoeller DA, Edwards J, Young VR, Oh SH, Dietz WH. Energy expenditure during carbohydrate overfeeding in obese and non-obese adolescents. *Am J Physiol* 1989;256:E357–67.

35. Roberts SB, Savage J, Coward WA, Chew B, Lucas A. Energy expenditure and intake in infants born to lean and overweight mothers. *N Engl J Med* 1988;318:461–6.

36. Griffiths M, Payne PR. Energy expenditure in small children of obese and non-obese parents. *Nature* 1976;260:698–700.

37. Griffiths M, Payne PR, Stunkard AJ, Rivers JPW, Cox M. Metabolic rate and physical development of children at risk for obesity. *Lancet* 1990;336:76–8.

38. Dietz WH, Gortmaker SL. Do we fatten our children at the television set? Obesity and television viewing in children and adolescents. *Pediatrics* 1985;75:807–12.

39. Epstein LH, Smith JA, Vara LS, Rodefer JS. Behavioral economic analysis of activity choice in obese children. *Health Psychol* 1991;10:311–6.

40. Garn SM, Clark DC. Trends in fatness and the origins of obesity. *Pediatrics* 1976;57:433–56.

41. Garn SM, Bailey SM, Higgins ITT. Effects of socioeconomic status, family line, and living together on fatness and obesity. In: Lauer RM, Shekelle RB, eds. *Childhood prevention of atherosclerosis and hypertension.* New York: Raven Press, 1980;187–204.

42. Grilo CM, Pogue-Geile MF. The nature of environmental influences on weight and obesity: a behavior genetic analysis. *Psychol Bull* 1991;110:520–37.

43. Plomin R. *Development, genetics and psychology.* Hillsdale, NJ: Lawrence Erlbaum Associates, 1986.

44. Rowe DC, Plomin R. The importance of nonshared (E_1) environmental influences in behavioral development. *Dev Psychol* 1981;17:517–31.

45. Epstein LH, Koeske R, Wing RR. The effect of family variables on child weight loss. *Health Psychol* 1986;5:1–12.

46. Epstein LH, Wing RR, Koeske R, Valoski A. Effects of parent weight on weight loss in obese children. *J Consult Clin Psychol* 1986;54:400–1.

47. Sobal J, Stunkard AJ. Socioeconomic status and obesity: a review of the literature. *Psychol Bull* 1989;105:260–75.

48. Rolland-Cachera MF, Deheeger M, Pequignot F, Guilloud-Bataille M, Vinit F. Adiposity and food intake in young children: the environmental challenge to individual susceptibility. *Br Med J* 1988;290:1037–8.

49. Rolland-Cachera MF, Bellisle F. No correlation between adiposity and food intake: why are working class children fatter? *Am J Clin Nutr* 1986; 44:779–87.

50. Wahler RG, Dumas JE. Attentional problems in dysfunctional mother-child interactions: an interbehavioral model. *Psychol Bull* 1989;105:116–30.

51. Compas BE. Coping with stress during childhood and adolescence. *Psychol Bull* 1987;101:393–403.

52. Downey G, Coyne JC. Children of depressed parents: an integrative review. *Psychol Bull* 1990; 108:50–76.

53. Dietz WH. Family characteristics affect rates of weight loss in obese children. *Nutr Res* 1983; 3:43–50.

54. Wagner ME, Schubert HJP, Schubert DSP. Sibship constellation effects on psychosocial development, creativity, and health. In: Reese HW, Lipsitt LP eds. *Advances in child development and behavior,* vol 14. New York: Academic Press, 1979;58–155.

55. Epstein LH. Clinical issues: retrospective essay on the behavioral treatment of obesity. In: Stricker EM, ed. *Handbook of behavioral neurobiology.* New York: Plenum, 1990;61–73.

56. Epstein LH, Valoski A, Wing RR, McCurley J. Ten-year follow-up of behavioral, family-based treatment for obese children. *JAMA* 1990;264:2519–23.

57. Israel AC, Stolmaker L, Andrian CAG. The effects of training parents in general child management skills on a behavioral weight loss program for children. *Behav Ther* 1985;16:169–80.

58. Aragano J, Cassady J, Drabman RS. Treatment of overweight children through parental training and contingency contracting. *J Appl Behav Anal* 1979;12:449–66.

59. Graves T, Meyers AW, Clark L. An evaluation of problem-solving training in the behavioral treatment of childhood obesity. *J Consult Clin Psychol* 1988;56:246–50.

60. Brownell KD, Kelman SH, Stunkard AJ. Treatment of obese children with and without their mothers: changes in weight and blood pressure. *Pediatrics* 1983;71:515–23.

61. Wadden TA, Stunkard AJ, Rich L, Rubin CJ, Sweidel G, McKinney S. Obesity in black adolescent girls: a controlled trial of treatment by diet, behavior

modification, and parental support. *Pediatrics* 1990;85:345–52.

62. Epstein LH, Wing RR, Koeske R, Ossip DJ, Beck S. A comparison of lifestyle change and programmed aerobic exercise on weight and fitness changes in obese children. *Behav Ther* 1982;13:651–65.

63. Epstein LH, Wing RR, Koeske R, Valoski A. A comparison of lifestyle exercise, aerobic exercise and calisthenics on weight loss in obese children. *Behav Ther* 1985;16:345–56.

64. Sasaki J, Shindo M, Tanaka H, Ando M, Arakawa K. A long-term aerobic exercise program decreases the obesity index and increases the high density lipoprotein cholesterol concentration in obese children. *Int J Obes* 1987;11:339–45.

65. Reybrouck T, Vinckx J, Van Den Berghe G, Vanderschueren-Lodeweyckx M. Exercise therapy and hypocaloric diet in the treatment of obese children and adolescents. *Acta Paediatr Scand* 1990;79:84–9.

66. Becque MD, Katch VL, Rocchini AP, Marks CR, Moorehead C. Coronary risk incidence of obese adolescents: reduction by exercise plus diet intervention. *Pediatrics* 1988;81:605–12.

67. Dietz WH, Hartung R. Changes in height velocity of obese preadolescents during weight reduction. *Am J Dis Child* 1985;139:705–7.

68. Epstein LH, McCurley J, Valoski A, Wing RR. Growth in obese children treated for obesity. *Am J Dis Child* 1990;144:1360–4.

69. Epstein LH, Kuller LH, Wing RR, Valoski A, McCurley J. The effect of weight control on lipid changes in obese children. *Am J Dis Child* 1980;143:454–7.

70. Piscano JC, Lichter H, Ritter J, Siegal AP. An attempt at prevention of obesity in infancy. *Pediatrics* 1978;61:360–4.

71. Nader PR, Baranowski T, Vanderpool NA, Dunn K, Dworkin R, Ray L. The Family Health Project: cardiovascular risk reduction for children and parents. *Dev Behav Pediatr* 1983;4:3–10.

72. Nader PR, Sallis JF, Patterson TL, et al. A family approach to cardiovascular risk reduction: results from the San Diego Family Health Project. *Health Educ Q* 1989;16:229–44.

73. Coates TJ, Jeffery RW, Slinkard LA. The heart health program: introducing and maintaining nutrition behavior change in children. *Am J Public Health* 1981;71:15–23.

74. Killen JD, Telch MJ, Robinson TN, Maccoby N, Taylor CB, Farquhar JW. Cardiovascular disease risk reduction for tenth graders: a multiple factor school-based approach. *JAMA* 1988;260:1728–33.

75. Epstein LH. Family-based treatment for preadolescent obesity. In: Wolraich ML, Routh D, eds. *Advances in developmental and behavioral pediatrics.* Greenwich, CT: JAI Press, Inc., 1985;1–39.

76. Wolfle JA, Farriet SC, Rogers CS. Children's cognitive concepts of obesity: a developmental study. *Int J Obes* 1987;11:73–83.

77. Birch LL. Obesity and eating disorders: a developmental perspective. *Bull Psychonomic Soc* 1991;29:265–72.

78. Birch LL, Marlin DW. I don't like it; I never tried it: Effects of exposure on two-year old children's food preference. *Appetite* 1982;3:353–60.

79. Birch LL, Zimmerman SI, Hind H. The influence of social affective context on the formation of children's food preferences. *Child Dev* 1980;51:856–61.

80. Birch LL, Deysher M. Caloric compensation and sensory specific satiety: evidence for self regulation of food intake by young children. *Appetite* 1986;7:323–31.

81. Birch LL, Birch D, Marlin DW, Kramer L. Effects of instrumental consumption on children's food preference. *Appetite* 1982;3:125–34.

82. Epstein LH, Wing RR, Valoski A, Penner B. Stability of food preferences in 8–12 year old children and their parents during weight control. *Behav Modif* 1987;11:87–101.

83. Brownell KD, Marlatt GA, Lichtenstein E, Wilson GT. Understanding and preventing relapse. *Am Psychol* 1986;41:756–82.

84. Dietz WH, Schoeller DA. Optimal dietary therapy for obese adolescents: comparison of protein plus glucose and protein plus fat. *J Pediatr* 1982;100:638–44.

85. Archibald EH, Harrison JE, Pencharz PB. Effect of a weight-reducing high-protein diet on the body composition of obese adolescents. *Am J Dis Child* 1983;137:658–62.

86. Wadden TA, Sternberg JA, Letizia KA, Stunkard AJ, Foster GD. Treatment of obesity by very low calorie diet, behavior therapy, and their combination: a five-year perspective. *Int J Obes* 1989;13:39–46.

87. Wadden TA, Stunkard AJ, Liebschutz J. Three-year follow-up of the treatment of obesity by very low calorie diet, behavior therapy, and their combination. *J Consult Clin Psychol* 1988;56:925–8.

Obesity: Theory and Therapy, Second Edition,
edited by A. J. Stunkard and T. A. Wadden.
Raven Press, Ltd., New York © 1993.

19

Surgery

Edward E. Mason and Cornelius Doherty

Department of Surgery, University of Iowa College of Medicine, Iowa City, Iowa 52246

Surgery is widely recognized as the treatment of choice for severe or "morbid" obesity. Obesity of this severity is rare, however, about 0.5% of the population (1). Do physicians need to know about such treatment if they are not directly involved in it? If so, why? Physicians and indeed other helping professionals should know about the surgical treatment of severe obesity for at least four reasons:

1. There are many severely obese patients in this country. Although the prevalence is only 0.5% of the general population, this means that 1.5 million Americans suffer from this disorder.

2. Severe obesity detrimentally affects the quality of life, the length of life, and the development of complications such as diabetes, hypertension, gallstones, hernias, degeneration of weight-bearing joints, endometrial cancer, and sudden death.

3. There is such a large number of patients who have already undergone surgery for their obesity and they are so widely scattered that many physicians, other than the surgeon who performed the operation, will be called upon to assist.

4. Physicians will be approached by an occasional severely obese person for advice about treatment. A physician well informed on the surgical treatments is in an excellent position to advise the patient about whether or not to undertake surgical treatment and where to go to receive it.

A TESTIMONIAL

The following testimonial introduces some of the complications of severe obesity and their correction by surgical treatment:

I am a 59-year-old male with a life-long history of severe chronic obesity. I weighed more than 200 lb by the time I was a sophomore in high school, and never weighed less than that until recently. I am a physicist by training, with a graduate degree from a major university and I currently manage a $150 million dollar per year high-technology business in a major medical diagnostic imaging company. I quit smoking 10 years ago and stopped overnight. I routinely smoked three packs of cigarettes a day and have never touched one since. I include this background information solely to establish that I am of at least average intelligence and possessed of some amount of will power.

Despite these attributes, however, I struggled with my weight problem for more than 40 years with very limited success. At times in my life I have lost as much as 110 lb on a single "diet episode" only to follow that up with a 180-lb weight gain. The "lose-gain" syndrome is undoubtedly known to everyone who has ever dieted. In the course of that time I tried innumerable diets, some of which were prescribed by physicians and some of which were offered by highly advertised national weight-loss clinics in one form or another. The end result was inevitably the same.

Five years ago I reached a crisis time in life. I weighed 475 pounds. I took more than 200 units of insulin a day to deal with the diabetes brought upon by this severe level of obesity, and I had such serious orthopedic problems that I could no longer walk without the aid of a cane, and at times required a pair of crutches. My existence was so miserable that I sought psychiatric counseling on the occasion of my annual physical exam. After a 2-hour interview session with a staff psychiatrist, his summarization was as follows: "You have as little self-esteem as anyone I have ever met. I would like to offer you hope that continued psychiatric counseling could effect significant change, but in truth, I cannot. I have never had significant success in dealing with this problem, nor has anyone else on the staff. I believe that your only hope is obesity surgery, and I further believe that you have less than 1 year to take action."

I was terrified by the prospect of any form of major surgery. At that weight I felt that I was a poor surgical risk. Nevertheless, I also knew that despite the fact that my weight problem was the bane of my existence, and the one thing in my life that I wanted most desperately to change, nothing else had worked for me. Through the efforts of a good friend, who is also a very fine surgeon in his own right, I was introduced to a bariatric surgery program and had a vertical banded gastroplasty on March 3rd of 1987. Today I weigh 163 lb, and my fasting blood sugars are typically 70 to 80 without insulin. I no longer need a cane to walk. In fact, many a Sunday morning I walk a 7-mile route and find it very pleasant to do so. When I reached 300 lb, as my weight came down, I joined the YMCA and now exercise regularly three times per week. Included in my exercise routine is at least 20 minutes of aerobic conditioning. I also joined a support group. I happened to choose Overeater's Anonymous, but I am sure there are others that are equally effective. It still helps very much at times to talk to other people who, like myself, could only deal with their emotional stresses in a very destructive way: by eating.

I believe that all three of the major changes in my life (the bariatric surgery, the exercise program, and the support group) are almost equally important. The bariatric surgery, however, was the critical change. It was a most important mechanical limitation on my ability to eat excess amounts of food, and thereby the means of providing a bridge to a far healthier life style.

My weight dropped consistently for more than 3 years following the surgical procedure, and in fact, I have been at my current weight of 163 lb for only about 8 months. My friend the surgeon, in one conversation when he was trying to persuade me to have the bariatric surgery, made the remark that, if I ever had it done, I would kick myself for not having done it 5 years earlier. He was wrong. I wish I had it done 20 years earlier.

I am sure that there are all levels of effectiveness of bariatric surgery depending upon the patient's level of motivation, but I feel reasonably confident that most would tell you that it had significantly improved their health and the quality of their life. It would seem reasonable to me that a study correlating the effectiveness of bariatric surgery with a comprehensive analysis of personality traits could identify those factors that make the procedure more effective in one patient than in another. In my own case, I strongly suspect that intense frustration with the weight problem over a period of years made me more willing to make the life-style changes necessary to enhance the effects of the surgery. Ironically, even the personality trait that contributed so much to the problem to begin with, that of being a very compulsive or a "driven" kind of person, has played a major positive role in my determination to "make the surgery work for me," having had it done. I am sure there are people far more capable than I am of evaluating success factors, and perhaps such studies have already been done. It may even be possible to enhance those positive factors in prospective bariatric surgery candidates through presurgical psychiatric care or counseling. Today I enjoy significantly improved health and a life style far more pleasant than I ever imagined I could have. For me, bariatric surgery was the critical element in this positive change.

Comment

This man was typical of his gender in that men tend to seek an operation only when they can no longer work. Men tend to be older and heavier, and to have complications of their obesity. Women tend to come earlier and to be more concerned about their appearance. Motivation to control eating is high. There is often a feeling of guilt or shame about the need to consider an operation for something that would seem to be so simple to control. There have usually been repeated failures of weight control even though there may be evidence of ability to control other injurious habits. Medical practitioners have failed to provide the life-long effective treatment that is required for severe obesity and do not attempt treatment because they recognize their ineffectiveness.

Weight loss after a gastric reduction operation usually occurs within the first year, but a normal weight is seldom reached. The above patient appears to have derived an added benefit from his exercise and support programs. His success in his professional life and in his management of his life after the operation show a compulsive intensity of effort that is a part of his personality. He was fortunate that there was not more damage from the 40 years of excessive weight, diabetes, and loss and gain of so much weight over the years. He has recently had a mild stroke from which he has had a nearly complete recovery with minimal residual effects. He would have derived benefit from an earlier operation. He mentioned that he might not have been so highly motivated if he had undergone the operation earlier in life. He knows now how much he missed in life because of his obesity and how important it is to maintain his normal weight.

SOME COSTS OF SEVERE OBESITY

Severe obesity is a costly disorder. The national medical effects of severe obesity in 1986 were calculated by Colditz (2) to have cost $39.3 billion or 5.5% of the entire cost of medical care. This large sum is even more remarkable in that it is the cost of a condition that is not often considered a disease, and is not listed as one of the big killers like cancer, heart disease, or stroke. However, the complications of severe obesity contribute significantly to well-recognized diseases such as insulin-dependent diabetes, myocardial damage, renal failure, irreversible hypertension, and even sudden death. These complications can be prevented by prompt treatment.

Treatment must be effective over the long term, as well as prompt. Fluctuation in weight may have negative health consequences independent of obesity and the trend of body weight over time according to Lissner et al. (3). Men and women with highly variable weights had increased total mortality as well as increased morbidity and mortality from coronary heart disease. Adverse outcome from weight fluctuation was strongest in the youngest cohort examined (ages 30 to 44), which was also noted to be the group least likely to have other diseases and the most likely to be dieting.

Obesity is far more common among persons of lower socioeconomic status; thus the costs of obesity and its complications fall disproportionately upon the poor, who are largely dependent on publically funded insurance for treatment. Despite their real medical need, failure to obtain approval for operations for severe obesity has prevented treatment of a segment of our population. In a recent report regarding the basis for their determination whether to approve operations for obesity, an agency wrote that "The long term success (of operations for obesity) remains largely the responsibility of the patient and the willingness (of the patient) to make permanent life style changes. . . . Compliance to dietary restrictions is very important in achieving a good weight loss." It has been customary for this agency to deny the use of operations for the treatment of obesity unless they receive evidence of at least 2 years of supervised dietary treatment of obesity. There is nothing in the medical literature to support a requirement for 2 years of supervised dietary treatment for those patients, who have already demonstrated inability to control their weight. That is why gastric reduction operations were developed for the treatment of severe obesity.

The reluctance to provide support for the surgical treatment of severely obese persons may appear to save money. Regrettably, this policy denies the natural history of a disease that is life-threatening, chronic, and often progressive. A recent surgical outcome study (4) disputes this policy. It indicates that surgical treatment can return some unemployed persons to the work force. Martin et al. (4) concluded that "the benefit from a reduction in weight for patients of lower socioeconomic class is significant, since approximately 45% of those receiving public assistance can decrease their level of support." In an editorial that followed Martin et al.'s paper, Civetta (5) observed: "Before we choose what not to pay for, we must learn to measure what we consider important. Current desires to control costs may adversely affect other societally desirable outcomes."

DO OPERATIONS ADDRESS THE ETIOLOGY OF OBESITY?

The experience of the last two decades with gastric reduction operations has revealed that the imposition of a limited capacity to eat a meal is not only well tolerated but is welcomed by the severely obese (6). Some of the early proponents of intestinal bypass, which permitted a large food intake, predicted that these patients would not be able to tolerate the limited intake imposed by a gastric reduction operation. The severely obese were thought to require large meals to preserve emotional stability. Studies of the emotional sequelae of gastric reduction operations revealed the fallacy of this prediction. Stunkard visited the University of Iowa Hospitals and Clinics (UIHC) in 1978 and worked with us in designing a questionnaire that was given to 80 of our Roux gastric bypass patients. A striking finding of this study (7) was that patients with gastric bypass, like the patients with intestinal bypass studied earlier (8), are able to lose weight without the depression that occurred when dietary reduction was attempted without an operation. This surprising finding raises the possibility that these surgical techniques do more than simply interfere mechanically with food intake; they may actually affect the etiology of obesity in some as yet undetermined manner. These and other favorable consequences of surgical reduction procedures led Stunkard et al. (9) to propose that the effect of these procedures is to lower the body weight set point.

Another etiologic effect of gastric reduction procedures is suggested by an observation volunteered by many patients: they never felt full before their operations but now know when they are full. Schachter in 1967 (10) summarized studies indicating that the severely obese lack internal cues. They are less aware of hunger, or fullness, and satiety is not within their experience. Their eating is accordingly governed by external cues such as the presence of food on the table, the clock showing that it is meal time, etc. An effective gastric operation provides patients with an internal cue of fullness after a small meal. Once these operations are reversed, most patients return to their original or a higher weight. However, as long as the pouch is small and the outlet is controlled so that the intestinal cue of fullness is maintained, they seem to be relieved of their compulsion to eat.

PROCEDURES

Vertical Banded Gastroplasty

Vertical banded gastroplasty (VBG) evolved from earlier forms of gastroplasty (11). Gastroplasty implies a change in the configuration of the stomach without resection and without any bypass of stomach, duodenum, or intestine. The initial gastroplasty was horizontal (Fig. 1) and established a fundic pouch. This configuration has been abandoned because the fundus stretched too much and frustrated weight loss. The VBG, designed with a lesser curvature, vertical pouch, is less distensible. It serves as an internal cue for satiety and is more effective for sustained weight loss. This operation requires adherence to described technique and to measured quality control values for safety and efficacy.

Vertical banded gastroplasty (Fig. 2) is a precise but simple procedure that reduces the capacity for a meal by 100-fold. A window is created with an instrument that removes two small, circular pieces of anterior and posterior stomach wall while it places two circular

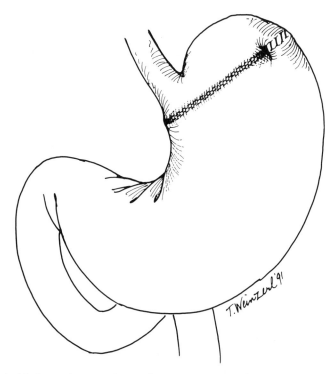

FIG. 1. Horizontal gastroplasty. Copyright held by The University of Iowa.

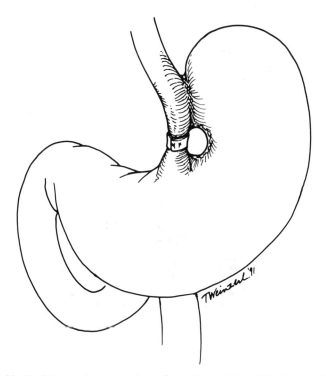

FIG. 2. Vertical banded gastroplasty. Copyright held by The University of Iowa.

rows of staples. The resultant window through the stomach allows stapling vertically, parallel with the lesser curvature to the angle of His, on the left side of the esophagogastric junction. This creates a 14-ml, vertical pouch. This window is then used to place a 5-cm circumference collar of Marlex mesh around the outlet of the pouch, which stabilizes it at an inside diameter of 11 to 12 mm. The collar is sewn to itself and not to the underlying stomach wall. Thus bacteria are not carried from the lumen out into the mesh. The mesh is rapidly incorporated by connective tissue and forms a new outer layer of the stomach, which protects it from infection. Marlex mesh collars are well tolerated.

Vertical banded gastroplasty functions solely to limit the amount of food that can be ingested at any one time. The pouch is emptying as it is being filled from the esophogus so that within a few months of the operation as much as a cup of food can be ingested in 20 minutes. The bites must be small and well chewed so that there are no chunks of fibrous meat or stringy vegetables that will block the passage. Liquids pass more quickly, and can be taken in larger amounts, which allows adequate hydration. What is ingested is digested in the stomach, duodenum, and intestine in a normal sequence, and is fully absorbed so that there is minimal risk of malnutrition.

Patients walk in the hall on the day of the operation. They require no nasal gastric tube and are given intravenous fluids from the night before operation and for 1 or 2 days following. They begin clear liquids the first day following operation and pureed foods on the second day. They leave the hospital most commonly on the fourth day. The midline upper abdominal incision seldom becomes infected (less than 2%); when such infections occur, they are so minor as to increase the median postoperative stay in the hospital by only 1 day. The most serious complication is a perforation of the digestive tract, which has occurred in 0.6% of patients and results in a median postoperative stay of 12 days. This finding compares with the 4-day median postoperative stay for the uncomplicated patient. Early detection of a perforation, followed by an emergency operation and closure, or drainage, usually results in rapid recovery. The diagnosis of perforation may be difficult and delayed, with consequent peritonitis and more complicated or lethal course. The mortality rate from all causes after VBG is less than 0.3%.

The experience at UIHC, 5 years after VBG (Fig. 3) and using a 5-cm collar, is that 15% of patients sustain a loss of 75% of their excess weight without need for a revision and can be considered to have an excellent result. Another 33% have a good result in that they lose 51% to 75% of their excess weight without further surgery. Another 30% achieve a fair result, sustaining a loss of 25% to 50% of their excess weight for at least 5 years and without revisional surgery. There were 22%

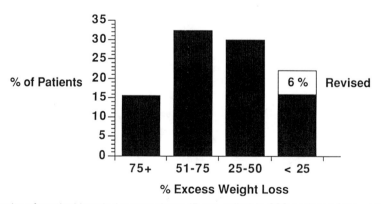

FIG. 3. Results of vertical banded gastroplasty (5-cm collar) in 303 patients followed for 5 years.

who were considered failures because they either required a revision operation (6%) or lost less than 25% of their excess weight (16%). These figures probably underestimate what can be accomplished with VBG (5-cm collar) since they represent the earliest patients. There have been changes during this decade of experience with VBG. A smaller pouch size, formed with a vertical four-row stapler, now provides a more secure partition.

Roux-en-Y Gastric Bypass

Roux-en-Y gastric bypass (RGB; Fig. 4), introduced by Griffen et al. (12), is the second most frequently used operation for treatment of obesity today. The original loop gastric bypass (LGB; Fig. 5) was introduced in 1967 as an analog of Billroth II gastric resection (13). The latter operation had been in use for over half a century for the treatment of acid peptic disease and cancer of the stomach. Weight loss, which was an undesirable side effect of resection, was used empirically for the treatment of severe obesity. The loop of jejunum that was used to drain the small upper stomach pouch allowed bile and pancreatic juice to enter the upper stomach and lower esophagus. This led to a modification in which one limb of a Y-shaped reconstruction of jejunum was used to drain the stomach pouch while the bile and pancreatic juice entered from a separate limb of the Y. Irritating digestive juices were thus excluded from the upper stomach. The exclusion of Y-

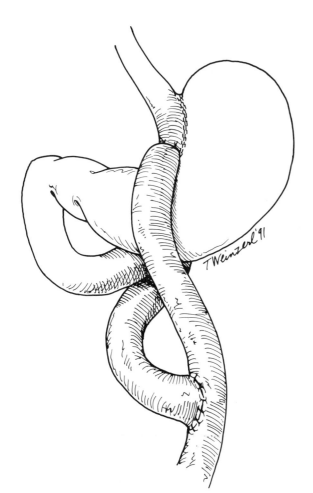

FIG. 4. Roux-en-Y gastric bypass. Copyright held by The University of Iowa.

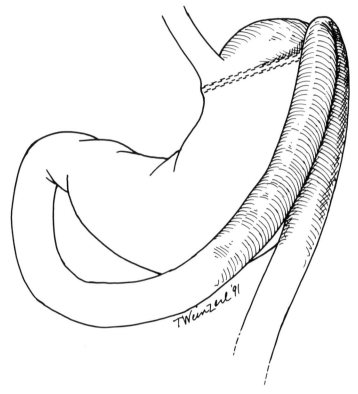

FIG. 5. Loop gastric bypass. Copyright held by The University of Iowa.

shaped jejunal reconstruction made the operation more complex and examination of the excluded stomach and duodenum more difficult.

Roux-en-Y gastric bypass carries a somewhat higher operative risk and increases the potential for long-term complication from bowel obstruction and acid peptic ulceration. These latter risks are low but remain for the life of the patient. Bypass of the pylorus allows stomach contents to empty into the small bowel without the normal control of osmoreceptors in the duodenum. Normally the duodenal contents remain isotonic with body fluids. Hypertonic fluids entering the small bowel may result in weakness and sweating after meals, which is referred to as the dumping syndrome. This has been cited as an advantage in weight control because it discourages the ingestion of sweets. If the stoma draining the pouch is as small as is recommended in most gastric reduction opera-

tions, there is less dumping. With a larger opening, the dumping may help in discouraging ingestion of sweets, but this is usually a temporary effect. There are patients who defeat these operations by continually snacking, and for them RGB is no better than VBG.

One of the disadvantages of bypass of the duodenum is malabsorption of iron and calcium. Iron deficiency anemia is common if there is a chronic loss of blood, as in heavy menses. The bone disease that is seen in postmenopausal women is likely to be exaggerated or to appear earlier than in women with a normal passage of food. The greatest disadvantage of gastric bypass is that over time the pouch, stoma, and adjacent jejunum increase in size, allowing the patient to eat a larger than needed meal. This in turn allows a return to an excessive weight and the need for another operation. In recent years all revisions of RGB at University of Iowa Hospitals and Clinics have been conversions to VBG (14).

Beginning early in the use of gastric bypass, efforts were made to simplify the operation. Many of the reasons for abandonment of gastric resection for the treatment of peptic ulcer disease have also been reasons for seeking a simpler and more physiologic operation for the treatment of severe obesity. Vertical banded gastroplasty may not produce as much weight reduction in early years as RGB, but it has many advantages for lifetime use.

Gastric Banding

Gastric banding (Fig. 6) involves the placement of a plastic collar around the entire circumference of the stomach with a small portion of the stomach left above the band, as the meal sizing reservoir. Since there is no stapling there is no risk of breakdown of a staple line. The problems with gastric banding have been related to the use of pouches that were too large (often unmeasured as well) and the difficulty in calibration of the passage between the upper and lower stomach. Reoperations were frequently required to remove, or reduce the tension of, a band that was too tight. Further enlargement of a pouch that was too large to begin with also resulted in obstruction, which was another reason for removal of the band.

Kuzmak (15) has introduced an adjustable collar with a bladder on the inside so that the stoma size can be changed by injection into a subcutaneous port. This operation is in use by a limited number of surgeons who are working under a protocol to determine the efficacy, advantages, and disadvantages of the technique.

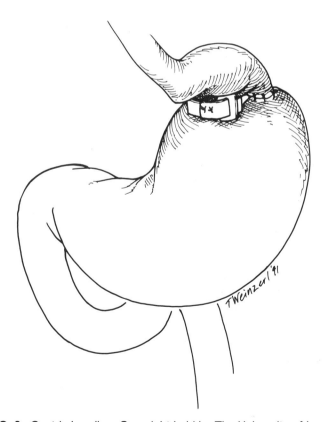

FIG. 6. Gastric banding. Copyright held by The University of Iowa.

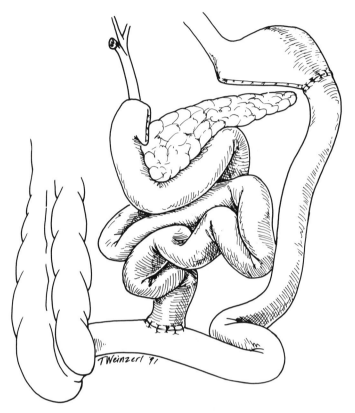

FIG. 7. Biliopancreatic bypass. Copyright held by The University of Iowa.

Biliopancreatic Bypass

Biliopancreatic diversion (BPD) (Fig. 7) is an operation designed to bypass much of the intestine without introducing the complications from overgrowth of bacteria in the bypassed bowel. There is no segment of small bowel that does not have either food or digestive juices washing through to decrease the concentration of bacteria. Biliopancreatic diversion has the configuration of RGB, but the limbs are much longer and much of the stomach is removed to decrease the risk of stomal ulcer. BPD was introduced by Scopinaro (16) to answer the objective of reducing weight to a normal level. It does not produce many of the complications of intestinal bypass, but it does cause protein malnutrition unless the patient makes a conscious effort to eat large amounts of protein. The procedure shares many of the disadvantages of RGB. Some surgeons have attempted to use BPD with a gastric bypass instead of gastric resection. This probably increases the incidence of stomal and duodenal ulcer. Biliopancreatic bypass requires intensive follow-up, with a considerable array of laboratory work. Since any operation for treatment of obesity must be present and effective for a lifetime, the use of a complex operation that requires ingestion of large amounts of protein and indefinite and expensive follow-up should not be used unless the patient can understand and afford these requirements and be willing to have the operation reversed later in life if the requirements cannot be met.

PSYCHOLOGICAL AND SOCIAL ASPECTS

A major contribution of the surgical treatment of obesity has been the light that it has thrown on the origins of the psychological problems that afflict severely obese persons.

For many years it had been believed that psychological problems were root causes of obesity; the corollary of this belief was that the more severe the obesity the more severe the psychological problems.

It is true that severely obese persons often have severe psychological problems, but experience with surgical treatment of severe obesity has made it clear that these psychological problems are largely secondary to the obesity. Rand and Macgregor (17) studied the perceived liability of morbid obesity in patients 3 years after successful obesity surgery and found that the perception of these patients was quite different from that of patients with other medical problems. The formerly obese would choose a major handicap such as deafness, dyslexia, diabetes, legal blindness, very bad acne, heart disease, or amputation of one leg, in preference to resumption of severe obesity. These answers are in marked contrast to those of people with other physical disabilities. People with these disabilities almost always find the familiar condition to be preferable to some other condition with which they have had no experience. In addition, all patients expressed a preference for being of normal weight and of modest means as compared with the imagined choice of being a morbidly obese multimillionaire.

Rand and Macgregor (18) have also investigated the conditions that have given rise to the derogatory views obese people have of themselves, beginning with Gluttony, one of the seven deadly sins listed by the early Christian church. Even today severely obese persons suffer from prejudice and discrimination. They are frequently and erroneously considered to be lacking in will power, lazy, and emotionally unstable. Many physicians share this attitude toward the severely obese.

After operation and weight loss these patients perceived little or no prejudice in their daily lives. The only exceptions were members of the medical profession and insurance companies. Self-insured formerly obese persons often cannot obtain insurance at the rates charged to normal weight adults even though they have a normal weight following a gastric reduction operation.

It might be expected that an operation that markedly reduced weight would have an effect on marriage. Neil et al. (19) thought there was a destabilizing effect. Rand et al. (20), however, cast a far more favorable light on the marital consequences of gastric restriction surgery. They found a relatively high frequency of divorce, but only among couples in conflicted marriages, in which divorce might be viewed as a positive step. In unconflicted marriages there was increased marital satisfaction. All studies agree that sexual satisfaction is improved. Hafner and Rogers (21), studying the adjustment of husbands to wives' weight loss, found that patients became more assertive and their husbands less assertive, and more dissatisfied.

One new development deserves mention. Many of the patients who have come to us for surgical treatment of obesity have confided that they were sexually abused as children. This information is surprising in that it has been volunteered without specific questioning by a physician. Felitti (22) has reported an increased prevalence of severe obesity among members of a health insurance organization who, during their annual medical examination, answered yes to the question "Have you ever been raped or sexually molested?" Patients answering in the affirmative had a fourfold higher incidence of severe obesity (25% were more than 100 lb over estimated ideal weight). The onset of obesity came subsequent to the sexual event and was most often proximate.

PREDICTION OF OUTCOME

It would be highly desirable if one could predict the outcome of surgery for obesity, both in terms of weight loss and of general well-being. A number of attempts at prediction have been made, with indifferent success. By far the most powerful predictor of total weight loss is initial weight, as has been noted repeatedly in patients with lesser degrees of overweight. Barrash et al. (23) confirmed the value of this predictor for 138 severely overweight patients treated with VBG. In this group initial weight correlated with weight loss ($r = 0.60$, $p < 0.0001$), accounting for 36% of the variance in weight loss at 1 year. The addition of age and various items on the Minnesota Multiphasic Personality Inventory to a full regression model increased the variance accounted for to 54.7%.

Attempts at prediction of weight loss from psychological testing, primarily the Minnesota Multiphasic Personality Inventory, have proved disappointing. Barrash et al. (23) found that the three personality clusters that had been reported by Duckro et al. (24) did not predict weight loss at 1 year and the ten clusters that he identified as of some predictive value were not replicated by subsequent investigators.

Valley and Grace (6) found that the simple measure of a history of psychiatric hospitalization was the strongest predictor of medical and psychological complications from, and satisfaction with, the type of horizontal gastroplasty that they were using at the time. Neither a history of psychiatric hospitalization nor other psychological measures, however, predicted weight loss.

There is today no basis for requiring routine psychological testing of patients before they are selected for treatment for obesity with an operation. Psychological testing might influence the decision to operate upon a patient whose weight was of borderline severity. It might be of greatest use to identify patients for whom special care could be provided in an effort to reduce the risk of medical and psychological complications and to ensure satisfaction with the operation.

When do patients choose to have an operation for severe obesity? They are usually at their highest lifetime weight and it might be concluded that they reach a degree of stress from the severity of obesity that causes them to elect this drastic action. Most of them have tried and failed diet and other nonsurgical means. Rand et al. (25) found that there were significantly more stressful life events during the 1- and 3-year period before gastric bypass for obesity than occurred in a control group of adults. These events included a major illness of a family member, major personal illness, major financial difficulties, a move to another city, or a new person in the household. Rand suggested that clinicians consider whether a patient was seeking an operation because of added life-stressful events, when in less stressful times the patient might seek other, safer means of weight control. An operation might be temporarily deferred, but there is no effective, safer means of weight control. The safest course for most severely overweight patients is still an effective weight-reducing operation.

CONCLUSIONS

More than 1.5 million people in the United States are candidates for surgical treatment of obesity. Such severe obesity is morbid and lethal. There is no effective treatment other than an operation. Early effective treatment can prevent irreversible complications that may otherwise develop. Vertical banded gastroplasty is the simplest and safest operation. It is well tolerated and forces most patients to eat small portions, chew well, and stop eating before overflow of the 100-fold reduced capacity. Patients achieve a new and more rewarding life as a result of the weight reduction.

REFERENCES

1. Kuczmarski RJ: Prevalence of overweight and weight gain in the United States. *Am J Clin Nutr* 1992;495S–502S.
2. Colditz GA. Economic costs of severe obesity. *Am J Clin Nutr* 1992;503S–7S.
3. Lissner L, Odell PM, D'Agostino RB, et al. Variability of body weight and health outcomes in the Framingham population. *N Engl J Med* 1991; 324:1839–44.
4. Martin LF, Tan TL, Holmes PA, et al. Preoperative insurance status influences postoperative complication rates for gastric bypass. *Am J Surg* 1991; 161:625–34.
5. Civetta JM. Editorial. *Am J Surg* 1991;161:634–5.
6. Valley V, Grace DM. Psychosocial risk factors in gastric surgery for obesity: identifying guidelines for screening. *Int J Obes* 1987;11:105–13.
7. Halmi KA, Stunkard AJ, Mason EE. Emotional response to weight reduction by three methods: gastric

bypass, jejunoileal bypass, diet. *Am J Clin Nutr* 1074;33:446–51.

8. Mills MR, Stunkard AJ. Behavioral changes following surgery for obesity. *Am J Psychiatry* 1976; 133:527–31.

9. Stunkard AJ, Stinnet JL, Smoller JW. Psychological and social aspects of the surgical treatment of obesity. *Am J Psychiatry* 1986;143:417–29.

10. Schachter S. Cognitive effects on bodily functioning. Studies of obesity and eating. In: Glass D, ed. *Neurophysiology and emotion.* New York: Rockefeller University Press, 1967;117–44.

11. Mason EE. Vertical banded gastroplasty for obesity. *Arch Surg* 1982;117:701–6.

12. Griffin WO, Young VL, Stevenson CC. A prospective comparison of gastric and jejunoileal bypass procedures for morbid obesity. *Ann Surg* 1977; 186:500–6.

13. Mason EE, Ito C. Gastric bypass in obesity. *Surg Clin North Am* 1967;47:1345–51.

14. Mason EE, Scott DH. Reoperations for failed gastric bypass procedures for obesity. *Surg Clin North Am* 1991;71:45–56.

15. Duzmak LI. Stoma adjustable silicone gastric banding. *Surgical Rounds* 1991;14:19–28.

16. Scopinaro N, Gianetta E, Civalleri D, Bonalumi U, Bachi V. Two years experience with bilio-pancreatic bypass for obesity. *Am J Clin Nutr* 1980;33:506–14.

17. Rand CSW, Macgregor AMC. Successful weight loss following obesity surgery and the perceived liability of morbid obesity. *Int J Obes* 1991;15 [*in press*].

18. Rand CSW, Macgregor AMC. Morbidly obese patient's perceptions of social discrimination before and after surgery for obesity. *South Med J* 1990;83:1390–5.

19. Neill JR, Marshall JR, Yale CE. Marital changes after intestinal bypass surgery. *JAMA* 1978;240: 447–50.

20. Rand CSW, Kuldau JM, Robbins L. Surgery for obesity and marriage equality. *JAMA* 1982;247: 1419–22.

21. Hafner RJ, Rogers J. Husbands' adjustment to wives' weight loss after gastric restriction for morbid obesity. *Int J Obes* 1990;14:1069–78.

22. Felitti VJ. Long-term medical consequences of incest, rape, and molestation. *South Med J* 1991; 84:328–31.

23. Barrash J, Rodriguez EM, Scott DH, Mason EE, Sines JO. The utility of MMPI subtypes for the prediction of weight loss after bariatric surgery. *Int J Obes* 1987;11:115–28.

24. Duckro PN, Leavitt JN, Beal DG, Chang AF. Psychological status among female candidates for surgical treatment. *Int J Obes* 1983;7:477–86.

25. Rand CSW, Robbins L, Kuldau JM. Stressful life events and the decision for surgery for obesity. *Psychosomatics* 1983;24:534–9.

Obesity: Theory and Therapy, Second Edition,
edited by A. J. Stunkard and T. A. Wadden.
Raven Press, Ltd., New York © 1993.

20

Obstetrical Problems in the Obese Patient

Joy D. Steinfeld and Arnold W. Cohen

*Department of Obstetrics and Gynecology, Division of Maternal-Fetal Medicine,
University of Pennsylvania Medical Center, Philadelphia, Pennsylvania 19104*

Obesity is one of the most common problems confronting the obstetrical team. Although obesity has been associated with increased maternal and fetal morbidity and mortality, there are few guidelines available to assist those caring for the obese patient. In this chapter, the patterns of weight gain and nutrition in pregnancy will be reviewed for both the normal weight and obese patient. The obstetrical complications associated with obesity will be identified and discussed, and management plans outlined.

DEFINITION

There is no universally accepted definition of obesity in pregnancy, so it is difficult to evaluate and compare the data that exist. Some authors define obesity using an absolute number, while others use height–weight relationships. Obesity has been defined as a prepregnancy weight greater than 200 lb or 90 kg (1). *Overweight* has been described as 120% of normal weight for height, and *obese* as 135% of normal weight for height (2). The body mass index (BMI) is calculated in metric units as weight/height², with obesity defined as a BMI > 29.0 (3). Peckham classified as obese any pregnant patient weighing more than 169 lb (4). Matthews defined extreme obesity in pregnancy as 200 lb or greater (5), and Tracy proposed 250 lb as the lower limit for massive obesity (6).

Because no standard definition of obesity exists, there is no truly accurate estimate of its prevalence. The prevalence rate in several studies varies from 3 to 10% (1,7,8).

NORMAL NUTRITION AND WEIGHT GAIN IN PREGNANCY

Pregnancy places an increased nutritional burden on the mother, as she must meet her own metabolic demands as well as those of the growing fetus. The dietary recommendations for pregnancy should allow for the proper regulation of maternal weight, promote fetal growth, and prepare the mother for labor, birth, and lactation. Approximately 300 extra kcal must be consumed daily in a typical pregnancy. Other daily nutritional requirements for a normal pregnancy include an additional 30 g of protein, 30 to 60 mg of elemental iron, and 300 μg of folic acid.

The recommended weight gain in pregnancy is calculated from the necessary increases from the fetus (7.5 lb), placenta (1.5 lb), amniotic fluid (2 lb), uterus (2.5 lb), mammary glands (1 lb), increased maternal blood volume (3.5 lb), interstitial fluid (2.5 lb), and maternal fat stores (5 to 8 lb). Therefore, current recommendations for weight gain in pregnancy for women of normal pregravid weight vary only slightly. The National Academy of Sciences recommends a

25 to 35 lb weight gain (3), while the American College of Obstetricians and Gynecologists advises a weight gain of 30 lb (9). A 1- to 2-lb gain is expected in the first trimester, and an 11- to 12-lb gain in each of the subsequent trimesters. If the gravida has a low prepregnancy weight, a slightly higher target weight gain is recommended, i.e., 28 to 40 lb. The suggested weight gain for a twin gestation is 35 to 40 lb over the course of the pregnancy.

Appropriate weight gain necessary for maternal or fetal well-being in an obese gravida is not the same as in the nonobese woman. A lower target range of 15 to 25 lb is generally accepted. Even with minimal weight gain in obese patients, fetal growth is not impaired, nor is fetal outcome adversely affected (10). Obese gravidas should not undertake weight reduction diets during pregnancy because pregnant women more easily progress to ketonuria and ketonemia under starvation conditions as a result of catabolism of fat stores (2). Extreme cases of maternal starvation, as observed during the siege of Leningrad in 1942 and the Dutch famine in 1945, demonstrated that poor maternal nutrition produced increased premature deliveries and perinatal mortality (11). There was also an increased incidence of low-birth-weight infants. These unfortunate historical events showed that a state of near starvation must be induced to establish a clear difference in the outcome of pregnancy. The pregnant patient who is obese prior to pregnancy protects both herself and her fetus from the effects of nutritional deprivation during pregnancy.

While weight gain in a normal pregnancy varies widely, the widest variation is seen in obese women. One of the clinical measurements that has been found to be of value in assessing fetal growth is prepregnancy weight for height, and serial weight measurements during the pregnancy (3). As prepregnancy weight increases or as gestational weight gain rises, fetal somatic growth increases (1). Thus one of the tools used to assess fetal growth and the general well-being of the pregnancy is lost in the obese gravida and in patients with abnormal patterns of weight gain.

Obese and nonobese patients whose weight gain during pregnancy does not follow the normal pattern present a problem. A steady, progressive weight gain generally represents a gain of lean as well as fat tissue, whereas an erratically high weight gain is likely to represent lean and fat tissue, plus fluid retention. When a pattern of inappropriate weight gain is suspected or established, gestational diabetes and other pathological conditions (e.g., preeclampsia) must be ruled out. If no pathological process is occurring, the patient should receive dietary counseling. Excessive weight gain in pregnancy is a risk factor at delivery, even in the nonobese patient. A very high gestational weight gain is associated with an increased rate of large for gestational age (LGA) infants. LGA babies have an increase in the risk of fetopelvic disproportion, operative delivery (instrumental delivery or cesarean section), birth trauma, perinatal asphyxia, and mortality (3). These increased risks are primarily related to the increased rate of fetal macrosomia in obese gravidas. Spellacy and coworkers (12) documented an increase in macrosomia due to weight alone of 5.6% in gravidas weighing more than 90 kg and 10% in gravidas weighing more than 112.5 kg. Of all infants in their series weighing more than 4,500 g, 44.6% were born to mothers weighing more than 90 kg, and 22.5% to mothers weighing more than 112.5 kg. These associations are more pronounced in short women, so a lower ceiling on weight gain for shorter women may be advisable. High gestational weight gain is also associated with increased postpartum weight retention and subsequent obesity (13).

OBSTETRICAL COMPLICATIONS IN THE OBESE PATIENT

Diagnosing pregnancy can be difficult in the obese patient. Irregular menses are more common in obese women, and pelvic examination to document the size of the uterus can be difficult or impossible. Auscultation of fetal heart tones transabdominally is less successful at early gestational ages than in the nonobese patient, resulting in an increased need for early pregnancy ultrasounds to establish whether a viable, intrauterine pregnancy exists. Transabdominal ultrasound in the obese patient is technically more difficult and less sensitive. The development of transvaginal ultrasound techniques offers a tremendous improvement in early pregnancy diagnosis and evaluation in the obese as well as nonobese patient. Diagnosis of pregnancy in an obese patient, even with the use of transabdominal ultrasound, could not be made in some cases until late in the first trimester. Using transvaginal ultrasound, a gestational sac can now be visualized at 5 to 6 weeks, a fetal pole at 6 to 7 weeks, and the fetal heartbeat at 7 to 8 weeks.

Maternal serum α-fetoprotein (AFP) levels are measured at approximately 16 weeks of gestation to screen for neural tube defects and other abnormal fetal conditions. Serendipitously, an association between low AFP levels and Down syndrome was noted after the test was in use (14). Obese gravidas need to have their serum AFP levels adjusted in order to compensate for their increased plasma volume (15), or they will have falsely lowered AFP levels, erroneously raising a question of a fetal trisomy and the need for amniocentesis. Should there truly be a need for genetic diagnosis, amniocentesis, chorionic villus sampling, and percutaneous umbilical blood sampling are technically more difficult to perform in the obese patient (16,17). Not only is there the problem of decreased resolution for these ultrasound-guided procedures, but the longer needles necessary to traverse the additional subcutaneous fat in these patients are not as precisely manipulated.

Monitoring fetal growth and well-being is also more challenging in the obese gravida. Sizing the uterus and assessing fundal height may continue to be a problem. In the nonobese patient, between 18 and 32 weeks gestation there is good correlation between the height of the uterine fundus in centimeters (measured as the distance over the abdominal wall from the top of the symphysis pubis to the top of the fundus) and the gestational age of the fetus in weeks (18). This correlation and the normal pattern of weight gain are no longer usable as tools to assess fetal growth in the obese patient. As the pregnancy progresses, the decreased resolution of transabdominal ultrasound in these patients may detract from the ability to detect and follow fetal anomalies or growth disturbances. Visualization decreases with a body mass index greater than the 90th percentile, with the most marked decrease for the fetal heart, spine, and umbilical cord (19). Many of the fetal structural defects missed on ultrasound are missed in obese patients (20). A relatively new but increasingly relied upon test for fetal status is the fetal (in utero) echocardiogram. This has become a virtually requisite test in numerous clinical situations (e.g., fetal arrhythmia, maternal insulin-dependent diabetes, drug exposure, or a previous child with a cardiac anomaly). Unfortunately, this study has decreased accuracy and resolution in the obese patient, with a higher rate of "unsatisfactory" studies (21).

Some maternal complications prior to delivery are more common in the obese patient. There is an increased incidence of urinary tract infection and pyelonephritis, phlebitis (22), and gallbladder disease (23) in obese patients compared with nonobese patients. Low back pain, which is common in pregnancy, may also be exacerbated in the obese gravida. Obesity may cause a delay in the diagnosis of some surgical emergencies as the obese patient's abdominal exam may be more difficult and less revealing. Obese patients are more likely to suffer from hypertension prior to pregnancy, and preeclampsia during it (24), both of which are associated with increased maternal and fetal morbidity and mortality. The reported incidence of superimposed preeclampsia ranges from 10 to 50%, depending on the degree of hypertension at the onset of pregnancy (25). They are also more likely to have impaired glucose tolerance and gestational diabetes (26). Horger et al. (27) observed that the frequency of abnormal glucose tolerance tests increases with increasing maternal weight (27). No patient weighing less than 100 lb had an abnormal glucose tolerance test before or at the time of delivery, but the number of patients demonstrating glucose intolerance progressively increased with increasing weight. Of patients weighing 250 lb or more, 100% of those tested prior to delivery and 55% of those tested at the time of delivery displayed abnormal glucose tolerance.

If the patient has had bypass surgery for morbid obesity, she will generally conceive after the period of maximal weight loss has occurred (6 months or more postoperatively). This is associated with the reversal of menstrual abnormalities associated with massive obesity (28). There may be chronic problems postoperatively with electrolytes and metabolism, and there is a high incidence of reoperation for complications of prior obesity surgery, including bowel obstruction, intraabdominal sepsis, and gastrointestinal bleeding. Over a 3-year period at the University of California at Los Angeles, 32 such patients underwent 76 reoperations for complications of prior obesity surgery. Following the initial revision, 23 patients required surgery for major complications, and 4 additional patients died (29).

A host of problems may present at the time of delivery. Monitoring the fetal heart rate via external fetal monitor at any time during the pregnancy, and particularly during labor, is less easily accomplished in the obese gravida. It is also more difficult to trace contractions in an obese patient using an external tocodynamometer. Use of an internal monitor and intrauterine pressure catheter can help overcome these difficulties during labor. Although more difficult in the obese parturient, assessment of fetal status via scalp sampling in labor may prove helpful.

In addition to the problems encountered with fetal heart rate monitoring and assessing the contraction pattern, discerning the fetal presentation and position is more difficult. There is some question of an increase in the incidence of abnormal presentations in the obese gravida, although this is not clearly documented in current obstetrical literature.

Prolonged labors and difficult deliveries are more common in obese patients (30), but whether this is primarily accounted for by those patients with macrosomic fetuses is unclear. There is an increased incidence of macrosomia in obese patients, and a sequential increase in the incidence of macrosomia with increasing pregravid weight (31). In one series, 38% of infants weighing over 4,000 g were born to mothers weighing 200 lb or more (32). Between 15 and 33% of infants born to obese mothers at term weigh more than 4,000 g, compared with 4 to 5% of leaner women's infants (1). Macrosomia, obesity, and abnormal glucose tolerance put the fetus at increased risk of shoulder dystocia, a potentially devastating complication at delivery (33). Golditch and Kirkman (34) noted a 3% incidence of shoulder dystocia in infants with birth weights of 4,100 to 4,500 g, and an 8.2% incidence in infants over 4,500 g at birth. Gross and coworkers reported a rate of 8.6% for infants between 4,000 and 4,499 g, and an astonishing 35.7% rate of shoulder dystocia in infants weighing 4,500 g or more (35).

Maternal positioning at the time of delivery assumes increased importance in the obese parturient. Padding the stirrups may help to decrease the incidence of nerve compression injuries. Adequate exposure in order to visualize the cervix and vaginal vault, and assess and repair lacerations, is also more difficult but crucial.

Should the obese gravida require a cesarean delivery, she will be subject to increased morbidity and mortality. Obese patients are more difficult to anesthetize, particularly with general anesthesia. Obese patients more rapidly become hypoxic during induction of anesthesia (36), in addition to presenting problems with positioning, intubation, and ventilation. Diminished cardiopulmonary reserve, concurrent systemic disorders such as hypertension and diabetes, and difficulty with surgical procedures despite muscular relaxation also contribute to management problems (37). Although it is not clearly demonstrated in the literature, some anesthesiologists feel that placement of regional anesthetics (e.g., epidural) is also more difficult in the obese patient.

Adequate surgical exposure may be a problem, especially if a large pannus is present, and influences the type of incision made. Although a vertical incision provides better exposure, facilitates delivery, and may prevent the incision from being under the moist pannus postoperatively, it is more uncomfortable for the patient, and is subject to higher rates of disruption. Regardless of the type of incision made, there is an increased incidence of wound infection and dehiscence in obese patients. In a series of 107 obese women delivered by cesarean section, Wolfe and coworkers (38) documented a 15% incidence of wound infection. In an attempt to decrease wound complications in the obese gravida, some surgeons have suggested alternative types of incisions, such as a transverse periumbilical incision (39) or a supraumbilical upper abdominal midline incision (40). These alternative incisions avoid attempts to elevate the pannus intraoperatively as is necessary when performing a Pfannenstiel's incision, avoid making an incision through the panniculus, and avoid the incision being under the pannus postoperatively, all of which are associated with increased rates of infection.

Wound closure must be scrupulous in the obese patient. Drains should be used more liberally, especially in the subcutaneous fat layer, and the type of closure chosen should be modified. The wound should be closed like any compromised patient's wound (e.g., steroid-dependent patients, or those with malignancies). Interrupted sutures on the fascial layer or a Smead-Jones type of closure for vertical incisions may be prudent. Sutures should be slowly dissolving or permanent on the fascial layer. Use of a nonabsorbable single-layer technique has also been shown to be successful in patients with midline vertical incisions at high risk for wound disruption (41).

Obese patients have increased operative times and increased blood loss, both of which contribute to increased postoperative morbidity and mortality (30,42). Not surprisingly, obese patients have longer postoperative hospital stays due to their increased rate of complications. In 588 patients weighing 250 lb or more who underwent cesarean section, estimated blood loss exceeding 1,000 cc, operating time of more than 2 hours, and postoperative wound infection were all more common (30,43). Use of prophylactic antibiotics has been shown to decrease the postoperative wound infection rate in obese patients (44), and their use is advised. Other factors contributing to the more morbid postoperative course in the obese patient are the increased rates of pulmonary complications (including atelectasis and pneumonia) and embolic events. Along with prolonged operative time (greater than 4 hours) and advanced age (greater than 70 years), obesity is a leading risk factor for pulmonary complications (45). The risk of postoperative pulmonary complications is correlated with the degree of the patient's obesity (46). Postoperative prophylactic heparin should be used more liberally in the obese postpartum patient, especially since the hypercoagulable effects of pregnancy do not resolve for several weeks after delivery. Unfortunately, obese patients undergoing abdominal surgery are more likely to fail low-dose heparin and experience thromboembolism than are patients with a normal body mass index (47). In addition to the higher rate of surgical complications, maternal mortality is increased by the higher rates of antepartum, intrapartum, and postpartum complications in the obese parturient. There was a 3.6% mortality rate reported by Abdel-Moneim (48) in obese surgical patients, but most of them had other complicating conditions including hypertension and diabetes. Unfortunately, it is not possible to separate the effects of obesity from other complicating factors in order to establish what the increase in maternal mortality is, if any, solely from obesity.

Are there any benefits derived from obesity? There is a decreased incidence of anemia in these patients (49), as well as some protection from osteoporosis (50). The incidences of low birth weight, infant prematurity, and intrauterine growth retardation are decreased. There is conflicting evidence regarding the rate of perinatal mortality in the obese population. Garbaciak et al. (51) noted a significant increase in perinatal mortality as a function of maternal weight only when other antepartum complications were present. In patients without antepartum complications, there was no significant difference in perinatal mortality regardless of weight (51), a conclusion supported by Rahaman et al. (52). Naeye (53), however, noted an increase in perinatal mortality with increasing maternal weight that was only partially explained by other factors. Thin subjects had a perinatal mortality rate of 37 in 1,000 offspring, which progressively increased to 121 in 1,000 in offspring of obese subjects ($p < 0.001$).

GENERAL MANAGEMENT PLAN

Optimal care of the obese patient should begin prior to pregnancy with family planning and nutritional counseling. The patient's weight should be stable and her diet well balanced. Oral contraceptives may be used for birth control, except in patients who have had gastrointestinal bypass surgery for morbid obesity. Steroid absorption in this group of patients may be inadequate to provide reliable contraception (54). Barrier methods and the intrauterine device are acceptable. In the morbidly obese patient, there may be a decrease in the efficacy of Norplant (55), so another method may be preferable.

Once pregnant, the patient should be seen early in gestation in order to date the pregnancy reliably using the menstrual history and pelvic examination. Transvaginal ultrasound is a useful adjunct to confirm dating early. A screening urine culture should be obtained. The patient should be counseled on good nutrition during pregnancy. A target weight gain of 15 to 20 lb, rather than 25 to 30 lb is sought. Little weight gain is expected during the first trimester. Weight should be gained progressively at the rate of approximately $\frac{1}{2}$ lb a week after the first trimester. Patients should be seen every 2 weeks and their weight recorded. Maternal fat stores of about 5 to 8 lb are usually deposited during early pregnancy, and provide an important energy source during lactation. Accumulation of this reserve would not be necessary in the obese gravida (56).

In the second trimester, an ultrasound examination should be scheduled to verify dates and evaluate fetal anatomy. The patient's baseline blood pressure should be established, and readings carefully followed during the course of the gestation. A screen for gestational diabetes should be planned by 24 to 28 weeks if there is no other indication for earlier testing (e.g., glycosuria). This evaluation is generally performed by administering 50 g of oral glucose to the nonfasting patient and obtaining a blood sugar 1 hour later. A 1-hour plasma glucose level of 140 mg/100 ml or greater is considered positive (2). A 3-hour oral glucose tolerance test should follow a positive screening test. To confirm normal fetal growth, serial ultrasound examinations should be done. If the patient has hypertension or diabetes, antenatal testing should be initiated at about 28 weeks gestation.

The patient's progress must be carefully followed once she is in labor. Direct monitoring using a fetal scalp electrode and internal pressure catheter will facilitate evaluation of progress. Anesthetic consultation to ensure adequate pain relief is appropriate, as conduction anesthetic techniques and intubation and ventilation are more difficult in these patients. Shoulder dystocia should be anticipated, and the patient's legs should not be strapped down prior to delivery to facilitate rapid manipulation should shoulder dystocia occur.

Postpartum care must be aggressive, with early ambulation and attention to pulmonary status encouraged. Consideration should be given to prophylactic heparinization, which should be continued until full ambulation is achieved. The amount of vaginal bleeding should be followed carefully, as the obese abdomen may mask uterine hypotonus.

FUTURE CONSIDERATIONS

Additional information from further research will improve management approaches in the pregnancy complicated by obesity. Careful definition of the problem and assessment of the prevalence of this condition should be sought. The actual incidence of concomitant hypertension, diabetes, and thromboembolic complications should be established. With a broader knowledge base and enhanced understanding of these patients, their care can be optimized.

REFERENCES

1. Kliegman RM, Gross T. Perinatal problems of the obese mother and her infant. *Obstet Gynecol* 1985;66:299–306.
2. Creasy RK, Resnik R. *Maternal-fetal medicine: principles and practice,* 2nd ed. Philadelphia: WB Saunders, 1989.
3. The Subcommittee on Nutritional Status and Weight Gain During Pregnancy and the Subcommittee on Dietary Intake and Nutrient Supplements During Pregnancy. *Nutrition during pregnancy.* Washington, DC: National Academy of Sciences, 1990.
4. Peckham CH, Christianson RE. The relationship between prepregnancy weight and certain obstetric factors. *Am J Obstet Gynecol* 1971;111:1.
5. Matthews HB, Der Brucke MG. Normal expectancy in the extremely obese pregnant woman. *JAMA* 1938;110:554.
6. Tracy TA, Miller GL. Obstetric problems of the massively obese. *Obstet Gynecol* 1969;33:204.
7. Edwards LE, Dickes WF, Alton IR, et al. Pregnancy in the massively obese: course, outcome, and obesity prognosis of the infant. *Am J Obstet Gynecol* 1978;131:479.
8. Petry JA. Obesity with pregnancy. *Obstet Gynecol* 1956;7:299.
9. Visscher HC, Rinehart RD (eds). *ACOG guide to planning for pregnancy, birth, and beyond.* Washington: The American College of Obstetricians and Gynecologists, 1990.
10. Ratner RE, Hamner LH 3d, Isada NB. Effects of gestational weight gain in morbidly obese women: II: Fetal outcome. *Am J Perinatol* 1990;7:295–9.
11. Smith CA. Effects of maternal undernutrition upon the newborn infant in Holland (1944–1945). *Am J Obstet Gynecol* 1947;30:229.
12. Spellacy WN, Miller S, Winegar A, Peterson PQ. Macrosomia—maternal characteristics and infant complications. *Obstet Gynecol* 1985;66:158–61.
13. Parham ES, Astrom MF, King SH. The association of pregnancy weight gain with the mother's postpartum weight. *J Am Diet Assoc* 1990;90:550–4.
14. Merkatz IR, Nitowsky HM, Macri JN, Johnson WE. An association between low maternal serum alpha-fetoprotein and fetal chromosome abnormalities. *Am J Obstet Gynecol* 1984;148:886.
15. Drugan A, Dvorin E, Johnson MP, Uhlmann WR, Evans MI. The inadequacy of the current correction for maternal weight in maternal serum alphafetoprotein interpretation. *Obstet Gynecol* 1989;74:698–701.
16. McGahan JP, Tennant F, Hanson FW, Lindfors KK, Quilligan EJ. Ultrasound needle guidance for amniocentesis in pregnancies with low amniotic fluid. *J Reprod Med* 1987;32:513–6.
17. Boulot P, Deschamps F, Lefort G, et al. Pure fetal blood samples obtained by cordocentesis: technical aspects of 322 cases. *Prenat Diagn* 1990;10:93–100.
18. Cunningham FG, MacDonald PC, Grant NF (eds). *Williams obstetrics,* 18th ed. Norwalk: Appleton and Lange, 1989;257–75.
19. Wolfe HM, Sokol RJ, Martier SM, Zador IE. Maternal obesity: a potential source of error in sonographic prenatal diagnosis. *Obstet Gynecol* 1990;76(3 Pt 1):339–42.
20. Pijlman BM, deKoning WB, Wladmiroff JW, Stewart PA. Detection of fetal structural malformations by ultrasound in insulin-dependent pregnant women. *US Med Biol* 1989;15:541–3.
21. Shime J, Bertrand M, Hagen-Ansert S, Rakowski H. Two dimensional and M mode echocardiography in the human fetus. *Am J Obstet Gynecol* 1984;148:679–85.
22. Krauer VF. Die Ubergewichtige Frau—ein Problem in der Geburtshilfe. *Gynaecologia* 1967;164:343.
23. Calhoun R, Willbanks O. Coexistence of gallbladder disease and morbid obesity. *Am J Surg* 1987;154:655–8.
24. Abrams B, Parker J. Overweight and pregnancy complications. *Int J Obes* 1988;12:293–303.
25. Anderson GD, Sibai BM. Hypertension in pregnancy. In *Obstetrics: normal and problem pregnancies.* New York: Churchill Livingstone, 1986.
26. Al-Shawaf T, Moghraby S, Akiel A. Does impaired glucose tolerance imply a risk in pregnancy? *Br J Obstet Gynaecol* 1988;95:1036–41.
27. Horger EO III, Miller MC III, Conner ED. Relations of large birth-weight to maternal diabetes mellitus. *Obstet Gynecol* 1975;45:150.
28. Printen KJ, Scott D. Pregnancy following gastric bypass for the treatment of morbid obesity. *Am Surg* 1982;48:363–5.
29. Cates JA, Drenick EJ, Abedin MZ, Doty JE, Saunders KD, Roslyn JJ. Reoperative surgery for the morbidly obese. A university experience. *Arch Surg* 1990;125:1400–4.
30. Johnson SR, Kolberg BH, Varner MW, Railsback LD. Maternal obesity and pregnancy. *Surg Gynecol Obstet* 1987;164:431–7.
31. Larsen CE, Serdula MK, Sullivan KM. Macrosomia: influence of maternal overweight among a low-income population. *Am J Obstet Gynecol* 1990;162:490–4.
32. Kirshon B, Wait RB. Incidence of gestational diabetes: effects of race. *Tex Med* 1990;86:88–90.
33. O'Leary JA, Leonetti HB. Shoulder dystocia: pre-

vention and treatment. *Am J Obstet Gynecol* 1990;162:5–9.

34. Golditch IM, Kirkman K. The large fetus—management and outcome. *Obstet Gynecol* 1988;52:26.

35. Gross TL, Sokol RJ, Williams T, Thompson K. Shoulder dystocia: a fetal-physician risk. *Am J Obstet Gynecol* 1987;156:1408–18.

36. Jense HG, Dubin SA, Silverstein PI, O'Leary-Escolas U. Effect of obesity on safe duration of apnea in anesthetized humans. *Anesth Analg* 1991;72:89–93.

37. Singh O. Evaluation of problems associated with obese patients during general anesthesia. *Middle East J Anesthesiol* 1985;8:241–7.

38. Wolfe HM, Gross TL, Sokol RJ, Bottoms SF, Thompson KL. Determinants of morbidity in obese women delivered by cesarean. *Obstet Gynecol* 1988;71:691–6.

39. Krebs HB, Helmkamp BF. Transverse periumbilical incision in the massively obese patient. *Obstet Gynecol* 1984;63:241–5.

40. Greer BE, Cain JM, Figge DC, Shy KK, Tamimi HK. Supraumbilical upper abdominal midline incision for pelvic surgery in the morbidly obese patient. *Obstet Gynecol* 1990;76(3 Pt 1):471–3.

41. Shepherd JH, Cavanagh D, Riggs D, Praphat H, Wisniewski BJ. Abdominal wound closure using a nonabsorbable single-layer technique. *Obstet Gynecol* 1983;61:248–52.

42. Wolfe HM, Gross TL, Sokol RJ, Bottoms SF, Thompson KL. Determinants of morbidity in obese women delivered by cesarean. *Obstet Gynecol* 1988;71:691–6.

43. Deleted in proof.

44. Forse RA, Karam B, MacLean LD, Christon NV. Antibiotic prophylaxis for surgery in morbidly obese patients. *Surgery* 1989;106:750–6.

45. Mircea N, Constantinescu C, Jianu E, Busu G. Risk of pulmonary complications in surgical patients. *Resuscitation* 1982;10:33–41.

46. Okeson GC. Pulmonary dysfunction and surgical risk. How to assess and minimize the hazards. *Postgrad Med* 1983;74:75–83.

47. Wille-Jorgensen P, Ott P. Predicting failure of low-dose prophylactic heparin in general surgical procedures. *Surg Gynecol Obstet* 1990;171:126–30.

48. Abdel-Moneim RI. The hazards of surgery in the obese. *Int Surg* 1985;70:101–3.

49. Luke B, Dickinson C, Petrie RH. Intrauterine growth: correlations of maternal nutritional status and rate of gestational weight gain. *Eur J Obstet Gynecol Reprod Biol* 1981;12:113–21.

50. Kelsey JL. Risk factors for osteoporosis and related fractures. *Public Health Rep* 1989;104[Suppl]:14–20.

51. Garbaciak JA Jr, Richter M, Miller S, Barton JJ. Maternal weight and pregnancy complications. *Am J Obstet Gynecol* 1985;152:38–45.

52. Rahaman J, Narayansingh GV, Roopnarinesingh S. Fetal outcome among obese parturients. *Int J Gynaecol Obstet* 1990;31:227–30.

53. Naeye RL. Maternal body weight and pregnancy outcome. *Am J Clin Nutr* 1990;52:273–9.

54. Woods JR Jr, Brinkman CR III. The jejunoileal bypass and pregnancy. *Obstet Gynecol Surv* 1978; 33:69.

55. Sivin I. International experience with Norplant and Norplant-2 contraceptives. *Stud Fam Plann* 1988;19:81–94.

56. Hytten FE, Leitch I. *The physiology of human pregnancy,* 2nd ed. Oxford: Blackwell Scientific, 1971.

Obesity: Theory and Therapy, Second Edition,
edited by A. J. Stunkard and T. A. Wadden.
Raven Press, Ltd., New York © 1993.

21

Public Health Approaches to Weight Control

*C. Barr Taylor and †Albert J. Stunkard

**Department of Psychiatry, Stanford University School of Medicine, Stanford, California
94305-5490; and †Department of Psychiatry, University of Pennsylvania,
Philadelphia, Pennsylvania 19104-2648*

Public health approaches to the control of disease have a long and successful history. In the 19th century, when infection was the most common cause of disease, public health approaches were about the only way to save lives. In 1854, for example, when a cholera epidemic was killing thousands of London residents, John Snow, a London physician, traced the origins of the epidemic to users of the Broad Street water pump. When he removed the pump handle, he stopped the epidemic and demonstrated that community intervention could save the lives of many people. Such interventions need not even be targeted at disease: the control of tuberculosis in the last two centuries has been due almost entirely to the increase in the standard of living.

Just as the increase in the standard of living has decreased the impact of infectious disease, so has it increased the impact of disorders of life style and personal habits. By one estimate, two-thirds of all deaths and years of life lost before age 65 are attributable to life style and can be prevented (1). The leading causes of premature death are all related to life style: tobacco, alcohol, injuries, high blood pressure, and overnutrition. Each of these life style factors would seem to be an important focus for public health interventions. Public health approaches to life style focus on populations at risk versus individ-

uals with identifiable disease. Such approaches also consider the best setting and method of delivery to achieve change. The focus of this chapter is on how public health approaches can be used to reduce the prevalence of obesity in America.

THE COMMUNITY

One approach to preventing and reducing the prevalence of obesity would be to focus on the whole population within a community, defined as where we live and work, and the values, customs, traditions, and laws that bind us together. There are many reasons and advantages for such an approach. Rose (2) has recently shown that the whole distribution of body mass index (BMI) behaves like an entity: as seen in Fig. 1, a shift in the mean weight of a population occurs across the entire distribution. By inference, a mean reduction in weight loss would reflect a change across the entire curve toward a lower weight. Americans are among the most obese populations in the world, with estimates of 20 to 50% of the adult population being obese, depending on the definition used (3,4). While biologic factors account for part of this problem, life style factors make an important contribution. The US diet is characterized by high fat intake, high refined sugar intake, and

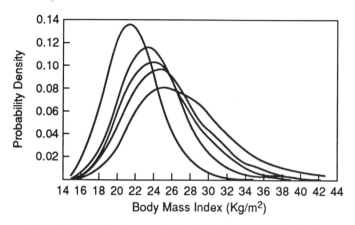

FIG. 1. Frequency distributions of body mass index in 10,079 individuals (men and women aged 20–59 years), arranged in five groups according to the median levels of their parent populations. (From ref. 2, with permission.)

relatively low cost. High-fat, high-caloric, inexpensive, readily available foods are heavily marketed to willing consumers. Furthermore, Americans become less active as they age, a tendency that might also contribute to obesity.

Community approaches to weight reduction have mostly been part of broader educational campaigns focused on cardiovascular risk reduction and on helping individuals adopt a healthier life style rather than changing the environment. The goal of community-wide cardiovascular risk reduction programs is to achieve at least a little change in most people in a particular geographic area. To achieve this goal, a variety of coordinated strategies are used to reach the whole population. In addition, specific interventions are developed for special segments of the population, and these interventions are delivered through multiple media and community channels and in multiple settings. The basic assumption of this strategy is that such an orchestrated effort will result in long-term behavioral change across a diverse population at relatively low cost. The interventions used in community-wide health education efforts derive from social learning theory, social marketing, mass communication, community organization, and diffusion theory (5).

Two pioneering studies begun in the early 1970s demonstrated the feasibility and effectiveness of community-wide interventions. The Stanford Three-Community Study attempted to reduce coronary risk factors in two small towns in California through a health promotion program that relied in great measure upon an intensive media campaign (6). Over the 2 years of the intervention, the program produced a marked reduction in coronary risk factors in the two experimental towns as compared with a control town. A project with similar goals was begun at about the same time in North Karelia, Finland (7,8). Finland has one of the highest rates of cardiovascular morbidity and mortality in the industrialized world. This project also reduced coronary risk factors. For the period 1974 to 1979, the reduction in age-standardized male coronary heart disease (CHD) mortality was 22% in North Karelia compared with 12% in the reference community. There was some evidence that the Stanford Three-Community intervention had an impact on reducing weight gain in the intervention communities, even though weight reduction was not a major goal for the project. The control town gained 0.45 kg during the 2-year program and 1-year follow-up, compared to no weight gain in the intervention towns. Weight reduction was not a goal for the North Karelia project and there were no apparent significant differences between the intervention and control populations on weight changes.

The Stanford Five-City Project followed on the results from the Three-Community Study. The Stanford Five-City Project had the goal of achieving community-wide change in risk factors through a comprehensive, integrated program of community organization and health education (9,10). In this very bold study, two intervention communities in northern California with a total population of about 123,000 were selected for the intervention, and two cities of about 198,000, also in northern California, served as controls. Changes in knowledge of risk factors, blood pressure, plasma cholesterol level, smoking rate, body weight, and resting pulse rate were assessed in a representative cohort and a cross-sectional survey at baseline and in four later surveys. Morbidity and mortality data are being monitored in these four and an additional city. The two educational cities received continual exposure to general education, punctuated by four to five separate risk factor education campaigns per year. Education was carried out through television and radio, newspapers, and other mass distributed print media and direct education. Community organizers led many seminars and workshops, facilitated worksite programs and competitions, organized community events such as walkathons, and attempted to ensure that the mass media and print materials were consistent with community values and rules. After 5 years there was a significant increase in knowledge about cardiovascular risk factors in the intervention compared with the control cities. There were also significant differences in percent reduction favoring treatment in blood cholesterol (2%), blood pressure (4%), resting pulse rate (3%), and smoking rate (13%) in the cohort sample. In the independent sample there was net reduction in community averages favoring treatment for blood cholesterol (2%) and blood pressure (4%), but no differences for smoking.

The results for BMI in the Five-City Project were modest. In the independent survey, adults in the intervention communities gained less weight than subjects in the control communities (0.57 kg compared with 1.25 kg) (11). In the cohort there were no significant differences. The greatest differences in the independent survey between intervention and control towns were observed in women aged 35 to 44, in whom the net gain was 2.28 kg in the control and 0.53 in the intervention towns. The intervention did not seem to stop the well-known increase in weight with aging, as seen in Fig. 2.

Perhaps the most impressive finding in this study is the remarkable overall gain in weight over time in both the independent and cohort samples. The weight gains in these two samples represent somewhat different phenomena. In the 6 years from the first to last independent survey, there was an increase in body mass index across almost all age groups for males and females and for intervention and control communities. A person surveyed in 1978-1979 was 2 to 5% lighter than a person of the same age surveyed in 1985-1986. In the independent sample, which reflects secular trends, both men and women showed an increase in body weight. The shift toward severe obesity in both the independent and cohort samples and in intervention and control towns was also striking. In the cohort sample the percentage of females 40% above ideal body weight increased by 3.5% in the intervention and 1.6% in the control. Even greater shifts were evident in the independent survey. Other studies have found similar increases in weight in the American population over time, at least in women (12,13). Furthermore, the shift occurred across the whole population, much as Rose (2) would have predicted.

Two other large community-wide interventions designed to reduce cardiovascular risk factors are now under way, one in Minnesota and another in Pawtucket, Rhode Island (14,15). The effects on weight loss or prevention of weight gain have not yet been reported. The Minnesota Heart Health Pro-

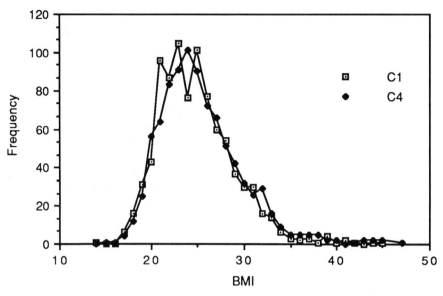

FIG. 2. The change in body mass index (BMI) from the first cohort (C1) in 1979/1980 to the fourth cohort (C4) in 1984/1985 for 903 subjects in the Stanford Five-City Project (11). There is a slight shift in the curve to the right.

gram included a program called "A Pound of Prevention," designed to recruit near-normal weight individuals to lose weight (16). Of about 6,000 individuals identified as being of eligible weight (<1.15 BMI), a random sample of 3,000 was sent an initial recruitment letter. Of those eligible, about 13% enrolled. Participants were asked to return a postage-paid postcard indicating their weight. Those in the intervention group received a monthly newsletter for 1 year that included information relevant to weight control. There were also financial incentives for weight maintenance. Subjects had $10 drawn from the account each month, to be returned with interest if they did not weigh more than they had at the initial weigh-in. At the end of a year the intervention group had lost a mean of about −1.0 kg compared to a gain of −.01 kg in the control group, a significant difference. If all the near-normal weight individuals had participated in the program, the Pound of Prevention program would probably have had a major impact in the community. However, lack of change in weight in the control group probably represents, at best, the weight changes in the 87% of subjects who did not

enroll and suggests that, at least in this segment of the population, little or no weight loss had occurred.

In order to reach a large number of people, the Pawtucket Heart Health Program (PHHP) devised a monthly city-wide weigh-in (17). This program allowed individuals to set a weight-loss goal and pledge a monetary incentive toward it. The activity was widely promoted and supported by the community. The City of Pawtucket Division of Parks and Recreation cosponsored the event and provided sites for weigh-ins and associated community events. A local dairy donated low-calorie frozen food to participants and gave coupons for a free half-gallon of low-fat milk to all weigh-out participants. The local daily newspaper provided space for a weekly column on weight loss, written by the PHHP staff nutritionist, during the 10-week period between the weigh-in and the weigh-out. PHHP distributed 7,500 flyers throughout the community. Altogether, 213 people enrolled. Of these, 129 returned for weigh-outs and lost on average about 3.7 kg. Although the weight loss for those completing the weigh-outs was substantial, the overall community participation rate was small, and the program was unlikely to have had a major impact on the community-wide BMI.

Determination of the effectiveness of community-wide approaches for weight reduction awaits final reporting of data from the Minnesota Heart Health Project and the Pawtucket Heart Health Program. However, the modest changes observed in the Stanford Three-Community Study and Five-Cities Project, the apparent lack of results from North Karelia, the small changes observed in the Pound of Prevention pilot project reported above, and the limited participation in the "weigh-in" suggest that the community-wide effects of the kind thus far undertaken are modest at best.

Perhaps the interventions would have been more effective if they had placed a greater emphasis on weight loss, which was not the primary aim. However, the recommended interventions that are part of these multifactorial risk reduction trials (increase in physical exercise, decrease in fat consumption, decrease in total caloric intake, increase in complex carbohydrates, etc.) should also reduce weight. Given the high prevalence of dieting already occurring in a community, it might even be naive to assume that a community-wide effect could exceed the effort and effects of commercial programs designed to attract potential dieters into their programs. Americans love to try to lose weight. In 1991, expenditures on weight control were estimated to be $17 billion (17a)! Of this, 38% went to fitness clubs, 11.9% to weight-loss centers, 11.7% to low-calorie foods, 9.5% to hospital/MD-based programs, 9.2% to residential spas, 8.7% to artificial sweeteners, and 7% to diet books and video- and audiotapes. A survey of dieting in the upper Midwest in 1980-1981 showed a lifetime prevalence of 44% in men and 72% in women (18). The Centers for Disease Control Behavioral Risk Factors Surveys conducted in 1981–1983 estimated that current dieting ranged from 5 to 9% in underweight men and women to 37 to 52% in overweight men and women (19). In a survey of dieting to lose weight in a population of over 4,500 men and women employed in 32 worksites in the upper Midwest, the lifetime prevalence of this behavior was estimated to be 47% in men and 75% in women, and point prevalence was 13% and 25% in men and women, respectively (20). The lifetime prevalence of participation in organized weight-loss programs was 6% in men and 31% in women, and point prevalence was 1% in men and 6% in women. *The New York Times* estimated that in 1986 as many as 65 million Americans were on a diet for at least part of the year, a figure that dropped to 45 million in 1991 (17a). Given the extent of dieting and the popularity of commercial weight-loss programs, it is somewhat surprising that weight continues to increase in the community-wide population. This fact alone suggests how difficult it is to lose and maintain weight loss.

COMMERCIAL WEIGHT-LOSS PROGRAMS

A dramatic development in recent years has been the rise of commercial weight-loss programs. The origins of this commercial movement can be traced to two prior developments—the rise of lay-led self-help groups for obesity and the introduction of behavioral technologies. The most prominent of the self-help groups is Take Off Pounds Sensibly (TOPS), which was founded in 1948 by a Milwaukee housewife based on her understanding of Alcoholics Anonymous. At the height of its influence TOPS enrolled more than 300,000 members in 12,000 chapters in all parts of the country. Its characteristics, which have been carefully studied (21), foreshadowed those of the commercial groups that followed it.

The membership of TOPS is almost exclusively female, white, and middle class. The average member is a 42-year-old woman whose ideal weight is 53.5 kg, and who entered TOPS weighing 80 kg, or 58% overweight. The effectiveness of the organization is difficult to assess because of the very high drop-out rate. TOPS' membership at any one time consists of a relatively small pool of longer term members and a much larger pool of members who have been in the organization for only a short period of time. The short-term members lose only small amounts of weight. The longer term members lose larger amounts of weight (an average of about 10 kg) and then slowly regain it, even though they remain in TOPS.

Although the founders of TOPS believed that they were modeling it on Alcoholics Anonymous, another self-help group, Overeaters Anonymous, has more firmly adhered to the precepts of Alcoholics Anonymous. The requirement of anonymity has made evaluation of the outcome of Overeaters Anonymous as difficult as that of Alcoholics Anonymous, and there are no firm data on outcome. The attempts to understand eating within an addictive framework is fraught with problems (22), and it is the impression of one of the authors (A.J.S.) that Overeaters Anonymous appeals more to persons suffering from bulimia than from obesity as such.

In contrast to Overeaters Anonymous, TOPS places major emphasis on weight change, and the weekly weigh-in is a key aspect of TOPS meetings. Early in its history TOPS made use of dramatic rewards (Crowning of the Queen) and punishments (Pig in the Pen) that were contingent upon weight loss and gain. When criticism of such punishments led to their abandonment, no comparably stimulating activities took their place and the content of the meetings was left to the ingenuity of individual groups. Discussion of the difficulties of dieting and the sharing of recipes came to fill a major part of the meeting time, not always with salutary consequences. In recent years TOPS has seen a marked decline in membership, and its role in weight control has been supplanted by commercial organizations. To the weigh-ins and group support that had been pioneered by TOPS, these organizations have added important new elements.

One of the new elements was behavior therapy. The feasibility of combining behavior therapy with group support had been demonstrated in a study of 298 members of 16 TOPS chapters in which the introduction of a behavioral program significantly reduced the drop-out rate and increased weight loss (23). TOPS did not capitalize upon this demonstration, but commercial organizations were not slow in incorporating behavioral components into their programs. Foremost among these organizations was Weight Watchers.

Weight Watchers was also founded (in 1961) by a housewife, but it rapidly developed into a commercial venture, and its original program, which relied heavily on inspirational lectures given by successful members, was supplemented by a carefully designed nutritional program and the aforementioned behavior therapy. When the company was purchased by H.J. Heinz in 1978, the sale of Weight Watchers foods increased significantly, and they were used as an optional portion control element of the program. Rigorous cost control measures have maintained Weight Watchers as the most economical of the commercial weight loss programs; in 1991 the cost of registration was $20, followed by $10 each for the weekly meetings. Weight Watchers has been rewarded by a large and probably expanding membership, with 16,000 meetings reaching a million people a week in the United States alone.

The full potential of lay-led weight control groups may not have been realized in the United States. In Norway a program that has enrolled 80,000 persons (of a population of 4 million at the time of the study) reported drop-out rates of less than 20% and weight losses averaging 6.4 kg, with the aid of follow-up sessions (24).

The late 1980s saw an explosive growth of commercial weight-loss programs, of which the best known are Diet Center, Jenny Craig, Nutri System, and Optifast. These programs are more ambitious than Weight Watchers, requiring a greater commitment from members, including substantial initial charges as well as purchase of the food that is part of the program. As a result, they are considerably more expensive than Weight Watchers—from $1,000 to $3,000 for a 6-month program. These four organizations have a total of at least 4,500 outlets with more than a million customers and revenues estimated at $3 billion a year.

A very recent development in the commercial weight-control field has been the explosive growth in the sale of products that had formerly been considered dietary supplements and that are now being marketed as meal replacements. The prototype of these products is Slim Fast and its 1988 update, Ultra Slim Fast, the sales of which have increased at least tenfold in the past 3 years, to reach numbers of customers estimated as high as 10–15 million. Part of the appeal of Ultra Slim Fast is its simplicity of use. A serving of Ultra Slim Fast, usually prepared as a milkshake, contains 220 calories, with 25% protein, 73% carbohydrates, and negligible amounts of fat. There is extensive vitamin supplementation and a large amount of fiber. For weight reduction, customers are advised to use Ultra Slim Fast two to three times a day, to replace two meals, and to eat one regular meal, either lunch or supper. For maintenance of weight loss, they are advised to use Ultra Slim Fast once or twice a day, replacing only one regular meal.

What accounts for the explosive growth in the commercial weight loss field? It has not been the result of clinical trials that have demonstrated either efficacy or safety. Instead, the growth is the result of intensive marketing campaigns that have dwarfed any previous such efforts in this field: Ultra Slim Fast alone is believed to have expended $80 million on advertising during 1990. The advertising messages have been short and unambiguous, in effect promising rapid, safe, and effortless weight loss, with extensive use of testimonials from celebrities.

Commercial weight-loss programs have been notoriously reluctant to report, or even to assess, the results of their programs. Much of what we know about these results has been obtained by investigators not connected with the programs. The problem of drop-outs from treatment by Weight Watchers was the focus of one series of studies. One of these studies found that 50% of enrollees dropped out within 6 weeks of entry into the program and a total of 70% by 12 weeks (25). Figure 3 shows the results of this and four other studies of commercial weight-loss programs (26). Note the striking similarity in the drop-out rates of programs conducted on three continents with different procedures and different clientele. Drop-out rates of this magnitude make it difficult to assess reports of weight loss by the survivors and explain why these organizations have been reluctant to report their results.

Fortunately, some commercial organizations have begun to assess their results and to publish the findings. In a retrospective study of 15 sites providing the Optifast program, Blackburn (27) reported that 24% of patients completed the 26 weeks of treatment. Better results were reported by Wadden and his colleagues in a prospective study of 18 Optifast sites enrolling 517 patients (28). In this study, 55% of patients completed the 26-week treatment, at which time men had lost 32 kg and women 20 kg. A 1-year follow-up showed that patients regained about one-third of the weight that they had lost.

Wadden's study shows that commercial weight-loss organizations can conduct careful assessment of their results and thereby strengthens the argument for full disclosure. Such disclosure is likely to reveal that these programs deliver far less than their advertising has promised. Awareness of the limitations of these programs should radically reduce the enthusiasm for their services and products. Disclosure will, however, permit patients and their doctors to make informed choices about treatment. Without information about the results achieved by a commercial weight-loss program, prospective customers of that program would be well advised to heed the dictum *caveat emptor.* There seems reasonable hope, however, that such information about programs will become

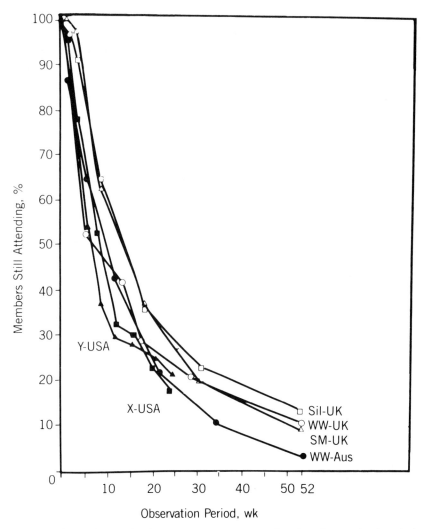

FIG. 3. Life table of participants in six treatment programs showing drop-out rates during the first year of membership, recalculated assuming the subjects not responding to the questionnaire had dropped out of treatment. (From ref. 25, with permission.)

available and that an informed public will be enabled to make decisions about treatment on the basis of facts, not advertising fantasies.

SPECIAL AT-RISK POPULATIONS

Many public health interventions focus on at-risk populations living within a community. An at-risk population is one that is particularly likely to develop a disease or problem. A number of such populations come to mind.

The Economically Disadvantaged

Socioeconomic status is strongly related to obesity (29,30). The first evidence of this special patterning of obesity within the population was obtained by the Midtown study of a population of 110,000 adults in an area of Manhattan selected so that it represented extremes in socioeconomic status from extremely high to extremely low (31). In this study, fully 30% of women of lower socioeconomic status were obese, compared with 16% of those in the middle-status and no more than 5% in the upper-status group. In a recent comprehensive report, Sobal and Stunkard (30) reviewed 144 published studies on the relationship between socioeconomic status and obesity. There is a strong inverse relationship between women and obesity in developed societies: women of higher socioeconomic status are thinner. The implication of this study for community-wide interventions is that education resources might be best focused on the less well educated and economically disadvantaged, women in particular.

Hispanics and Blacks

Ethnicity interacts with socioeconomic status (SES) to create some populations at great risk for becoming obese. Hispanic and black women tend to be much heavier than white women even when SES is accounted for. About 48% of adult black women are 20% or more overweight (32,33). By ages 45 to 75, 60% of black women are obese. Black women are twice as likely as white women to become overweight. Hispanics, the second largest (and fastest growing) minority population in the United States, are heavier and have greater truncal obesity than non-Hispanic whites (34).

The Community Health Assessment and Promotion Project, based in Atlanta, was designed to help one such ethnic group, obese black women who were also hypertensive, to lose weight (35). Participants attended 20 2-hour sessions for 20 weeks. The sessions included time spent engaging in moderate-intensity physical activity as well as instruction in weight control. The nutrition information was targeted to the customary buying and eating habits of the participants. The exercise program was tailored to the special needs of this population with respect to safety (e.g., security escorts were provided for groups walking in dangerous neighborhoods) and privacy (e.g., curtains were installed on windows in the exercise room to ensure privacy). In addition, free transportation and child care were offered and home visits undertaken to encourage participation. The prelim-

inary results were encouraging, at least as far as demonstrating that such a specially designed program can lead to reasonably high attendance. In a sample of the approximately 400 women who have participated, 49 of 70 attended 10 or more of the 20 sessions. The average weight loss was a little over 1 kg.

The Zuni Diabetes Project is an example of a community-based (versus community-wide) intervention that attempted to reduce weight in another special ethnic group at risk for obesity and also diabetes (36). Non-insulin-dependent diabetes mellitus (NIDDM) is a major risk factor for cardiovascular disease, and obesity is a major risk factor for NIDDM. The Zuni Indians of western New Mexico are one of a number of tribes whose prevalence rates of NIDDM are high: in Zunis aged 35 the rate is 28%. The Indian Health Service initiated a community-wide exercise and weight-control program designed to instruct and motivate Zunis with and without NIDDM to increase their levels of physical activity, lose body fat, and achieve or maintain normal body weight. Exercise classes were offered 5 days a week, several times daily, in a variety of sites in the Zuni community. Participants in the community exercise program were recruited through personal invitations, recommendations from physicians and nurses, and a general community advertisement campaign. Since 1985 the program has been sustained with the leadership and support of 15 to 20 Zuni volunteers working under direction of the Zuni Wellness Center, a tribally owned program. A number of exercise-oriented events such as foot races are offered throughout the year. In 1987 a weight-loss competition was incorporated into the program. Eight groups, four associated with the aerobic classes, three from worksites, and one from another tribe, began the program. Total weight loss for each team was graphically illustrated on display boards that were posted in four community locations. Each week average weight loss for each team's members was also calculated so participants could follow team standings. Ninety-two percent of those who signed up finished the 10-week program. A retrospective analysis found that 45% of the enrollees finished and lost the goal of 2.3 kg. Assuming that the rest did not lose any weight, the overall mean weight loss would be about 1 kg. Assuming that 7/8 of the participants were Zunis, then about 230 Zunis participated in the competition, or about 6% of the adult Zunis. The authors were able to attract males and sedentary females into the program. The overall results were not likely to have impacted the population weight, but they demonstrate the effectiveness of a weight-loss competition within a community targeted at certain groups or organized in community settings.

Another potential target for a community-wide intervention is young people who are already overweight and who have familial risk factors for obesity. At least one very long-term study has shown that a family-based intervention was associated with long-term weight loss (37). Young people with obesity can also be identified through the schools and then referred to special intensive programs (38,39).

REACHING POPULATIONS THROUGH SPECIAL SETTINGS

Schools

Since obesity begins early in life, interventions in the school would seem to be highly appropriate. In theory, schools are a convenient place for such interventions, the interventions can be sustained throughout much of the child's life, and knowledge related to healthy weight regulation can be combined with exercise during physical education and sports and with nutrition through school lunch programs. Most of the school-based programs have focused on changing knowledge, attitudes, and behavior, confirmed usually by self-report (40), and most have shown some modest benefit from the intervention. The results of one school-based program targeted at overweight children was

quite successful. In this study, 48 overweight children in grades 2 to 5 participated in a peer-led intervention compared with 42 control children from another school (41). The 12-week program consisted of counseling and social support provided primarily by older, well-liked peers. The counselors were trained to weigh the children, to check lunch boxes for nutritious foods, and to recommend changes in eating and exercise. After 12 weeks, the children in the experimental school lost 0.15 kg and reduced their percentage overweight by 5.3%, whereas those in the control school gained 1.3 kg and increased their percentage overweight by 0.3%. Most school studies have found weight losses of 2% to 5%. Weight stabilization, not weight loss, may be a realistic goal for school programs.

Changes in physical activity and diet may be more readily achieved than weight loss. For instance, in Texas, two of four elementary schools were assigned to an intervention condition that consisted of classroom health education, vigorous physical exercise, lower fat school lunches, and a curriculum designed to teach the importance of nutrition and exercise. Analysis of school lunches showed a decline from baseline to posttest in the two intervention schools of 15.5% and 10.4% for total fat. At posttest the percent of time children engaged in moderate-to-vigorous physical activity increased from 10 to 40% (42). By their self-report, students in the intervention consumed less total fat than students in the control group.

Worksites

One community institution has particular attractiveness for health promotion in general and weight loss programs in particular. It is the worksite. Many of us spend more of our time at work than at any other activity, and our relationships with our fellow workers are often among the most important of our lives. Interactions with fellow workers, worksite policies and incentives, the worksite environment itself, and the provision of facilities for exercise all speak to the strengths of the worksite as a place for health promotion. Health promotion programs at the worksite keep to a minimum time lost from work, and the worksite provides access to large numbers of persons who can be reached at relatively low cost. Finally, the worksite provides elements to which social learning theory ascribes primary importance in the control of behavior —its cues and its consequences, modeling, and (perhaps most important) an environment in which behavioral change can be maintained.

The logic of the worksite for health promotion has led to a large and growing number of efforts to capitalize upon the potential of this resource. Worksite programs designed to control problems such as hypertension and smoking have been highly successful. By contrast, the results of programs of weight control at the worksite have been consistently disappointing, even at sites where other health problems have been successfully addressed. These results probably tell us more about obesity than they do about programs of health promotion, attesting to the remarkable resistance to control that is noted in other chapters of this volume.

The limited effectiveness of worksite programs of weight control is not due to any limitation in the energy or creativity of those who have designed them. Indeed, the history of these programs reveals a systematic and imaginative effort that is the equal of health promotion programs devoted to any other disorder. As was true of most worksite programs of the time, those devoted to weight control 10 years ago were basically clinical, devised for office use in the treatment of highly motivated patients.

An early example was the program developed for the United Store Workers Union in New York (43). This union had already sponsored a highly successful program of hypertension control at the worksite (44) and was strongly supportive of the weight-control program. Over a period of 4 years three cohorts

comprising 172 women were treated in a series of 16-week behavioral programs adapted from clinical use (45). Information from the treatment of each cohort was utilized to improve the program for the next cohort and the attrition rate dropped appreciably; members and officers of the Union were enthusiastic about the program. As has occurred often in worksite programs, the results belied the enthusiasm.

Recruitment into the program was extremely limited—172 of 15,000 union members. Attrition, the bane of so many clinical programs, averaged 42%, approximately the same as that of other worksite weight-control programs of the period (46–48). Figure 4 shows a pattern of attrition similar to that of commercial weight-loss organizations. Finally, even among the select (and biased) sample of persons who completed the program, weight loss averaged no more than 3.6 kg.

Far better results were obtained when the same behavioral program was delivered in a way that took advantage of the special characteristics of the worksite. One such characteristic is the opportunity for competition provided by the worksite. Competition is embedded in the American Way of Life, driving many persons to surpass their own expectations and motivating health behavior change.

The first description of a weight-loss competition was reported by the vice-president of the Colonial Bank of Chicago in 1980 (49). The competition was initiated by a challenge from the Colonial Bank to two other banks, and the program was carried out by a commercial weight-loss organization. Members of the Colonial Bank lost half a ton of fat and nevertheless lost the competition, but few details of the intervention were provided.´

A systematic assessment of the use of weight-loss competitions at the worksite was carried out over a period of 5 years under the auspices of the County Health Improvement Program (CHIP) (50). CHIP was a community-based, multiple-risk-factor program designed to reduce mortality and mor-

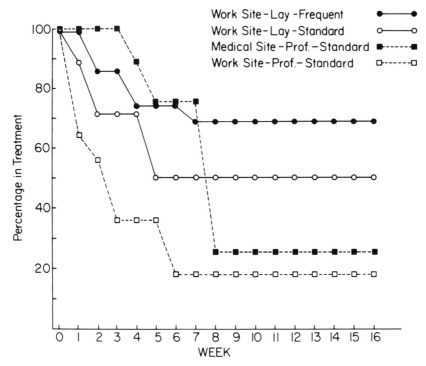

FIG. 4. Life table of participants in first cohort of weight-loss program conducted by the United Store Workers Union. Three programs were carried out at the worksite and one, for contrast, at a medical site. Two programs were conducted by union leaders (lay), while two were conducted by a psychologist (professional). One program met four times a week (frequent), while three met once a week (standard). Note the high drop-out rate in each of these four variants of the basic behavioral program during the 16-week treatment period (43).

bidity from cardiovascular disease in a rural county in north-central Pennsylvania. A centerpiece of CHIP was its health behavior competitions, of which those involving weight loss were the most prominent.

The first CHIP weight-loss competition took place among three banks and the results immediately made clear the potential of the method (51). Recruitment was extraordinarily high—all employees were invited to participate and almost all did. The attrition rate was extraordinarily low (0.5%), unusual even in the best clinical programs, and the weight loss, (5.5 kg in the 12-week program) was significantly greater than the 3.6 kg of the 16-week Store Workers program.

The program was oriented around the weekly weigh-ins, in a central location of the bank, accompanied by considerable local publicity and a high level of employee inter-

est. Weight-loss goals were kept modest in order to discourage crash dieting. Participants paid $5 to enter the program and the pool was awarded to the winning bank. At each weigh-in employees were given an installment of the same weight-loss manual that had been used in the Store Workers program. The results were recorded weekly on a large, prominently placed bulletin board, similar to a United Way thermometer. Professional time devoted to this first program was minimal, confined to planning, preparation, and initial implementation.

Studies of weight-loss competitions over the subsequent years determined the effective elements of weight-loss competitions (43, 52,53). Team competitions were more effective than either team cooperation or individual competitions for men and more effective than individual competition for women. The combination of cooperating with one's peers against an out-group seems to be the essential element in team competitions. Furthermore, the motivation of women appears to be somewhat different from that of men, cooperation being more important and individual competition less important.

The development of a manual for health promotion competitions greatly reduced the time and effort required to mount these programs and made it possible for companies to carry them out with their own personnel. The resulting ten competitions at 15 worksites recruited essentially every overweight employee in each worksite—1,177 or 21% of all employees. Furthermore, these competitions attracted two groups that have traditionally shunned health promotion programs—men and blue-collar workers of either sex. Finally, the average weight loss was just as great as that of the first competitions—6.3 kg for men and 4.4 kg for women.

Programs for the control of obesity are increasingly scrutinized from the standpoint of their cost effectiveness. The very low costs

and the reasonable effectiveness of weight-loss competitions suggest that they should show a highly favorable ratio and such is the case. Costs of weight-loss competitions at the CHIP worksites were estimated according to standard methods and effectiveness by percentage loss in body weight rather than by amount of weight lost. Using percentages makes it possible to compare the treatment of persons with widely varying body weights, and 1% per week is the desirable weight loss of patients in conservative programs, irrespective of their starting weight. Figure 5 shows that the cost of $0.92 for a 1% loss of body weight by competitions compares very favorably with the results of other weight-loss programs for which such a measure is available.

Maintenance of weight loss is the final, critical element in programs of weight control and it has been on the rock of maintenance that clinical programs have foundered. Weight-loss competitions have fared no better. Efforts to evaluate the maintenance of weight loss following three competitions were flawed by less than perfect follow-up, with

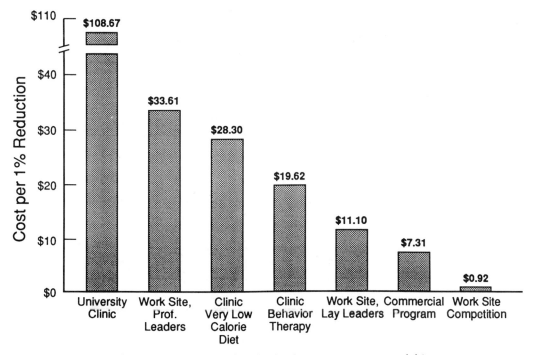

FIG. 5. The cost per 1% reduction in percentage overweight.

rates of from 58% to 87%. Even in the samples thus biased in favor of maintenance, a 6-month follow-up found only 54% of the weight loss had been maintained, while 8-month and 1-year follow-ups of two other programs found values of no more than 51% and 27%, respectively.

The transitory nature of weight lost during worksite programs has nowhere been better demonstrated than in the landmark Healthy Worker Project, a large 2-year randomized trial of worksite intervention for weight control and smoking cessation (R. W. Jeffery, *personal communication, 1991*). This trial had been preceded by extensive pilot studies that had developed methods for coping with the critical problems of recruitment and attrition in health promotion programs. Relying on a special feature of the worksite, Jeffery and his colleagues used payroll deductions as incentives to successfully recruit employees and also to reduce attrition in weight-loss programs to 21% (54) in one study and to 6% in another (55). In the Healthy Worker Project, payroll deductions were combined with state-of-the-art behavioral programs for weight loss and smoking cessation. Participation in both programs was high, and the degree of behavior change was positively correlated with the rate of employee participation in both programs.

After 2 years the net effect of the weight-loss program was negligible, whereas there were significant results in the smoking cessation program. The reasons for the apparent ineffectiveness of the weight-loss program are unclear, but one possibility is that, although some weight loss was achieved over the short term, it was not maintained well enough to be reflected in the long term. Once again, a weight-control program was far less successful than another health promotion program at the same worksite, perhaps further testimony to the refractoriness of obesity.

Further evidence of the long-term ineffectiveness of worksite weight-loss programs has recently been reported from an Australian program in which ambulance stations were randomized to four conditions (56). At 6 months, two programs with behavioral components had outperformed the other two programs. At 1 year, however, the average weight of members in each of these programs was slightly greater than at baseline.

It is clear that worksite weight-control programs are limited by poor maintenance of weight losses. Although disappointing, this limitation is not surprising. Weight losses achieved in clinical programs are also poorly maintained (57), and in comparison with clinical programs, those at the worksite have notable advantages, particularly their far lower costs. Their resulting very favorable cost effectiveness described above suggests that this modality deserves continuing study and support.

INEXPENSIVE INTERVENTIONS

Because the principles of behavior modification for weight loss and increasing exercising have been well specified, and because many such programs include considerable information (e.g., on basic nutrition, the amount of fats in various foodstuffs, etc.), it would seem possible to use inexpensive mediated programs and materials for weight loss. Such inexpensive interventions would be of great use to community-wide weight reduction or weight-gain prevention programs. Even a relatively ineffective intervention spread over a large population can have an important public health effect. The previously mentioned program, A Pound of Prevention, developed by the Minnesota Heart Health Project, is an example of one such relatively inexpensive approach. The Stanford Five-City Project incorporated a Weight-Loss Kit, consisting of 4 pages of weight-loss information sent to all households in the community. An unpublished evaluation of the kit done at a worksite found that the kit produced about 1 kg weight loss over 6 months (J. Flora, *personal communication*). The kit was more effective when the material was sequenced and combined with a performance contract. Recently, videotape and computer weight-loss programs have been used to produce weight loss. Table 1 shows the 6-month weight loss results from three studies done at Stanford to evaluate low-cost, but relatively intensive interventions. In the first intervention, 90 mildly to moderately overweight women participated in a study examining the potential utility of a hand-held computer. The study compared the use of a computer with one introductory session and the computer with four additional group support sessions, and a therapist-conducted weight-loss group. The mean weight losses in all three groups were modest (less than 3 kg at 6 months); the computer-alone group was much more cost effective (58). The authors then investigated the utility of combining an even more intensive intervention with the computer therapy and one that required weight loss before using the computer (59). The latter group proved much more effective than the former, with a 6-month posttreatment weight loss of 3.8 kg compared with essentially no change in the computer-only group (0.9 kg).

Videotape weight-loss programs would also seem promising, particularly if well conceived, produced, and combined with an exercise segment, as was the case of the program developed by Nestlé. However, in an evaluation of this program in a controlled study, Saylor (60) found that the effects were modest, with weight losses of less than 3 kg in the video-only group. On the assumption that participants might have trouble adhering to the video program, Saylor also included a group that was provided a self-help program designed to enhance compliance with the use of the videotapes. This group did better than the videotape-only group, and even continued to lose weight after the 6-month follow-up period, an unusual finding in such studies. Computer, video, correspondence courses, and self-help materials all have an effect on weight loss, but a modest one. This small effect spread across populations would seem to confer some public health benefit, but it is important to remember that in the Five-City study, most of the households in the community received the weight-loss kit, which produced no measurable effect in the community. It is also not clear that the new, fancy, and sometimes very impressive computers and videotapes and now emerging multimedia interventions are much better than a well-done book or pamphlet.

CHANGING THE FOOD SUPPLY

A more intensive effort, and one directed to at-risk populations like the very obese and the poor, with interventions occurring at the workplace and perhaps in the school, might very well enhance the effects of community-wide interventions. However, none of these interventions may address an important underlying cause of obesity in America—our readily available, high-caloric, high-fat diet. The consumption of high-calorie fast foods may partly explain a rise in BMI found in the Five-City Project. For instance, between the first and final samples, subjects in the control cities increased the number of reported times they ate fast food by about 57%, while subjects in the intervention cities increased by about 29%. If this self-report is accurate, this

TABLE 1. *Computer and video weight-loss interventions*

	Weight loss (kg)	
Intervention	Posttreatment	4–6 Month follow-up
Computer only	2.3	1.4
Computer + group support	2.6	2.1
Behavior therapy (58)	2.2	2.7
Pocket computer only	3.1	0.9
Computer following weight loss through low-fat diet (59)	5.3	3.8*
Video program	2.1	1.8
Video program plus guided help program	2.9	3.2*
Control (60)	1.4	1.5

* $p < 0.05$, compared with control.

increased consumption of fast foods might represent a significant increase in calories. One survey notes that 40 to 50% of the calories in most fast-food meals comes from fat and that fast foods are generally high in caloric content (61). The US National Restaurant Association estimates that on a typical day, 45.8 million people—a fifth of the American population—are served at fast-food restaurants (62). Every second an estimated 200 people in the United States are served a hamburger (63).

If increase in fast-food consumption is part of the explanation for the increase in weight, and a well-thought-out and well-instituted community-wide education effort had little effect, then the data suggest that community-wide efforts might be more successful if they addressed the quality of food itself (64). In doing so, community-wide efforts become much closer to traditional public health interventions, in which emphasis is placed on reduced exposure to environmental hazards. This type of intervention is like removing the handle of the Broad Street pump.

One environmental intervention would be to alter food at the point of sale towards the preparation of less caloric, less fatty foods. In recent years, some fast-food chains have responded to community pressures to make such changes by altering how food is prepared. For instance, some fast-food restaurants have switched from animal to vegetables oils for cooking, and others have developed low-fat, low-calorie menu items. Proctor & Gamble has introduced Milky Way II, a candy bar that has fewer calories and 50% fewer calories from fat, yet is the same size as the traditional Milky Way. It uses caprenin, a fat substitute derived from fat molecules found in coconut, palm kernel, and rapeseed oils.

The National School Lunch Program, started 45 years ago, serves an estimated 24 million children every day. According to the Center for Scientific Study, the average school lunch is 37% saturated fat. In recent years, the program has been trying to improve by purchasing such things as fruits canned in juice rather than syrup, tuna packed in water, reduced-fat ground beef, and low-fat ground turkey. Peanut butter using tropical oils has been eliminated. On the other hand, some school districts contract with fast-food chains like Pizza Hut to provide school lunches. The State of California required its Department of Education to develop and maintain nutrition guidelines for school lunches and breakfasts and for all food sold on public school campuses. The guidelines, which are being developed, will limit fat, cholesterol, and sodium contents of school lunches. Changes in the school lunch program face a number of obstacles, however. According to school lunch nutritionists, the fast-food generation demands school-based foods that have the appeal of fast foods. Federal support of the program has been dramatically reduced. In real inflationary terms, schools receive half as much for a school lunch today as they did in 1946. The food available is also related to the US Department of Agriculture (USDA) commodity program, which supplies food to schools from its surpluses. A recession, drought, or change in crops can strongly impact the available food.

A second environmental intervention would be to regulate the advertising and promotion of certain kinds of foods. An American child is exposed to thousands of food commercials in a year, many of which promote high-sugar cereals. Experimental studies with children have demonstrated direct effects of exposure to advertising for high-calorie foods on actual snack choices and consumption (65,66), which is of course the point of advertising. Legislation ensuring that labels on foods are easily read and understood might help consumers select low-fat, or low-sugar foods.

A third environmental approach to obesity would be to alter economic policies regarding food. Such policies would examine the economic subsidization and taxation of various foodstuffs. The rate of consumption of even such highly addicting substances as alcohol and cigarettes has been shown to be related to price (64). The State of California has recently introduced a tax on snack foods (partly defined by the sugar content); the effects of this tax on consumption will be important to monitor. Although such approaches are of great public health importance, they may be relatively much more costly to the poor. Accordingly, a strategy that is already a part of farm subsidies would be to ensure that "healthy" foods are available at very low cost to impoverished people.

SUMMARY

Public health approaches seek to reach large populations with the hope that even small changes in individuals will produce significant results in a population. Such an approach seems well suited to the control of obesity. However, the results of public health efforts for weight control have been modest. The few large-scale community interventions (with control or prevention of obesity at least as a secondary goal) have had little effect on interrupting the relentless trend toward increased body weight in the population. Even efforts directed toward more restricted populations have had limited success. One of the largest such populations has been the clients of commercial weight-loss programs. The best of these programs may rival the best treatment under medical auspices, but many are clearly ineffective, and the field is flooded with organizations that do not reveal their results and substitute testimonials for data.

Worksite programs have attracted increasing attention, and efforts to make use of the special characteristics of the worksite, such as weight-loss competitions, have improved the results. Schools should be promising sites for weight control, but few school-based programs have been developed and evaluated. Programs are beginning to be targeted at populations at high risk, e.g., black women and Zuni Indians, a reasonable strategy. Technical innovations are being introduced in an effort to individualize treatment while controlling costs. The early results of the use of hand-held computers and videotapes warrant further study of these methods.

What may well be the most promising public health measures are only now beginning to be explored. These are policy options such as improving the quality of food served in school lunch programs, regulation of the advertising of junk foods, labeling of processed food, and the ultimate social reinforcer—subsidization of the production of healthy foods and taxation of the production of unhealthy foods.

Public health approaches to weight control have so far achieved only modest success, perhaps because they have not placed enough emphasis on environmental change. Education combined with environmental change may achieve greater effects than either alone.

REFERENCES

1. Amler RW, Dull HB, eds. *Closing the gap: the burden of unnecessary illness.* New York: Oxford, 1987.
2. Rose G. Population distributions of risk and disease. *Nutr Metab Cardiovasc Dis* 1991;1:37–40.
3. Millar WJ, Stephens T. The prevalence of overweight and obesity in Britain, Canada, and the United States. *Am J Public Health* 1987;77:38–41.
4. Shah M, Jeffery RW. Is obesity due to overeating and inactivity, or to a defective metabolic rate? A review. *Ann Behav Med* 1991;13:73–81.
5. Farquhar JW, Fortmann SP, Flora JA, et al. Effects of community-wide education on cardiovascular disease risk factors: the Stanford Five-City Project. *JAMA* 1990;264:359–65.
6. Farquhar JW, Maccoby N, Wood PD, et al. Community education for cardiovascular disease. *Lancet* 1977;1:1192–5.
7. Puska P, et al. Ten years of the North Karelia project: results with community-based prevention of coronary heart disease. *Scand J Soc Med* 1983;11:65–8.
8. Puska P, Nissinen, Tuomilehto J, et al. The community-based strategy to prevent coronary heart disease: conclusions from the ten years of the North Karelia Project. *Annu Rev Public Health* 1985; 6:147–93.
9. Farquhar JW, Fortmann SP, Maccoby N, et al. The Stanford Five-City Project: design and methods. *Am J Epidemiol* 1985;122:323–4.
10. Farquhar JW, Fortmann SP, Flora JA, et al. Methods of communication to influence behaviour. In: Holland W, Detels R, Knox G, eds. *Oxford textbook of public health,* vol 2, 2nd ed. Oxford: Oxford University Press, 1990;331–44.
11. Taylor CB, Fortmann SP, Flora J, Kayman S, Barrett DC, Jatulis D, Farquhar JW. Effect of long-term community health education on body mass index. *Am J Epidemiol* 1991;134:1–15.
12. Harlan WR, Landis JR, Flegal KM, et al. Secular trends in body mass in the United States, 1960–1980. *Am J Epidemiol* 1988;128:1065–74.

13. Williamson DF, Kahn HS, Remington PL, et al. The 10-year incidence of overweight and major weight gain in US adults. *Arch Intern Med* 1990;150:665–72.
14. Blackburn H, Luepker RV, Kline FG, et al. The Minnesota Heart Health Program: a research and demonstration project in cardiovascular disease prevention. In: Matarazzo JD, Miller NE, Weiss SM, et al, eds. *Behavioral health: a handbook of health enhancement and disease prevention.* New York: John Wiley & Sons, 1984;1171–8.
15. Lasater T, Abrams D, Artz L, et al. Lay volunteer delivery of a community-based cardiovascular risk factor change program: the Pawtucket experiment. In: Matarazzo JD, Miller NE, Weiss SM, et al, eds. *Behavioral health: a handbook of health enhancement and disease prevention.* New York: John Wiley & Sons, 1984;1166–79.
16. Forster JL, Jeffery RW, Schmid TL, Kramer FM. Preventing weight gain in adults: a pound of prevention. *Health Psychol* 1988;7:515–25.
17. Lasater TM, Sennett LL, Lefebrvre C, DeHart KL, Peterson G, Carleton RA. Community-based approach to weight loss: the Pawtucket "weigh-in." *Addict Behav* 1991;16:175–81.
17a. *The New York Times* 1991 Nov 24:F5.
18. Jeffery RW, Folsom AR, Luepker RV, et al. Prevalence of overweight and weight loss behavior in a metropolitan adult population: the Minnesota Heart Survey Experiment. *Am J Public Health* 1984;74:349–52.
19. Forman MR, Trowbridge FL, Gentry EM, Marks JS, Hogelin GC. Overweight adults in the United States: the Behavioral Risk Factor Surveys. *Am J Clin Nutr* 1986;44:410–6.
20. Jeffery RW, Adlis SA, Forster JL. Prevalence of dieting among working men and women: the Healthy Worker Project. *Health Psychol* 1991;10:274–81.
21. Garb JR, Stunkard AJ. Effectiveness of a self-help group in obesity control: a further assessment. *Arch Intern Med* 1972;134:716–20.
22. Wilson GT. The addiction model of eating disorders: a critical analysis. *Adv Behav Res Ther* 1991;13:27–72.
23. Levitz LS, Stunkard AJ. A therapeutic coalition for obesity: behavior modification and patient self-help. *Am J Psychiatry* 1974;131:423–7.
24. Grimsmo A, Helgesen G, Borchgrevink CF. Short-term and long-term effects of lay groups on weight reduction. *Br Med J* 1981;283:1093–5.
25. Volkmar FR, Stunkard AJ, Woolston J, Bailey BA. High attrition rates in commercial weight loss programs. *Arch Intern Med* 1981;141:426–8.
26. Ashwell M. Commercial weight loss programs. In: Bray G, ed. *Recent advances in obesity research: II.* London: Newman Publishing, 1978;266–76.
27. Blackburn GL. Perspectives on obesity: Sandoz OPTIFAST Program health and obesity study. Sixth Annual Sandoz Nutrition Optifast Postgraduate Meeting, Orlando FL, May, 1988.
28. Wadden TA, Foster GD, Letizia KA, Stunkard AJ. A multi-center evaluation of a proprietary weight reduction program for the treatment of marked obesity. *Arch Intern Med* 1992;152:961–6.
29. Goldblatt PB, Moore ME, Stunkard AJ. Social factors in obesity. *JAMA* 1965;152:1039–42.
30. Sobal J, Stunkard AJ. Socioeconomic status and obesity: a review of the literature. *Psychol Bull* 1989;105:260–75.
31. Srole L, et al. *Mental health in the metropolis: the Midtown Manhattan Study.* New York: McGraw-Hill, 1962.
32. Kumanyika S. Obesity in black women. *Epidemiol Rev* 1987;19:31–50.
33. Williamson DF, Kahn HS, Byers T. The 10-year incidence of obesity and major weight gain in black and white US women aged 30–55 years. *Am J Clin Nutr* 1991;53:1515S–1518S.
34. Joo SK, Mueller WH, Hanis CL, Schull WJ. Diabetes Alert Study: weight history and upper body adiposity in diabetic and nondiabetic Mexican American adults. *Ann Hum Biol* 1984;11:1161–71.
35. Lasco RA, Curry RH, Dicson VJ, Powers J, Mense S, Merritt RK. Participation rates, weight loss, and blood pressure changes among obese women in a nutrition-exercise program. *Public Health Rep* 1989;104:640–6.
36. Heath GW, Wilson RH, Smith J, Leonard BE. Community-based exercise and weight control: diabetes risk reduction and glycemic control in Zuni Indians. *Am J Clin Nutr* 1991;53:1642S–1646S.
37. Epstein LH, Valoski A, Wing RR, McCurlex J. Ten-year follow-up of behavioral, family-based treatment for obese children. *JAMA* 1990;264:2519–23.
38. Mellin LM, Slinkard LA, Irwin CE. Adolescent obesity intervention: validation of the Shapedown program. *J Am Diet Assoc* 1987;87:333–8.
39. Wadden TA, Stunkard AJ, Rich L, Rubin CJ, Sweidel G, McKinney S. Obesity in black adolescent girls: a controlled clinical trial of treatment by diet, behavior modification, and parental support. *Pediatrics* 1990;85:345–52.
40. Jackson MY, Proulx JM, Pelican S. Obesity prevention. *Am J Clin Nutr* 1991;53:1625S–1639S.
41. Foster GD, Wadden TA, Brownell KD. Peer-led program for the treatment and prevention of obesity in the schools. *J Consult Clin Psychol* 1985;53:538–40.
42. Simons-Morton BG, Parcel GS, Baranowksi T, Forthofer R, O'Hara NM. Promoting physical activity and a healthful diet among children. Results of a school-based intervention study. *Am J Public Health* 1991;81:986–91.
43. Brownell KD, Stunkard AJ, McKeon PE. Weight reduction at the worksite: a promise partially fulfilled. *Am J Psychiatry* 1985;141:47–51.
44. Alderman MH, Schoenbaum EE. Detection and treatment of hypertension at the worksite. *N Engl J Med* 1975;293:65–8.
45. Brownell KD. *Behavioral therapy for obesity: a treatment manual.* Philadelphia: University of Pennsylvania Press, 1979.
46. Abrams DB, Follick MJ. Behavioral weight loss intervention at the worksite: feasibility and maintenance. *J Consult Clin Psychol* 1983;51:226–33.
47. Fisher EB Jr, Lowe MR, Levenkron JC, Newman A. Reinforcement and structural support of maintained risk reduction. In: Stuart RB, ed. *Adherence, compliance and generalization in behavioral medicine.* New York: Brunner/Mazel, 1982;145–68.
48. Follick MJ, Fowler JL, Brown R. Attrition in worksite interventions: the effects of an incentive procedure. *J Consult Clin Psychol* 1984;52:139–40.
49. Hynes O. Presentation on the Colonial Bank of Chicago Weight Loss Program at the Healthy American

Conference on the Corporate Commitment to Health, Washington, DC, June 9–10, 1980.

50. Stunkard AJ, Cohen RY, Felix MRJ. Mobilizing a community to promote health: The Pennsylvania County Health Improvement Program (CHIP). In: Rosen JC, Solomon LJ, eds. *Prevention in health psychology.* Hanover, NH: University Press of New England, 1985;143–90.

51. Brownell KD, Stunkard AJ, Felix MRJ, Cooley NB. Weight loss competitions at the worksite: impact on weight, morale and cost-effectiveness. *Am J Public Health* 1984;74:1283–5.

52. Cohen RY, Stunkard AJ, Felix MRJ. A comparison of three worksite weight loss competitions. *J Behav Med* 1987;10:467–79.

53. Stunkard AJ, Cohen RY, Felix MRJ. Weight loss competitions at the worksite: how they work and how well. *Prev Med* 1989;18:460–74.

54. Forster JL, Jeffery RW, Sullivan S, Snell MK. A work-site weight control program using financial incentives collected through payroll deduction. *J Occup Med* 1985;27:804–8.

55. Jeffery RW, Forster JL, Snell MK. Promoting weight control at the worksite: a pilot program of self-motivation using payroll-based incentives. *Prev Med* 1985;14:187–94.

56. Gomel M, Oldenburg B, Simpson JM, Owen N. A randomized trial of worksite cardiovascular risk reduction: comparison of risk factor assessment, risk factor education, behavioral counseling and incentive strategies [*submitted*].

57. Brownell KD, Jeffery RW. Improving long-term weight-loss: pushing the limits of treatment. *Behav Ther* 1987;18:353–4.

58. Agras WS, Taylor CB, Feldman DE, Losch M, Burnett KF. Developing computer-assisted therapy for the treatment of obesity. *Behav Ther* 1989;21:99–109.

59. Taylor CB, Agras WS, Losch M, Plante TG, Burnett K. Improving the effectiveness of computer-assisted weight loss. *Behav Ther* 1991;22:229–36.

60. Saylor KE. *Enhancing a videocassette weight-loss program through self-directed adherence training* [dissertation, Stanford University School of Education, 1987]. *Dissertation Abst Int* 1988;49/03-B:0920.

61. Massachusetts Medical Society Committee on Nutrition. Fast-food fare: consumer guidelines. *N Engl J Med* 1991;321:752–5.

62. Brown M. Fast foods are hazardous to your health. *Sci Dig* 1986;94:31–6.

63. Harris M. The revolutionary hamburger. *Psychol Today* 1983;17:6–8.

64. Jeffery RW. Population perspectives on the prevention and treatment of obesity in minority populations. *Am J Clin Nutr* 1991;53:1621S–1624S.

65. Gorn GJ, Goldberg ME. Behavioral evidence for the effects of televised food messages on children. *J Consum Res* 1982;9:200–5.

66. Jeffrey DB, McLellarn RW, Fox DT. The development of children's eating habits: the role of television commercials. *Health Educ Q* 1982;9:78–93.

Obesity: Theory and Therapy, Second Edition,
edited by A. J. Stunkard and T. A. Wadden.
Raven Press, Ltd., New York © 1993.

22

Talking with Patients

Albert J. Stunkard

*Department of Psychiatry, University of Pennsylvania,
Philadelphia, Pennsylvania 19104-2648*

It seems fitting to close this volume on obesity with a chapter on talking with patients, particularly with women patients. The emphasis on women is because they constitute the vast majority of persons seeking treatment for obesity and because they bear the psychological wounds that result from the pervasive derogation of obesity in our society. Paradoxically, men—who are at far higher risk of complications of obesity—rarely seek treatment. Talking with them is easier and will be discussed briefly.

Some of our talk with obese women will concern the treatment of their obesity but much of it will not. We sometimes forget that obese women have all of the medical needs of nonobese persons (and often more), and they may not wish to try losing weight and may not be able to, even if they try. Far too often our patients' obesity colors all of our contact with them, and far too often we focus our attention on treatment of their obesity. The poor results of treatment hardly warrant this focus and it forecloses the more useful alternative of talking with our patients. This alternative contrasts dramatically with what obese patients have come to expect.

Most of us know that obese persons are subject to prejudice and discrimination, but few realize the extent of these evils (1). Children as young as 6 years of age describe silhouettes of an obese child as "lazy . . . dirty . . . stupid . . . ugly" (2). When shown drawings of an obese child and of children with severe handicaps, such as missing hands

and facial disfigurement, both children and adults rated the obese child as the least likeable of all (3). Poignantly, obese persons manifest exactly the same kind of prejudice.

It would be reassuring to learn that physicians and other helping professionals are immune to this stereotyping, but this is not the case. A survey of physicians revealed that they saw their obese patients as "weak-willed, ugly and awkward" (4). Such attitudes are not lost on our patients; another survey of obese persons quantified their perceptions. When asked how often they had been "treated with disrespect by the medical profession because of my weight," 46% reported "always" and 40% reported "usually" (4).

It has been argued that physicians' demeaning attitudes toward obese persons derive from disappointment over the poor results of their treatment. Physicians are just frustrated, the argument goes. This explanation seems plausible until we realize that these attitudes are present in house officers, long before they have experienced the frustrations of treatment. It seems more likely that physicians have simply assimilated the demeaning attitudes of our society.

The suffering of obese persons from these societal attitudes has one redeeming feature. Having come to expect rejection and disparagement, obese persons are favorably surprised when they receive the consideration that physicians usually accord their patients. Here is a golden opportunity. As with any chronic illness, we rarely have an opportunity to cure. But we do have an opportunity to treat the patient with respect. Such an experience may be the greatest gift that a doctor can give an obese patient; it compares favorably with the modest benefits of our programs of weight reduction. How can we go about talking with our patients in such a way as to confer this gift? A convenient framework is the first visit of an obese patient to the doctor, and this chapter will be organized according to this framework, starting with the chief complaint.

THE CHIEF COMPLAINT

A history of the present illness traditionally begins with the chief complaint, and there seems no reason to make an exception for obese patients. It is critical, however, to remember that the real chief complaint is defined by the patient, not by the physician. To the clinician the patient's obesity may be her most salient feature and so all too often it becomes her chief complaint, whether she wishes it to be or not.

Obese patients are so familiar with this redefinition of their concerns that it may not be the liability that it would be with other patients. Nevertheless, it is a liability that is best avoided. Clinicians who take their obese patients seriously enough to accept their definition of the problem may experience an unexpected gratitude, and even a measure of tolerance for the mistakes that they will surely make along the way. Obese patients often say that their dissatisfaction with doctors began when a physician assumed that their obesity was the reason they had sought medical help and had ignored their chief complaint. This disregard even caused obese persons not to seek medical help for disorders that they know require such help. They do not want to experience once again the disregard of their request and, implicitly, of their worth, by a physician redefining their chief complaint.

The patient's chief complaint may well be something other than her obesity. In this case it is well to proceed as with a nonobese patient. If the obesity need not be considered in taking a history of the present illness, don't consider it. If it needs to be considered, as, for example, with a patient presenting with diabetes or arthritis of the weight-bearing joints, it is well to ask only as much as is necessary to understand the other illness.

There is no danger that the problem of obesity will never come up, but there is merit in waiting until the patient raises the issue. It is a rare obese person who has not been distressed by her obesity, by her inability to control it, and by the prejudice that it has aroused. Even if the patient has come for another problem, when she feels sufficiently confident of her doctor, she will raise it. At that point a simple, "tell me about it," is sufficient.

Occasionally an obese patient will reach the end of an initial interview without ever having mentioned her obesity. At such a time it is reasonable to ask "has your weight been much of a problem for you?" If the patient wants to talk about it, this is all the encouragement she will need; if she does not, further questions are not likely to be useful. Obesity is not a secret; both you and the patient know it is a problem for her and the diagnosis does not require the probing that may be necessary in the case of bulimia or alcohol abuse. If the patient chooses not to talk about it, respect her privacy. The meager benefits that we can offer are hardly a reason to reopen old wounds.

HISTORY OF THE PRESENT ILLNESS

If the patient responds to the invitation to discuss her obesity, or if she has defined it as her chief complaint, obesity becomes the subject of the present illness. History-taking presents the physician with excellent opportunities to provide emotional support by, among other things, helping the patient bring order out of chaos. All too frequently chaos characterizes patients' understanding of their obesity. Such an outcome is not an unreasonable result of the seemingly endless sequence of losing and regaining weight and the daily round of slights and rebuffs, prejudice and discriminations. A quiet, thoughtful inquiry helps to put things in perspective and to reduce the emotional turmoil. As the patient and physician construct the history, they can make it coherent and reasonable and alleviate the ill-defined menace and despair evoked by the history the patient had used to explain her condition.

Lifetime Weight History

There are a number of ways to take a history of a patient's obesity, but a reasonable one is to begin with a lifetime history of the patient's weight, beginning with her birth weight. Occasionally knowing the birth weight is useful; a very high birth weight suggests a family history of diabetes, or a very low weight suggests a difficult pregnancy. This question, however, is primarily designed to help establish a therapeutic alliance. After all, this is the kind of question that doctors ask patients. It starts history-taking in a professional way; birth weight is a neutral topic, with none of the pejorative associations that so many later weights will have.

The next question can be about weight as a baby. Most patients can report whether they were "chubby" or "thin" or that their weight was not unusual. Certain conclusions can be drawn about someone who was chubby as a baby and has remained overweight. Such a person can be expected to have a stronger genetic predisposition to obesity (5), to be heavier as an adult, and to have encountered more social stress than persons whose obesity began during adult life. Despite earlier beliefs, persons with juvenile onset obesity probably do not have a harder time losing weight in treatment, but they are likely to have a hard time maintaining their weight losses.

The first day in school is a reasonable next topic of inquiry. Can the patient remember having been considered fat? This is the first time when social interactions become painful and patients may remember having been teased about their weight. Unpleasant experiences at this age do not seem to have the deleterious long-term consequences that they do during adolescence, but it can be useful to patients to remember these events and any pain that they caused.

Adolescence is a critical period in psychosocial development, and it deserves special attention in taking a history of obese persons (6,7). Does the patient remember having been overweight during this time? Useful milestones are graduation from eighth grade and from high school. It is during this period that the devastating impact of rejection is first incorporated by obese girls into the disparagement of their body image. It is also frequently a time of their first reducing diet, with all of the attendant pain—mother's distress, an uncaring doctor, the short-lived pride in losing weight, and the long-term discouragement when it is regained. It is worthwhile asking about the first attempt at weight loss and what kind of diet it involved (strict or liberal), the extent of supervision, the use of appetite-suppressant medication, and, finally, the patient's weight at the beginning and end of the diet and how much weight was lost. These facts give the physician a feeling for important events in the patient's life and establish a pattern of inquiry into later attempts at weight reduction.

Information about past efforts at weight reduction helps to estimate the likelihood of success in the future. Some histories can give a fair warning against further attempts. The patient who has made several attempts in what appear to be good programs and who has either failed to lose weight or has rapidly regained it is not likely to fare better under your care. If such a patient has no indications for weight reduction, as is often the case, you may be most helpful to her by dissuading her from another attempt, no matter how convincing a case she may make. It is far better not to repeat the familiar history of disillusionment and failure, and the reassurance that her doctor sees no pressing need for weight reduction may be enough to persuade the patient to call off the attempt and not to feel badly about doing so. If weight reduction is indicated, on the other hand, a careful history will highlight the strengths and weaknesses that the patient brings to it.

Further inquiry into the history of the patient's weight follows the pattern already established: determining weights at the time of various life events—entry and graduation from college, time of the first job, events in the life of the patient's children. One event is particularly worthy of note—pregnancy. A common history among obese patients is weight gain with each pregnancy followed by only partial loss of the weight that had been gained. Rössner (8) has recently documented this marked vulnerability of obese women; in contrast to a mean weight increase of 1 kg a year after delivery among women of normal weight, already obese women averaged a gain of 9 kg a year after delivery (8).

Periods of Weight Change

Having established a general outline of a patient's lifetime weight history, the clinician can move to a more detailed analysis of periods of weight change and the emotional ups and downs with which they are associated. The patient is more likely to describe the emotional downs, and these can prove instructive. What kind of event in the past has led to weight gain or to the breaking of a diet? If similar events are occurring now, or are threatening to occur, the patient might best deal with them before beginning a weight-loss program.

Patients do, of course, have emotional ups, and they are often associated with weight loss, even when the patient makes no special effort to lose weight. Falling in love may be the most powerful stimulus for weight loss, but anything that elevates the patient's self-esteem helps her to lose weight. When things are going well the patient has a better chance of losing weight and avoiding the ill effects of dieting.

Dieting does have ill effects, and this may be the time to inquire into them. The most serious complication is the so-called "dieting depression," a relatively uncommon outcome but one to be avoided (9). Any history of depression or other emotional disturbance during weight reduction should be taken seriously, and patients with such a history should attempt weight loss cautiously, if at all.

After completing the history of the patient's weight, the clinician may ask about her food intake. There has long been uncertainty over the validity of obese patients' reports of their food intake. This uncertainty has now been resolved by research that utilized doubly labeled water, a precise measure of energy expenditure. This research has shown that self-reports grossly underestimate the energy intake (with which the energy expenditure is in equilibrium) (10). Obese people eat more and report less than do persons of normal weight (and even the latter underreport their caloric intake).

This information is useful in avoiding arguments with patients about how much they eat. It is enough to ask what they eat and when and how much. If the amount seems small, note the fact and ask the patient how much she eats at times when she is gaining weight. Nod approvingly as she recovers additional items, and it may be possible to reconstruct a reasonable account of the type of food she eats and the pattern of food intake. What is learned about the pattern is likely to be more useful than what is learned about the amount.

Patterns of Food Intake

The most clearly defined pattern of food intake is binge eating, which has recently been recognized by the formal diagnosis of "binge-eating disorder" (11). This pattern is characterized by the rapid and uncontrolled consumption of large amounts of food in a short period of time. During the binge the patient feels out of control and after it expresses guilt and remorse. Binge eating is believed to be associated with emotional disturbance and with a poor outcome of attempts at weight reduction. Surveys within the last few years indicate that the problem is far more widespread than we had believed and that it exists in from 25 to 50% of obese persons applying to weight reduction programs (11).

Binge-eating disorder is the same as bulimia nervosa except that the person does not vomit. This lack of vomiting means that the large amount eaten during binges makes a substantial contribution to the excess calories of the obese binge eater. It is helpful to discuss their eating with binge-eaters and to find out how often and under what circumstances the binges occur. Understanding these circumstances may help to alleviate the anxiety and distress that accompany binge eating. It is not yet possible to prescribe more specific treatments for binge eating disorder, although psychiatric referral may be indicated and cognitive behavioral treatment and antidepressant medication are currently being explored.

Other patterns of food intake are less dramatic but no less important. Overeating in association with excessive alcohol intake can be a serious problem, particularly among men. Alcohol has two undesirable effects. First is the excess calories contributed by the alcohol; second is the associated disinhibition of dietary restraint, leading to overeating. These effects make alcohol troublesome in social situations, at parties, and when dining out. Thoughtful questioning can often delineate such problems with sufficient clarity that the patient can consider means of coping with them.

Two other eating patterns contribute to excessive food intake—snacking and the consumption of large meals. The consumption of large meals may be the easier of the two patterns to control, since it is a decision that need be made only three or four times a day, and one in which others can help the patient. Thus if a homemaker can be persuaded to decrease the size of meals, everyone in the home will benefit. Snacking, on the other hand, requires a more thorough change in personal habits and life style. Although people can make such changes on their own, most will require outside help, perhaps in the form of a weight reduction program with a heavy behavioral emphasis.

Body Image Disparagement

One problem of obese persons is sufficiently widespread and sufficiently distressing to deserve special attention. It is disparagement of the body image (6,7). Persons with this condition view their bodies as grotesque and loathsome, and feel that others view them with hostility and contempt. They are preoccupied with their obesity, and weight is their overriding concern, often to the exclusion of any other personal characteristic. They see the entire world in terms of body weight, dividing society into people of greater or lesser body weight and then responding to them in terms of this division—envy towards anyone thinner and contempt for those who are fatter.

One might expect that body image disparagement would occur in all obese persons, but such is not the case. It occurs in only a minority of obese persons and only in those who had been obese during adolescence, apparently a critical period for development of the disorder. Body image disparagement is affected only modestly by weight loss but has been alleviated by psychoanalytic treatment (12).

If the disorder is of only limited intensity, many patients will be relieved that their doctor recognizes it and reassured by discussing it. If it is more severe the clinician can serve a useful function by letting the patient know that body image disparagement is not a necessary accompaniment of her obesity. She may not believe it at first, but such information can help to ease the pain, and it can prepare the way for more formal interventions. Psychoanalytic treatment has relieved body image disparagement (12), suggesting that psychotherapy may be helpful; two new approaches deserve attention. One is cognitive-behavioral treatment, which is now under active investigation. The other is the feminist therapies that seek to free women from the tyranny of the cultural stereotypes that they have incorporated into their views of themselves.

Family History

Taking a family history is often a perfunctory matter, carried out more from habit than from conviction. Such should not be the case with an obese person. Recent research has revealed a strong genetic contribution to human obesity (13,14). The presence of obesity among family members provides an excellent starting point for a discussion of this contribution as noted below.

The Physical Examination

The physical examination of obese persons involves several important considerations, but we will focus on just one—the body fat distribution. Recent research has revealed that medical complications of obesity are closely linked to the distribution of body fat (15,16). Upper body fat (particularly "visceral" fat, that within the abdominal wall) presenting as a "pot belly" conveys most of the risk associated with obesity. Lower body fat (around the hips and thighs), on the other hand, is accompanied by fewer medical complications.

Laboratory tests

After the history and physical examination the physician will discuss with the patient the laboratory tests that are needed. It is a measure of our ignorance of the causes of obesity that the outcome of these tests rarely influences our understanding of why the patient is obese. Instead they indicate the extent of the complications of the obesity and the urgency with which they require control. The most effective measure of control is surely weight reduction and the extent of the complications will indicate how urgently weight reduction

should be considered. In the vast majority of cases urgent measures are not required. In some instances, however, sleep apnea and congestive heart failure among them, immediate treatment in the hospital may be indicated. The problems of severely obese people merit special attentions.

Special Problems of Severe or "Morbid" Obesity

Occasionally the physician will be consulted by a severely obese person, weighing at least 100% over standard weight. These patients have usually experienced the most severe prejudice and discrimination and they deserve the physician's deepest concern. Most of them are thoroughly disillusioned with standard programs of weight control, and their valuation is usually correct.

For them the treatment of choice is surgical, and Mason's chapter (*this volume*) describes the surprisingly good results of surgical treatment of severe obesity, when carried out by experienced hands. Nevertheless, even here, there is merit in getting to know the patient before prescribing treatment. These patients need the detached concern of a good doctor. Some arrive at the doctor's office demanding surgery, others are unrealistically frightened of it, and few have the kind of information that would permit a rational choice. It is thus helpful to describe the risks and benefits of surgical treatment and leave the decision as to pursuing it up to the patient. A surprising number of patients return after months and even years, having made up their minds to ask for surgical treatment.

The Patient's Understanding of Her Obesity

At this point in the history, it is time to ask the patient how she understands her affliction. The history-taking will already have touched upon this understanding and some patients may already have discussed it. If not, this is a good time to pursue the topic. To what does the patient attribute her obesity, her difficulty in losing weight, the pressure to regain lost weight? From the answers to such questions the clinician should be able to construct a general idea of how the patient views her obesity. It is then useful to reflect back to her your understanding of her view and to modify any misconceptions that you may have. Then reflect with the patient on various derogatory explanations that she has come to accept and highlight them for further discussion. If she is not particularly forthcoming, it will take little more than mention of some of the common explanations to bring them to mind—defective impulse control, a lack of will power, gluttony, fat slob. . . .

SUMMING UP

The most important component of the patient's first visit is the summing up. After the patient has told her story to a sympathetic listener she will be receptive to new ideas. This is a time to correct her misapprehensions about her obesity and to help her to revise some of her self-defeating ideas. It is well to signal the beginning of this important task, perhaps by laying down any notes, pushing back one's chair, and generally indicating that there will be a change in the nature of the interview.

An important task is helping the patient to a new understanding of her obesity, beginning with a disconfirmation of her derogatory explanations. A start can be made by simply identifying and rejecting them. New genetic findings can be introduced in their place. The strength of genetic influences is still not widely known nor is the lack of influence of the early family environment (13,14). The first of these findings provides a nonjudgmental explanation of the patient's tendency to gain weight. The second finding can help an obese woman by redefining her mother's role in the disorder. Her mother didn't cause the obesity through the faulty child-rearing practices that have been blamed in the past. Instead, her contribution was transmitted through her genes and if she is

herself obese, as she probably is, she is as much a victim of her genes as is her daughter. She may have failed as a mother in many ways but these failures did not cause the patient's obesity. These facts may help the patient reevaluate her mother, transforming her from scapegoat to fellow sufferer.

Discussion of genetic issues in obesity requires a delicate balance. The patient should learn enough about genetic issues to reduce the guilt from which she suffers. At the same time the strength of genetic influences should not be exaggerated or cause the patient to lose hope. Many obese persons, who by definition are genetically predisposed to obesity, have lost weight and maintained their weight losses.

A second area in which new information can be profitably shared with obese women concerns the risks associated with body fat distribution, since the excess body fat of most women is located around their hips and they are accordingly at low risk of complications. As they struggle with their heavy social and psychological burdens, they can at least know that the medical problems with which they have been threatened, often by physicians, may be largely insignificant.

TALKING WITH MEN

Just as research on body fat distribution can reassure many women about their obesity, it has sounded the alarm for obese men whose obesity is usually of the upper body type. They are often at significant risk, often do not know it, and rarely seek treatment. The physician is on firm ground to approach obese men in a far different manner from the approach to obese women. It is entirely appropriate to stress to men with upper body obesity, particularly those with hypertension, impaired glucose tolerance, and hyperlipidemias, the risks they run and the benefits of treatment.

Just as talking with obese women requires concern for the psychological trauma they have experienced, so talking with obese men requires attention to their denial. One measure of this denial is the scarcity of men in weight reduction programs. Despite the health risks from their obesity, men consistently number less than 20% of persons enrolled in commercial weight-loss programs. One deterrent has been the almost exclusively female enrollment in these programs and the perception by men that weight reduction is primarily the cosmetic problem that it tends to be for women. Even the disappointing results of weight-loss efforts among women need not be a barrier. Men, who have so seldom seriously attempted weight reduction, may well be more successful than women. Clearly a shift in efforts at weight reduction from women to men should be a major goal of those involved in the treatment of obesity.

OBESITY AS A LIFETIME PROBLEM

A general principle that is usefully conveyed during the first interview with obese patients, and repeated in subsequent ones, is that obesity is a lifetime problem. Furthermore, it is a lifetime problem not because of any defect in the patient but because of defects in our treatment. In this regard it is no different from disorders such as hypertension and diabetes, which also require lifetime attention. The goal, accordingly, is to help the patient to think in terms of years and not in terms of the next reducing diet.

A skillfully done interview may well dissuade an obese woman from undertaking a weight reduction program and if she can do this without regret, it is frequently the best course of action. If, however, she still wants to undertake treatment, if there are at least modest prospects of success, and if treatment is medically indicated, the options can be described. With obese men, on the other hand, it is appropriate for the physician to adopt a more aggressive approach.

A DISCUSSION OF TREATMENT

Physicians today rarely treat their obese patients for their obesity. If their patients do receive such treatment it is usually from commercial weight-loss programs, and the patient has made the arrangements herself. This scenario is not widely acknowledged but it should be. The availability of commercial weight-loss programs can be the basis for a revision of traditional views of the relationship between the doctor and the obese patient. The first step is for the doctor to learn enough about weight-loss programs to be able to make appropriate recommendations. Two kinds of information are required—the elements of a good weight reduction program and the character of specific programs.

The elements of a good weight reduction program are nutrition education, group support, measures to increase physical activity, self-monitoring of body weight and food intake, stimulus control, and other behavioral measures. They are described in Wadden's chapter (*this volume*) and in greater detail in Brownell's *LEARN Manual* (17).

Commercial weight-loss programs vary widely in the intensity of their treatment (and in their cost). Conservative programs like Weight Watchers include the measures described above, delivered in a large group format. They are relatively inexpensive and produce a slow rate of weight loss. More expensive programs, such as Nutri System, add an effort at portion control achieved through the purchase of packaged foods. Programs such as Optifast use very-low-calorie diets, which achieve more rapid weight loss but require medical monitoring at considerably increased expense. Data on short- and long-term weight loss of these programs are unfortunately in short supply.

A major problem with weight-loss programs is that, no matter how good they are in conception, many are poorly implemented, as described in Taylor and Stunkard's chapter (*this volume*). Some years ago Volkmar and his colleagues (18), studying an apparently well-planned Weight Watchers' program in California, found that 50% of the persons who entered the program dropped out within the first 6 weeks and another 20% dropped out in the following 6 weeks. No matter how well designed, programs that are not attended cannot help.

A FINAL WORD

The ascendance of the commercial weight reduction programs can mean, as we have noted, a major change in the relationship of the doctor with the obese patient. Physicians no longer need feel impelled to undertake a treatment with which they have justifiably felt uncomfortable. Instead, by deferring weight reduction to the commercial programs, the physician can attend more broadly to the patient's needs. If an attempt at weight reduction seems justified, the physician can help guide the patient to the most appropriate program and stand by, welcoming her success, supporting her if she fails. If an attempt at weight reduction appears unjustified, the physician may be able to help the patient avoid another experience of failure. Most of all, the new relationship can be one in which talking with patients assumes once again its traditional role, uniting the doctor and patient in their sacred enterprise.

REFERENCES

1. Stunkard AJ, Wadden TA. Psychological aspects of severe obesity. *Am J Clin Nutr* [*in press*].
2. Staffieri JR. A study of social stereotype of body image in children. *J Pers Soc Psychol* 1967;7:101–4.
3. Goodman N, Dornbusch SM, Richardson SA, Hastorf AH. Variant reactions to physical disabilities. *Am Sociol Rev* 1963;28:429–35.
4. Maddox GL, Liederman V. Overweight as a social disability with medical implications. *J Med Educ* 1969;44:214–20.
5. Price RA, Stunkard AJ, Ness R, et al. Childhood onset (age < 10) obesity has high familial risk. *Int J Obes* 1990;14:185–95.
6. Stunkard AJ, Mendelson M. Obesity and the body image: I. Characteristics of disturbances in the body image of some obese persons. *Am J Psychiatry* 1967;123:1296–300.
7. Stunkard AJ, Burt V. Obesity and the body image: II. Age at onset of disturbances in the body image. *Am J Psychiatry* 1967;123:1443–7.
8. Öhlin A, Rössner S. Development of body weight during and after pregnancy. In: Björntorp P, Rössner S, eds. *Obesity in Europe 88*. London: John Libbey, 1989;115–20.
9. Stunkard AJ. The "dieting depression." Incidence and clinical characteristics of untoward responses to weight reduction regimes. *Am J Med* 1957;23:77–86.
10. Bandini LG, Schoeller HN, Dietz WH. Validity of reported energy intake in obese and nonobese adolescents. *Am J Clin Nutr* 1990;52:421–5.
11. Spitzer RL, Devlin M, Walsh BT, et al. Binge-eating disorder: a multisite field trial of the diagnostic criteria. *Int J Eat Disord* 1992;11:191–203.
12. Rand CSW, Stunkard AJ. Obesity and psychoanalysis. *Am J Psychiatry* 1978;135:547–51.
13. Stunkard AJ, Sorensen TIA, Hanis C, et al. An adoption study of human obesity. *N Engl J Med* 1986;314:193–8.
14. Stunkard AJ, Harris J, Pederson N, McClearn GE. The body-mass index of twins who have been reared apart. *N Engl J Med* 1990;322:1483–7.
15. Lapidus L, Bengtsson C, Larsson B, Pennert K, Rybo E, Sjöström L. Distribution of adipose tissue and risk of cardiovascular disease and death: a 12 year follow up of participants in the population study of women in Gothenburg, Sweden. *Br Med J* 1984;289:1257–61.
16. Larsson B, Svardudd K, Wilhelmsen L, Bjorntorp P, Tibblin G. Abdominal adipose tissue distribution, obesity and risk of cardiovascular disease and death: 13 year follow-up of participants in the study of men born in 1913. *Br Med J* 1984;288:1401–4.
17. Brownell K. The LEARN Manual. Dallas: American Health Publications, 1991.
18. Volkmar FR, Stunkard AJ, Woolston J, Bailey BA. High attrition rates in commercial weight reduction programs. *Arch Intern Med* 1981;141:426–8.

Subject Index

•